ORTHOPAEDIC NURSING AND REHABILITATION

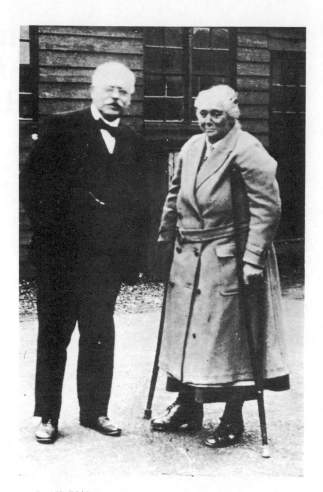

*Despite a life-long physical handicap, Dame Agnes Hunt
(1867–1948), seen here with Sir Robert Jones, became a
trained nurse, and founded at Baschurch what was to
become, under the influence of Robert Jones and herself,
the first orthopaedic hospital. Later, they founded the first
training college for the disabled in this country.
From her remarkable vision, energy, and love for suffering
humanity was born our present service for orthopaedic
patients, and with it, the principles of nursing care which
are the heritage of orthopaedic nurses today.*

ORTHOPAEDIC NURSING AND REHABILITATION

MARY POWELL OBE SRN MCSP Orthopaedic Nursing Certificate

Formerly Matron, Robert Jones and Agnes Hunt Orthopaedic Hospital,
Oswestry, Shropshire, United Kingdom

Foreword by Robert B. Duthie MA MB ChM FRCSE FRCS

Nuffield Professor of Orthopaedic Surgery, Oxford University;
Honorary Consultant Surgeon to the Nuffield Orthopaedic
Centre and Accident Department, John Radcliffe Hospital, Oxford;
Consultant Adviser in Orthopaedic and Accident Surgery to the
Department of Health and Social Security;
Member of the Royal Commission on Civil Liability and
Compensation for Personal Injury.

NINTH EDITION

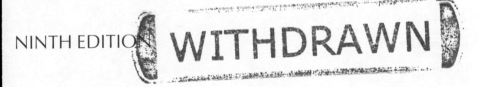

Churchill Livingstone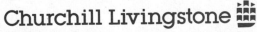

EDINBURGH LONDON MELBOURNE AND NEW YORK 1986

CHURCHILL LIVINGSTONE
Medical Division of Longman Group Limited

Distributed in the United States of America by
Churchill Livingstone Inc., 1560 Broadway, New York,
N.Y. 10036, and by associated companies, branches
and representatives throughout the world.

First edition 1951
Second edition 1956
Third edition 1959
Fourth edition 1962
Fifth edition 1965
Sixth edition 1968
Seventh edition 1976
Eighth edition 1982
Ninth edition 1986

ISBN 0 443 03238 6

British Library Cataloguing in Publication Data
Powell, Mary
    Orthopaedic nursing and rehabilitation.—9th ed.
    1. Orthopedic nursing
    I. Title
    610.73'677   RD753

Library of Congress Cataloging in Publication Data
Main entry under title:
Orthopaedic nursing and rehabilitation.
    Bibliography: p.
    Includes index.
    1. Orthopedic nursing. 2. Physically handicapped—
Rehabilitation. I. Powell, Mary. |DNLM: 1. Orthopedics
—nursing. 2. Rehabilitation—nurses' instruction.
WY 157.6 077|
RD753.P6   1986   610.73'677   85–26957

Printed in Great Britain at The Bath Press, Avon

Foreword

Three years have passed since the last edition of this outstanding contribution to orthopaedic nursing and it is a great pleasure to welcome this new one. Miss Powell has obviously improved several parts of the text by rewriting and indeed by expanding certain sections. Her distinguished contributors have written well and maintained a uniformity of language which makes reading so pleasing and comprehensible. There is a constant and important emphasis upon caring for the orthopaedic patient—indeed the titles or headings for each of the chapters are entitled 'care' of the injured patient, 'care' of the paralysed patient etc. This to me epitomised Miss Powell's contribution to her profession—it always has been directly concerned with the patient and the quality of nursing care. Not for Miss Powell has been the increasingly non-concerned, professional administrative nurse of modern times who is more concerned with the administrative role or the nursing process. The emphasis throughout this most important book is how to manage and care for the orthopaedic patient totally.

In the introduction there is given a well accepted explanation about the derivation of the word 'orthopaedic'. 'Paedios' meaning the child but a further origin could easily be from the Greek word 'paedeau' which Sayre explained many years ago as being 'to teach'. Miss Powell has been an outstanding teacher and this new edition will sustain this reputation for many years to come.

R. B. D.

*Dedicated to
the orthopaedic team—
everywhere*

Preface to the ninth edition

The eighth edition of this book was a major revision, so that the ninth, following closely on its heels, is not so much a re-write as an update. Nevertheless, some important items have been added. The section on passive movements of joints in Chapter 1 is included because in some parts of the world physiotherapists are not available for this essential treatment and it must be carried out by nurses. A new chapter (Ch. 2) deals with aspects of infection control, of special significance in orthopaedic surgery and, therefore, in orthopaedic nursing. Chapter 8, which deals with operating theatre technique has been completely rewritten, as has Chapter 23 dealing with spinal injuries.

I am most grateful to my contributors and to other people for advice and help, notably Professor Brian T. O'Connor and Mr G. K. Rose. Mr Gwyn Evans has given me valuable assistance with Chapters 14 and 15 and Mr John Patrick also assisted me with a section in Chapter 14. My erstwhile colleagues at Oswestry have, as always, given me their loyal support—Marion Tidswell, Gerald Briffett, Pat McNulty, Gwilym Jones, Sydna Colbert, Jill Jones, Marie Carter and David and Joyce Jones have been most helpful.

Finally, I would like to thank Professor Robert Duthie for writing the Foreword, the publisher, editor and staff at Churchill Livingstone for their kind efficiency and the printers for their important contribution.

In conclusion, I must mention my family and friends, whose loud groans and cries of 'What, again?' accompany the production of each new edition.

Castle Pulverbatch, 1986   M. P.

Contributors

J. A. Bentley MCSP ONC
Superintendent Physiotherapist, Robert Jones and Agnes Hunt
Orthopaedic Hospital, Oswestry

J. L. Brennan MD(Lond) MRCP FRCPath
Consultant Pathologist, Robert Jones and Agnes Hunt
Orthopaedic Hospital, Oswestry

R. Geoffrey Burwell BSc MD FRCS (Eng)
Professor of Human Morphology and Experimental
Orthopaedics, University Hospital and Medical School,
Nottingham; Honorary Consultant in Orthopaedics,
Nottinghamshire Area Health Authority (T),
Nottingham

A. K. Clarke BSc MB BS MRCP
Consultant in Rheumatology and Rehabilitation, Royal
National Hospital for Rheumatic Diseases, Bath

Stephen Clarke
Disablement Resettlement officer, Employment Division, MSC,
Oswestry Job Centre, Shropshire

Michael W. J. Davie MA MD MRCP
Consultant Physician and Director of Research, Charles Salt
Centre, Robert Jones and Agnes Hunt Orthopaedic Hospital,
Oswestry

Christine Davies
Theatre Sister, St Luke's Hospital for the Clergy, London

Michael W. Elves MSc PhD FIBiol FRCPath
Director, Mammalian Biology Division, Glaxo Group Research
Ltd, Greenford, Middlesex

Barbara Goff ONC MCSP DipTP
Formerly Teacher, Oswestry and North Staffordshire School of
Physiotherapy, Oswestry

Michael Frederick Highfield SRN ONC
Assistant Director of Nursing Services, Royal Shrewsbury
Hospital, Shrewsbury

John Rodney Hughes MSc SRN ONC DN(Lond)
District Nursing Officer, Shropshire Health Authority. Former
Charge Nurse, Midland Spinal Injuries Unit, Oswestry

Elizabeth A. Jenner SRN DipN(Lond)
Senior Nurse, Infection Control/Research, Paddington and
North Kensington Health Authority, St Mary's Hospital,
London

J. G. Kendall MB FRCS
Medical Director, Derwen Training College for the Disabled,
Oswestry

R. Kershaw FPS
Principal Pharmacist, Robert Jones and Agnes Hunt
Orthopaedic Hospital, Oswestry

Vivien Lawson BA(Hons) CQSW DipSocWork
Senior Social Worker, Robert Jones and Agnes Hunt
Orthopaedic Hospital, Oswestry

Ian William McCall MB ChB DMRD FRCR
Consultant Radiologist, Robert Jones and Agnes Hunt
Orthopaedic Hospital, Oswestry

John P. O'Brien PhD FRCS(Edin) FACS
Honorary Consultant Orthopaedic Surgeon, The London
Hospital, Whitechapel, London; Visiting Professor,
Bioengineering Unit, Strathclyde University, Glasgow;
Recently, Director, Department for Spinal Disorders,
Orthopaedic Hospital, Oswestry

Myra Christine Peacock BA DipSpEd CE
Head Teacher, Robert Jones and Agnes Hunt Orthopaedic
Hospital Special School, Oswestry

E. G. Gerald Roberts BSc MB BCh FRCP(Lond)
DCH(Eng) MRCS
Formerly Consultant Paediatrician, Chiyd Area Health
Authority; Formerly Honorary Consultant Paediatrician, Robert
Jones and Agnes Hunt Orthopaedic Hospital,
Oswestry

J. B. D. Rogers ONC MCSP DipTP
Formerly Assistant Principal, The Oswestry and North
Staffordshire School of Physiotherapy, Oswestry

Eryl Thomas SRN ONC
Plaster Room Sister, Robert Jones and Agnes Hunt Orthopaedic
Hospital, Oswestry

Patricia M. Wood MCSP DipTP
Senior Teacher, School of Physiotherapy, Withington Hospital,
Manchester

B. P. Wordsworth MB MRCP(UK)
Honorary Senior Registrar in Rheumatology and Rehabilitation,
Nuffield Orthopaedic Centre, Oxford

Contents

SECTION ONE

Comprehensive care of the orthopaedic patient

Comprehensive patient care
The orthopaedic team
Orthopaedic nursing

Introduction

The word 'orthopaedic' was coined by a French Surgeon, Nicholas Andry in 1741. It is derived from two Greek words: *orthos* meaning 'straight', and *paedios*, meaning 'of a child', and has therefore been taken to mean 'the rearing of straight children'. In modern times, it means much more. Roaf and Hodkinson in their book *A Textbook of Orthopaedic Nursing* give a historical survey of the development of orthopaedic surgery and interesting speculations on the future of this speciality. Noon (1984) writing in the *Nursing Mirror* discusses modern advances in orthopaedic treatment and care. Many readers will be familiar with Dame Agnes Hunt's book, (1983) *This is my life* in which she describes the birth of orthopaedic nursing as a speciality and the founding of the centre which bears her name.

Orthopaedic surgery has been defined as 'concerning the study of the form and function of the human frame; its attack is directed against those affections that deform the architecture or arrest the balanced mechanism of mans body and injuries of bones, muscles, nerves and soft structures which result in loss of form or function are thus its legitimate objective' (Sir Walter Mercer).

When these words were written the 'legitimate objective' included large numbers of patients suffering from those great scourges of yesteryear, skeletal tuberculosis, osteomyelitis and poliomyelitis, and at that time these cases formed the bulk of what is spoken of as 'cold' orthopaedics (a loose term used to describe 'chronic' conditions, as opposed to recent injuries). The attack on these 'affections that deform the architecture' has largely succeeded, due mainly to major advances in surgery, in drug therapy and in vaccines but also to social and economic advances with improved standards of living, not to mention the introduction of that great piece of social legislation the National Health Service, now reorganised with the object of integrating hospital services with preventive and social services in the community, together with a shift of emphasis from the treatment of hospital-centred illness to preventive measures. There is also emphasis on treating patients in their own homes whenever possible, because, it is said, care in the community is better than in an institution unless very special circumstances are present—e.g. nobody available at home to care for the patient—or very special treatment techniques are required which are available only in a hospital; moreover, people prefer to be in their own homes rather than in an institution, and when cared for in the community do not run the risk of being institutionalised, i.e. depressed, apathetic, and unnecessarily dependent upon others for the ordinary acts of daily living. Finally, community care is said to be cheaper than maintaining patients in a hospital setting.

But as old enemies retreat, new ones emerge; the 'affluent society' brings its own problems, associated with the life style of the people; economic advance does not necessarily mean a healthy way of life despite the wide publicity given to health education; for example, many people eat more food than they need and 'dig their graves with their teeth', (Baly, 1973) take insufficient exercise and suffer from psychological problems due to the stress of their way of life, not to mention the high incidence of addiction to tobacco, alcohol and drugs. Moreover, although medical advance and social change has eliminated many of the infectious diseases of the past, there are increasing hazards due to noise, violence, vandalism, road accidents and pollution of the environment by chemicals and other substances. In recent times, unemployment has given rise to new problems.

Social change, improved medical care and economic advance has, however, ensured longer expectation of life, so that we are now faced with increasing numbers of aged patients suffering from degenerative conditions of bones and joints which become the 'objective' seen all too often in ortho-

paedic practice. Another important development of modern times is the large number of patients who in the past would not have survived but who now do so because of advances in medicine and surgery. Many of these patients cannot look for 'cure' but will need 'care' for the rest of their lives. This in turn led to new legislation and to the development of social services for disabled people and to improvements in the design and manufacture of equipment to assist nurses and others in the care of patient both in the hospital and in the home. Notable advances have also been made in aids to daily living and in means of transportation for disabled people. Indeed, there is new emphasis on their rights, benefits and services. Other important developments are the establishment of day-centres and the proliferation of self-help groups representing almost every disabling condition from birth to old age. Most of these groups produce their own literature, often written by members themselves and who describe their own experiences. For example *So you're paralysed*, by Bernadette Fallon (Spinal Injuries Association), and *Patient's Prospect*, by Ann Armstrong (Invalids at Home).

Orthopaedic surgery, in common with other specialised forms of surgery has been immeasurably strengthened, not only by the advances in drug therapy mentioned earlier, but by advances in anaesthesia, in radiography and other investigations, in bio-engineering, in methods of resuscitation and in the medical management of patients who sustain multiple injuries and of those undergoing major operations. Moreover, the patient is not only treated for his orthopaedic condition, as a 'body', but as a person with emotional, psychological, spiritual, social and economic needs. Further, his family and his place in the community are considered as part and parcel of his total care. Patients both in hospital and in the community are encouraged to become involved in their own care more freely than in the past. For example, a method of reporting and 'handing over' at the bedside has been reported (Rowe & Perry, 1984) with patient participation. There has been a great advance in the care and welfare of vulnerable groups, including children and the aged. Smith (1984) writes on the ailments and management of the latter group in relation to orthopaedics.

As for children, they not only receive special

consideration, including immigrant children (Ford, 1979; Aslam & Healy, 1982), but their parents also, especially in relation to admission to hospital (Glen, 1982). It is interesting to note here, however, that despite great improvements in maternal and child care, infant mortality in the United Kingdom (11.7 per 1000 live births) is greater than all but one other advanced country. (WHO Annual Statistical Report).

It should also be noted that immigrants to Britain have posed new problems for nurses, who, in order to give appropriate total care must learn about cultures other than their own.

Important developments in nursing also influence patient care, including introduction of the Nursing Process.

This has important implications for nursing despite the fact that one writer (Jayrain, 1984) expresses his 'despair at the confusion and uncertainty that exists about the nursing process' and suggests that 'the people who are expected to teach it to learners sometimes do not understand it themselves'. This writer goes on to suggest 'radical treatment' to tackle this problem and so put an end to the 'prevailing state of confusion'.

There is new emphasis on research in nursing (Hunt, 1984) and it has been reported that nurses are becoming familiar with computers. Watt & Kenny (1984) quote Professor Ronald of New York State University as saying 'Learning about computers and their use in nursing is a significant challenge for nurses throughout the world'.

There are also new challenges because of advances in organ transplantation and in genetic engineering.

For the purpose of this book, we will define orthopaedic practice as including the following:

1. *'Cold' orthopaedics*, a term used to describe chronic, congenital, degenerative and non-traumatic disorders, as opposed to acute conditions due to
2. *Trauma*, which includes all injuries to the neuro-musculo-skeletal system. In this connection however, it is important to remember that concomitant injuries to other body structures may threaten life and require treatment which takes precedence over those with which we are directly concerned.

3. *Rehabilitation*. This is not a treatment in itself and indeed it is true to say that all medical, surgical, nursing and para-medical activities are part of rehabilitation; it is a process aimed at the preservation or restoration of independence, which begins with promotion of positive health and prevention of disease and injury at community level, and continues in hospital by means of prompt and effective treatment and nursing care. It is complete only when the patient is restored to the maximum physical, psychological, social and economic independence commensurate with his condition.

In this connection, this book shows many 'aids to function'. It should be stressed that aids and adaptations are advised only when the patient cannot use normal everyday equipment, e.g. feeding utensils, or toilet fixtures.

COMPREHENSIVE PATIENT CARE

This describes a concept, already referred to in a previous paragraph, of the care of the patient as a whole person rather than as a 'case'. It arises from the fact that treatment of the physical condition is not enough; social problems are equally important. Preservation or restoration of social and economic independence is not only good medicine but good sense, since such independence means fewer claims on scarce and expensive national health and welfare resources.

THE ORTHOPAEDIC TEAM

For the nurse an outstanding facet of caring for orthopaedic patients is the recognition of the work of other team members; in many instances, comprehensive care may be difficult to attain without their expertise. In most situations this team is led by the doctor, whether orthopaedic surgeon, accident surgeon, orthopaedic physician, rheumatologist, or rehabilitation specialist. On the other hand, we know that there are shifts of leadership according to the situation; indeed, nursing leadership has assumed new importance in modern times because direct patient care is so often given by members of staff who may have had only minimal professional training. Other team members with whom we are closely associated are the physiotherapist, occupational therapist and social worker; indeed, in some instances the nurse has to assume some of their functions in a modified way, if only because she is the only team-member who is with the patient 24 hours of every day. This is not to say that the nurse can replace these specialised workers, but she needs an understanding of their functions in order to work closely with them in the general *management* of the patient and in achieving the objective of comprehensive patient care. Other team members include the orthotist-/prosthetist, the bio-engineer, the manufacturer and supplier of orthopaedic equipment and appliances, the radiographer, the medical secretary, the laboratory technician, the pharmacist, the nutritionist, and sometimes the speech therapist, and the school teacher; workers in other disciplines of medicine and surgery are called in from time to time. The nurse also requires a working knowledge of the general organisation of the hospital and the role of those whose administrative functions provide the rails on which the nursing and other services run, not forgetting the part played by workers in portering, catering, domestic and other developments which form part of the complex organisation of the hospital in which she works. Moreover she must learn the function of the Health and Welfare Community Services which will ensure that health care begins and ends in the patient's home.

ORTHOPAEDIC NURSING

This term is a misnomer; rather, we should call it 'nursing applied to orthopaedic patients' because the principles of nursing apply to these patients as to all others. It has been said that 'Nurses have long recognised that basic orthopaedic principles are applicable to all areas of nursing, not just to the patient who has a bone fracture or some other pathological skeletal change' (Wolff et al, 1978). On the other hand the skills to be acquired by the so-called 'orthopaedic nurse' are expert knowledge of the patients condition, of his particular needs and, most important, of how these are to be met and how complications are prevented.

In addition to a sound knowledge of the principles of orthopaedic treatment and nursing care, the nurse must develop an 'orthopaedic eye'—an acute awareness of correct body posture and mechanics—so that nothing that interferes with the patient's treatment will escape her notice.

Prevention of complications is a vital part of orthopaedic nursing—indeed it has been said that 'much orthopaedic nursing care is of a preventive nature' (Luckman & Sorenson, 1980).

A patient with an acute abdominal condition may be in hospital for a few days or weeks; a patient with an orthopaedic condition may be in hospital for many days or weeks or occasionally for months; this can give rise not only to physical problems but social ones as well. As she grows in knowledge and experience the nurse will learn to 'take the long view' since many orthopaedic conditions tend to run a prolonged course. It is important to remember that while we take a professional view of plaster casts, splints and different appliances such as those used for traction purposes, they are nevertheless unnatural encumbrances to the patient and, indeed, even 'instruments of torture'; although a patient wearing a splint or other device for treatment or an orthopaedic condition may be otherwise healthy, he is as deserving of our care, sympathy and attention as any other patient.

In this connection we would stress the *importance of observation*: mention of the importance of observation of the patient may seem superfluous in any nursing situation; it is stressed here because tragedies have occurred in orthopaedic practice and patients have lost life or limb because watchfulness has been defective. Moreover, it is not enough to be watchful oneself; junior staff, ancillary staff, patients and their relatives must be *taught* this essential discipline. It is notable that dramatic, acute and unusual problems which present an exciting challenge to the therapeutic team are usually accurately observed and handled well; many orthopaedic conditions however, are not dramatic and often tend to run a prolonged course so that it is all too easy to overlook clinical signs which might indicate that all is not well with the patient. Moreover the fact that the patient may not be 'ill' in a medical sense, in so far as his main problem is often a diseased, deformed, degenerated or injured limb does not cancel out the essential nature of educated, acute and continuous nursing observation.

The orthopaedic field not only requires the training and ability to nurse the very ill, but as often as not, the very uncomfortable as well. Moreover, in a day and age when patients in general hospitals who have had major abdominal surgery are allowed up from bed shortly afterwards, the orthopaedic patient is often completely confined to bed because weight-bearing on a limb is not permitted. Though modern treatment and surgery, especially day-surgery, has greatly reduced in-patient time, orthopaedic patients are still relatively 'long stay'. This gives the orthopaedic nurse great scope in the practice of bedside nursing in its widest sense, particularly with regard to the *prevention of complications* which may hinder the patient's recovery or even cause permanent disability and loss of independence.

On the other hand, we must not over-nurse nor over-protect the patient who for his final rehabilitation must learn to do things for himself; the intelligent management of patients suffering from a wide range of orthopaedic conditions and who, perhaps undergo complex processes leading to full rehabilitation for life and work is at the same time one of the most challenging and satisfying branches of her profession open to the nurse of today.

Nursing of whatever kind is the art and science of tending the sick; though the scientific aspect has assumed new importance in this technological age. James Smith (1982) writes that 'there is more to the art than science alone' and points out that 'clinical judgments and professional insights' are not necessarily always dependent on a scientific basis but on 'the fruits of experience'.

In another publication Rowden (1984) says 'Nursing cannot be defined as a science in the purest form; we draw on a host of sciences to form a body of knowledge that is relevant to caring for people'. This author goes on to suggest that giving care entails a good measure of intuition, and that nursing is also an art.

Nursing is essentially practical and cannot be learned from books alone. This book is written in the hope that it will assist the orthopaedic nurse to a deeper knowledge of the needs of her patients, so that she can develop her expertise to the highest degree. It is slanted towards care of the patient in hospital; however, reorganisation of the National Health Service will facilitate communication and cooperation between personnel in hospital and their counterparts in the community, and complete the network needed to convert 'comprehensive patient care' from concept to reality.

BIBLIOGRAPHY

Aids for the home 1983 Nursing Times Community Outlook, Pull-out supplement, 13 April

Aslam, Mohamed, Healy M 1982 Present and future trends in the health care of British-Asian children. Nursing Times, 11 August

Baly M E 1973 Nursing and Social Change. London: Heinemann

Chilman A, Thomas M 1986 Understanding Nursing Care, 3rd edn. Edinburgh: Churchill Livingstone

Computers in nursing 1984 The Journal of the British Computer Society Nursing Specialist Group. Nursing Times, 5 September

Consumer Publication 1974 Coping with Disablement. London: Consumer's Association

Davies B M 1975 Community Health and Social Services. London: English Universities Press

Department of Health and Social Security 1976 Prevention and Health: Everybody's business. London: HMSO

DI ISS and Welsh Office 1977 Help for Handicapped People. Leaflet HB1. 1977 Aids for the Handicapped. Leaflet HB2 September 1977. London and Cardiff

Disability Rights Handbook for 1984. London: The Disability Alliance ERA

Glen S A 1982 Hospital admission through the parents' eyes. Nursing Times, 4 August

Guide to the Social Services 1978 London: Macdonald and Evans, for the Family Welfare Association Ltd

Hunt Dame Agnes 1938 This is my Life. Exeter: A Wheaton and Co

Hunt J 1984 The outlook is promising. Nursing Mirror, 18 July

International Classification of Impairments, Disabilities and Handicaps 1980. Geneva: World Health Organization

Jayrain R 1984 Radical treatment indicated. Nursing Mirror, 18 July

Luckman J, Sorenson K C 1980 Medical-Surgical Nursing. New York: W B Saunders

Morris A, Butler A 1972 No Feet to Drag—Report on the Disabled. London: Sidgwick & Jackson

National Association for the Welfare of Children in Hospital, 7 Exton Street, London SE1 8VE

Noon S 1984 Orthopaedic care. Nursing Mirror Clinical Forum, 18 January

Roaf R, Hodkinson L J 1976 Textbook of Orthopaedic Nursing. Oxford: Blackwell Scientific Publications

Roper N 1982 Principles of Nursing, 3rd edn. Edinburgh: Churchill Livingstone

Roper N, Logan W W, Tierney A 1985 The Elements of Nursing, 2nd edn. Edinburgh: Churchill Livingstone

Roper N, Logan W W, Tierney A 1981 Learning to Use the Process of Nursing. Edinburgh: Churchill Livingstone

Rowden R 1984 The nursing process debate. 2. Doctors can work with the nursing process. Nursing Times, 9 May

Rowe M A, Perm A 1984 Don't sit down nurse—it's time for report. Nursing Times, 2 June

Smith C 1984 Orthopaedics and the elderly. Nursing Times, 11 April

Smith J P 1982 Graveyards are full of indispensable people. Nursing Mirror, 6 January

Watson-Jones R 1948 Dame Agnes Hunt. Journal of Bone and Joint Surgery, 30: 709–713

Watt S, Kenny G 1984 Appliance of Science in A and E. Nursing Mirror, 18 July

Wolff L, Weitzel M H, Fuerst E V 1978 Fundamentals of Nursing. Philadelphia, New York, Toronto: J B Lippincott Co

1

Principles of treatment of orthopaedic patients

INTRODUCTION

Methods of treatment vary in different centres, but *underlying principles remain unaltered*; a sound grasp of the principle enables us to understand differences and variations in methods of treatment. 'Understanding fundamentals makes a subject more comprehensible' (Bruner, 1960). Variations in treatment often result from the experience of a doctor, nurse, or paramedical worker who has found such a method successful in his or her hands.

TREATMENT OF THE PATIENT AS A WHOLE

We have already discussed the concept of comprehensive patient care and indicated that this implies an attempt to meet not only physical needs by psychological and socio-economic needs as well; further, we cannot divorce the patient from his family, his community and from society as a whole. Help with social problems is not always easy to obtain or easy to give, which highlights our dependence on those resources where advice, help and support for the patient can be offered in areas outside our own particular sphere.

Treatment of an orthopaedic condition includes investigation into the state of the general health and active treatment where indicated. Moreover it is important to remember that conditions which impair the general health often lead to orthopaedic conditions; for example, obesity adds to the effort required by the heart and lungs and overloads the joints as well; cardio-vascular disorders lead to falls, and falls result in fractures; finally we remember the vast numbers of old or ageing members of the community who present with such degeneration of the musculo-skeletal system that orthopaedic treatment is necessary.

DEFINITION OF ORTHOPAEDIC TREATMENT

Broadly speaking, orthopaedic treatment falls into three categories (Adams, 1971) as described below.

1. *No treatment* other than reassurance and advice (Fig. 1.1). A patient may seek medical

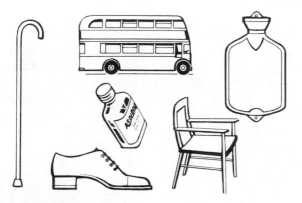

Fig. 1.1 Osteoarthritis—conservative treatment. Simple measures to relieve pain in osteoarthritis of the hip: analgesics, warmth, a raised heel and a stick; 'don't stand when you can sit, don't walk when you can ride'. (From Apley, G. A. *A System of Orthopaedics and Fractures*, 4th edn, p. 57. Butterworths.)

advice simply because he fears he may have cancer or tuberculosis or some other serious condition, and merely requires assurance that his fears are groundless. Then there is the patient with some chronic condition for which no active treatment is indicated but who may need advice regarding, perhaps, aids to daily living so as to retain his independence. Similarly, a disabled child might not require active treatment but his parents might need advice, reassurance and support, sometimes over a long period.

2. *Conservative treatment.* This includes advice (Fig. 1.1) as well as enforced rest, both general and local, various forms of traction, splints and plaster casts, manipulation with or without anaes-

thesia, drug therapy, physical treatment by means of physiotherapy and occupational therapy, and in certain cases, radiotherapy.

3. *Operative treatment.*

OPERATIVE TREATMENT (SURGERY)

Orthopaedic surgery is of two main types:

1. *Emergency surgery*, mainly required by the victims of trauma; it may be life-saving; the operation is not a planned procedure in the sense that it is an unexpected event; this however does not prevent the nurse from anticipating surgery when the patient is admitted and commencing preparations, nor does it prevent the surgeon from planning the operation as soon as he is cognisant of the condition of the patient.

2. *Elective surgery* is deliberately planned and performed at a pre-arranged time; sometimes the patient who has undergone emergency surgery requires elective procedures at a later stage of treatment. For discussion here we shall confine ourselves to the broad principles of elective orthopaedic surgery. Broadly speaking, orthopaedic operations are performed:

   a. for the relief of pain;
   b. for improvement of function;
   c. for correction of deformity;
   d. for improvement of appearance (cosmetic reasons).

Sometimes two or more objectives are required by the same patient, for example, operative treatment in osteoarthritis of the hip relieves pain, corrects deformity, and improves function. It is important to remember that every operation is a serious matter and one not lightly undertaken; the orthopaedic surgeon will give due consideration not only to the orthopaedic condition, but to the age, general health, social conditions and occupation, intelligence, emotional status and degree of cooperation to be expected from each individual patient before embarking on the procedure, having in mind the regime to be followed afterwards. In the case of children the attitude of the parents is also taken into consideration.

Operations will not be described here and the

reader is referred to the textbooks of orthopaedic surgery listed in the bibliography. Roaf & Hodkinson (1971) give a summary of orthopaedic operative procedures, and whilst it is unnecessary for the nurse to know every detail of a specific operation, she must understand its purpose and the broad principles of the procedure. It is essential that nurses accompany their patients to the operating theatre, if not on every occasion, at least from time to time, because if an operation is never seen one cannot visualise the nature and extent of the surgical procedure in relation to the tissues of the patients body. For example, the nurse who has seen various hip operations is obviously in a better position to understand the after-care of the patient than the one who has not; moreover, having once witnessed the use of saws, hammers and chisels on sensitive bone, one can more easily appreciate and evaluate the patient's post-operative pain.

THE NEED FOR KNOWLEDGE OF ANATOMY AND BODY MECHANICS

Since orthopaedic work is concerned with derangements of the form and function of the body, the student must gain a sound knowledge of the position, structure and function of bones, joints and muscles, especially those which are of special significance in the work she is doing. It is quite unnecessary for her to know the detailed structure of every bone in the body or the attachments and nerve supply of each individual muscle, but she cannot nurse her patient intelligently if she does not carry in her mind's eye a picture of his broken bone, diseased joint or severed tendon; moreover she cannot recognise and report on the onset of complications, such as a drop-foot from pressure on the common peroneal nerve, or the onset of radial palsy in a patient using crutches.

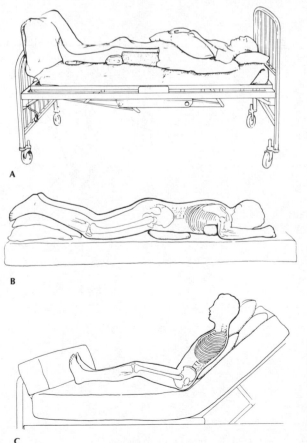

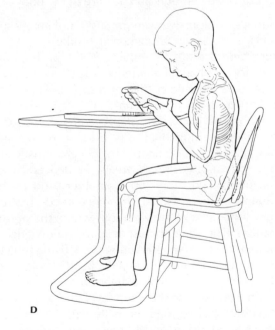

Fig. 1.2 A. Pillow supports maintain good alignment. Note roll to hold hand in position of function. Forearm may be placed in extension or supination without change in shoulder position. Support may be rearranged to place humerus in neutral position. Outer thigh roll prevents outward rotation. Regular change of position is physiologically important. For hemiplegia patients an inner thigh roll is needed to prevent adductor contractures. **B.** Prone position. **C.** Semi-supine position in bed. **D.** Seated position.

The study of orthopaedics cannot therefore be separated from study of the anatomy applied to the part of the body which is involved, and related to the condition under discussion. Reference has already been made to the 'orthopaedic eye'; students are urged to cultivate their powers of observation in a positive sense for the benefit of their patients and the advance of their own knowledge and experience.

Anatomy is best learnt, not in isolation but in relation to particular patients and particular conditions; Roaf & Hodkinson (1971) give anatomy relevant to various orthopaedic conditions and the work of Riddle (1977) is well known in this field.

Body landmarks are important because in common with landmarks elsewhere they tell us where we are. Moreover, body landmarks are often 'pressure areas' as well, for example the sacrum, the great trochanter, the malleolus.

The surface contours and posture of the body

Surface contours vary enormously in different subjects, despite the fundamental similarity of structure, and are greatly influenced by the muscular development and the amount of subcutaneous fat. There are also great differences of habit in what is known as posture, meaning the attitude or carriage of the body. The *stance* and *gait* also vary in different individuals, as evidenced by one's ability to recognise people by a characteristic attitude or walk. Posture is greatly influenced by the balance of one joint upon another, and by the 'build' of the individual, difference in bodily structure producing many variations within the normal pattern. The student must acquire a knowledge of normal posture by observation of the living subject. It is said to be present when the head is held erect, the chin in, the spine straight and presenting its normal curves; the shoulders level, the pelvis level, the chest arched, and the belly flat; the hips and knees in extension, and the feet in the plantar-grade position.

Posture and the nurse

The orthopaedic nurse must be acutely aware of her own posture and that of her colleagues and her patients. In her patients, a knowledge of what

their posture should be, both in bed and afoot, enables her to carry out the surgeon's orders. From observation of her colleagues, she will learn the infinite variations in posture which are present in normal individuals. In herself, the maintenance of good posture prevents fatigue and strains of the feet and back, and helps to preserve a high standard of general health and mental alertness. In most schools of nursing, student nurses are given postural exercises and education in walking. They are also taught the correct method of lifting and turning heavy patients and of helping them in and out of bed. This subject is well covered in a booklet *The handling of patients—a guide for nurse managers*, published jointly by the Back Pain Association and the Royal College of Nursing. Other important publications on this subject are listed in the Bibliography, and are aimed not only at showing efficient lifting techniques but at protecting the lifters' backs from injury. Nursing procedures such as bed-mak-

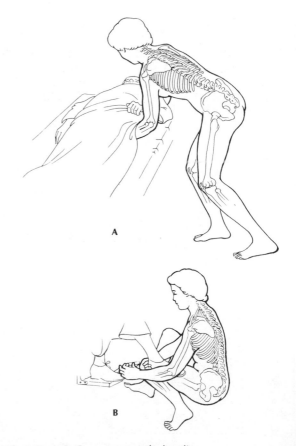

Fig. 1.3 A, B. Correct posture for bending.

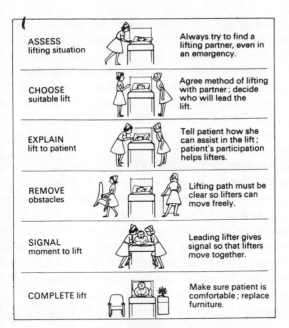

ASSESS lifting situation		Always try to find a lifting partner, even in an emergency.
CHOOSE suitable lift		Agree method of lifting with partner; decide who will lead the lift.
EXPLAIN lift to patient		Tell patient how she can assist in the lift; patient's participation helps lifters.
REMOVE obstacles		Lifting path must be clear so lifters can move freely.
SIGNAL moment to lift		Leading lifter gives signal so that lifters move together.
COMPLETE lift		Make sure patient is comfortable; replace furniture.

Fig. 1.4 Team-work is essential to lift a patient safely.

1. Never stand when it is possible to sit—e.g. when feeding a helpless patient. If the standing position is imperative, raise one foot on a stool, or place one foot in advance of the other and shift the bodyweight from one foot to the other at frequent intervals.

2. When lifting a heavy patient, flex the hips and knees so that the strain is taken on the muscles of the legs, abdomen and hips rather than on those of the back. *Never* lift a weight, whether it be an object off the floor or a baby from his cot with the knees straight (Figs. 1.3, 1.4, 1.5).

3. Concentrate on learning the correct method of lifting, bed-making and 'turning', as taught in the class-room. Do not make heroic attempts to perform these tasks alone (Fig. 1.4); bed-making, for example, requires two nurses working in unison; single-handed efforts can only lead to discomfort for the patient and fatigue and overstrain for the nurse.

ing are also taught with emphasis on coordinated team work so as to reduce strain to a minimum. The nurse with an upright graceful carriage, who performs her tasks in a smooth effortless manner is a joy to watch and an example to all around her (Figs. 1.3–1.5).

In carrying out nursing duties, fatigue and strain (particularly of the lower back) can be avoided by observing the following rules:

The normal curves of the body

The spine. This presents four antero-posterior curves, viz.: the thoracic and pelvic curves, concave forwards, and the cervical and lumbar curves, concave backwards. The thoracic and pelvic curves are developed first; the cervical curve appears as the growing baby raises his head, and the lumbar curve as walking commences. The lum-

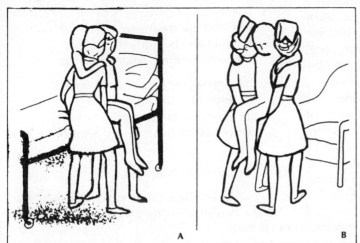

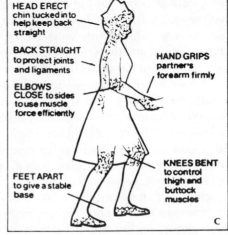

HEAD ERECT chin tucked in to help keep back straight

BACK STRAIGHT to protect joints and ligaments

ELBOWS CLOSE to sides to use muscle force efficiently

FEET APART to give a stable base

HAND GRIPS partner's forearm firmly

KNEES BENT to control thigh and buttock muscles

A   B   C

Fig. 1.5 **A, B.** A method of lifting a patient from bed to chair. **C.** Key factors in lifting. (Drawings 1.4 and 1.5 from the Eothen Films lifting and carrying patients teaching programme.)

bar curve is always more marked in females than in males due to the greater forward tilt of the pelvis.

The pelvis. This is normally held so that the anterior superior iliac spines are level and in the same vertical plane as the symphysis pubis. The female pelvis is wider and its forward inclination more marked than in the male.

The lower limbs. The femur inclines slightly inwards and presents a mild forward bowing. The inward inclination is accentuated in females owing to the greater width of the pelvis. The tibia inclines very slightly forward and outwards. In the normal subject both knees and both malleoli touch in the standing position, and the feet should point straight forwards.

The upper limbs. The height at which the shoulders are carried varies in different individuals, but normally both shoulders are held at the same level. At the elbow, the forearm bones make an angle of 10 degrees to 15 degrees with the humerus when the joint is held in extension. This results in an arc, convex inwards, which is called the 'carrying-angle'. It is greater in females than in males to allow the arm to swing clear of the wider pelvis.

MUSCLE ACTION

Movement is produced by a strong contraction of muscles, due to a rapid and synchronous discharge of impulses from the nervous system. The extent of muscular contraction required to produce a movement depends on the forces which must be overcome, such as the force of gravity, or there may be other obstructing forces within the body, such as insufficient relaxation of opposing muscles. Each muscle or group of muscles performing a given function is balanced by its 'opponent' or 'antagonist', having the opposite function; for example, flexion of the elbow is carried out mainly by brachialis, biceps and brachio-radialis, whilst the opponent or antagonist is the extensor of the elbow, i.e. the triceps muscle. Thus every normal movement involves *group action* of a number of muscles, with lengthening of some muscles and shortening of others. For instance, in the example given above, on bending the elbow there is contraction and shortening of the flexors of that joint and relaxation and lengthening of the extensors.

The antigravity muscles are those which are concerned with maintaining the upright position, i.e. the erector spinae.

Paralysis of muscles which is due to a lesion of the lower motor neurone resulting in loss of tonicity is spoken of as 'flaccid paralysis'. Lesions of the upper motor neurone produce an increase in muscle-tone which is spoken of as 'spastic paralysis' (Chs 14, 17, 18, 23 and 24).

Muscle spasm is a state of tonic contraction, not under control of the will, and is Nature's way of protecting a diseased or injured part of the body, e.g. spasm of the thigh muscles in fracture of the femur, or of the lumbar muscles in prolapse of an intervertebral disc. Muscle spasm is also seen where there is interruption of normal control of impulses from the brain and spinal cord, as in Pott's paraplegia (Ch. 17), spinal cord injury (Ch. 23) or strokes (Ch. 24).

JOINTS

The bones of the skeleton are connected to one another at different parts of their surfaces, and such connections are termed joints or articulations. These are beautifully constructed mechanisms, clothed and lubricated by synovial membrane and fluid, surrounded by capsules, and bound together by ligaments. It is important for the nurse to remember that muscles and tendons acting upon and surrounding a joint also act as supporting structures. The degree of movement of which each joint is capable and the means by which it is normally limited should also be studied.

Limitation of joint movement is due to:

1. the shape of the constituent bones;
2. the restraint of the ligaments;
3. the resistance of muscles;
4. contact of the part moved with other structures.

This is described as follows:

Flexion or bending; *extension* or straightening.

Abduction or drawing away from the mid-line of the body.

Adduction or drawing towards the mid-line of the body.

Internal (medial) and external (lateral) rotation,

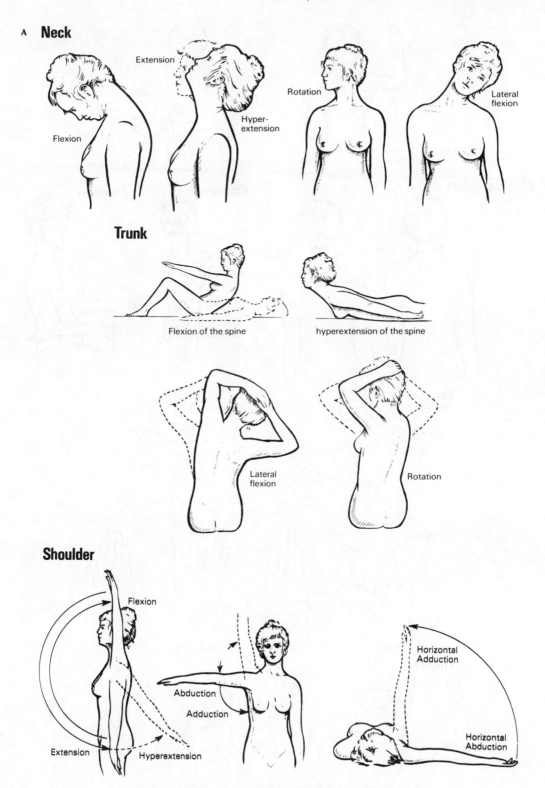

A **Neck**

Extension

Flexion

Hyper-extension

Rotation

Lateral flexion

Trunk

Flexion of the spine

hyperextension of the spine

Lateral flexion

Rotation

Shoulder

Flexion

Horizontal Adduction

Abduction

Adduction

Horizontal Abduction

Extension

Hyperextension

Fig. 1.6   Movements of joints. **A.** Spine. **B.** Upper extremity. **C.** Lower extremity

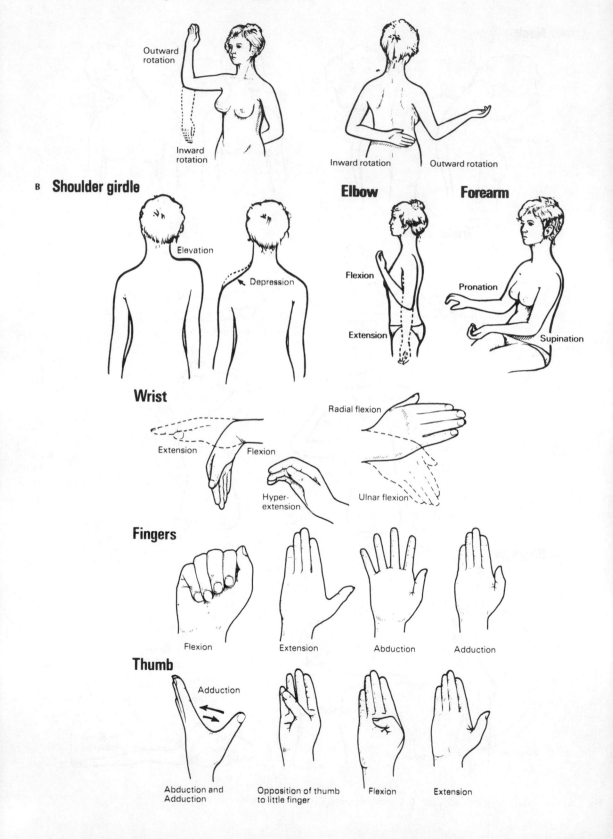

Outward rotation

Inward rotation

Inward rotation   Outward rotation

B **Shoulder girdle**

Elevation

Depression

Elbow

Flexion

Extension

Forearm

Pronation

Supination

Wrist

Extension   Flexion

Hyper-extension

Radial flexion

Ulnar flexion

Fingers

Flexion   Extension   Abduction   Adduction

Thumb

Adduction

Abduction and Adduction

Opposition of thumb to little finger

Flexion

Extension

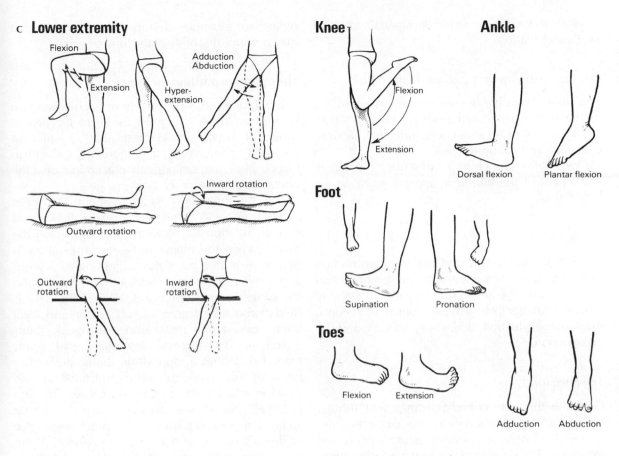

c **Lower extremity**

Flexion
Extension
Hyper-extension
Adduction
Abduction
Outward rotation
Inward rotation
Outward rotation
Inward rotation

Knee

Flexion
Extension

Ankle

Dorsal flexion
Plantar flexion

Foot

Supination
Pronation

Toes

Flexion
Extension
Adduction
Abduction

or rolling towards or away from the mid-line of the body.

Circumduction is a combination of all these movements.

Individual joints will now be considered.

The spine

This is a flexible rod capable of a wide range of movement: flexion, extension, side-bending and rotation.

The shoulder joint

This is a ball and socket joint and its movements are greatly aided by the movements of the scapula on the chest-wall, as seen by the comparatively wide range of movement which can be developed when the joint is fixed, e.g. by arthrodesis. The glenoid cavity is shallow and does not enclose the humeral head firmly, so that the joint is easily dis-

located, especially if its muscular supports are lost, as for example in poliomyelitis. Movements permitted are flexion, extension, abduction, adduction, rotation and circumduction.

The elbow joint

This is a hinge joint permitting flexion and extension.

Supination, turning the forearm palm upwards, and *pronation*, turning the forearm palm downwards, occur at the superior and inferior radio-ulnar joints. For this movement to be pure, it must be performed with the arm held to the side, and the elbow flexed to the right-angle, otherwise rotation occurs at the shoulder joint.

The wrist joint

This joint allows of flexion, or *palmar-flexion* (i.e. in the direction of the palm) and extension or *dorsi-*

flexion; abduction or *radial deviation*; adduction or *ulnar deviation*.

The first carpo-metacarpal joint of the thumb

This joint is capable of very free movement owing to the shape of the articulating surfaces. Movements permitted are abduction, adduction, flexion, extension and circumduction.

Opposition ('pinch-grip') describes the rotary movement of the thumb in approximating to the little finger.

The hip joint

This is a ball and socket joint similar in construction to the shoulder joint except that the femoral head fits firmly into the acetabulum, so that its stability is much greater. Movements consist of flexion, extension, abduction, adduction, rotation, and circumduction.

The knee joint

Generally this is described as a hinge joint, though some degree of rotation can occur when the joint is flexed. Otherwise movements are flexion and extension. The stability of this joint is greatly dependent on the surrounding musculature, notably the quadriceps.

The ankle joint

This is formed between talus below and the mortice of the tibia and fibula above. Movements are flexion or *dorsiflexion*, i.e. bending towards the body, and extension, or *plantar-flexion*, i.e. bending towards the ground.

The joints of the foot

These produce *inversion*, or turning up the inner border of the foot, and *eversion*, or turning up the outer border of the foot.

Abduction or *adduction* of the foot also occurs at these joints.

The joints of the body are interdependent, in that deformity or limitation of movement of one joint often imposes unnatural mechanical strains on others; for example, dysfunction of the hip-joint may produce disability of the lumbar spine.

The optimum position for joints

The optimum position for a joint is considered to be that in which it is most useful to the patient should it become ankylosed, that is, stiff. An inflamed or injured joint is therefore splinted in this position, and deliberately placed in it after the operation of arthrodesis.

Thus the shoulder is placed in about 70 degrees of abduction, 30 degrees of forward flexion and enough rotation to allow the hand to reach the mouth when the elbow is flexed. The elbow is placed in a little more than right-angled flexion, and the forearm in mid-rotation, depending upon the patient's occupation and wishes. The wrist is held in about 30 degrees of dorsiflexion and slight ulnar deviation; metacarpo-phalangeal joints flexed at 90 degrees; interphalangeal joints extended; thumb in opposition. Some authorities consider this position extreme and advocate the position adopted in grasping a tumbler. The hip is usually placed in extension, unless the lumbar spine or opposite hip is also stiff, when some degree of flexion may be of benefit to the patient. About 15 degrees or 20 degrees of abduction and external (lateral) rotation is considered useful. The knee is placed in a position just short of full extension, and the ankle joint is held so that the foot is at a right angle to the leg. The joints of the foot are placed in the neutral position as regards inversion–eversion, abduction–adduction.

Wherever possible, the normal physiological curves of the body are preserved, as for example in the spine and in the palmar and plantar arches.

DEFORMITY

A deformity is a malformation of the body or limb. It may be:

1. *Congenital*, that is, present at birth, and due to a developmental error or to some factor in the maternal environment (Ch. 14).
2. *Acquired*, that is, due to disease or injury.

A postural deformity. This is due to habitual bad

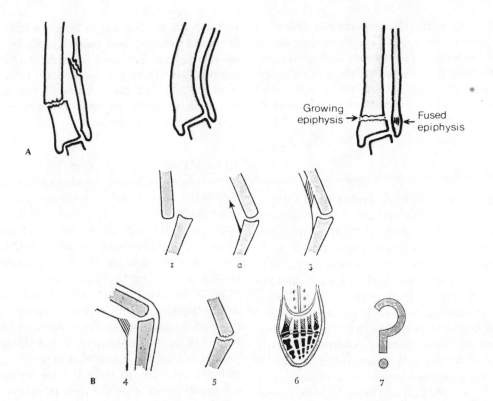

Fig. 1.7 A. Three causes of deformity arising in a bone: 1. Fracture; 2. Bending of softened bone; 3. Uneven epiphysial growth. **B.** Seven causes of deformity arising at a joint: 1. Dislocation; 2. Muscle imbalance; 3. Tethering of muscle or tendon; 4. Soft-tissue contracture; 5. Arthritis; 6. Posture; 7. Idiopathic (cause unknown). (Adams)

position and is capable of being voluntarily corrected by the patient.

A structural deformity. This is due to architectural changes in the part involved, and cannot be voluntarily corrected by the patient.

Postural deformities may become structural, as in course of time soft tissues adapt themselves to position and become contracted, and skeletal changes eventually follow.

Compensation for deformity

The body weight must always be kept over the centre of gravity. In order to achieve this, a shift of one part of the body will be accompanied by a shift of another part in the opposite direction, for example, if one leg is shorter than the other, the pelvis on that side will be tilted downwards to allow the foot to reach the ground. A corresponding curve of the lumbar spine will follow, and this may be compensated for by a thoracic curve in the opposite direction. Thus it will be seen that each part of the body is mechanically dependent upon the rest.

The treatment of deformities is described in later pages; as a general rule, mild deformities due to changes in soft tissues may be amenable to correction by conservative means, but those due to bony changes require operative interference. Moreover, the treatment is influenced by the extent to which a deformity interferes with *function*; a patient may seek treatment for a deformity for cosmetic reasons only; on the other hand it is important to remember that as time goes on any part of the musculo-skeletal system which is no longer perfect will show signs of stress and will wear out faster than normal parts, for example, a hip joint damaged by slipping of the upper femoral epiphysis or by Perthes' disease may become the seat of osteo-arthritic change earlier than might occur in a comparable but undamaged hip joint. It is also important to remember that deformities in children are influenced by *growth*; for example, a neglected clubfoot will produce most growth on the side of the foot on which there is least pressure, i.e. on the lateral aspect of the foot, so that as growth proceeds so does increase of the deformity.

REST

We are all familiar with our body's need for rest, and the benefit we derive from it; it is Nature's way of healing our ills, particularly when it is combined with change of environment and of daily occupation, as on a holiday. In general, the only time we do not enjoy rest is when it is forced upon us by extraneous circumstances, such as illness, accident, unemployment, or even imprisonment. In normal circumstances, the need for rest varies in different individuals and is governed not only by variations in physical make-up but by mental attitudes, for example, a holiday spent lying on a beach in the sun may be one person's idea of Heaven and, to another, the last word in boredom. In the same way, our patients vary in their reactions when enforced rest is ordered as a definite therapeutic measure, with the following aims in view:

1. To provide the best possible condition for
   a. the body's natural powers of resistance to be brought to bear on disease processes, and
   b. for full use of the natural recuperative powers of the body in adjusting its metabolism after injury or following operative interference.
2. To provide immobility of the body as a whole and so inhibit the activity of vital organs, as for example in disorders of the heart or lungs.
3. To relieve pain by removing the strain of weight-bearing and of the pull of gravity on the body or part of the body, as in patients suffering from pain in the back.
4. To prevent strains in the region of a diseased part or where a wound is present, and so promote healing of body tissues, as for example, after an operation.

In addition there are patients who require rest in bed for a combination of the conditions outlined above, for example, a patient with osteomyelitis

of the tibia is confined to bed not only because he has a diseased and painful limb, but because he also has a generalised illness with a raised body temperature. There are also patients who are completely confined to bed because there is no alternative, as for example, the patient who is unconscious following a head injury.

GENERAL REST

Before the advent of modern drugs and of modern orthopaedic surgery, rest was often 'enforced, uninterrupted and prolonged' (Hugh Owen Thomas). *General rest* for the whole body and *local rest* provided by some form of splintage, is still regarded as a mainstay of treatment in orthopaedic practice despite the fact that it can be described as a two-edged sword; in many cases it is essential to relieve pain and to allow damaged tissues to heal, but at the same time it is a danger to the patient because it leads to degenerative changes in body structure, to stasis in vital organs, and to unnatural pressure on soft parts or on body prominences.

Dr R A Ascher (1947) wrote on 'the dangers of going to bed' as follows:

Look at a patient lying long in bed—what a pathetic picture he makes; the blood clotting in his veins, the lime draining from his bones, the scyballa stacking up in his colon, the flesh rotting from his seat, the urine leaking from his distended bladder and the spirit evaporating from his soul.

Controlled rest and local rest

An example is seen in the patient with a fracture of the femur who is confined to bed (*controlled rest for the whole body*) and his injured limb is immoblised in a Thomas bed-splint (*local rest*). This regime helps the patient's own recuperative powers to overcome the effects of his injury, prevents pain on movement of the injured limb, and immobilises it in a good anatomical position while healing takes place. At first, the patient is allowed only limited activity and will require nursing care on the lines about to be discussed, but as healing takes place and the pain and swelling of the limb subsides, he will gradually be able to undertake more and more of his own care; exercises for all parts of his body and muscle contractors for the injured limb will be introduced. In due course, the splint is removed and the patient begins to move the limb under supervision, though weight-bearing is not permitted until the bone is soundly united. At this stage, the patient is encouraged to carry out his own care and progresses gradually to full active exercises until he is allowed up, sometimes with local protective splintage, such as a caliper. Programmes of intensive and strenuous exercises are sometimes necessary as a prelude to his return to work, but such programmes include periods of *controlled rest* to avoid both general fatigue and undue strains of the injured part. A gradual return to sporting activities is also used as an introduction to heavy work. Thus it will be seen that controlled rest is used therapeutically throughout the patient's treatment from the moment he enters the hospital until his return to normal life.

Balance between rest and activity

In many conditions, and in patients who are at a 'half-way house' stage between complete rest and full activity, an important part of our duties is to control, on the one hand, the amount of rest which the patient needs for his recovery, and on the other, his activity which is aimed at the restoration of function. This often requires sophisticated judgement which can only be learned by experience; moreover not only the nurse but all members of the orthopaedic team play their part, including the surgeon whose orders lay down the general pattern of the programme of treatment, the physiotherapist and often, the occupational therapist as well.

Factors which prevent rest

Some of these are so obvious as to seem unworthy of mention, but they all influence our patient—management and must not be taken for granted; avoidance of these factors, listed below, by all the means in our power is an essential part of good nursing.

1. An uncomfortable bed; a hard, lumpy mattress; insufficient pillows; tight or inadequate bed-clothes; 'umbilical' beds; rubber or plastic sheets; creased or rucked-up sheets or draw-sheets; patched sheets; wet beds; food crumbs.

2. Cold, especially cold feet; over-heating; draughts.
3. Pain; skin irritation; inability to move from an uncomfortable position or from the rays of strong light or sunlight.
4. Hunger and thirst; disturbances of bowel or bladder function; 'indigestion'.
5. Cough; interference with respiration.
6. Noise; the telephone; transistor radios; television; heavy footsteps; loud voices; 'things that go bump in the night'; snores.
7. Too many visitors, especially those we do not wish to see.
8. Insecurity in the ward situation; an uneven pattern of nursing care; lack of confidence in one's attendants.
9. Fear; anxiety; boredom; grief.

Some other observations on rest in bed

Lying in bed continuously is not a natural state; most people soon tire of it and long for nothing so much as to get up. Moreover our body metabolism is designed for alternating rest and activity so that enforced and continuous rest interferes with this, particularly in relation to nitrogen balance. Acceptance of enforced rest is governed not only by the patient's normal activity of body but by his activity of mind and by his temperament. People with boundless physical and mental energy are the worst sufferers, and many of our patients only submit cheerfully to rest in bed by a definite effort of will. Those whose mental endowment is such that they cannot appreciate the need for rest in bed are particularly poor subjects, and we have all met the patient who, on his first day out of bed will, if unsupervised, attempt a marathon walk and then complain of pain and fatigue; the answer is to *make haste slowly*, deliberately increasing activity each day and accepting some degree of fatigue or even discomfort as a natural sequence. Patients do not always appreciate the fact that it *takes time* to 'get over' the effects of disease, injury or operation; for example a woman who has had her bunions corrected may be bitterly disappointed because her feet do not feel normal on her first day out of bed; in fact it may be several weeks or months before she can take her 'new feet' for granted.

The bed-pan. This deserves special mention in

relation to continuous, enforced rest in bed since there is evidence to suggest that patients find the use of bed-pans very worrying (Anderson, 1978), because of embarrassment and loss of dignity. The nurse must preserve the patient's privacy and sense of dignity as far as possible, and whenever indicated, seek the doctors permission to get the patient out of bed on to a bedside commode or to the lavatory on a wheelchair or sani-chair. It can be claimed that in some cases the effort and strain involved in the use of a bed-pan causes more pain, more discomfort and certainly more anxiety than the once-daily use of a commode or sani-chair, as for example, in some patients with low back pain.

Another important method of avoiding the spectre of the bed-pan to some degree is *the use of a urinal for female patients as well as males*; further reference to this will be found later. The patient whose splint or plaster cast might be contaminated by urine or faeces requires special attention; such contamination represents a failure in nursing care.

The complications of rest in bed (Fig. 1.8)

Although rest in bed is ordered as a therapeutic measure, there are patients to whom it is actually harmful, hence the term 'controlled rest'. For example, aged patients may deteriorate rapidly and die

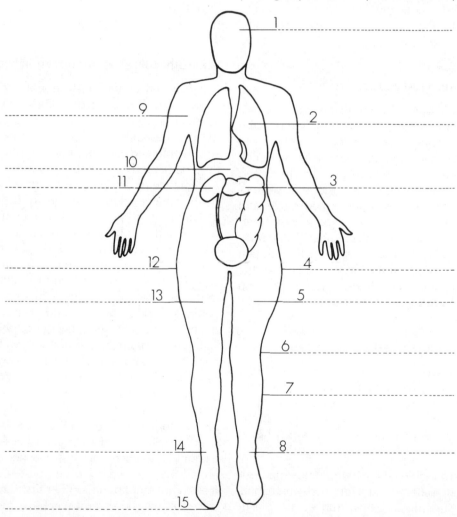

Fig. 1.8 The complications of rest in bed. The student should fill in the blank spaces beside the numbers and refer to the table overleaf.

The complications of rest in bed

Problem	Objective	Nursing Action	Response
General: Loss of independence.	For the patient to be as independent as possible.	Treat as a guest. Give encouragement. Provide aids to independence. Allow patient to make own decision as far as possible.	
Loss of self-respect.	To maintain self-respect.	Ensure adequate explanations are given with regard to condition, treatment, care and prognosis.	Observe and report/record mental state.
Boredom.	To maintain interest.	Encourage visiting. Encourage patient/staff conversation.	
Apathy.		Encourage interaction between patients. Play, for children. Diversional Therapy for all patients. Provide/suggest: reading material, TV, Radio, Portable telephone, Education.	
Affecting Respiratory System. Chest Infection.	To ensure adequate ventilation of lungs.	Discourage smoking if patient smokes, explaining reasons for this. Support in upright position with provision of heart table if possible. Encourage and supervise breathing exercises as instructed by physiotherapist. Encourage expectoration of sputum if appropriate. Provide sputum carton and tissues. Ensure adequate fluid intake. Give steam inhalation. Oxygen if required. Give analgesia as prescribed as pain may inhibit deep breathing exercises and expectoration of sputum.	Observe cough, character of sputum, measure and record. Observe and record effect.
Digestive System. Anorexia.	To stimulate appetite, and to provide suitable diet.	Help the patient to choose suitable diet from menu. Present food attractively; served at right temperature. Mouth-care. Regular opportunity for cleaning teeth and using mouthwash.	Observe and report on diet taken.
Excessive weight gain.		Provide prescribed diet containing required calories and nutrients.	
Constipation.	Regular bowel action.	Provide: Diet containing bran roughage, fruit. Adequate fluid intake. Privacy and comfort for defaecation at time which habit dictates. Help with cleansing afterwards. General exercises while in bed and mobilisation as early as possible. Laxatives, suppositories, enemata as prescribed.	Observe, report and record bowel action.
Affecting Renal Tract. Retention of Urine. Stasis. Urinary Tract Infection. Renal Calculi.	To ensure adequate urinary excretion of waste products.	Encourage patient to take adequate fluids. Explain reason for increased intake, and discuss preference for drinks. Provide privacy for urinal or bed-pan when required. Support in the best position which condition will allow.	Fluid Balance Chart.

(cont'd)

Complications of rest in bed (cont'd.)

Problem	Objective	Nursing Action	Response
		Run taps into adjacent hand-basin. Warm compress lower abdomen. Intermittent catheterisation or indwelling catheter as requested by doctor if patient unable to pass urine. 4-hourly catheter toilet if indwelling catheter. Turn patient regularly where recumbent position has to be maintained. Give drugs to prevent and/or treat infection as prescribed.	Save specimen of urine and do ward test. Send specimen to laboratory for culture and sensitivity. 4-hourly record of temperature, pulse and respiration. Record position changes. Record and note effect.
Circulatory System. Slowing of Venous Return. Deep Vein Thrombosis. Pulmonary Embolism.	To keep blood circulating. To prevent deep vein thrombosis.	Avoid pressure on calves of legs especially during operation. Teach and encourage deep breathing and leg exercises regularly. Elevate foot of bed. Give analgesia as prescribed if pain inhibiting patient doing exercises. Ensure adequate fluid intake. Provide aids to improving venous return as advised by doctor e.g. Flowtron boots, elastic stockings. Administration of anticoagulant drugs as prescribed.	Observe and report and record: Calf tenderness. Pain in leg. Oedema. Pyrexia. Pain in chest. Cough. Blood-stained sputum.
Loco-Motor System: Joint Stiffness. Muscle Wasting. Deformity.	To maintain a full range of joint movement with no muscle wasting or deformity.	To encourage regular active exercises as instructed by physiotherapist of perform regular passive movements. Careful positioning of patient. Provide bed-cradle to prevent pressure from bed-clothes.	Note movement of limbs and trunk.
Local/General Osteoporosis.	To endeavour to minimise osteoporosis as a result of lack of activity.	Encourage exercise.	
Skin. Pressure Sores.	To maintain skin intact and free from soreness.	Regular alteration of position. Provision of hand-grip to facilitate patient altering own position where possible. Avoidance of friction. Careful lifting. Care when giving and removing bed-pans. Prevent patient sliding down bed. Ensure cleanliness and careful drying of skin. Adequate nutrition. Adequate hydration. Use of aids—e.g. sheepskin pads, bed cradle. Ripple mattress. Waterbed/mattress. Mobilisation as soon as possible.	Observe skin state. Record position changes.
Formation of thick hard skin and thickening of nails on feet.		Frequent washing with immersion of feet in water if possible. Oil application. Chiropody.	

before their time if simply left in bed to do so; on the other hand, the decision to keep such a patient in bed is made on medical grounds and must be accepted. In addition there are patients who for psychological reasons develop a great fondness for bed, and in general any measure which will allow patients out of bed at an early stage in treatment, if only for a limited period and if only in a wheelchair, is worthy of serious consideration. Modern techniques in orthopaedic surgery are also directed to this end; for example, the patient who sustains a fracture of the femur may be treated by means of internal fixation with a metal plate or nail, thus avoiding the prolonged rest in bed referred to in a previous paragraph.

Complications are outlined in the form of a simplified list (see below); in practice they are often found to be inter-related, and their implications are discussed further in subsequent chapters in relation to conditions in which they are most likely to occur.

The complications of prolonged rest in bed will be discussed as a problem-solving approach to nursing care, each complication being identified as an actual or potential problem for each patient. The nursing action should be planned for each patient on an individual basis and the response to care evaluated by careful observation and recording.

Sexual frustration. Though not listed as a complication of rest in bed, patients in hospital who are accustomed to an active sex life can feel very deprived. One patient reported (Macmillan, 1980) 'I miss the old cuddle in bed with the wife. We became strangers, know what I mean?'

Patients who have suffered some permanent physical impairment may worry about their future in sexual relationships. This problem is discussed in an article in the *Nursing Mirror* (Leonard, 1981) 'Understanding Sexuality: talking through a taboo'. Other publications deal with the sex life of the paralysed patient (Ch. 23).

Conclusion

Rest in bed is a valuable therapeutic measure in utilising the patient's natural resources; it is up to us to exercise such control, judgement and attention to nursing detail as to use it to the best possible advantage and to avoid the complications outlined in the previous paragraph.

LOCAL REST

Local rest is ordered to relieve pain, or to allow diseased or damaged tissues to heal after injury or operation.

It is achieved by immobilisation of the body or part of the body by means of a splint, a plaster cast or a traction device; supporting bandages and arm slings are also used.

SPLINTS, BRACES AND APPLIANCES (ORTHOSES)

All devices applied to the body are *appliances* in the sense that they serve a use or purpose, but in general we use the word 'splint' when we refer to a device which is applied to protect and/or immobilise a part and to restrict movement; a *brace* is also a splint but in general this term refers to a device which is used to assist weight-bearing; braces are also called calipers or leg-irons and some spinal supports come under this heading, for example, the Milwaukee brace. Sometimes the patient's bed can be regarded as a splint, for example a child with suspected transient arthritis of the hip may be ordered strict rest in bed with the specific purpose of resting the hip; then there are mobile, 'active', 'working' or 'dynamic' splints which allow certain movements, for example an active splint ordered for a radial nerve lesion; a wheelchair can also be regarded as a 'working' splint. There are also certain splints which allow controlled movement, such as a jointed caliper (long-leg brace). Further information on splints, braces and appliances will be found in Ch. 7.

Other purposes of splintage

Apart from providing local rest by limiting movement, splints are also used for the following purposes:

1. For first aid in injuries.
2. To provide fixed traction (the Thomas bed splint) (Fig. 1.10).
3. To prevent deformity, or, to retain correction when it has been achieved, to correct *mild* deformity, for example, an inside iron outside T-strap (short leg brace) is used for an inverted foot in hemiplegia (Fig. 7.7A, B, C). Corrective retentive splintage is also applied in clubfoot. A Milwaukee brace is used in the treatment of scoliosis (Fig. 15.6A, B, C, D) and maintains continuous extension of the spine so that further deformity is prevented and may even correct itself as the child grows.

4. To relieve weight, as in a weight-relieving caliper (brace with ischial seat) or Thomas patten-ended caliper (Fig. 7.2C).
5. To stabilise joints and to protect weak muscles, as in poliomyelitis or muscle weakness from some other cause, for example, spinal cord injury.
6. To maintain extension of the spine and/or hips and knees for maintenance of the erect position with weight-bearing, as in the examples given above or in allied conditions; for example, spina bifida.

Splints are fabricated by a splint-maker (orthotist) usually employed by a commercial undertaking. In the past splints were made mainly of leather or metal or a combination of both and were often heavy and cumbersome; though some splints of this description are still used, other materials such as various forms of plastic are now available which are light in weight, durable and less conspicuous in appearance than those of the past.

Various splints are described in Ch. 7. Kennedy, Day and Stewart give comprehensive and up-to-date surveys of orthopaedic splints and appliances.

In general, nurses are not expected to measure patients for splints except for those taken from hospital stock, notably the Thomas bed-splint, Braun splint and perhaps a metal cock-up wrist splint.

Home-made splints such as plaster shells for the foot or a cock-up splint for the wrist are usually made in the outpatient department or the plaster room; physiotherapists and occupational therapists often show great ingenuity in the design and fabrication of simple and inexpensive home-made splints (Figs 22.4, 22.6). Plaster spinal jackets and other spinal supports also come into this category for example, Nicholls *et al.* (1966), describe an 'instant body corset' made from Tubigrip body bandage combined with plaster of Paris. Cervical collars are frequently ordered and if required immediately, might be made of sorbo rubber or some other soft material or from other materials such as plastics (Kennedy, 1974).

Notes on the nursing management of patients wearing splints

1. A splint must fit perfectly, otherwise it will be uncomfortable or ineffective or both.

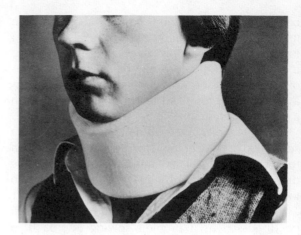

Fig. 1.9 An example of a cervical collar. (Raymed Division of Thackaray.)

2. It must perform the purpose for which it is ordered; an inefficient splint is a waste of time and money.
3. A splint must be reasonably comfortable or the patient will not wear it; however it is important to remember that it takes time and perseverance for a patient to get used to wearing a splint; patients vary in their reactions in that some have low tolerance to any form of splint or appliance and the nurse must be prepared to give advice in this connection.
4. It must be worn according to the doctor's orders; a splint discarded against advice does not help the patient and again, wastes time and money.
5. The splint should be as light in weight, unobtrusive, inconspicuous, and inexpensive as possible.
6. Good personal hygiene is imperative; the skin and the splint itself must be kept clean and dry.
7. The splint must be maintained in good repair; where splintage is to be worn for a long period, a second splint should be available for use while the first one is repaired.
8. In children, splintage must not become outgrown. N.B. Include *footwear* in your observations.
9. The patient or his relatives must be taught the management of the splint; clear instructions are given as to whether or not it can be removed at any time, and whether it is worn under or over the clothing; in this connection

the patient is warned that any form of splintage, including a plaster cast, produces abnormal wear and tear of clothing.
10. A splint must not interfere with circulation or nerve supply to the limbs.
11. Non-immobilised joints must be exercised regularly.

Nursing examination of a patient wearing a splint

Does the *patient* look happy and comfortable? What is the general state of health? What is the splint supposed to do? Is it doing it? Does it fit well? Is it clean, in good repair, with all parts functioning correctly? In a child, is it becoming outgrown? Is the skin intact and healthy? Is there incipient deformity of some part? Is there any sign of pressure on blood vessels or nerves, such as oedema, muscle weakness, or sensory disturbances such as tingling or numbness? Are all non-immobilised joints moving freely? Are the doctors' instructions being followed? Does the patient and/or his relatives understand the management of the splint? Finally, is the patient at work/school? If not, why not? If she is a housewife/mother, is she able to cope with her domestic duties?

Other specific questions will arise in connection with each individual patient.

Individual splints for different purposes are discussed in Ch. 7.

The complications of local rest

Like those of general rest, complications are linked to degenerative changes in body tissue, to stasis in vital organs (e.g. blood vessels) and to unnatural pressure on soft parts or on bony prominences. These changes can affect not only the immobilised limb but other parts as well, e.g. stiffness of the shoulder in Colles' fracture.

Prevention is achieved by:

1. Active exercises and, where possible active use of all joints not immobilised; setting (isometric) exercises for joints which cannot be moved e.g. quadriceps drill for the immobilised knee.
2. Prevention of oedema by avoiding dependency of a limb and by elevation when indicated.
3. Avoidance of exposure of the part to extremes of temperature.
4. Care of the splint, plaster cast or other device used for immobilisation (Chs 6 and 7).
5. Care of the skin (Chs 6 and 7).
6. Prompt reporting of any sign of neuro-vascular involvement, including numbness, 'pins and needles', pain and swelling, or deformity of a non-immobilised part.

PLASTER OF PARIS

Plaster casts are used progressively less often nowadays because modern techniques of orthopaedic surgery employ internal fixation of certain fractures and artificial replacement of certain joints; nevertheless plaster is still an important and easily available method of immobilisation.

Plaster technique is described in Chapter 6; Roaf & Hodkinson (1971) also describe the chemistry of plaster of Paris and give a resume of the objectives of application of a plaster of Paris splint.

Who applies the plaster cast? In some centres, plaster casts are applied only by doctors, whilst in others a technician is specially trained for the task; in others nurses are expected to apply plasters. The nurse manager in charge of the outpatients department or plaster room must be well versed in plaster technique. It does not matter who applies the plaster provided it does the patient no harm and in any event *the care of the patient and the prevention of complications is an important nursing responsibility.* In this connection the importance of *observation* cannot be overstressed; nursing vigilance may save a patient's limb, if not his life.

Special vigilance is required in conditions where the circulation is already deficient, for example in cardio-vascular or metabolic disease, or in neurological conditions. All members of the staff and where appropriate, the patient and/or his relatives must be taught essential observations. In the conscious patient beware of intractable *pain; it may be the only sign of imminent vascular catastrophe.*

TRACTION

Traction is used for the following purposes:

1. To gain or maintain bony alignment, as in a dislocation or fracture.
2. To secure immobilisation of an inflamed or injured joint.

3. To relieve pain.

4. To correct *mild* deformity.

Principles of traction. 'Two strong men will suffice by making extension and counter-extension' (Hippocrates 350 BC). 'For every action there is an equal and opposite reaction' (Newton's third law of motion).

Traction on a limb requires a fixed point from which to work, or an equal counter traction in the opposite direction.

Continuous traction is that which is maintained without interruption. This entails not only maintaining the traction, but the counter-traction as well. Unless otherwise ordered, all traction applied in the ward is maintained continuously. Examples are seen in many parts of this book.

Intermittent traction is applied from time to time. For example, patients on head-halter traction for pain in the neck may be allowed to remove the halter for meals or toilet purposes. Similarly, patients treated for low back pain by leg or pelvis traction may be allowed to release it at intervals, especially for toilet purposes (Ch. 28). Intermittent traction is also used in the Physiotherapy Department in the treatment of these conditions.

1. *Manual traction* is applied by the hands, as when a doctor reduces a fracture.

2. *Fixed traction* is traction between two fixed points. For example, in the Thomas bed-splint, traction is exerted by extension tapes tied to the end of the splint, while counter-traction is supplied by the pressure of the ring against the ischial tuberosity (Fig. 1.10). Another example of fixed traction is that supplied by the Jones abduction frame, in which the pull of skin extensions made from strapping are tied to extension bows is countered by the pressure of a groin strap (Fig. 1.11).

3. *Balanced traction* (sometimes called 'sliding traction') is traction exerted against a weight (Fig. 1.12A, B, C). *Pugh's traction* is a simple example, when strapping skin extensions are tied to the raised foot-end of the bed (Fig. 1.12A). *Weight and pulley traction* is a form of balanced traction when extension tapes are tied to a cord which carries a weight running over a pulley fixed to the elevated foot-end of the bed; counter-traction is provided by the patient's body-weight. It is seen in Fig. 1.12B.

In Fig. 1.12C balanced traction is supplied by a cord from a skeletal pin carrying a weight over

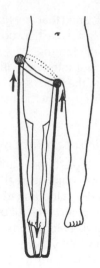

Fig. 1.10 Fixed traction is supplied by the pull of extension tapes tied to the end of a Thomas bed-splint, countered by pressure of the ring against the ischial tuberosity (Watson Jones).

the pulley attached to a Braun's splint. *Russell traction* is a special example of balanced traction, in which a canvas sling is placed beneath the knee and attached to a weighted cord running over four pulleys, as shown in Fig. 1.13. A modification of this type of traction is described in Chapter 27. An essential feature of this type of traction is the 'monkey pole', or trapeze.

Balanced traction with suspension is shown in Figs 21.22, 21.23. Note that continuous traction

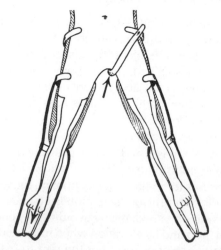

Fig. 1.11 In the abduction frame the pull of skin-extension tied to the bows of the frame is countered by the pressure of a groin strap (Watson Jones).

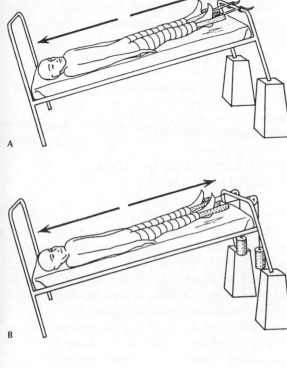

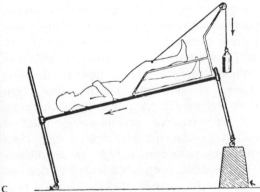

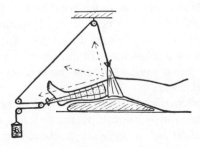

Fig. 1.12 Balanced traction (see text) (Watson Jones).

Fig. 1.13 Hamilton Russell traction (Watson Jones).

is applied by means of a skeletal pin and countered by the patient's body weight. The limb is immobilised in a Thomas bed-splint combined with Pearson flexion-piece, and this apparatus is suspended by means of cords, weights and pulleys in such a way that the patient's body and splinted limb move as one unit. As in Russell traction an essential adjunct to this arrangement is the 'monkey pole', trapeze or patient-helper device (not well shown in this picture) which the patient uses to raise himself from the bed and change his position. This method of applying traction is effective and comfortable and the relative mobility of the patient helps to prevent the complications of rest in bed and of immobilisation already discussed.

Methods of applying traction

1. In *skin traction* the traction force is applied to the skin, from where it is transmitted to the muscles and then to the bone. Skin extensions are made from strapping, either elastoplast extension strapping, Leslie's Holland Strapping, Taylor's perforated zinc-oxide strapping, or Unna's paste (a mixture of zinc-oxide, glycerine, gelatine and water). Collodion covered by ribbon gauze may also be used. Commercial extension packs are in common use in most centres.

2. In *skeletal traction*, traction is applied directly to a bone; a metal pin is driven through the bone and attached to a stirrup to which the traction is exerted by means of weights. The pin may be a Kirschner wire, a Steinmann pin, or ice-tong calipers (see Figs 21.14B, 21.15, 23.14, 23.15A and B).

3. In *pulp traction* a suture is placed through the pulp of a finger or toe and fastened to an extension piece incorporated in a plaster cast. This is rarely used nowadays.

Halo-pelvic traction is seen in Fig. 15.8A, B.

Dangers and complications of traction

1. Skin traction

a. Discomfort, especially from sweating in a hot environment; itching beneath the skin extensions, or an unpleasant prickling sensation when hairs begin to grow on shaved skin; skin reactions, varying from mild erythema to severe generalised reaction.

b. Localised sores, especially where bandages and/or extension material causes pressure, for example, above the heel.

c. Oedema indicates interference with circulation and may be caused by tight bandages or tight bands in extension strapping.

d. Drop foot, from pressure on the lateral popliteal nerve. Other deformity, either at a joint or in a bone or associated with some other part, for example, hyperextension of the knee joint.

e. Muscle wasting.

f. Joint stiffness.

g. Insufficient traction force, i.e. loosening or slipping of skin extensions causing a joint irritation or redisplacement of bone at a fracture site.

NB. The application of skin traction is contraindicated in the presence of a skin condition such as eczema or psoriasis, where there are varicose veins, or where there is loss of normal skin sensation or indeed, any neuro-vascular deficit. It is also important to remember that a child's skin is delicate and that that of an old person is often thin, friable and easily damaged. Prolonged cortisone therapy also undermines the resilience of the skin.

2. Skeletal traction

a. Infection at the site of insertion of the skeletal pin.

b. Cutting out of the skeletal pin from the bone, with displacement at the fracture site.

c. Over-distraction at a fracture site leading to delayed or non-union.

d. Deformity, joint stiffness and muscle wasting as in (1) above.

e. Disturbance of bone growth (in children).

In general, it is true to say that although skeletal traction looks formidable, it is far more comfortable than that applied to the skin; moreover if the traction force is required for a long period (for example, for 8–12 weeks in fracture of the femur) it is not only more comfortable but more effective, less liable to disturbance and more fool-proof than skin traction, which in general, is only suitable for relatively short periods of immobilisation in adults, and for longer periods in children, because spasm of powerful muscles which may exist in the adult and which must be overcome are not so well-developed in the child. This is the reason why the classical treatment of fracture of the femur by means of continuous fixed skin traction in a Thomas bed-splint is, generally speaking, suitable only for children or for thin young adults. Combined with this factor is that of the relatively rapid rate of union of a fracture seen in the child (Ch. 21).

Finally, in discussing the use of traction we note that patients immobilised by this means for any length of time are liable to develop concurrent complications of rest in bed.

THE ROLE OF DRUGS IN CURRENT ORTHOPAEDIC PRACTICE

The revolutionary advances in the field of pharmacology and therapeutics over recent years have been significantly reflected in orthopaedic practice but it is outside the intended scope of this book to discuss in other than general terms what has become a major influence in both prophylaxis and therapy of many orthopaedic conditions.

In addition to the drugs specifically prescribed for the particular orthopaedic condition it is increasingly common to find the patient requiring drug therapy for unrelated concurrent disease so that it becomes evidently necessary for the orthopaedic nurse to be aware of the potency and consequently conversant with the toxic side effects of a wide range of medicines and to observe recording procedures and attendant safety measures. There is need for vigilance for the possibility of abnormal reaction, hypersensitivity and interaction (such as potentiation of certain drugs by alcohol, or the dietary limitations with certain types of antidepressants). It is obvious that such a wide and detailed subject cannot be incorporated in a general textbook on orthopaedic nursing and there are many excellent volumes devoted to pharmacology and therapeutics. Recommended supplementary reading must include the redesigned British National Formulary which is a pocket sized, readily available booklet normally kept on every hospital ward. It is an invaluable source of information and guidance covering a wide range of drugs, their implications and cost.

The following classes of medicinal agents of particular relevance to orthopaedic practice is therefore offered as a general guidance to further reading.

GROUP 1. MEDICINES USED TO RELIEVE PAIN

Analgesics, with or without anti-inflammatory properties, account for quite the highest percentage of prescribed medicines and drug cost in the Health Service and new preparations or re-presentation of established drugs are constantly introduced.

Aspirin still holds a remarkable place in treatment and remains a valuable drug, possessing analgesic, anti-inflammatory and anti-pyretic properties. Prolonged use or the high dose levels often necessary in rheumatological conditions may produce undesirable side effects, notably indigestion, nausea, tinnitus and the less easily detectable bleeding from the gastric mucosa. Many attempts have been made to overcome these problems by producing soluble derivatives, enteric coating and change in chemical structure, often at high cost, e.g. Benoral, Dolobid.

Paracetamol has less analgesic property than aspirin but does not cause gastric mucosal bleeding though hepatic damage can result from high dosage. Paracetamol overdosage has become the most common poisoning encountered in emergency departments.

Combined with dextropropoxyphene as Distalgesic it is widely prescribed for less than severe pain and some concern is being expressed about the accumulating evidence of both toxicity and dependence, the former in particular with concurrent intake of alcohol. Both aspirin and paracetamol are frequently combined with other analgesics such as Compound Aspirin and Codeine tablets, Paracodol, Paramol.

Centrally acting analgesics

Dihydrocodeine (DF118) has a potency intermediate with codeine and morphine and is valuable, providing nausea and dizziness are not encountered. The injectable form is classed as a controlled drug.

Centrally acting analgesics are generally less effective in musculoskeletal pain than peripherally acting agents.

Buprenorphine is being increasingly used both as injection and as a sublingual form.

Pentazocine (Fortral) finds frequent usage in severe pain where it is not considered prudent to prescribe narcotics. There are conflicting opinions on its value. The search for the ideal powerful analgesic devoid of addictive properties continues.

Morphine-like analgesics. Preoperatively, combined with atropine, and for severe post-operative pain morphine remains pre-eminent and together with diamorphine (heroin) finds major usage in the relief of pain in the terminally ill patient. The more recent trend has been to give much higher dosage than in the past.

Papaveretum is sometimes preferred and the synthetic narcotic pethidine is often adequate without possessing the potency of the opiates. These are, of course, controlled drugs and produce dependence.

MST is a slow release form of morphine claimed by the makers to sustain adequate control with a twice daily dosage. It is many times more expensive than simple morphine mixtures.

Local anaesthetics are extensively employed, lignocaine hydrocholoride in strengths from 0.5 to 2 per cent, plain or with adrenaline, and for longer action bupivacaine (Marcain) is preferred.

GROUP 2. DRUGS USED IN RHEUMATOLOGICAL CONDITIONS

Where aspirin and other mild analgesics have proved unsuitable or ineffective a number of alternative drugs are available and these have been discussed in the section devoted to rheumatology.

Indomethacin has now been long established and is a powerful anti-inflammatory agent. Experience of the many side effects, some serious, has resulted in discreet prescribing, and the need to discontinue the drug often occurs. It is now available in a sustained release form designed for bedtime dosage to reduce morning stiffness and suppositories can reduce the gastro-intestinal upset.

Efficacy of a particular drug varies very considerably and the most effective medicine or combination of medicines is determined often by individual patient response. An entirely effective remedy has not been found and this accounts to some extent for the continuous flow of new preparations on to the market; ibuprofen, ketoprofen and flubiprofen are generally less potent than indomethacin and like naproxen and mefenamic acid offer alternative and effective therapy with a wider margin of freedom from toxicity.

Piroxicam is the most frequently used non-steroidal anti-inflammatory drug world wide.

Phenylbutazone has now been withdrawn from the market except for use in ankylosing spondylitis.

Corticosteroids are powerful anti-inflammatory agents but the initial enthusiastic use has been tempered in the light of experience of the dangerous side effects. The generally accepted principle is to use the smallest possible maintenance dose and prednisolone is often the drug of choice to allow critical dosage to be obtained.

Methylprednisolone and triamcinolone as depot preparations for intra-articular administration produce sustained local relief from pain and stiffness and are very extensively used.

Suppressive anti-rheumatic treatment with slow-acting remission-inducing drugs such as gold, penicillamine or antimalarials is used in patients with persistently active symptomatic disease which has not responded to non-steroid anti-inflammatory drugs.

GROUP 3. ANTIBIOTICS

The 40 years or so that have passed since the availability of penicillin has seen the development of a powerful armoury of chemotherapeutic agents with extensive application to orthopaedics. The antibiotics have revolutionised the treatment of such conditions as osteomyelitis, septic arthritis, tuberculosis of bone and joint and many other infective processes. The value of penicillin has been substantially reduced with the emergence of resistant organisms but derivatives of the basic penicillin nucleus play an important role.

Ampicillin and amoxycillin are wide spectrum antibiotics whilst cloxacillin and flucloxacillin are particularly applicable to the treatment of penicillin resistant strains of gram positive organisms especially staphylococci. Ampicillin and cloxacillin are often combined as a prophylactic in hip replacement and other major surgery as are the cephalosporins (cephradine, cephalexin, cephaloridine). A new generation of cephalosporins are emerging which are not inactivated by β lactamase produced by gram negative organisms (β lactamases are enzymes capable of nullifying the effi-

cacy of the antibiotic). Cefotaxime, cefuroxime and ceftazidime are finding increasing use.

Advantage is taken of the synergistic effect of antibiotics such as that shown by a sodium fusidate/erythromycin combination in osteomyelitis. Gentamycin, colomycin and piperacillin are normally reserved for infections due to gram negative bacteria and are particularly effective against pseudomonas species resistant to other antibiotics. Gentamycin has been recently incorporated into bone cement for use with prostheses and this finds increasing acceptance by many surgeons. The antibiotic is released slowly into the immediate tissue. Otherwise the local application of antibiotic is avoided because of the enhanced risk of resistance developing, an exception being the irrigation of infected wounds with a sterile solution of antibiotic in combination with a medically acceptable non-irritant detergent.

Urinary infections common in spinal injury patients often require antibiotic therapy determined by laboratory isolation of the responsible organisms and subsequent sensitivity test, though other chemotherapeutic agents such as nitrofurantoin, nalidixic acid and particularly co-trimoxazole are often preferred. These are generally more toxic than the antibiotics but have the advantage that resistance does not develop so readily.

Where anaerobic organisms are the cause of the condition, metronidazole is the drug of choice and can be given intravenously, orally or rectally.

Streptomycin is now usually confined to the treatment of tuberculosis but always in combination with other anti-tubercular drugs, again to prevent the emergence of resistance. Following the conclusive trial of some ten years ago by the British Thoracic and Tuberculosis Association, streptomycin has been replaced to some extent by rifampicin in combination with ethambutol and isoniazid.

GROUP 4. DRUGS USED IN SPECIFIC ORTHOPAEDIC CONDITIONS

Osteoporosis

The theraputic regime depends greatly on the severity and calcium and vitamin D BPC plus Sandocal is often used initially. In severe conditions calcium infusion (as gluconate) is given. Sodium fluoride

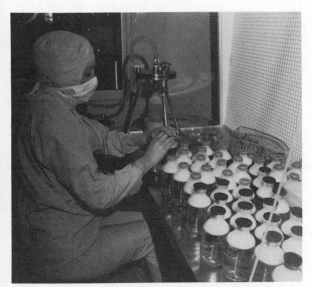

Fig. 1.14 Sterile fluids being prepared in the pharmacy.

plus vitamin D plus calcium has been shown to reduce incidence of acute vertebral collapse but there is evidence that sodium fluoride increases the risk of fracture of neck of femur.

Osteomalacia

Vitamin D therapy is adequate in the majority of cases. For severe conditions higher dosage of calciferol is required and in certain types phosphate or calcitriol may be necessary.

Paget's disease of bone

Adequate control can still be sometimes achieved by aspirin. Salmon calcitonin can achieve a reduction of pain and is given by injection in initially high dose followed by lower maintenance levels. Mithramycin can also dramatically reduce pain and the acute effect can be used to determine whether pain is due to Paget's disease or osteoarthritis. Diphosphanates have been shown to be effective in patients with polyostotic Paget's.

Malignancy of bone

The cytotoxic agents used in other forms of malignant growth find similar use in tumour of bone. Methotrexate and other folic acid antagonists are used, together with certain antibiotics which have been shown to inhibit growth of tumours (Adria-

mycin, actinomycin). Thiotepa and other cytotoxic drugs are occasionally used locally.

Chymopapain (Discase) is a revolutionary treatment in patients with sciatic pain secondary to herniation of intervertebral discs of the lumbar spine who are unresponsive to conservative treatment, including those who would be candidates for surgical removal of the discs. The exact mechanism by which it relieves pain is not known.

Anti-spastic agents

Advances in the drug control of spasm associated with spinal injury and other conditions have occurred with the introduction of baclofen (Lioresal) and dantrolene (Dantrium). Because Dantrium is a peripherally acting drug it would be logical to assume that it would be the drug of choice in complete spinal cord lesion, but baclofen, diazepam and other centrally acting drugs still find some advocates. Diazepam possesses certain anti-spastic properties but has some disadvantage in the tendency to produce drowsiness at the relatively high dosage necessary.

PHYSIOTHERAPY

Physiotherapy has a prominent role in the treatment of orthopaedic patients and it is essential for the nurse to know more about it than in any other speciality because the effects of the best physiotherapy can be nullified by lack of follow-up in the ward or home situation. Moreover, the physiotherapist may visit the ward, or the patient the appropriate department, once or twice during the day, but treatment—for example, free active exercises or passive movements—must be continued in the ward in order to be effective. To give a simple example, in leg injuries 'quadriceps drill' (Ch. 21) should be performed by the patient five minutes of every waking hour. Moreover, a physiotherapist may not be immediately available to teach the patient simple free exercises, as for example, following operative treatment or injury where early movement of fingers or toes is imperative; the nurse, on the other hand, in one form or another is in constant attendance and must be prepared to assume the responsibility of initiating simple physiotherapeutic activities in the ward and in the emergency/outpatient department. Indeed, in the latter case, teaching simple free active exercises and giving advice to patients regarding activities of daily living and, perhaps, elevation of an injured limb is *imperative*; for example, in the case of a patient with a Colles' fracture treated in a plaster cast, the nurse must be prepared to teach the patient essential finger, elbow and shoulder exercises.

On the other hand, it has been noted by Hockey (1980) that 'the pressures on the nurse's role from paramedical professions occur because nurses still fill gaps. They are on duty for 24 hours a day, seven days a week; they take on all the functions which other people relinquish at unsocial hours. Therefore, a nurse can be a physiotherapist at the weekend, but it is a specialised physiotherapist role on a weekday, which causes conflict and unhappiness within the nursing profession.' Another area of conflict is that since physiotherapy is such an essential part of orthopaedic treatment, the patient might come to regard the physiotherapist as the sole agent in his/her recovery. The present author recalls vividly a farewell scene when a lady was being discharged from hospital and both the ward sister and the physiotherapist were present. The patient indicated the latter and said 'This is the lady who *really* helped me—she taught me to walk'. It happened that the sister had seen the patient through a particularly stormy post-operative period which appeared to have been forgotten! If conflicts arise they can only be avoided by the closest co-operation and exchange of knowledge between the two disciplines involved and by the respect which each profession should feel for the other.

It should be stressed here that although the physiotherapeutic measures described in this book relate to patients suffering from disorders of the locomotor system, the physiotherapist, in common with other team members, will treat the patient as a whole person so that other body systems may require treatment at the same time. Moreover the physiotherapist often has unique opportunities to talk with the patient alone and may uncover other areas where the patient needs help, for example, with financial or social problems.

Before proceeding further with this discussion we would point out that excellent advice to nurses on the subject of physiotherapy is contained in the publication *Lifting, Handling and Helping Patients* (Downie & Kennedy, 1980).

The importance of team-work

In many cases, physiotherapeutic treatment cannot succeed without the co-operation of the nursing staff. For example, it is futile for an elderly or heavily-handicapped patient to attend the physiotherapy department several times a day for exercise sessions or to begin to learn to walk, if for the remainder of the the day he is simply left to lie in bed, or worse still, to sit in a chair; constant co-operation between the physiotherapist and the nurse is required so that physiotherapeutic treatment is supported by purposeful activity in the ward. In addition there are patients whose physiotherapy must be timed to fit in with nursing treatment, as for example in patients suffering from spinal cord injuries (Ch. 23), when treatment for the limbs and often, for the chest as well, is carried out when the patient is turned. Other patients requiring close co-operation between the nurse and physiotherapist are those with chest injuries or with thoracotomy or tracheostomy, especially those requiring special chest manipulations to loosen secretions which are then removed by suction.

Children require special consideration and their treatment must often be timed not only to fit in with nursing programmes but with their education.

The importance of controlled rest

It is also most important that the nurse and physiotherapist work together not only in the matter of the patient's active treatment, but to ensure that he gets sufficient rest, and also to ensure that physiotherapeutic treatment is constantly adjusted to the age and condition of the individual patient so that he is not taxed beyond his strength.

Specialised physiotherapeutic treatment will be discussed in later pages; here we shall deal briefly only with those aspects which directly concern the nurse.

EXERCISES

Broadly speaking, exercises are ordered for the following purposes:
1. *To retain movements* in joints and normal tone in the muscles controlling them, so that stiffness is prevented, as for example in patients who are confined to bed for long periods.

2. *To restore movements* which have been lost owing to disuse, injury or disease of joints.
3. *To redevelop muscles* and to *restore muscle balance* after disuse, disease or injury, so that joint movement is controlled.
4. *To retain memory of movement patterns and to regain functional control* in general, and in particular with regard to the patients' occupational and recreational needs.

1. *Free active exercises* are performed by the patient himself. They are designed to gain or retain joint movement and to strengthen muscles; moreover, movement of joints and contraction of muscles stimulates the circulation, helps to prevent venous stagnation, promotes healing and improves the nutrition of the part.

2. *Isometric (setting) exercises* (static contractions) are performed by the patient himself and consist of muscular contractions without movement of the underlying joint; they are *essential* in the immobilised patient for the maintenance of muscle tone and nutrition of the part. Effects are similar to those of active exercises.

3. *Active assisted exercises* are active movements performed by the patient but assisted by the physiotherapist or by some mechanical device; or occasionally by the patient's sound limb (auto-assisted).

4. *Resisted active exercises* are performed against resistance, either supplied by the physiotherapist or by some mechanical device, such as a weight attached to the limb.

5. *Breathing exercises* are given to preserve lung expansion, encourage the interchange of gases, to prevent consolidation of the lungs, to encourage coughing; in certain cases, nurses are taught chest manipulations by the physiotherapist, for example in high spinal cord lesions (see Ch. 23).

The dangers of free active exercises. Broadly speaking, free active exercises are not dangerous provided they are performed regularly and correctly within the limits of pain and within the tolerance of the individual patient. It is better for the patient to perform a few simple exercises correctly than a dozen incorrectly; over-exercise might exacerbate an inflammatory condition, and any *forced* movement is definitely contra-indicated; post-operative conditions and recent injuries are approached with care and caution. In general, setting (isometric) exercises, i.e. static muscular contractions can be taught quite safely, with the reservations referred to above; the nurse will be guided by the individual case, the orders of the doctor and the advice of the physiotherapist.

Importance of convincing the patient of the value of free active exercises. In some cases the patient does not believe that exercises will help him; he finds the constant repetition boring and would prefer to undergo some form of treatment which is done 'to' or 'for' him, rather than try to improve by his own efforts. For this reason every member of the orthopaedic team must be trained to teach and supervise simple exercises to the extent that they are taken for granted as part and parcel of every patient's treatment and as an integral part of ward routine and of outpatient practice. To the patient, routine daily performance of his exercises should come as naturally as breathing.

Exercise classes. When possible, exercises are given in classes; the patient feels that there are others in the same boat as himself, the competitive spirit is encouraging, and boredom is avoided. Exercises are often performed to music, and games are used as well as formal exercises, especially in children.

Cases which require careful re-education of muscles or groups of muscles are treated individually, though they may graduate to classes during later treatment for exercises of a general nature.

A passive movement is not an exercise and is performed not by the patient but by some other agency, usually the nurse or the physiotherapist. In certain circumstances other workers or a patient's relatives are taught to give passive movements; (see Chs 23 and 24) they are given *only in the case of paralysed or unconscious patients*, to retain joint movement, prevent contracture and subsequent deformity, to maintain the circulatory flow and nutrition of the limbs, and to retain the patient's memory of movement patterns.

PASSIVE MOVEMENTS

This section is taken from *Lifting, Handling and Helping Patients* by Patricia A. Downie and Pat Kennedy by kind permission of the authors and publishers.

The normal range of movement in a joint or the extensibility of muscle is maintained by active movement, that is, movement carried out consciously by the person himself. When someone is either unconscious or not able to move because of disease such as poliomyelitis, polyneuritis, multiple sclerosis, motor neurone disease or because of injury to the nerves following a spinal injury as in paraplegia and tetraplegia, tightness and contractures to both joints and muscles can occur.

These can be prevented in most cases by the physiotherapist and the nurse giving regular passive movements to the affected joints and by the careful positioning of the limb(s). Any nurse who is caring for such patients continually will be shown exactly what is required, and how best to achieve it, by the physiotherapist; in many cases the two professions will work together to combine their care at stated times of the day and night.

Tightness and contractures are caused by shortening of the soft tissues, i.e. the capsule of the joint and other ligaments and muscles which surround and control the joint. The difference between tightness and contracture is one of degree. When only 'tightness' is present, the soft tissue changes are reversible and a full range of movement can be obtained, and then maintained by passive movements of the affected joints, followed by active movement if and when this becomes possible. A 'contracture' is an irreversible shortening of the tissues and, unless slight, a full range of movement will not be regained; joints will become deformed, and if the knee joints or hip joints are affected then walking will be extremely difficult. Contractures are preventable by constant vigilance on the part of all concerned with the care of the patient.

Points to be observed when giving passive movements

Before giving passive movements to a patient the nurse must place herself in such a position that she is able to move without strain and without losing her balance. Even if the patient is apparently unconscious, the nurse must explain to the patient exactly what she is going to do, giving confidence by her approach and manner. She must not be in a hurry. She must, whenever possible, face the patient.

The patient should be in a comfortable position and relaxed. Clothes and bedclothes which may restrict the movement should be loosened or removed. They must be replaced at the end of treatment.

1. It is necessary (for the nurse) to know the normal range of movement in every joint to appreciate the abnormal. Passive movements are given to maintain normal range of movement; if the range is exceeded the joint may be damaged and irreparable harm done.

2. The part to be moved should be supported by the hands of the nurse. The grip should be gentle but firm, with the hands moulded to the part and avoiding any bony prominences. The fingers must not dig into the patient.

3. In order to limit the movement to the joint which is to be moved, the bone proximal to the joint must be fixed either by one hand or by the position into which it is placed before the movement is carried out; the other hand must grasp as near as possible distal to the joint. It is important to ensure that movement does not take place at other joints, resulting in excess movement at joints which are already mobile, at the expense of a stiff joint remaining stiff.

4. The movement should commence with gentle traction of the joint surface and then the movement itself should be performed in a slow, smooth and rhythmical manner. It must not cause pain nor elicit spasm.

5. The movement should be given three times in each direction, at least two or three times a day. It is far better to give treatment little and often. If there is limitation of range of movement, it is better to aim at gaining range over a period of time rather than forcing the range in one treatment. If the soft tissues are overstretched or torn, inflammation will be set up and the joint will become stiffer and more painful due to the formation of adhesions and a protective resistance to pain.

6. Any increase of pain or any decrease of range of movement should be reported immediately to the doctor.

Technique of massive movements for individual joints

Upper limb

Fingers

Movements possible: Flexion, extension, abduction, adduction and combination movements.

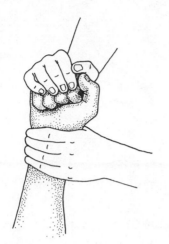

Fig. 1.15 Flexion of the fingers. The fingers should be directed towards the thumb. The wrist is fixed by the lower hand.

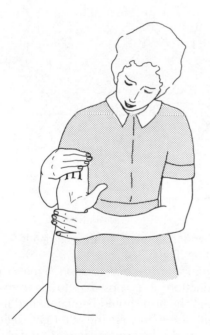

Fig. 1.16 Extension of the fingers.

Grip: The fingers are fixed at the head of the metacarpals with one hand and the other hand flexes and extends the interphalangeal joints collectively; similarly each finger may be moved individually. The fixing hand should then be moved lower to fix the wrist and the movement repeated to include the metacarpo-phalangeal joints, i.e. making a fist (Figs 1.15 and 1.16). To achieve abduction and adduction each finger must be moved separately while the others are fixed.

Thumb

Movements possible: Flexion, extension, abduction, adduction, circumduction and opposition.
Grip: As for fingers.

Wrist

Movements possible: Flexion, extension and circumduction.
Grip: The arm is bent at the elbow and supported on a pillow with the hand at 90 degrees to the pillow; the lower forearm is fixed firmly with one hand while the patient's hand is held with the other; with slight upward traction the wrist is moved into flexion and extension (Fig. 1.17); it can then be moved laterally into radial and ulnar deviation; finally a combination of all these movements will produce circumduction.

Radio-ulnar joints (inferior and superior)

Movements possible: Pronation and supination.
Grip: The elbow is bent to 90 degrees, one hand fixes the elbow above the joint while the other holds the hand as for a hand shake and rotates the forearm into supination and pronation. The wrist should be maintained in the mid-position.

Elbow

Movements possible: Flexion and extension. Elbow flexion is vital for eating. When flexion is given as a passive movement it must be given also in the direction of the mouth, i.e. combined shoulder flexion and abduction.
Grip: The upper arm should be supported; one hand should hold above the elbow on the posterior aspect and the other hand should hold the forearm just above the wrist to prevent movement, usually the fingers in front and the thumb behind (Fig. 1.18). The elbow is then flexed and extended; flexion will be limited by the contact of the flexor surfaces and as the elbow is extended care must be taken not to hyperextend—to prevent this it is wise to slide the upper hand down so that it can 'feel' the extended joint. Finally, the upper arm should be lifted in slight abduction and shoulder flexion and the elbow flexed toward the mouth.

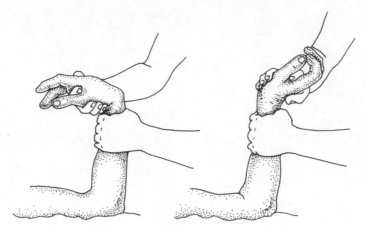

Fig. 1.17 (a) Flexion of the wrist. (b) Extension of the wrist.

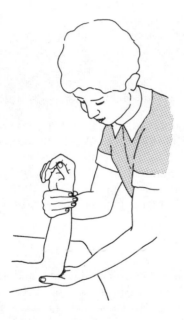

Fig. 1.18 The starting position for flexion and extension of the elbow.

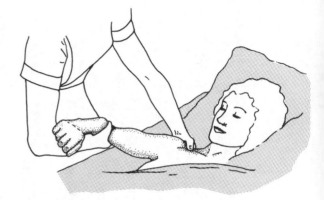

Fig. 1.19 Abduction of the shoulder.

Shoulder

Movements possible: Flexion, extension, abduction, adduction, elevation, internal rotation and external rotation.

Grips: The patient may be in sitting, half lying or lying; the lower arm, i.e. from the elbow down, is allowed to rest on the nurse's own arm; her other hand is used to fix the shoulder girdle by placing it over the acromion and coracoid process, thumb in front and fingers behind; the arm is then lifted sideways and upwards to approximately 90 degrees abduction (Fig. 1.19).

Internal and external rotation: From a position of abduction it is possible to perform limited rotation. The arm should be maintained in abduction with the elbow resting at a right angle on the bed; the arm is then rotated forward and backward.

Another method is to start with the arm into the side with the elbow resting on the bed at right angles; the operator fixes the elbow above the joint with one hand and with the other holds the wrist; the arm is then rotated at the shoulder joint by bringing the forearm across the body (internal rotation) and then away from the body (external rotation) (Fig. 1.20). The upper arm must remain in contact with the body at all times and the elbow likewise must be flexed at right angles.

Flexion and extension: This is carried out using

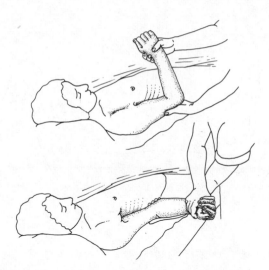

Fig. 1.20 Upper: internal rotation of the shoulder. Lower: external rotation of the shoulder. Note that the upper arm is alongside the trunk and the elbow flexed to a right angle—this is necessary to localise the movement to the shoulder.

the same grip as for abduction and it may be continued upwards and forwards to become elevation of the shoulder. Finally the arm should be carried across the body, i.e. the hand should be taken towards the opposite shoulder.

Lower limb

Toes

Movements possible: Flexion, extension, abduction, adduction and combination movements.

Grip: The toes are fixed at the head of the metatarsals with one hand and the other hand flexes and extends the toes at the interphalangeal joints collectively. Each toe may be moved individually by fixing each metatarsophalangeal joint and moving each interphalangeal joint. Abduction and adduction is most easily performed for the great toe. A gliding movement is possible between the metatarsal joints but is usually only carried out by the physiotherapist—it is not essential to the prevention of deformity. Extension and flexion is essential to prevent curling of the toes and a flexion contracture of the toes can be extremely disabling.

Ankle

Movements possible: Dorsiflexion and plantar flexion.

Grip: One hand fixes the ankle above the joint while the other holds the foot—the heel resting in the flexed fingers and the foot lying along the lower forearm (Fig. 1.21). The foot is then moved

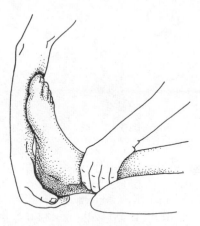

Fig. 1.21 Dorsiflexion of the ankle. In this diagram the left hand grips just above the malleoli; the heel of the foot rests in the palm of the right hand and the foot rests along the forearm. The pillow prevents hyperextension of the knee joint.

upwards to a right angle (dorsiflexion) and downwards (plantar flexion). When giving dorsiflexion it is essential that the movement is carried to its extreme and where there is a feeling of tightness, then the movement should be gently pushed beyond the easy range; if this is not done, the tendo Achilles will shorten and walking will become very difficult. The tendo Achilles can become tight and shorten in an insidious fashion—nurses must be aware of this and be especially vigilant.

Inversion and eversion take place at the midtarsal joints; one hand should restrict the ankle movement while the second hand grasps the foot at its mid-point (Fig. 1.22). The foot is then moved into inversion, i.e. turned inwards, and then into eversion, i.e. turned outwards. A combination of dorsiflexion, eversion, plantar flexion and inversion will produce circumduction. Inversion and eversion movements are important for they help the foot to accommodate to walking over rough surfaces.

Knee

Movements possible: Flexion and extension.

Grip: One hand holds the foot as for ankle dorsi-

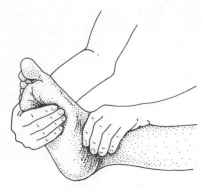

Fig. 1.22 Inversion of the foot. The upper hand grips just below the malleoli and prevents movement in the ankle joint.

flexion while the other is placed at the back of the knee, in the popliteal fossa, to prevent the knee joint falling into hyperextension (Fig. 1.23). The knee is then fully flexed with the hand at the back of the knee being brought to the front to give added assistance in the flexion (Fig. 1.24); the knee is then extended and the hand is returned to the popliteal fossa to prevent hyperextension by support.

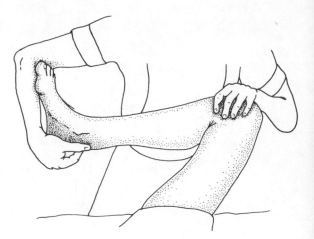

Fig. 1.24 Flexion of the knee joint and the hip joint.

in a straight position on the operator's arm and then the leg is lifted upwards—the hand on the buttock/lower lumbar region prevents the movement taking place in the lumbar region (Fig. 1.25).

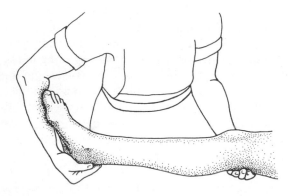

Fig. 1.23 Extension of the knee. The upper hand supports the knee and prevents hyperextension.

Hip

Movements possible: Flexion, extension, abduction, adduction, internal rotation, external rotation and circumduction.

Grip: Flexion of the hip can be said to have been combined with knee flexion (Fig. 1.24); extension of the hip needs to be carried out either with the patient lying prone or on his side. If the patient is prone, one hand is placed over the buttock, the other arm supports the leg which is allowed to lie

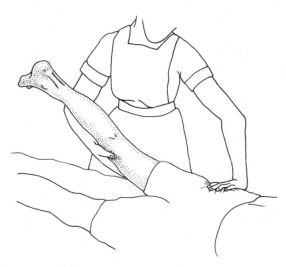

Fig. 1.25 Extension of the hip joint with the patient in the prone position. The pelvis must remain flat on the bed—the hand on the pelvic rim will feel immediately there is movement in the lumbar region. The ankle of the opposite leg should be supported on a pillow, keeping the toes off the bed.

If the movement is carried out in side lying, the under leg should first be placed in a full flexed position—this helps to prevent the movement taking place in the lumbar region. Using grips similar to those used in prone lying, the upper leg is carried into extension with the hand on the lower lumbar region being used to prevent lumbar movement.

Abduction of the hip is carried out in the lying position; the leg opposite to that which is to be moved should be placed in a fully abducted position (Fig. 1.26)—this helps to prevent side flexion

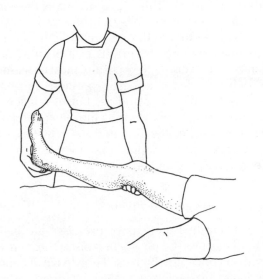

Fig. 1.26 Abduction of the hip. This diagram shows the movement being performed with the pelvis fixed by placing the other leg in full abduction.

taking place at the lumbar region—and the leg is then carried sideways. Alternatively, the nurse supports the whole leg on her lower arm and places her other hand on the crest of the ilium and then carries the leg sideways to its fullest range before movement, caused by the tilting of the pelvis, is felt at the lumbar region. The leg is then carried back to the mid-position and finally across the midline into adduction.

To achieve internal and external rotation the legs should be placed slightly apart and then by placing the hands, one on the lower leg and one on the thigh, the whole leg can be rolled inwards and then rolled outwards. If it is preferred, the leg can be flexed to a right angle and the leg rolled inwards, i.e. towards the other leg, and outwards, i.e. towards the mattress of the bed. The foot must remain flat on the bed.

Dangers of passive movements. Unlike free active exercises, passive movements are fraught with danger, particularly in the hands of anyone other than the orthopaedic surgeon or the physiotherapist whose special training teaches them 'how far to go' in manipulating different parts of the body. On

the other hand, regular passive movements are essential for the unconscious patient and for the paralysed, but they must be given with the utmost care and gentleness; each joint is carried through its full range once or twice daily but over-stretching in any one direction should be avoided; it is important, however, to maintain the full range of joint movement, for example even a mild degree of flexion contracture of the knee joint might prevent a paralysed patient from wearing a caliper (long leg brace) for walking; conversely hyperextension of the knee joint leads to instability and predisposes to joint effusion. Moreover, the bones of patient deprived of weight-bearing for a long period become atrophic and can be fractured by relatively trivial violence. Another hazard associated with over-energetic passive movements is ectopic bone formation in adjacent muscle-groups, which can form a bony block and a hindrance to joint movement especially at the elbow and hip joints.

Passive stretching of any joint which is stiff because of disuse, disease or injury is *absolutely forbidden* and is performed *only* by an orthopaedic surgeon or by a physiotherapist working to his specific orders. Nurses and others must avoid the idle passive stretching one sometimes sees being perpetrated during examination of the fingers and toes of patients wearing splints or plaster casts; by all means *feel* the fingers and toes but *do not manipulate them*. Further, do not allow patients to manipulate their own fingers or toes, (unless of course there are paralysed digits when the patient will be deliberately taught the procedure).

In the case of children, parents and others are forbidden to apply passive stretching to any joint stiff from disuse, disease or injury. On the other hand, in certain conditions—e.g. club-foot, cerebral palsy—the parents or guardians of a child, especially one suffering from paralysis from any cause, may well be taught manipulations to prevent deformity and at the same time, be warned of the attendant dangers.

Treatment by manipulation. As already stated, forced passive stretching of any part of the body is never undertaken by nurses, parents or others except where it is specially ordered by and supervised by the doctor; the physiotherapist however uses special techniques to stretch contracted structures, again under specific orders from the doctor.

Manipulation with or without anaesthesia for example, of the spine or the shoulder may be performed by the doctor and followed up immediately by physiotherapeutic treatment.

Teaching patients to transfer from one situation to another and to walk is an important part of physiotherapeutic treatment; in general, and where a physiotherapist is readily available, the patient's initial attempt at transfer activities and at walking is taught by the therapist; in her absence however, or on subsequent occasions these must be carried out by the nurse. A useful book on handling disabled patients is published by the Chartered Society of Physiotherapists.

Pre-operative exercises. In hospital the physiotherapist visits every patient before operation, to make his acquaintance, to gain his co-operation and to assess his physical condition and personality, so that plans can be made for the subsequent *post-operative* treatment. Since *breathing exercises* are always given post-operatively it is helpful to the physiotherapist to know the state of the patient's lungs beforehand; moreover for obvious reasons breathing control and coughing is more easily learned by the patient before operation rather than afterwards, as are any specific exercises which will be required post-operatively, for example, quadriceps drill in lesions of the semi-lunar cartilage. *Manipulation* of a joint under anaesthesia is always followed by physiotherapeutic treatment, so that the physiotherapist requires an accurate assessment of the pre-operative condition.

Post-operative exercises. It is important for the nurse to remember that post-operative exercise is aimed not only at the restoration of functions of a particular joint, but at the *prevention* of serious complications such as bronchitis, pneumonia or circulatory disturbances such as deep vein thrombosis. Although it is the duty of the physiotherapist to teach the appropriate exercises, it is the nurse's duty to see that they are carried out regularly.

Home exercises. These should be simple and foolproof. Wherever possible, written or tape-recorded instructions are given. Patients suffer from emotional as well as physical trauma so that they easily forget the most simple exercises. It is better for the patient to perform three exercises correctly than a dozen incorrectly. The patient is also instructed in such active use as is fitted to his condi-tion, for example, a patient with a wrist immobi-lised in plaster for a Colles' fracture should carry out any light work which does not involve wetting the plaster.

Postural training. This is given to restore the poise and balance of the whole body. The aim is to establish a new postural reflex, to break old habits and introduce new ones by means of a planned programme of exercises. New posture must be learned not only in relation to static positions in lying, kneeling, sitting and standing, but in relation to the carriage of the body during movement. *Relaxation* exercises are often required and activities such as dancing and swimming may form part of the re-educative programme.

Neurophysiological techniques

Many interesting systems of exercises are being increasingly used by physiotherapists. These are all based on concepts which use knowledge of neuro-physiology to facilitate movement or to reduce excessive muscle tone.

The use of apparatus

Many appliances have been devised as aids to physiotherapy. The ones in general use include walking machines, stationary bicycles and rowing machines, and various elaborate arrangements of slings and pulleys.

Other forms of physiotherapeutic treatment

Massage. This is not often ordered in orthopaedic practice, though it is useful in improving circulation, reducing oedema and for mobilising tissues after injury. It is usually enjoyed by the patient.

Electrotherapy. Muscle-stimulating currents may be used to evaluate the state of nerve and muscle, to delay fibrosis in a denervated muscle, or in the re-education of muscle of poor function. Other forms of electrotherapy such as diathermy may be ordered, but a description of such treatment is outside the scope of this book.

Radiant heat. This is frequently ordered for the relief of pain before exercises and the improvement of local circulation.

Ice. Ice is also used for the relief of pain and

improving circulation, as well as for facilitation of movement and reduction of excessive muscle tone.

Heliotherapy. Ultraviolet rays are ordered in the absence of natural sunlight in cases of rickets or of general debility. Local artificial sunlight may be ordered in the treatment of wounds.

Hydrotherapy (exercises in water). This is valuable for many orthopaedic conditions, for example, osteoarthritis (Ch. 27) and paraplegia (Ch. 23), and is usually enjoyed by the patient (Fig. 1.27). A medical examination is always conducted before 'pool' treatment is instituted in order to exclude contra-indications.

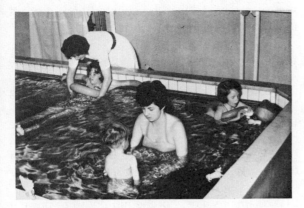

Fig. 1.27 Patients suffering from various orthopaedic conditions undergoing treatment by hydrotherapy. Note that the physiotherapist may enter the pool herself or work from the side.

Re-education in walking

When the function of walking has been interfered with by disease, injury or deformity of any part of the body, re-education is ordered. In all cases, it is essential that the patient is taught to *stand* unassisted before actual walking is attempted, especially if he has been bedridden for a long period. When balance is assured, the following instructions are given:

1. The bodyweight must be taken equally on both legs.
2. Steps must be short and of equal length.
3. The toes must point straight forward.
4. The heel strikes the ground first; at the moment weight is taken on the foot which is in front, the *knee is pressed back* by action of the quadri-

ceps, and the patient pushes off on the toes of the foot which is behind.
5. The knee on that side is then flexed to 'follow through' the step, but *it must be straight at the moment at which it takes the bodyweight*. The patient must practise this 'heel-and-toe' exercise in 'slow motion' until it becomes his habitual manner of walking. Extension of the knee must be insisted upon at every step, especially after knee injuries.

The use of crutches

Crutches must be of such length, and the hand-rests so placed, as to allow the weight to be taken on the hands and not in the axillae. A careful watch is kept for crutch palsy. If it occurs, the crutches are temporarily discarded. In children, the crutches must not become outgrown.

Elbow crutches are sometimes used, especially in cases in which they are required permanently.

Walking on crutches

General instructions. The patient learns to stand and balance on the crutches before attempting to walk. He is taught to lift first one crutch and then the other and if possible, to lift alternate legs. It is essential that the patient looks ahead and not at his feet. Always stand close *behind* patients learning to stand and walk and a belt (or substitute for a belt) should be worn round the patient's waist to be grasped by the therapist.

Types of gait

1. *Non-weight-bearing.* The affected limb is not put to the ground. The crutches are placed a short distance in front and the patient hops forward on the sound limb.
2. *Partial weight-bearing.* The crutches and the affected leg move forward together, most of the bodyweight being taken by the crutches.
3. *Four-point crutch walking.* When the patient is confident of his balance, instruct him to place the right crutch forward, then the left foot; the left crutch follows, and finally the right foot. One crutch is always kept forward to prevent the patient from falling. The crutches and the feet must be placed forward in short steps of equal length.

4. *Tripod walking.* In patients with extensive paralysis of the legs and trunk tripod walking is employed. The crutches are placed well forward and out to the sides, and the patient leans forward between them, so that the crutches form two arms of a tripod and the body a third. When balance is assured first the right and then the left crutch is placed a short distance forward and the legs are drawn towards them as one unit. In time, some patients learn to 'swing through', when the crutches are placed forward together and the legs are thrust forward between them. Patients with powerful upper limbs may achieve a fast crutch gait by this method.

Walking with sticks

This is ordered for patients who are not so disabled as to require crutches but who need support. In general, the patient requires two sticks when he first becomes ambulant. They are used in the same manner as crutches, placing the right stick forward, the left foot following, then the left stick and the right foot. One stick may then be discarded indoors, then outdoors, until the patient can dispense with this support altogether.

Walking in a caliper

If the caliper is 'long', that is, weight-relieving, the patient is tempted to clear the ground by swinging the caliper out sideways; this must not be allowed. 'Hitching', or lifting, of the pelvis is practised while the patient is still in bed, and a correct standing position is taught before walking is attempted; the patient is first taught to stand in the caliper; do not allow him to progress by clutching at the wall or the furniture; start off with the feet side by side and about six or eight inches apart, so that the body weight is evenly distributed over a wide base. Instruct the patient to *lift* the caliper forward, not swing it, to take a short step, and to bring the sound leg forward beside it. As confidence increases, the sound leg passes the splinted one in a short but even and normal step.

Method of negotiating steps

To go upstairs, the sound foot is placed on the step above, and the splinted foot is then lifted on to the same step. To go downstairs, the splinted foot is placed on the step below, then the sound one. The same instructions apply in any case in which splintage fixes the knee and/or the hip.

Sitting in splintage which fixes the hip

A high, hard upright chair is generally preferred to an armchair. The patient stands with his back to the chair, a little in front and to the side of the affected hip; he flexes the sound knee and lowers the buttock of the unaffected side on to the seat. Patients in splintage which fixes the hip and/or the knee can go to the cinema if they occupy the end seat of a row, so that the splinted limb projects into the centre aisle.

Rising from the sitting position

The patient stands with the back of the sound leg in contact with the chair; he leans forward by flexing the hips, and sits down. On rising from the chair, the sound knee is flexed so that the foot is behind the level of the affected one; the patient then *leans forward* and stands by extending the hips.

Permanent stiffness of the hip does not prevent the patient from leading a normal life. In one instance, arthrodesis of the hip has not prevented a young woman from training as a nurse; another patient with permanent stiffness of *both* hips is able to climb trees. In young subjects, the lumbar spine develops such a wide range of movement that stiffness of the hip passes almost unnoticed.

Stiffness of the knee is not more disabling, but it is more noticeable as the limb sticks out, for example, when travelling in public vehicles. This however does not prevent the patient from following normal pursuits.

Games and sports are used as a basis for physiotherapy in many conditions, notably for paraplegic patients (Ch. 23) and for children (Chs 11, 12, 14, 15, 16, 17, 18) and the aged (Ch. 21). In some centres, the physiotherapeutic/occupational therapy team is strengthened by the work of remedial gymnasts or of technicians who specialise in some form of remedial therapy.

Finally, the physiotherapist has a powerful influence on the morale of the patient and can give him the incentive to work out his own salvation for independent living. Moreover she often has opportunities to be alone with the patient and to talk freely with him about his problems.

OCCUPATIONAL THERAPY

In common with physiotherapy, an understanding of the role of the occupational therapist is essential to our own work; it is not enough to save a patient from the jaws of death; he must also be restored to independence and the measures used to achieve this require the understanding and co-operation of the whole team. In general, the physiotherapist tends to concentrate on restoring the function of the lower limbs, as in learning to walk; conversely the occupational therapist tends to concentrate on restoring the function of the upper limbs, as in learning to deal with feeding, the toilet and with other activities of daily living, for example, cooking, ironing etc. In practice, however, the work of both therapists tends to overlap because the aim of treatment is directed towards the rehabilitation of the whole patient—'who does what and to whom' varies in different centres depending upon the type of patient, the facilities and the expertise of the staff available, and on the direction of the doctor.

The occupational therapist is expert at using arts and crafts, games and other activities as a means of restoring function with particular emphasis, as outlined above, on activities of daily living. Moreover, activities directed towards re-training disabled individuals either to return to a previous job or to enter a new one is a vital aspect of her work; further references will be made to this important function under the heading *Rehabilitation* (Chs 34 and 35). Other important aspects of the work of the occupational therapist are advice on home adaptations and the design and utilisation of gadgets used as aids to independent living.

Finally, in common with the physiotherapist, the occupational therapist has an important influence on the patient's mental attitudes; Winifred Hector (1970) discussing occupational therapy in connection with psychiatric nursing says that occupational therapy 'should not be thought of only as a way of passing the time. It turns the patients' thoughts outwards, increases his morale and his motor skills'. This remark applies equally to patients suffering from orthopaedic conditions.

The physiotherapist and occupational therapist as teachers

This is a very important role in relation to both patient and nurse; for example, the physiotherapist who teaches the nurse how to assist coughing and expectoration in the paralysed patient may at the same time be teaching her how to save a life (Ch. 23). The orthopaedic surgeon might give orders for special treatment following an operation, for example, in hand surgery, where the nurse's full co-operation is required so that the effects of treatment are not nullified in the ward. The physiotherapist also teaches her special skills in handling, positioning and moving disabled patients and in helping them to move from one position to another; the occupational therapist teaches her special skills related to recovery of function in activities of daily living.

MEDICAL SOCIAL WORK

In the past the medical social worker was called a lady almoner and her work was largely directed towards solving the patient's financial problems. Today, while financial problems still loom large, the medical social worker in common with other team members is concerned with the total care of the patient so that emotional and social needs receive equal attention. Moreover the social worker is concerned not only with the patient himself but with his family, his work and his social background.

In hospital, and in ideal circumstances, the medical social worker interviews each patient who attends the out-patient/casualty department or who is admitted to a ward. She can then make an assessment of the patient's physical, mental, financial, social and emotional status; most important of all, she makes herself known to him and where possible, to members of his family. In common with the other team members, she can help the patient express and overcome his natural fears; even if it turns out that the patient requires no specific assistance, he should know that the social worker is there to help if the need arises. Moreover, many patients are helped simply by discussing problems with someone who is not directly involved in physical care.

If the social worker is unable to interview every patient she relies upon the other team members for referral of patients in need of her services. It is important for all the team members to appreciate the need for early recognition of conditions where medico-social help will be required; for example, in the case of an aged patient who is likely to present a 'disposal problem' on discharge, the social worker needs early warning of the situation. She is a vital link between the patient in hospital and the community outside.

In the community, she helps to resolve the problems of daily living encountered by the orthopaedically disabled patient. These might include not only finance but housing, jobs, transportation, education, and perhaps, social isolation. Further discussion of the work of the medical social worker will be found in Chapters 34 and 35.

REHABILITATION

Rehabilitation is discussed at some length in the final chapter of this book, simply for convenience in arranging material and not because it is an afterthought or terminal event in the patient's treatment; it is a process of restoring each patient to his highest level of physical, functional, social and economic independence, including all activities of daily living and of gainful employment. It is perhaps unfortunate that the word 'rehabilitation' is commonly associated only with restoration of independence in patients with permanent and irrevocable physical handicap, such as the paraplegic and the amputee. For this reason, nurses may mistakenly regard it as none of their business, and moreover, develop an attitude which envisages nursing duties only as comprising the care of the acutely ill so that the nurse will lose many opportunities of helping her patient towards a better life (Marshall & Mair, 1967). That is precisely what rehabilitation is all about—a better life for the patient. On the other hand, in defence of the nurse who regards only the care of the acutely ill as her special prerogative,

this too is the first line of defence against disablement and an essential part of the rehabilitation process, as is *prevention* of disease, injury and disability in the community.

For the purpose of discussion, patients are divided into *the temporarily disabled*, who are expected to make a full recovery in the course of time without significant physical disability, and *the permanently disabled*, who must cope with some form of disablement for the rest of their lives; it should be noted that an important aim of treatment and nursing care is:

1. to prevent temporary disablement from becoming permanent, and
2. to prevent the permanently disabled from developing such complications as might be a hindrance to their ultimate enjoyment of 'the better life' referred to in a previous paragraph.

Moreover, 'a better life' includes not only physical independence but socio-economic independence as well, and resettlement in a previous job or retraining for a new one is an essential part of the rehabilitation of both the temporarily and permanently disabled.

The rehabilitation of the temporarily disabled is achieved by maintaining a high level of general health, and by means of the avoidance of complications, including those of rest in bed and of immobility, supported by purposeful activity directed towards the restoration of personal independence in activities of daily living and job resettlement; last but not least, by constant encouragement, by cultivation of a positive attitude of mind and finally, by resolution of social problems where possible and by an early return to home and work. In this connection, the co-operation of personnel in the Community Health and Welfare Services may be required to complete the process of restoration of the patient to the physical, social and economic independence which is the whole object of the exercise.

The rehabilitation of the permanently disabled. This is a different story, because we face the fact that complete recovery from a disabling condition is impossible; on the other hand, partial or even complete restoration to physical, social and economic independence *is* possible, even in very severely disabled patients, for example, the paraplegic, the amputee, or the victim of rheumatoid arthritis. But even in these patients, re-training for a new job and resettlement in a new living situation and a vigorous approach to social problems can restore the patient to a measure of independence commensurate with his disability, although it may require more time, more money, more expertise, more people, and even more positive purposeful activity than that we have already outlined in connection with sufferers from temporary disablement.

Strong motivation of the patient himself is imperative; many of them put the able-bodied to shame by their example of tireless effort, ingenuity, perseverance and determination shown in overcoming their handicaps (Fig. 1.28).

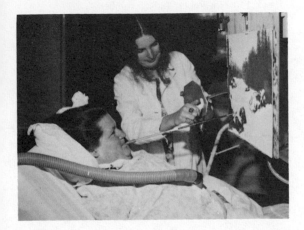

Fig. 1.28 Artist at work despite disability. (Courtesy of Mouth and Foot Painting Artists.)

Finally, for those disabled early in life from congenital or other conditions, modern education, transportation, rehabilitation facilities and techniques offer new hope and a new promise of a better life than was possible in the past.

BIBLIOGRAPHY

Adams J C 1971 Outline of Orthopaedics. Edinburgh: Churchill Livingstone

Anderson M I 1972 Physiotherapeutic management of patients on continuous traction. Physiotherapy, 58: 51–54

Ascher R A J 1947 The dangers of going to bed. British Medical Journal, 2: 967

Badawr, M 1982 The role of the hospital social worker. Nursing Mirror, 29 September

Bamford T 1982 Three cheers for social workers. Nursing Mirror, 10 March

Bleackley R (ed.) 1974 Despite Disability. Reading: Educational Explorers

Bradley D 1979 Checking a plaster, how and why. Nursing Times, 1 August, 710: 1190

British Medical Association and Pharmaceutical Society 1976–78 British National Formulary. London

Bruce C 1983 Are we being served? Nursing Times, 20 July

Bruner J S 1960 The Process of Education. New York: Pitman House

Chapman C M 1977 Sociology for Nurses. London: Balliere Tindall

Chartered Society of Physiotherapy 1975 Handling the Handicapped. London: Woodhead Faulkner

Chilman A M, Thomas N (eds) 1986 Understanding Nursing Care, 3rd edn. Edinburgh: Churchill Livingstone

Clarke F 1983 The changing scene in out-patients. Nursing Times, 4 May

Consumers' Association 1974 Coping with Disablement. London: Consumers' Association

Day B 1972 Orthopaedic Appliances. London: Faber & Faber

DI ISS and Welsh Office 1977 Help for Handicapped People. Leaflet HB1 March. Aids for the Disabled. HB2 September

Downie A, Kennedy P 1980 Lifting, Handling and Helping Patients. London: Faber & Faber

Family Welfare Association 1978 Guide to the Social Services. London: MacDonald & Evans

The handling of patients 1981. London: The Back Pain Association and the Royal College of Nursing

Hector W 1970 Modern Nursing—Theory and Practice. London: Heinemann

Hockey L 1980 Challenges for nursing. Nursing Times, 22 May

Hopkins S J 1977 Drugs and Pharmacology for Nurses. Edinburgh: Churchill Livingstone

Hunt P (ed.) 1966 Stigma. London and Dublin: Geoffrey Chapman

Jones B R 1975 Pharmacology for Students and Pupil Nurses. London: Heinemann

Iveson-Iveson J 1981 You're pulling my leg. Nursing Mirror, 7 October

Kakkar V V 1977 The prevention of acute pulmonary embolism. British Journal of Hospital Medicine 18: 32

Kennedy J M 1974 Orthopaedic Splints and Appliances. London: Ballière Tindall

Leonard C 1981 Understanding sexuality: talking through a taboo. Nursing Mirror, 29 July

Lindsay M 1981 Inside the outpatient department. Nursing Times, 13 October

Macmillan P 1980 Strange encounter. Nursing Times, 6 November

MacRae R 1976 Clinical Orthopaedic Examination. Edinburgh: Churchill Livingstone

Marshall J, Mair J 1967 Neurological Nursing. Oxford: Blackwell Scientific

Miller G A H 1977 The management of acute pulmonary embolism. British Journal of Hospital Medicine 18: 26

Morris G K, Mitchell J R A 1977 The aetiology of acute pulmonary embolism and the identification of high risk groups. British Journal of Hospital Medicine 18: 6

Moss B A 1981 What is occupational therapy? Nursing Times, 7 October

Nichols P R J et al 1966 Immediate lumbar supports. British Medical Journal 2: 707

Nuki G 1983 British Medical Journal 287: 39–43

Oakley C 1977 The diagnosis of acute pulmonary embolism. British Journal of Hospital Medicine 18: 15

Owen R 1972 Indications and contra-indications for limb traction. Physiotherapy 58: 44

Powell M 1972 Application of limb traction and nursing management. Physiotherapy 58: 46

Powell M 1973 Limb traction—some aspects of nursing management. Nursing Mirror, 27 July, 26

Rayner C 1967 Essentials of outpatient nursing. London: Arlington Books

Riddle J T E 1985 Anatomy and Physiology Applied to Nursing. Edinburgh: Churchill Livingstone

Roaf R, Hodkinson L J 1971 A Textbook of Orthopaedic Nursing. Oxford: Blackwell Scientific

Robinson W 1973 Sport and recreation for the mentally and physically handicapped. Nursing Times, 12th July, 895
   Orthotics—1
      Rose G K 1977 Total functional assessment of orthoses. Physiotherapy 63: 78
      Stallard J 1977 Mechanics allied to orthoses. Physiotherapy 63: 84
   Orthotics—2
      Davies J B 1977 Use of heart rate in assessment of orthoses. Physiotherapy 63: 112

Roper N 1982 Principles of Nursing, 3rd edn. Edinburgh: Churchill Livingstone

Roper N, Logan W W, Tierney A 1981 Learning to use the process of nursing. Edinburgh: Churchill Livingstone

Roper N, Logan W W, Tierney A 1985 The Elements of Nursing, 2nd edn. Edinburgh: Churchill Livingstone

Rowe J, Dyer L (eds) 1977 Care of the Orthopaedic Patient. London: Blackwell Scientific

Sears W G, Winwood R S 1975 Medicine for Nurses. London: Arnold

Sinclair D 1969 Human Growth after Birth. London: Oxford University Press

Smith J P 1981 Sociology and Nursing. Livingstone Nursing Texts. Edinburgh: Churchill Livingstone

Stewart J D M 1975 Traction and Orthopaedic Appliances. Edinburgh: Churchill Livingstone

Tucker W E 1969 Home Treatment and Posture. Edinburgh: Churchill Livingstone

Vasey J, Crozier L 1982 A move in the right direction. A neuromuscular approach. Nursing Mirror, series of articles 28 April, 5 May, 12 May, 19 May, 26 May, 30 June

Wilson-Barnett J 1981 Patients first. Nursing Mirror, 29 July

Wright B 1981 Lifting and moving patients. 1. An investigation and commentary. 2. Training and management. Nursing Times, 11th November, 18th November

Wright V 1977 Rheumatism for Nurses and Remedial Therapists. London: Heinemann

2

Aspects of infection control in orthopaedic nursing

Introduction

Infection control is a specialist subject and discipline in its own right. The principles of infection control do not vary; only the ways in which they can be applied. If the nurse understands the principles at the outset, procedures can be safely adapted to meet the patient's needs in any particular nursing situation. The intention of this chapter, therefore, is to highlight certain aspects of infection control which whilst important in any clinical situation, are particularly relevant when caring for orthopaedic patients.

HOSPITAL INFECTION

At any point in time about 20 per cent of all patients in hospital are infected (Meers et al, 1981). Half of these patients are already infected on admission and are said to have community-acquired infections. However, one in every ten patients develops an infection as a direct result of hospitalisation. These hospital-acquired infections are sometimes referred to as nosocomial infections. The most prevalent hospital-acquired infections are: urinary tract infection 30 per cent, respiratory tract infection 20 per cent, surgical wound infection 19 per cent, and infection of skin and soft tissue 13.5 per cent. The prevalence of these infections amongst orthopaedic patients is shown in Table 2.1. Nearly all of these infections are endemic and tend to be ignored. 2.5 per cent of all hospital acquired infections are infections of bones and joints.

Table 2.1 Prevalence of Hospital Acquired Infections (HAI) in orthopaedic patients (Meers et al, 1981)

	%
Nos. surveyed	2315
All HAI	13.1
Urinary tract	3.8
Wound	3.8
Skin	2.2
Lower respiratory	1.4

For the patient and family, hospital-acquired infection causes pain and distress. It prolongs hospitalisation, and may result in loss of earned income and even loss of employment. If treatment with antibiotics or surgery is necessary to cure the infection, the patient is at risk from the inherent dangers of such therapy. For the doctor and hospital, financial considerations include the expense of these treatments and the risk of litigation. It has been estimated that over half of hospital-acquired infections are preventable.

Infection may be endogenous or exogenous.

Endogenous: Self or auto infection

The patient develops an infection from his own micro-organisms, e.g. *E. coli* is the commonest aerobic gut commensal but if it ascends the patient's urinary tract in sufficient numbers, it will probably cause a urinary tract infection.

Exogenous or cross infection

The patient becomes infected from micro-organisms transmitted to him from another source, which may be animate, e.g. staff who do not wash their hands in between each patient care procedure, or inanimate, e.g. contaminated disinfectants. The principal sources of micro-organisms are shown in Fig. 2.1. The principal routes of transmission are shown in Fig. 2.2.

Infections can be caused by any of the following micro-organisms: bacteria, viruses, protozoa, fungi, chlamydiae, rickettsiae, mycoplasma. Most hospital-acquired infections are caused by bacteria. Twenty years ago, the Gram positive cocci, particularly *Staphylococcus aureus*, were the scourge of our hospitals. Today, however, 60 per cent of hospital-acquired infections are caused by Gram negative bacilli such as *E. coli*, klebsiella, pseudomonas, serratia, and acinetobacter spp.

This reflects the hazards associated with the kind of care we are giving our patients today, such as frequent instrumentation of the urethra, particularly the increased use of the indwelling catheter, and the increased use of humidifiers and nebulisers for respiratory therapy.

However, the Gram positive cocci do still cause problems. *Staphylococcus aureus* remains the bacterium most frequently isolated from hospital-

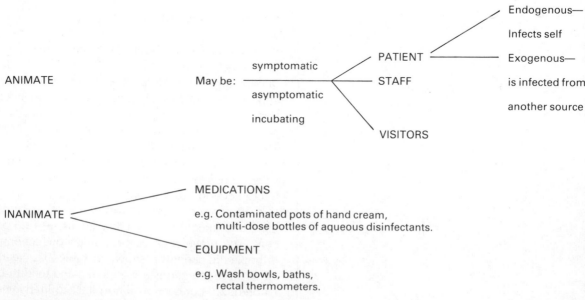

Fig. 2.1 Principal sources of micro-organisms.

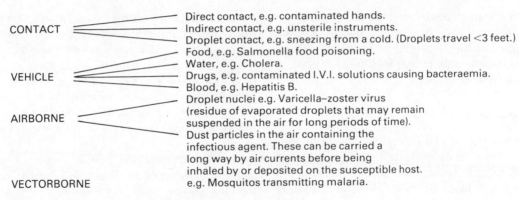

Fig. 2.2 Principal routes of transmission of micro-organisms.

acquired wound infections (Jenner, 1983). *Staphylococcus epidermidis* was once dismissed as a skin commensal of no consequence, but its pathogenicity is now well recognised especially in patients with prosthetic implants. Similarly, *Staphylococcus saprophyticus* is now well recognised as a urinary pathogen, particularly in catheterised patients.

Risk factors

The orthopaedic patient is particularly vulnerable to infection for several reasons and may be classified as a 'high risk' patient.

Length of hospitalisation

Many orthopaedic conditions necessitate a prolonged period of hospitalisation. The longer a patient is in hospital, the greater his chances of acquiring an infection.

Length of pre-operative hospitalisation

Similarly, the length of pre-operative hospitalisation is recognised as a factor associated with an increased risk of post-operative wound infection. Therefore, patients should whenever possible be investigated pre-operatively on an out-patient basis. Admission to hospital can then be planned for the day before surgery. This ideal can often be achieved: for example, patients undergoing a total hip replacement. On the other hand, there are many orthopaedic conditions which necessitate prolonged pre-operative hospitalisation and these patients are at increased risk of infection.

Pre-existing infection

A patient who is already infected is at risk of wound contamination with micro-organisms carried on the skin scales or from the actual lesions. If possible, therefore, elective surgery, particularly orthopaedic operations, should be postponed until the patient is free from infection.

Age

Patients at either end of the age spectrum are at increased risk of infection. In the very young, the immune defence mechanism may not be adequately developed, and the very old have declining powers of tissue repair. So, the child undergoing surgery for congenital hip dislocation and the elderly lady with a fractured neck of femur are both particularly vulnerable.

Mental attitude

Patients who understand what will be involved pre- and post-operatively seem to acquire fewer wound infections than those who have received inadequate psychological preparation and who do not realise what the operation entails. Once again, therefore, children and elderly, confused patients are at special risk.

Nutrition and metabolism

Fat patients are prone to infection because adipose tissue is relatively easily invaded by micro-organisms. Very thin patients are also at risk because starvation has a deleterious effect on many of the body's natural defence mechanisms.

Patients with diabetes mellitus are predisposed to infection because they have a neuropathy and vasculopathy and decreased white blood cell activity. A diabetic patient may well have to undergo an orthopaedic operation.

Chemotherapy

Patients on steroids or other immunosuppressive drugs have seriously impaired immune defences. The rheumatoid patient on steroid therapy who requires corrective surgery for deformities will be immunocompromised and therefore be at increased risk of infection. A patient with cancer and bony metastases may require admission to an orthopaedic ward following a pathological fracture. Such a patient is likely to be on cytotoxic drugs and may therefore have a reduced white blood cell count and so an increased susceptibility to infection.

Foreign bodies

The implantation of prostheses such as hip joints is associated with a high risk of infection which is likely to have disastrous results and will be extremely difficult and costly to treat.

Bone

Bone is a hard substance and in certain areas is deficient in blood supply. If it does become infected, it is liable to become the seat of chronic infection unless treated promptly with appropriate antibiotics.

Urinary catheters

Orthopaedic patients are frequently catheterised. Almost 4 per cent of patients with hospital-acquired urinary tract infections are to be found on orthopaedic wards. In 1978, a urinary tract infection in an orthopaedic patient cost £775 and extended the stay from 24–41 days (Davies & Cottingham, 1979).

INFECTION CONTROL PROGRAMME

The majority of District Health Authorities have an Infection Control Committee and an Infection Control Team. All have an Infection Control Officer.

The District Infection Control Committee is a strategic group consisting of 10–30 members, most of whom are heads of departments. The frequency of meetings varies from monthly to twice a year. Each meeting is a forum for the exchange of information and for ratification of policies and procedures.

The District Infection Control Team is regarded as the spearhead of the Infection Control Committee. It consists of the consultant microbiologist (who usually assumes the role of Infection Control Officer), Registrars training in the speciality of microbiology and one or more Infection Control Nurses. Occasionally a senior medical laboratory scientific officer is also a member of the team and of course, there is secretarial support.

The team is responsible for the monitoring, surveillance and investigation of infections and for advising on preventative and control measures. This is an advisory service which is available to all staff and patients within all health care facilities in the District, including the community. It is a practical and tactical team that meets twice a day to discuss current infection control problems and to plan future activities.

Most of the activity of the Infection Control Team lies in surveillance, control, teaching and research in the hospitals. A team which is clinically orientated, and spends most of its time on the wards, but liaises constantly with the microbiology laboratories, is better equipped to prevent or control cross-infection than one which spends most of its time in the laboratory.

SURVEILLANCE ACTIVITIES

The rapid identification of a patient who is a cross-infection risk is of paramount importance, because it allows appropriate infection control measures to be instituted promptly, so helping to prevent the spread of the infection. Such a patient may be suffering from an infection classically referred to as an 'infectious disease' or may have become infected or colonised with a multi-resistant strain of a hospital bacterium. Surveillance activities are carried out in both the microbiology laboratory and the wards/departments. The laboratory is regarded as a 'diagnostic service', but in practice it often serves to confirm the clinical impression—hence the importance of a two-pronged approach to surveillance. The Infection Control Nurse visits the laboratory at least twice a day to scrutinise, record and act upon laboratory reports as relevant.

All patients who are seriously ill because of an infection and all those who are in isolation should be visited daily by a member of the Infection Control Team. Units caring for patients who are particularly vulnerable to hospital-acquired infections are also visited regularly.

Having identified an infection control problem and advised on it, it is necessary to evaluate the recommended actions. Both prevalence and incidence surveys may be carried out: first, to identify problem areas, and secondly, to assess the effect of control measures which have been introduced.

CARE OF THE INFECTED PATIENT

Medical and nursing procedures are designed to prevent cross-infection. However, patients who are colonised or infected with multi-resistant organisms or those suffering from communicable diseases require special modifications to their management. Segregation and isolation precautions may be necessary when caring for these patients to limit the spread of infection.

Isolation presents certain disadvantages to both the patient and the hospital. Procedures may be time-consuming and may render visits by hospital staff inconvenient which in turn may discourage the best patient care.

The use of a single room is usually necessary, but segregation may have an adverse psychological effect on the patient and his visitors. It may also be necessary to restrict the patient's visitors and to exclude children.

In an attempt to balance the disadvantages of isolation against the risks of cross-infection, categories of source isolation have been devised.

CATEGORIES OF SOURCE ISOLATION

There are five categories: strict isolation, wound and skin precautions, respiratory precautions,

enteric/urine precautions, blood precautions. The appropriate category of isolation depends upon the virulence of the organism and the way in which it is spread.

Patients requiring strict isolation will have to be transferred to an isolation hospital and will not be considered further here. Others can be nursed in an isolation cubicle in a general hospital. In a few instances, patients can be cared for safely in the open ward, with only minimal modification to their management.

Responsibilities

It is the responsibility of the consultant-in-charge to place an infected patient on isolation precautions, to prevent the spread of infection to others.

It is the responsibility of the ward sister to ensure that isolation procedures are carried out correctly and that the appropriate isolation notice is displayed. Advice may be freely sought from any member of the Infection Control Team, and the ward sister should liaise with the Infection Control Nurse concerning the nursing care of infected patients.

All staff and visitors are responsible for complying with the isolation precautions and for pointing out to offenders, departures from accepted practice. Anyone failing to observe correct procedure will invalidate the efforts of all others.

In the interests of safety, the Infection Control Officer should be informed of any individual who persistently ignores recommended techniques.

Aim

The aim of source isolation is to contain the infection and prevent its transmission to other patients, staff and visitors.

Cohort isolation

Patients with the same infection can be nursed in the same room.

Wound and skin precautions

Aim

This is to prevent cross-infection of patients and other personnel from infection transmissible by direct contact with wounds and heavily contaminated articles.

Essential precautions in this category include:

proper hand disinfection before and after patient contact

safe handling and disposal of dressings and contaminated equipment

correct use of gowns and gloves.

Orthopaedic patients with surgical wounds, chronic wounds and skin conditions infected or colonized with the following bacteria should be isolated on wound and skin precautions.

Bacteria	Period of isolation
Streptococcus pyogenes (β haemolytic streptococcus Lancefield group A.)	For 48 hours from start of appropriate antibiotic. Ideally this is penicillin.
Staphylococcus aureus Multi-resistant strains and those that are of a particularly virulent phage type.	Until strain is eradicated. Suppress dispersal with antistaphylococcal topical agents (Table 2.3).
Gram-negative bacilli which are resistant to aminoglycocides.	Until strain is eradicated.

Respiratory precautions

Aim

This is to prevent transmission of organisms by means of droplets and droplet nuclei which are coughed, sneezed or breathed into the air. Some of the organisms responsible for illnesses in this category can be spread by freshly contaminated articles.

Essential precautions in this category include:

a single room, well ventilated with the door kept shut

proper hand disinfection after contact with contaminated articles

safe handling and disposal of secretions e.g. sputum and paper tissues

correct use of a high-efficiency filtration mask, when indicated.

Diseases referred to as 'childhood diseases' are included in this category. They sometimes occur in adults.

Orthopaedic patients who are suffering from the following infectious diseases should be isolated on respiratory precautions.

Infectious disease	Period of isolation
Active pulmonary tuberculosis.	If direct smear of sputum is positive for tubercle bacilli, isolate for 14 days after start of appropriate triple chemotherapy including rifampicin.
Chickenpox, German measles, measles, mumps, whooping cough.	Isolate for period of communicability.
Herpes zoster (shingles).	Isolate from immunocompromised patients and from staff and patients who have not had chickenpox, until lesions are dry and crusted.

Enteric/urine precautions

Aim

This is to prevent infections which can be transmitted through direct or indirect contact with infected faeces, urine and, in some instances, heavily contaminated articles.

Transmission of infection is by ingestion of the pathogen.

Essential precautions in this category include:

safe disposal of excreta

safe disposal or heat disinfection of bedpans and urinals

correct use of gloves and aprons

proper hand disinfection after contact with excreta, or contaminated objects.

The importance of handwashing in preventing transmission of enteric diseases must be stressed, not only for all hospital staff, but also for the patient who must be taught to wash his hands carefully, especially after defaecating and before handling food.

Orthopaedic patients who are suffering from the following conditions should be nursed on enteric or urine precautions as appropriate.

Condition	Period of precautions
Diarrhoea of unknown cause.	Until infective cause has been excluded.
Salmonella, shigella, campylobacter, rotavirus, enteropathogenic E. coli infections.	Until infective agent is no longer being excreted.
Hepatitis A.	Only during the pre-icteric phase.

Multi-resistant organisms in the urinary tract of incontinent or catheterised patients e.g. klebsiella, pseudomonas, acinetobacter, serratia spp.

Until patient is micturating normally.

It is impossible to distinguish with certainty between hepatitis A and hepatitis B on clinical grounds alone. Therefore, all viral hepatitis should be considered hepatitis A for purposes of isolation until diagnosed serologically.

Blood precautions

Aim

This is to prevent infections which can be transmitted through blood or blood products.
  Transmission is by inoculation of the pathogen. Essential precautions in this category include:

  safe handling of blood
  avoidance of 'needle stick' injuries
  correct use of gloves
  labelling specimens 'Bio-hazard'.

Orthopaedic patients who are suffering from the following conditions should only be isolated if bleeding heavily. Otherwise, the patient can be nursed safely in the open ward providing precautions are taken when handling the patient's blood.

Condition

1. Hepatitis B.
Those who are 'e' antigen positive are more infectious than those who are not.
2. Patients with Acquired Immune Deficiency Syndrome (AIDS).
The route of transmission of the virus that causes this syndrome is not yet fully understood, but it is thought to be spread primarily via the blood.

Note

The infectious conditions cited are only examples. Other, less common infective problems may also affect orthopaedic patients. Table 2.2 summarises the main infection control measures necessary to prevent cross-infection.

TUBERCULOSIS

For practical purposes, the only source of tuberculous infection is a person with pulmonary tuberculosis whose sputum is positive for tubercle bacilli on direct smear (Joint Tuberculosis Committee of the British Thoracic Society, 1983). Contacts are at greatest risk of acquiring the infection *before* the patient has started treatment. Once appropriate triple chemotherapy has begun, the risks of infectivity are negligible.

Patients with newly diagnosed pulmonary tuberculosis should preferably be treated at home. Results of well-supervised home treatment are as good as those attained in patients treated in hospital. If hospitalisation is essential, then the patient has to be segregated from other patients who may be particularly susceptible to infection because of lowered resistance due to illness or drugs. The infectious patient will be isolated in a single, well-ventilated room and respiratory precautions observed when caring for him. These infection control measures can usually be discontinued after the patient has had fourteen days' treatment of appropriate antibiotics. A commonly prescribed regimen today consists of rifampicin, isoniazid and ethambutol. Pyrazinamide is also sometimes used in combination. Treatment is usually continued for a total of nine months.

The annual notifications to the Office of Population Census and Surveys for *Mycobacterium tuberculosis* in England and Wales are falling:

  1981 Total number of isolates = 8128 (Respiratory isolates 5859)
  1982 Total number of isolates = 7406 (Respiratory isolates 5822)

In comparison, TB of bone and joints is rare in this country. In 1982 there were only 79 reports of *Mycobacterium tuberculosis* from this site made to the Communicable Diseases Surveillance Centre. This figure probably reflects 50 per cent under reporting, but it still illustrates the relative order of magnitude.

Amongst immigrants, TB is commonest in those from the Indian sub-continent and the Vietnamese Boat People. These patients may have a poor command of the English language and their practices of basic hygiene may differ from those of native-

Table 2.2 Infection control precautions for categories of source isolation

Precaution	Wound and skin	Respiratory	Enteric/urine	Blood
Single room	Usually necessary. Keep door shut.	Necessary. Keep door shut.	If incontinent or on urinary drainage.	Only if bleeding heavily.
Hands to be washed	Before and after contact with site. After contact with immediate environment.	After contact with sputum.	After contact with faeces. Before and after handling urinary drainage system.	After contact with blood.
Gloves to be worn: *Sterile*	Contact with infected site or dressing.			
Unsterile		Handling contaminated articles.		Handling blood.
Gown to be worn:	For direct patient contact and bedmaking.			
Apron to be worn:			Handling excreta.	Handling blood
Mask to be worn:	No.	By staff when entering room and by patient when leaving room if patient's sputum is positive for tubercle bacilli on direct smear. For first 14 days of triple antibiotic therapy.		
Linen		Discard gently into RED plastic alginate stitched bags. Seal before leaving room.		
Crockery and cutlery		Dishwashing machine or disposables.		
Equipment	Use disposables, or clean then disinfect or sterilize after use.			
Cleaning	Notify unit domestic manager. All isolation cubicles to be cleaned *daily* after all other ward cleaning has been completed. An isolation cleaning pack is used. A terminal clean with hot soapy water will also be required followed by a wipe over with,			
	A clear soluble phenolic		*A hypochlorite detergent*	
Comments	Isolate wound with occlusive dressing.		Check bedpan washer is reaching 80°C and is not leaking. Check macerator is functioning. Keep lid closed for one minute after cycle has finished.	Discard 'sharps' safely.
	Label specimens 'Bio hazard' and transport containers in sealed plastic bags.			

born British people. Therefore the nurse's educational role is an extremely important one. Patients must be taught to cover their mouth and nose when coughing and sneezing. They must be taught to expectorate into a disposable handkerchief or into a sputum pot with a lid. Such infectious waste should be discarded into plastic bags, sealed and incinerated. Patients with pulmonary tuberculosis whose sputum is negative on direct smear and patients with non-pulmonary disease do not need to be isolated and may be nursed in an open ward.

Non-pulmonary tuberculosis is non-infectious even though tubercle bacilli may have been cultured from specimens from the lesions.

Notification

All cases of tuberculosis, whether infectious or not, are statutorily notifiable in accordance with the Public Health Act 1981 for England and Wales. The Medical Officer for Environmental Health of the Borough in which the patient resides, must be informed, in writing, on the prescribed form.

ACUTE HAEMATOGENOUS OSTEOMYELITIS

As the name implies, this condition is caused by infecting bacteria spread by the blood stream from a skin lesion or other septic focus to a long bone, although any bone can be affected. When the infection is established, a small abscess forms in the metaphysis. This eventually leads to the formation of a sub-periosteal abscess and subsequent penetration of the soft tissue. Signs and symptoms vary in severity and sub-periosteal pus may be present without clinical signs of abscess. Treatment is usually conservative unless there are definite signs of abscess formation. If pus is obtained surgically, then this should be cultured along with blood and swabs from infected skin lesions and boils. The majority of cases are caused by *Staphylococcus aureus* although about 30 per cent are culture negative. As most staphylococci are now resistant to penicillin, a full antibiotic sensitivity profile must be done.

Penicillin is the drug of choice, but if the infecting organism is resistant, either cloxacillin, erythromycin or clindamycin, is given in combination with sodium fusidate. Apart from being particularly effective anti-staphylococcal antibiotics, these combined drugs have an additive effect. They penetrate both dead and viable bone and may also prevent or delay the emergence of resistant strains. One or other may be inactivated by pus—but rarely both.

If appropriate antibiotic therapy is commenced intravenously within three days of illness, 95 per cent of acute osteomyelitis patients will be cured conservatively. Drugs can be given orally once the septicaemic and toxaemic phases have passed. Therapy is usually continued for six weeks.

CHRONIC OSTEOMYELITIS

This infection is a complication of acute haematogenous spread, compound fractures and orthopaedic operations. Most sufferers of the disease are victims of delayed diagnosis and inadequate antibiotic therapy with or without surgery. Infected cavities develop, surrounded by sclerosed bone. Periosteum, muscle, fascia and skin may be involved. Even if the appropriate antibiotics are given, they cannot be sufficiently concentrated in the infected tissues to kill the infecting micro-organism. Dead bone must be excised so that the blood supply to the infected area is improved. Sequestrectomy and debridement with primary or delayed skin closure may be necessary. Bone grafting may also be required. The debris is cultured. Staphylococci are still the commonest infecting bacteria and flucloxacillin, erythromycin or clindamycin with sodium fusidate the antibiotic regimen of choice. The bone may also be irrigated with antibiotics by means of a closed suction system inserted in theatre.

JOINT INFECTIONS

These may be caused by staphylococci, haemolytic streptococci, and coliforms. Meningococci, gonococci, pneumococci, salmonella spp., brucella spp. and tuberculosis may also cause a septic arthritis. Joint fluid is aspirated and cultured along with blood and specimens from any infected focus on the skin, in the nasopharynx or genito-urinary system.

The choice of systemic antibiotic will depend upon the infecting organism.

Patients with advanced rheumatoid arthritis are particularly at risk of bacterial infections, especially if they are on large doses of steroids. There is a high mortality amongst those who develop a septic arthritis. Prompt diagnosis and swift use of systemic antibiotics are essential.

CONTROL ACTIVITIES

Control activities are often linked to surveillance activities as both are intrinsic components of an Infection Control Programme. Control activities range from liaising with the Occupational Health Department regarding infected staff to providing specialist advice to the district planning team in respect of upgrading and new building schemes. Planned preventative maintenance schedules need to be discussed with hospital engineers to avoid recurring problems such as malfunctioning bedpan macerators. The Infection Control Nurse liaises with the Supplies Officer and will be asked to advise on the infection control merits of various pieces of equipment prior to purchase. Such consultation often prevents the purchase of 'white elephants' and thus saves considerable sums of money. The Infection Control Nurse is usually a member of the Nursing/Supplies Liaison Committee and may represent nursing opinion at Regional Contract Supplies meetings. She is also usually a member of the Nursing Procedures Committee.

Infection control policies and procedures that have been agreed with nursing, domestic, laundry and catering staff need to be monitored and revised accordingly. Consultants who adopt a policy of 'never say "No" to an admission' may need to be reminded about the infection control hazards and practical difficulties which ensue from ward over-crowding. Adequate bedspacing and ventilation are still essential to the delivery of safe health care.

HAND DISINFECTION

Hand disinfection before and after each patient contact is the most important measure in the prevention of cross-infection. Organisms can be spread on staff hands by such a simple contact as taking the pulse. Hand disinfection is still essential even if gloves are worn and 'non-touch techniques' are used.

Nails should be kept short and clean. Wrist watches and rings (except wedding bands) should not be worn on duty. Apart from the fact that these might scratch the patient, their presence prevents effective hand disinfection.

Nailbrushes are not used for routine hand-cleaning. If using a nailbrush is essential, for example prior to carrying out an invasive procedure, a sterile brush from Central Sterile Supply Department must be used.

Social handwash

A social handwash is carried out before starting work, before handling food and drugs and before leaving the ward. The hands are washed after visiting the toilet, after handling patients and bedding, after handling bedpans, urinals and other contaminated equipment and whenever the hands are soiled.

Preparations

Liquid soap from wall dispenser e.g. Sterisol, *or* Plain tablet soap—stored dry in a soap dish which allows drainage of excess water.

Method

The hands are washed thoroughly with soap in free running water. They are then dried thoroughly on disposable paper towels. The whole process should last approximately 30 seconds.

Aseptic handwash

An aseptic handwash is carried out before aseptic techniques and after care of patients in source isolation.

Preparations

Chlorhexidine gluconate 4 per cent detergent (Hibiscrub)
Povidone-iodine 7.5 per cent detergent (Videne), *or* Hexachlorophane 3 per cent (Ster-Zac DC skin cleanser) if allergic to above.

When in use, the container must be put in its wall-mounted bracket. Correct procedure for dispensing the solution cannot be carried out if it is 'free standing' on the edge of the sink. When empty, the container is returned to the pharmacy department where it is cleaned and disinfected before being refilled. It is not 'topped up' on the ward.

Method

Using the elbows to regulate the taps, the temperature of the water is adjusted and the hands are wetted.

With the elbow, 5 ml of the preferred solution is dispensed into the palm of the hand.

The wash, in free running water, lasts one minute.

All surfaces are lathered thoroughly. Particular attention is paid to the tips of the fingers, thumbs and interdigital clefts.

After care of a patient in source isolation, the forearms are washed as well, up to the elbows.

The solution is rinsed off and the hands and fore-arms dried thoroughly on absorbent paper towels.

Sinks

Clinical sinks should be of a type approved by the consultant microbiologist. Those situated in isolation cubicles, treatment and clean utility rooms and the ward should be fitted with elbow or foot-operated taps. Plugs and overflows should be absent.

Towels

An adequate supply of soft, absorbent paper towels must be maintained to encourage thorough hand-drying and prevent chapped hands.

Aseptic handrub

An alternative method of disinfection for hands that are not grossly soiled, is an alcoholic handrub. Such a preparation is particularly useful when handwashing facilities are inadequate or absent and in high risk units, where such frequent hand disinfection is required that it becomes too time consuming.

Preparations

0.5 per cent Chlorhexidine in 70 per cent Isopropyl Alcohol + emollient (Hibisol), *or*
60 per cent Isopropyl Alcohol + emollient.

Method

3 ml of the solution is dispensed into the palm of the hand and rubbed to dryness with friction over all surfaces, especially the finger tips, thumbs and interdigital clefts.

N.B. it is important not to exceed the stated dose.

Handcream

Handcream to prevent dry hands is supplied in tubes because pots of cream are easily contaminated.

Skin rashes

If skin rashes or sensitivities occur, these should be reported to the Infection Control Nurse and Occupational Health Department.

CARE OF THE CATHETERISED PATIENT

Urinary tract infection is one of the most commonly encountered infections in orthopaedic wards. The main cause of urinary tract infection, and the commonest predisposing factor in life threatening Gram-negative septicaemia, is the use of an indwelling urethral catheter.

Morbidity and mortality can be reduced by:

1. avoidance of unnecessary catheterisation.
2. The use of an aseptic technique not only when

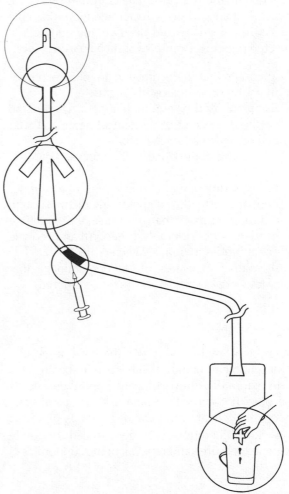

Fig. 2.3   Entry points for infecting bacteria in the catheterised patient.

inserting the catheter, but also in continued catheter care.

3. understanding the ways in which bacteria can enter the drainage system and directing infection control measures towards minimising the entry of bacteria at these points (Fig. 2.3).

4. removing the catheter as soon as possible because the prevalence of bacteriuria increases with the duration of catheterisation.

Urethral catheterisation should not be used routinely to obtain a urine specimen for microbiological examination, nor should it be used simply as a means of preventing skin maceration in the incontinent patient.

Abuse of catheterisation is no substitute for skilled nursing care; if catheterisation can be avoided, it should be. Greater attention to simple nursing measures would decrease the numbers of infected patients. Examples of such measures are:

5. adequate hand disinfection to prevent cross-infection of catheterised patients.

6. using a closed system for bladder irrigation and washouts instead of disconnecting the catheter and using a bladder syringe.

7. promoting continence in the confused elderly, by patience and habit training.

8. lifting women with broken hips onto slipper bedpans instead of catheterising them. Though this requires more than one nurse, the extra time needed is considerably cheaper than a course of antibiotics to treat a catheter infection.

Alternative measures of bladder drainage that carry fewer risks should always be considered.

Penile sheath

Incontinent males who do not have an outlet obstruction can be fitted with a penile sheath. This is an externally fitting appliance and therefore its use does not carry the same risks as an invasive procedure. Local complications such as phimosis and skin ulceration can be avoided by daily hygiene measures and renewal of the condom.

Suprapubic catheterisation

Patients requiring long-term drainage generally find

it much easier to cope with a suprapubic catheter than with a urethral catheter, particularly at home.

Intermittent catheterisation

Patients with spinal cord injuries do not usually have obstructive lesions of the urethra and so, because catheters can be passed with minimal trauma, their urinary incontinence can be managed by sterile intermittent catheterisation.

Post-operative patients

Those who fail to empty their bladder spontaneously, despite skilled nursing ploys, will require catheterisation with a non-retention catheter. However, if this procedure needs to be repeated more than two or three times, an indwelling catheter should be inserted and placed on free drainage.

Avoidance of re-catheterisation

This is one of the major principles in the prevention of urinary tract infection, because re-catheterisation increases the risks. The selection of the right catheter at the outset of the procedure is extremely important.

Selection of catheter

Catheters are made in different materials, lengths and widths. The size of the retention balloon also varies. Each has a specific use and the nurse must take time to consider which one will best meet her patient's needs. The smallest size capable of providing adequate drainage should be used.

Junction breaks

Once the catheter has been inserted aseptically the drainage system should not be interfered with unless essential, when an aseptic technique must be used. Accidental and deliberate disconnections of the catheter and drainage tube are a major cause of urinary tract infection. Junction breaks for bladder washouts and irrigations must be avoided. A closed system such as the Vygon Slade irrigation system should be used with a three-way catheter.

The safest form of bladder irrigation is to ensure that the catheterised patient has a high fluid intake.

Anchoring the catheter

Once connected, the catheter should be anchored to the inner aspect of the thigh. If this is not done, the catheter will tend to be pushed to and fro in the urethra when the patient moves. This piston effect increases the likelihood that pathogens will gain access to the space between the catheter and urethral mucosa.

Strapping the catheter also relieves the traction exerted by the balloon on the bladder neck, thus reducing trauma. Sufficient slack must be allowed to prevent the development of pressure sores on the scrotum.

Meatal care

The catheter meatal junction is one of the main entry points for bacteria into the urinary tract. Meatal toilet should be carried out aseptically once or twice daily to remove discharges and encrustations which form a nidus for infection. When bathing, patients on short-term catheterisation should, if possible, have a shower or blanket bath, because submerging the meatal junction in contaminated bath water, increases the risks of infection.

Retrograde spread

A large proportion of infections arise from the ascent of bacteria from the drainage bag, helped by the thin film of fluid that coats the drainage tube.

Reflux of urine can be prevented by ensuring that the bag is kept below the level of the bladder at all times. Unobstructed flow must be maintained and the system must be prevented from kinking.

Emptying the bag

This is an aseptic procedure. The hands must be disinfected before and after handling the outlet tube. Each bag must be emptied into a container or jug, which should either be a single-use disposable item or should be heat disinfected between each use. If the bedpan washer is functioning properly at 80 °C for one minute, this does the job.

Changing the bag at arbitrary fixed intervals is unnecessary and increases the infection risks. If the system is functioning well; leave well alone. If the junction is broken, a fresh sterile bag should be connected. A drainage bag is a pre-sterilised, single use item; it must never be disinfected and re-used.

Catheter specimen of urine

This should never be collected by disconnecting the catheter from the drainage tube as this junction break is an infection hazard. Neither should a specimen be collected from the bag via the outlet tube. Urine in the bag is stale and will not show the numbers of micro-organisms that are actually present in the bladder. A catheter specimen of urine is obtained aseptically by aspirating 5 ml of fresh urine with a needle and syringe via the self-sealing sampling port. The sampling port is first cleaned with an alcohol swab.

Spatial dispersion

Infection control measures are more easily implemented if catheterised patients are not nursed in adjacent beds. Spatial dispersion makes it easier to remember that the aseptic maintenance of a urinary drainage system is a vital part of the patient's individualised care.

CARE OF SURGICAL WOUNDS

Surgical wounds are classified according to the likelihood of their becoming contaminated and infected. This is an international system.

Classification

Category A—'Clean' wounds

These are wounds which have been made in an operation which did not transect the gastro-intestinal, genito-urinary or tracheo-bronchial systems, and which was not performed in the vicinity of any apparent inflammatory reaction, e.g. total hip replacement.

Blomgren et al (1982) report infection rates as high as 13 per cent for superficial infection and 5.4 per cent for deep joint infection after these operations whereas Lidwell et al (1982) report infection rates in joints as low as 0.2 per cent after total hip and knee replacements.

Category B—'Clean–contaminated' wounds

These are wounds which have been made in an operation which transected one of the three systems mentioned above where bacterial contamination could have occurred, but in an operation in which no actual evidence of bacterial contamination was available, e.g. cholecystectomy.

Category C—'Contaminated' wounds

These are wounds which were made during an operation transecting a system in which bacteria were known to be present, or in the vicinity of apparent inflammatory reactions, e.g. colonic operations. This category also includes wounds resulting from fresh trauma such as road traffic accidents.

Category D—'Dirty or infected wounds'

These are principally wounds in which pus was encountered during the operation or in which a perforated viscus was found. The implication is that at the time of the operation, the operative field was already heavily contaminated with the micro-organisms which caused the infection subsequently reported, e.g. drainage of an abscess.

An infected wound is defined as one showing signs of clinical infection plus a positive culture.

Pre-operative preparation

As most wound infections are theatre-acquired and endogenous, the importance of pre-operative skin preparation of both patient and staff and skilled surgical technique cannot be overstressed.

Hair should only be removed from the operative site if it is likely to interfere with the surgical incision or skin closure. The procedure should be performed as close to the time of surgery as possible and never the day before. Hair should be removed without damaging the skin because nicks and small abrasions will become heavily colonised with hospital strains of bacteria. Shaving increases the wound infection rate (Cruse & Foord, 1980). Depilatory creams or clipping are much safer.

A *shower*, bath or bedbath should be taken shortly before the operation. The patient puts on a clean theatre gown and cap and gets into bed made up with clean linen.

Total body washing with chlorhexidine gluconate has been researched recently. One Swedish study of 28 orthopaedic patients (Seeberg & Bergman, 1980) showed that *two* washes were effective in reducing the skin flora. The study was not designed to show whether this also reduced the incidence of post-operative wound infection. A more recent English study (Ayliffe et al, 1983), which included an orthopaedic hospital, showed that a *single* pre-operative bath with chlorhexidine detergent did not influence the incidence of post-operative infection in spite of a relatively high incidence of infection with skin organisms.

Skin disinfection

In hip operations and operations on limbs with impaired circulation, spore-forming organisms such as *Clostridium perfringens* present a particular hazard. In such cases a compress of 10 per cent povidone iodine may be applied and bandaged to the operation site, thirty minutes pre-operatively.

If the patient already has infected lesions such as pressure sores or varicose ulcers and it is not practical to postpone surgery, the lesions should be sprayed with povidone iodine and occluded with a fresh sterile dressing.

Another important aspect of skin disinfection is the way in which the alcoholic solution is actually applied to the skin immediately before incising. Lowbury & Lilly (1975) have shown that it is more effective to do this with a sterile gloved hand than to apply the solution with swabs held in forceps.

Recommended solutions for skin disinfection of both patient and staff are listed in Table 2.3.

Factors affecting the incidence of wound infection

Staff activity

The more people that there are in theatre, the greater the incidence of bacterial shedding.

One study has shown (Blomgren et al, 1982) that during a total hip replacement operation, up to eleven people were present in the theatre, thirteen people visited and the operating room doors open 173 times. These figures demonstrate lack of staff discipline and it is hardly surprising that there was

Table 2.3 Chemical disinfectants: summary of main uses

Use	Approved name	Proprietary name
Hands		
Aseptic technique	Chlorhexidine gluconate	
and care of	4% detergent	Hibiscrub
infected patients	Povidone-iodine	
	7.5% detergent	Videne
	Chlorhexidine 0.5% in	
	70% alcohol with emollients	Hibisol
Operation site	Chlorhexidine 0.5% in	
	70% alcohol	
	Povidone-iodine 10% in	
	30% alcohol	
	Iodine 1% in alcohol	
Skin cleaning		
Fresh trauma,	Chlorhexidine 0.25% ⎤ 100 ml	Savloclens 3%
A & E	Cetrimide 0.5% ⎦ sachet	
Urethral	Chlorhexidine 0.015% ⎤ 25 ml	Savlodil 1%
Catheterisation	Cetrimide 0.15% ⎦ sachet	
Injections	Industrial methylated	
	spirit 70%	
Staph. aureus protocol	Povidone-iodine 14 ml sachet	Steribath
	Hexachlorophane 3% liquid soap	Ster-Zac DC skin cleanser
	Hexachlorophane 0.3% powder	Ster-Zac powder
	Chlorhexidine hydrochloride 0.1% ⎤	Naseptin cream
	Neomycin sulphate 0.5% ⎦	
Fibreoptics e.g.	Glutaraldehyde 2%	Cidex
Arthroscopes		
Environment	Clear soluble phenolic	Hycolin 1.5%
(rarely necessary)	or	
	Hypochlorite	Chloros
	10 000 parts per million	
	Choice depends on organism	

NB. No disinfectant will work in the presence of dirt.

a high incidence of post-operative sepsis in patients operated on in these conditions.

Time

The duration of the operation and the length of the surgical incision are also important factors because the longer the tissues are exposed, the greater the chance of wound infection occurring. Blomgren et al (1982) report operating times for total hip replacements ranging from 108–468 minutes.

The air

Airborne bacteria are an important cause of joint infection following prosthetic implants.

The use of ultra-clean air systems has been shown to halve the sepsis rate of those operated on in a room ventilated conventionally with a posit- ive pressure air supply. If, in addition, a body exhaust suit is worn by the surgical team, the sepsis rate is more than halved again (Lidwell et al, 1982). Such expensive equipment cannot be afforded by many hospitals other than specialist centres. For those who do not consider this a high priority, the infection rate can also be substantially reduced by the judicious use of prophylactic antibiotics (Table 2.4).

Table 2.4 Influence of prophylactic antibiotics on rate of sepsis (Lidwell et al, 1983a)

		%of infected joints	
		Without prophylactic	With prophylactic
Ventilation	Clothing	antibiotics	antibiotics
Control	Conventional	3.4	0.85
Ultraclean	Conventional	1.7	0.42
Ultraclean	Body exhaust	0.76	0.19

Infecting bacteria

Many different types of bacteria cause joint infections after prosthetic surgery (Lidwell et al, 1983b). The commonest is *Staphylococcus aureus* and very small numbers are needed to cause an infection. The patient is at particular risk from staphylococcal carriers.

Staphylococcus albus, usually regarded as of low pathogenicity, is the second most commonly isolated bacterium from septic implants. The third most common group of organisms isolated from infected hip and knee joints are 'gut' organisms.

Prophylactic antibiotics

Over 30 000 joint replacement operations are now performed annually in the UK. Infection may lead to an unstable joint, which may have to be removed in a second operation. A Girdlestone may be required. Patients who have had previous hip operations are at increased risk of deep sepsis (2.6 per cent compared with 0.9 per cent for first operations). The prevention of infection in these operations is a high priority, and the benefit of prophylactic antibiotics has already been referred to. Infection that manifests soon after operation is usually caused by bacteria introduced directly into the wound at the time of surgery. On the other hand, some joints may not become infected for several years after the operation and these infections are usually caused by haematogenous spread of micro-organisms from elsewhere in the body, e.g. following dental treatment.

As infections may be of early or late onset, the optimum timing of antibiotic prophylaxis is uncertain. However, they are prescribed in 66 per cent of joint replacement operations.

Peri-operative cover with cloxacillin for no more than 24 hours is a commonly used anti-staphylococcal regimen (Emmerson, 1982) but this antibiotic is ineffective against 15 per cent of the infections which are caused by 'gut' organisms. The use of bone cement incorporating gentamicin is also favoured by some (Buckolz et al, 1979).

Instruments

Sterile instruments and drapes are essential if the skin or membrane is going to be cut. These are commonly supplied on the Edinburgh Tray System by the Theatre Sterile Supply Unit where heat sterilisation is achieved by autoclaving.

Trials of adhesive plastic drapes have failed to demonstrate a reduction in the incidence of post-operative wound infection.

Tissue handling

A surgical incision has breached the first line of defence against infection; the intact skin. Traumatised tissue is very vulnerable to infection.

Haemostasis must be complete because blood is a good culture medium. Excessive blood loss renders the patient more liable to infection from micro-organisms which have contaminated the tissues. The patient is also at increased risk of infection from prolonged anaesthesia or hypotension.

Wound drainage

Drained wounds are more likely to become infected than wounds without drains. Closed suction drainage such as Redivac carries a lower infection risk than open wound drainage such as a corrugated drain. The risk of infection is lowered if the drain is brought out through a separate stab wound and not via the main incision. It is safer if the theatre wound dressing is applied in such a way that the drain can be removed without having to take down the whole of the suture line dressing.

Wound closure

Tape closures are associated with a lower incidence of infection than clips, which in turn cause fewer infections than sutures. Clips and sutures are foreign bodies and are potential pathways for micro-organisms to enter the wound and produce an abscess. The numbers of sutures or clips and the tension they exert are also important aspects of surgical technique.

Wound dressings

Wounds should be covered post-operatively with some form of protective dressing. A plastic dressing which can be sprayed on is frequently all that is needed. Wounds without drains will be well sealed within 24–48 hours.

Discharging wounds should be re-dressed as soon as 'strike through' is evident. Ideally, dressings should be done in a properly ventilated treatment room, where there is a lower level of activity than in a busy surgical ward.

The dressing technique should be simple. The use of sterile gloves, instead of forceps, has much to commend it. Bulky dressings are easier to handle and learners are more dextrous. The wound can be dressed more quickly with the result that there is less heat loss, and the wound is not exposed to contamination by hospital bacteria for prolonged periods of time. The type of dressing used must be chosen to meet the needs of that particular wound. There are many products other than gauze.

Wound cleaning

Clean wounds do not require cleaning. The purpose of cleaning a wound is to remove the debris and discharge on which bacteria thrive. This is accomplished by the physical action of wiping a cotton wool ball along the incision, so discharging wounds can be cleaned with either a dry cotton wool ball or one moistened in normal saline. As this action does not allow a disinfectant sufficient contact time with the organisms in order to kill them, the use of disinfectants for this purpose is of very limited value.

A wound swab for culture and sensitivity testing should be pre-moistened in sterile saline or water. The swab should be rotated over the discharging site after the stale exudate has been cleaned away. A sample of pus is always preferable to a wound swab. This can often be obtained by aspirating with a sterile syringe.

Plaster of Paris

An outbreak of *Pseudomonas aeruginosa* post-operative wound infection after orthopaedic surgery has been described (Houang et al, 1981). The outbreak strain was shown to multiply and survive in plaster of Paris for at least three weeks.

The reservoir of these Gram-negative bacilli was the residual water in two plastic buckets used to prepare the plaster of Paris. The buckets were merely rinsed and covered with lids between use. As a result of this investigation, plaster of Paris is now made up with sterile water in an autoclaved stainless steel bucket, in some hospitals. This measure may well be justified when plaster of Paris is to be applied over a wound.

For application to intact skin, it is probably sufficient to dry the buckets thoroughly after use and to store them inverted. Plaster of Paris has also been implicated in other orthopaedic infections (Kozinn, 1962; Murray & Denton, 1949).

Chronic wounds

The prevention of pressure sores is a constant challenge to the nurse caring for orthopaedic patients, many of whom are immobile for prolonged periods of time, or elderly.

As with a surgical wound, it is important to determine whether the micro-organisms that have been cultured from the pressure sore are actually causing an infection or are merely harmless commensals. If, when on inspecting the wound, the nurse considers it necessary to dress it using a sterile technique, then the wound should not be irrigated first with bathwater since this is likely to be grossly contaminated.

Some pressure sores require radical surgical debridement and occasionally a rotation skin flap to buttock is performed. Such care is extremely costly and hazardous for the patient. Many infected pressure sores could be prevented.

PREVENTION OF CHEST INFECTIONS

The infection hazards associated with the use of respiratory therapy and anaesthetic equipment are well known. Patients receiving endotracheal suction, artificial ventilation, nebulisation or humidification are likely to be infected unless aseptic procedures are employed and equipment is safely decontaminated. All respiratory equipment including simple steam inhalers and oxygen humidifiers, should be cleaned and disinfected. Heat disinfection is the method of choice and this should be done every day and in between patients. Humidifiers should be refilled with sterile distilled water, never topped up.

Oxygen tubing and face masks should be changed at least daily. They are disposable and should not be re-used.

Physiotherapy is also a valuable means of preventing chest infections in patients who have undergone general anaesthesia. Pre-operative physiotherapy involves deep breathing and coughing exercises to encourage maximum respiratory function.

CARE OF INTRAVENOUS INFUSIONS

In the UK almost 40 per cent of surgical patients have a peripheral intravenous infusion for varying periods of time but it is a potentially dangerous procedure. There is a 15.1 per cent incidence of thrombophlebitis and a 0.5 per cent incidence of hospital acquired bacteraemia in these patients (Nyström et al, 1983).

Most intravenous infusion infections are caused by:

1. inadequate preparation and after care of the drip site.
2. indiscriminate manipulation of the intravenous system.

It is essential that both the patient's skin and the hands of the operators who handle the system are thoroughly disinfected with a suitable preparation (Table 2.2). A cursory wipe with an alcohol swab and failure to wash the hands are inexcusable.

The drip site should be inspected daily for signs of infection. If evident, the needle should be resited as soon as possible. A swab of the drip site should be taken and blood cultures should be obtained from the other arm if there are any signs of systematic infection.

Rigid containers must be vented by the appropriate airway with a non-wettable bacterial filter.

Giving sets should be changed aseptically every 48 hours and immediately after change over from blood to electrolyte solution. Additions of drugs to the infusion bag should be avoided because of contamination and drug interactions. Intravenous drugs are best given as bolus doses via the latex bung on the side arm unless dilution is required, when a burette should be used.

EDUCATION

Education of all hospital staff is a vital and continuing part of the control of infection: the more widely the principles are understood, the more effective and safer the care becomes. Infection control measures must be simple and practical if there is to be a high level of compliance.

Conclusion

In order to prevent and control hospital-acquired infections attention must be focused on:

1. The patient and his environment.
2. The staff and their practices.

Wherever there are patients and staff there is a need to develop an Infection Control Programme. Patients and staff congregate in wards and departments and the majority of hospital-acquired infections result from procedures and practices carried out on patients by staff. The control of infection is the responsibility of every individual who comes into contact with the patient.

BIBLIOGRAPHY

Ayliffe G A J, Noy M F, Babb J R, Davies J G, Jackson J 1983 A comparison of pre-operative bathing with chlorhexidine detergent and non-medicated soap in the prevention of wound infection. Journal of Hospital Infection 4: 237–244

Blomgren G, Hambreus A, Malmborg A 1982 Hygienic and clinical study of elective and acute hip operations. Journal of Hospital Infection 3: 111–121

Buckolz H W, Rottger J, Lodemkamper H, Engelbrecht E, Siegal A, Elson R A 1979 The management of deep infection involving joint implants. Journal of Bone & Joint Surgery 61B: 118

Cruse P J E, Foord R 1980 The epidemiology of wound infection. A 10-year prospective study of 62 939 wounds. The Surgical Clinics of North America 60: No 1, February

Davies T W, Cottingham J 1979 The cost of hospital infection in orthopaedic patients. Journal of Infection 1: 329–338

Emmerson A M 1982 Infections of bones and joints. The microbiology and treatment of life-threatening infections. Letchworth: Research Studies Press

Houang E T, Buckley R, Smith M, O'Riordan S M 1981 Survival of Pseudomonas aeruginosa in plaster of Paris. Journal of Hospital Infection 2: 231–235

Jenner E A 1983 Identification of the infected patient. Nursing November Supplement 1–3

Joint Tuberculosis Committee of the British Thoracic Society 1983 Control and prevention of tuberculosis: a code of practice. British Medical Journal 287: 1083–1156

Kozinn H A 1962 Clostridium welchii infections due to plaster of Paris after a shelf procedure of the hip. New England Journal of Medicine 267: 348–349

Lidwell O M, Lowbury E J L, Whyte W, Blowers R, Stanley S J, Lowe D 1982 Effect of ultraclean air in operating rooms on deep sepsis in the joint after total hip or knee replacement: a randomised study. British Medical Journal 285: 10–14

Lidwell O M, Lowbury E J L, Whyte W, Blowers R, Stanley S J, Lowe D 1983a Better ventilation in operating rooms. British Medical Journal 286: 1214–1215

Lidwell O M, Lowbury E J L, Whyte W, Blowers R, Stanley S J, Lowe D 1983b Bacteria isolated from deep joint sepsis after operation for total hip or knee replacement and the sources of infections with *Staphylococcus aureus*. Journal of Hospital Infection 4: 19–29

Lowbury E J L, Lilly H A 1975 Gloved hand as an applicator of antiseptic to the operation site. Lancet July 26 ii: 153–156

Meers P D, Ayliffe G A J, Emmerson A M et al 1981 Report on the national Survey of Infection in Hospitals 1980 Journal of Hospital Infection 2: 23–28

Murray E G D, Denton G D 1949 Plaster of Paris as source of infection in tetanus and gas gangrene. Canadian Medical Association Journal 60: 1–4

Nyström B et al 1983 Bacteraemia in surgical patients with intravenous devices: A European multicentre incidence study. Journal of Hospital Infection 4: 338–349

Seeberg S, Bergman B R 1980 Pre-operative total body washing with Chlorhexidine gluconate performed by patients undergoing orthopaedic surgery. Royal Society of Medicine International Congress & Symposium Series. No 23: 77–80

3

General management of orthopaedic patients

THE ENVIRONMENT OF THE ORTHOPAEDIC PATIENT

THE ORTHOPAEDIC CENTRE

This may consist of a hospital devoted entirely to the treatment of patients suffering from orthopaedic conditions or it may exist as part of a general hospital. In the past, patients suffering from diseases of bones and joints, particularly tuberculosis, who required a prolonged period of treatment in hospital were often segregated in country centres for 'fresh-air' treatment, while in urban areas the victims of trauma were treated in the wards of general hospitals. The loose term 'cold orthopaedics' has already been mentioned in Ch. 1 and refers to patients requiring conservative treatment or elective surgery, as opposed to the victims of trauma whose surgery is dictated by their injuries and which is often of an emergency nature. The tempo of a nursing unit full of patients suffering from 'cold' orthopaedic conditions will obviously be slower than one which is receiving the victims of accidents, but there are occasions when the patient who belonged initially to one category enters another, for example, a patient with a degenerative condition could undergo major surgery which would place him temporarily in the same category as the patient requiring resuscitation; similarly, the patient who is admitted as the result of an accident may eventually require elective surgery and a long period in hospital. For the purpose of nurse-training, experience in both 'cold' orthopaedic units and those devoted to the treatment of accidents is ideal and *visits* to special centres (e.g. for medical rehabilitation, spinal injury, limb-fitting) and to patients in their own homes is essential.

THE ORTHOPAEDIC WARD

When Florence Nightingale (1860) said 'a hospital should do the sick no harm' she had in mind the infections which were rife in the institutions of her time. Even to the present day a patient can enter a hospital for an elective operation and acquire an infection which may cause the operation to fail or even threaten his life. Moreover, any patient with an infected wound is a danger to others and, further, infection occurring in bone surgery is a dreaded complication because it can become deep-seated, difficult to eradicate and cannot always be cured by antibiotics, because bone is a dense structure not easily reached by antibiotics carried in the blood-stream. It follows therefore, that the nurse has special responsibilities in this regard, for example, in preparing the patient for surgery, and in carrying out wound dressings and other procedures. Control of many of the wider aspects of the patient's environment in hospital is outside the jurisdiction of nurses working at ward or departmental level; it is obvious that dust should be excluded, and where possible, air-conditioning probably provides the safest and most comfortable environment. In every hospital the environment should be such as to serve as a model to the community, and though such items as care and cleanliness of the environs, maintenance of buildings and of essential services are outside the control of the nurse, she must be aware of them as the essential background of her work.

At ward and departmental level, it is self-evident that services such as building maintenance, linen supplies, laundry, waste disposal and catering must be maintained at a high level of hygiene.

Cleanliness, achieved by means of hygienic cleaning methods is also self-evident, as is the exclusion of dust and dirt and control of vectors such as flies, rats, mice and cockroaches. A high standard of cleanliness is required not only for aesthetic reasons but for the control of infection (Ch. 2.)

Nurses—quite rightly—are no longer expected to carry out routine ward cleaning themselves but the fact that this is now 'a non-nursing duty' does not remove the responsibility of ensuring that this essential element of a safe environment is not neglected. Close co-operation with the hospital engineer, Control of Infection Officer (if available), and the domestic and catering managers and other personnel is essential, and the motivation and morale of all categories of staff is improved by a sense of belonging to the health team and by awareness of their important contribution to the patients' welfare. It has been said that hospital workers at the bottom of the hierarchy often suffer from the stress of being 'an under-valued cog in a large machine' (*The Guardian*, 2 Dec. 1983)

Control of noise. Whilst a certain amount of noise is inevitable, for example, from the telephone, it is very distressing to some patients, and every effort should be made to keep it to a minimum, especially at night. Source and levels of noise on a ward at night has been reported by Ogilvie (1980), who reports 'nurses were not very light-footed and chatted and giggled frequently (singing in the kitchen was overheard on one occasion)' To quote Miss Nightingale once more, 'unnecessary noise is the most cruel absence of care that can be inflicted on either sick or well'. Television sets and radio sets other than those with earphones must be banned from wards where the noise from them is extremely irritating to patients who do not want to hear it. There is no doubt that, apart from that emanating from the sources referred to above, and except perhaps in a childrens' ward (where *absence* of day-time noise is a cause for concern) the loudest and most continuous noise in hospital is made by the staff; careless handling of equipment is often to blame; for example trolleys for food and for conveyance of patients. But the most potent source of noise is the heavy footstep in hard-soled shoes, the loud voice and the loud laugh which can be a serious irritation to patients in a ward, and is to be deprecated in corridors and in areas accessible to the public. Moreover, people judge the hospital by the behaviour of the staff and it has been said that 'the image which any individual projects of himself when he appears before others will contribute to the viewer's conception of the place and its activities of which that person is a part' (Hewitt, 1981). The same author goes on to say 'We must become aware of the fact that others will place interpretations on our appearance and actions'.

It goes without saying that every hospital ward should be light, airy, warm, pleasantly decorated, quiet, and convenient for nursing purposes. In old buildings, it is sometimes none of these things, but it does not follow that a sub-standard ward means sub-standard treatment or nursing care. By and large, the patient most in need of skilled treatment and nursing care is one who cares least about his surroundings; his main interest is in the doctor and nurse who will give him the treatment, care, attention and sense of security that he needs. On the other hand, however, we often see the patient who though not actually very ill in the medical sense, is none the less very uncomfortable and is likely to be uncomfortable for a long time, for example, the heavy patient in a plaster jacket, the elderly patient on Russell traction, the child in a plaster hip spica for congenital dislocation of the hip. To these patients, pleasant surroundings *do* matter (Fig. 3.1), and as already stated in Ch. 1 the very uncomfortable are as much our special care as the very ill. We have also discussed the fact that patients suffering from orthopaedic conditions are often completely confined to bed because weight-bearing on a limb is not permitted; the nursing care required by these patients is discussed later in general terms and in greater detail in relation to specific orthopaedic conditions.

Since our patients are mostly confined to bed there are two factors in ward design which are most likely to cause distress to them and inconvenience to ourselves; they are (1) overcrowding and (2) lack of privacy. Overcrowding of wards means that there is insufficient accommodation for extra equipment such as Balkan beams, and insufficient space on each side of the bed for carrying out nursing procedures efficiently. Most important of all, the patient is at such close quarters with his neighbours that disagreeable sights, sounds and smells are inescapable. Over-crowding in itself means lack of privacy both for examination purposes, for nursing procedures and, most embarrassing of all, for toilet procedures.

For many years controversy has raged regarding the optimum size of a hospital ward, and indeed this has been discussed in a publication by Noble & Dixon (1978). More recently Burrows (1980), Billing (1982), and Williamson (1983) have discussed new approaches to ward design in the nursing press. If it is a large open unit of 30 to 40 beds

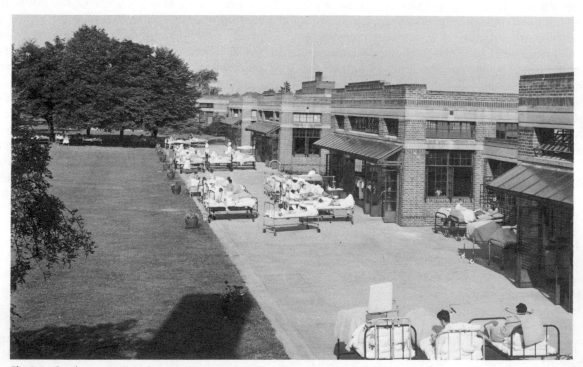

Fig. 3.1 Ready access to outdoors is enjoyed by patients who can be wheeled out in their beds.

there is often a strong feeling of camaraderie amongst the patients and overall nursing supervision is facilitated, but it is not always ideal for patient-care because it cannot be organised to suit the needs of a large number of patients who may range in age from the adolescent to the octogenarian and in condition from the very ill to the convalescent. There is a tendency nowadays to subdivide large units into open bays for four to six beds, but this has the disadvantage that a patient may find himself cooped up with another with whom he is not in sympathy. Small wards give greater flexibility in the use of hospital beds but are wasteful of nursing time; from the patient's point of view the thing that really matters is adequate space around his bed, cubicle curtains for privacy, and something to see (e.g. a view from a window) other than the ceiling, his neighbour or the patient opposite.

Toilet accommodation deserves special mention; baths and lavatories must be easily accessible to and specially adapted to the needs of disabled patients (Fig. 3.2A and B). A shower, and a bidet (if possible) are provided for patients unable to use a bath-tub.

Flooring must be 'non-slip' and wide doorways are required for the passage of beds and wheelchairs; where possible, steps are replaced by ramps.

Ground floor wards with ready access to outdoors are a great asset to patients who can be wheeled out in their beds (Fig. 3.1).

Wheeled beds allow long-stay patients in a suitable state of health to enjoy fresh air and sunshine; in some centres, visitors are permitted to push patients around the grounds in their beds, or they may attend outdoor sports. The privilege of being taken outdoors by visitors can be a boon to long-stay patients since it allows the luxury of private conversation; one of the features of hospital life is the inability even to post a letter without all and sundry knowing of it, or of exchanging a few words in private with one's nearest and dearest. In some long-stay patients this produces a feeling of helplessness, dependency, frustration and loss of identity.

The orthopaedic bed

A rigid base is essential and if not included in the construction of the bed a *fracture board* is required. Wheeled beds as described above are ideal for transportation of the patient to the X-ray and other departments and in some cases, to the operating theatre. A variable-height type of bed with trapeze (Fig. 3.3A and B) is excellent because when used at normal hospital height it facilitates delivery of nursing care, but can be lowered to enable patients not only to get *into* bed, but also to leave it, and moreover to sit on it with feet on the floor in order to get dressed. In the past, rehabilitation of patients in activities of daily living was often hindered by the height of a standard hospital bed.

Bed-making

Orthopaedic treatment and appliances often mean unconventional bed-making, and the nurse will learn to apply conventional methods to the needs of the individual patient; the main thing to remember is that the bed must be as *comfortable* as possible because 'beds are made for people, not for diseases' (Hector, 1970). Bedclothes are arranged so that the patient's body is covered but the affected limb is exposed (Fig. 10.23); draughts must be excluded but bedclothes must not be so tightly tucked in as to press upon the feet or any other part of the body; the extravagant use of pillows is often required, or other aids such as water beds, alternating pressure pads and sheepskins. The structure of the mattress varies with the condition of the patient; for example, a firm mattress must be used with a plaster bed. Special mattresses are being developed continuously, e.g. the Dyson flotation mattress, and the Clinitron device (*Nursing Times*, 23 April 1981). Some conditions require the patient to undergo several sessions of physiotherapeutic treatment during the day, so that it may be most convenient and helpful to make the top bedclothes into a pack which can be removed easily. Other requirements may be Balkan beams, tilting mirrors, back-rests, bed-elevators and bed-cradles. Various types of orthopaedic beds will be seen in the pages of this book; a feature of one type is that the bed-end is moveable so that patients lying in the prone position have their feet over the end of the bed (Fig. 3.4).

Special beds are continually being developed,

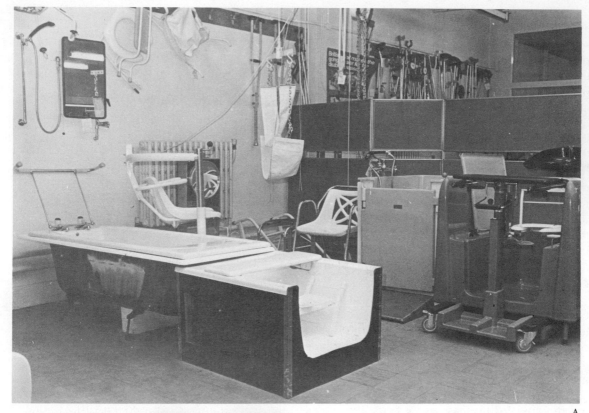

A

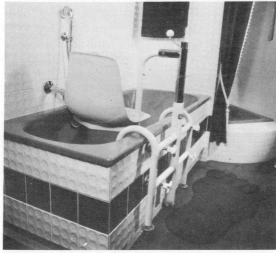

B

Fig. 3.2 A, B. Various bathroom adaptations seen at the Disabled Living Foundation.

Fig. 3.2B Bathroom adaptation (Meyra).

especially for patients with a high risk of pressure sores.

The net suspension bed shown in Fig. 3.5 is reported to be comfortable and has been used for home nursing; at the same time it has been pointed out that (in common with many other aids) it is no substitute for good nursing (Scott, 1977).

The low air loss bed shown in Fig. 3.6 has been reported as being the ultimate technical solution to pressure sore problems; it provides even distribution of body weight by means of a system of air sacs fed continuously with temperature-controlled air from a blower. It is reported to be labour-saving in that all nursing care can be carried out without

A

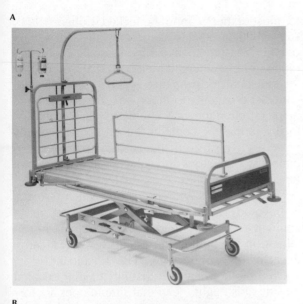

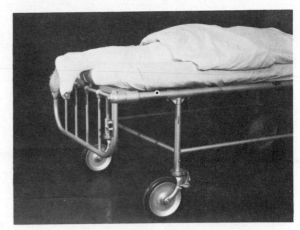

Fig. 3.4 Orthopaedic bed with adjustable rail to allow the feet to hang free over the end. The affected area is unencumbered by bedclothes.

B

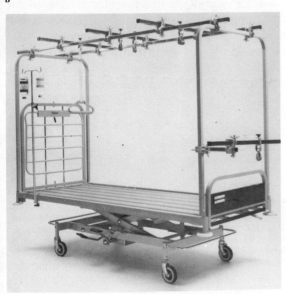

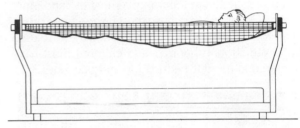

Fig. 3.5 Net suspension bed. The patient should show a clearly defined profile, with heels, thighs, buttocks and shoulders equally supported.

Fig. 3.3   A, B. 'King's Fund' variable height beds. **A.** Ellison Hospital Equipment. **B.** Hoskins Ltd.

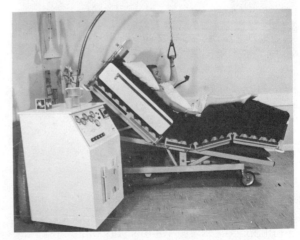

Fig. 3.6   Low air loss bed.

lifting the patient, and to be very efficient in the prevention and treatment of pressure sores. (Scales et al, 1974.)

At present, this bed is not in common use because of its cost and because it occupies two bed spaces in a hospital ward. In discussing its use, it has been said that 'in the end, however, a country that cannot afford enough nurses to care for the elderly will find it a good bargain to invest in more

and better apparatus'. (*British Medical Journal* (1978) 1: 1232.)

Many aids to function are shown in the pages of this book; it should be stressed here however, that aids should not be used until every effort has been made to help the patient manage with the normal items for everyday use.

Storage space for wheelchairs, and other equipment is essential; inadequate floor space for storage and manoevrability is the biggest single obstacle to their effective use (Norton, 1976). This author makes many other pertinent comments on the environment of the long-stay patient.

Storage space for personal possessions and clothing is also essential so that ambulant patients can wear their own clothes and shoes; in addition the patient confined to bed for any length of time needs occupation to pass the time pleasantly and profitably, and to 'work at something that provides a sense of accomplishment' (Henderson, 1969). Moreover, such activities might be therapeutic, for example, aimed at the improvement of hand function. This means that there must be adequate provision for the storage of materials such as those used in occupational therapy, and children must have material at hand for education and play (Fig. 3.7).

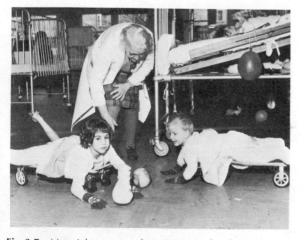

Fig. 3.7 Materials, space and opportunities for play are essential for young patients.

In this connection it is not unknown for complaints to be made regarding the 'untidy' appearance of an orthopaedic ward; yet this very untidiness may indicate activity aimed at maintaining high morale and retaining or restoring independence of mind and body; the meticulously tidy ward, like the meticulously tidy home, does not necessarily reflect the well-being or the happiness of the people in it.

The bedside locker. This term is a misnomer,

for most of them cannot be locked (Cohen, 1964), so that patients tend to keep their wallets, handbags or other treasured personal possessions under their pillows or elsewhere in their beds. Lack of security for personal possessions is very worrying for patients, especially to those who are disabled and helpless; often they are unable to reach a bedside locker so that the contents are at the mercy of any passer-by. This means that custody of the helpless patient's possessions and valuables is an important nursing responsibility.

The use of aids and equipment. Much research is devoted to the design and manufacture of appliances both as aids to nursing care in the hospital and in the home, and as aids to the patient in the activities of daily living. (Figs 3.8 and 3.10.)

On the other hand, availability of sophisticated nursing aids might mean that simple ones are forgotten; for example, a small electric torch is useful to the nurse for close examination of patients wearing splints and plasters, and for patients for self-examination; a hand-held mirror gives the immobilised patient an expanded view of his environment and can also be used for self-examination (Fig. 3.8).

Fig. 3.8 Availability of sophisticated nursing aids might mean that simple ones are often forgotten. A small electric torch is useful to the nurse for close examination of patients wearing splints and plasters, and for patient for self-examination. A hand-held mirror gives the immobilised patient an expanded view of his environment and can also be used for self-examination (Chapter 22).

In the hospital, training of staff members in the use of equipment is essential, if only because it is expensive (Fig. 3.9). It should be noted that special equipment which the patient and helper use in the hospital may also be required in the home, (Fig. 3.10) where it is chosen very carefully so that neither the State nor the patient and/or his family is put to needless expense.

Research into items of equipment and aids to function is continually being pursued and new materials are continually coming on to the market;

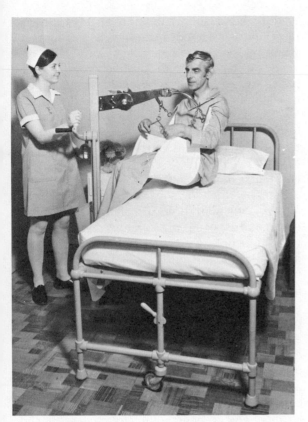

Fig. 3.9 The Ambulift is used to transfer to and from bed/bath (Mecanaid).

for example, a plastic substance called 'Gripkit' can be moulded like Plasticine to make handles for cutlery, pens and pencils, doorkeys etc., and also to attach extensions to taps, door handles, electric switches etc., for the use of patients with

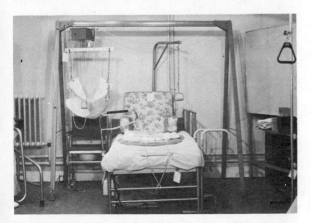

Fig. 3.10 Research into aids for the handicapped is conducted by the Disabled Living Foundation.

disturbance of hand function. It is claimed that no special training is required to use this substance in safety (*Nursing Times*, 1978).

Progressive patient care

This describes a system of nursing patients in groups in the same ward, or in a series of different wards according to their needs in respect of treatment and nursing care, rather than according to age, sex or allocation of beds to particular surgeons. Nursing staff is also allocated to the different groups according to the nursing care required, so that very ill patients receive skilled and unremitting nursing care at the hands of the most experienced staff available, while those at the other end of the scale whose condition and treatment is such that their main need is for hotel services may only require minimal over-all supervision. Moreover, patients whose preparation for discharge home includes the practise of self-care may be best treated in a ward devoted entirely to this purpose.

Intensive nursing care. This means what is says, and in general is also interpreted to mean that a patient requiring this standard of care needs a nurse at his bedside continuously. 'Monitoring' devices which record vital findings such as temperature, pulse and respiratory rates and blood pressure are also in use. It has been pointed out however that although monitoring apparatus can enhance the quality of nursing it is in no sense a substitute for a nurse, nor does it mean that a nurse's place is in a viewing room instead of at the bedside (London, 1966).

The late Dame Agnes Hunt, who pioneered orthopaedic nursing, was also a pioneer in another sense in that she established, as long ago as 1920, a ward adjacent to the operating theatre where patients were prepared for operation and where they were received post-operatively and nursed until pronounced fit to return to their wards. This was probably the first 'intensive care' unit to be established in this country and the concept of grouping patients according to their needs has since been widely developed.

Patient assignment. Agnes Hunt was also a pioneer in this connection since she advocated the system of holding one nurse personally responsible for the total care of a given number of patients, allocating easily managed ones to the inexperienced student who then graduated to more difficult ones as her knowledge and skills increased. This is an infinitely better and more satisfying way of both practising and teaching total patient care than the more familiar 'job-assignment' method, but it requires an efficient leader.

It is interesting to note modern interest in the development and indeed, extension of this system of nursing care, as discussed by Crow (1971) in *The Nursing Process* and in numerous other publications listed in the Bibliography at the end of this chapter.

Introduction of the Nursing Process has caused a great deal of discussion and, indeed, controversy, in which not only nurses but doctors have participated (Mitchell et al, 1984) (The Nursing Process Debate). When discussing the Nursing Process we should perhaps take heed of James Smith's words (1982) when he states that 'management systems are guide-lines, not tablets of stone'. Another publication (Faulkner, 1981) discusses the changes which implementation of the Nursing Process might lead to in connection with the rôle of the ward sister and the doctor–nurse relationship. Other writers discuss means by which the process is implemented (Johnson & Cavill, 1981), and a research project (Miller, 1984) shows that it is particularly relevant to the care of the long-stay patient.

Despite the controversy, implementation of the Nursing Process is seen by one writer as vital to the future of nursing as a profession (Scott, 1982). In another publication, Chapman (1977) suggests that organisational factors need to be overhauled, with less emphasis on task performance so that nurses are allowed to develop closer relationships with patients than was possible under a 'job-assignment' system.

Team-nursing means the division of a ward staff into different teams, each of which gives total care to a certain group of patients; again, efficient leadership is essential.

Categorisation of patients into groups according to their nursing needs is a valuable management tool.

SOME SPECIAL POINTS IN MANAGEMENT

Throughout this book frequent mention will be made of the fact that treatment of a patient is incomplete unless it includes consideration of him as a whole person and as a member of society.

The nurse will learn the channels through which patients are admitted to hospital and the facilities available for their care when they are discharged. Most important of all, she will bear in mind that to most people life in a hospital ward is far from normal. Some patients find simply being in hospital a frustrating, bewildering and painful experience—and much more so, if as so often happens, they are literally 'tied down' by some form of splintage. This is particularly true of children (who in any case require special consideration) and in energetic vigorous people who resent the subjugation of their personal life to the inexorable routine of a hospital ward. It is important that the patient in hospital feels that he is accepted as he is, but he in turn must accept his situation; we have all met the patient who 'kicks against the pricks' and rails against Fate, whilst at the same time making no effort to rehabilitate himself. It is he who fails to make a good recovery or to adjust himself to a disability. On the other hand, most patients show common sense, cheerfulness, fortitude and perseverance, and co-operate fully to a successful end-result of their treatment. Many patients actually enjoy their stay in hospital and make hosts of friends; for some it may well be a Heaven-sent rest.

The manner in which *new patients* are received is most important. It has been shown that the highest level of anxiety is shown by patients at the time of admission to hospital (Wilson-Barnett, 1978). Often they are filled with fears of the unknown, and a smile, a warm welcome and a sympathetic attitude will do much to reassure them. Patients must receive adequate information before admission regarding travelling directions, articles to be brought with them, visiting hours, etc.

Discipline

Although the rules which make for efficient management and the well-being of all must be carried out, discipline cannot be so strictly enforced as in a general ward. Long-stay patients are usually permitted more latitude as to visitors, personal possessions, outings, access to television, etc., than those in general wards, though these things must never be permitted to distress those not in a condition to enjoy them. The atmosphere of an orthopaedic ward should be busy, pleasant, and cheerful without being rowdy. Patients are encouraged to take a lively interest in their surroundings and an intelligent (but not morbid) interest in their conditions.

The nurse–patient relationship

Some orthopaedic patients are in hospital for many weeks, and this in itself calls for special qualities in the nurse; her approach is, in the nature of things, more personal and friendly than is customary in a general ward. A friendly approach, however, does not mean allowing herself to become involved in emotional situations which may react unfavourably on herself, on her patient and on his fellow-sufferers in the ward.

The nurse may often be in a position to receive a patient's confidences, and she should report any cause for anxiety, such as home or monetary difficulties, to the nurse in charge or the doctor.

Team work

This is more important in orthopaedics than in any other branch of nursing, because many procedures cannot be undertaken by one nurse alone. In large orthopaedic wards, bedpan 'rounds' should be shared by the nursing staff. Such an important nursing procedure should not be delegated to one solitary junior nurse or to an orderly; the modern tendency is to do away with the 'round', in favour of an 'on demand' system of giving bedpans.

Patients who require special consideration

Elderly patients present special problems; they may have no friends or relatives to care for them, and if unfit to live alone on discharge, special arrangements must be made by the medico-social worker. When attending these patients the nurse should remember the deference due to the aged, and be prepared to pander to old folks' fads and fancies. Small comforts mean a great deal and in caring

A

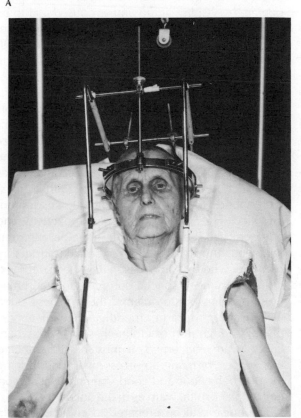

B

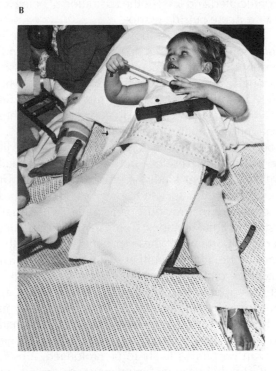

Fig. 3.11 A, B. Patients requiring special care—the old and the young, especially those who are immobilised by splints, plasters or traction devices.

for the aged, as in caring for children, one's watch-word should be to 'treat them as one's own'. In caring for the elderly, measures aimed at the pre-vention of complications which may slow down early discharge from hospital are essential. Scarce and expensive hospital beds, urgently required for other patients, may be 'blocked' by the elderly for want of a dynamic approach to their medical, nurs-ing and social problems. The care of the elderly patient is discussed further in later chapters.

Mature people in middle life usually fit in well in a hospital ward, except where there are problems such as the man who is worried about business matters or where there are domestic problems, for example, children who must be left in the care of a friend or relative. Physical amenities are impor-tant, such as unrestricted or flexible visiting hours, reasonable privacy, the provision of facilities such as radio and television, newspaper deliveries, a library service, adequate storage space for personal belongings, a trolley shop and a visiting hair-dresser. A trolley-telephone, if available, is much appreciated and lessens the frustration of being 'cut off' from the outside world.

Adolescents. These boys and girls are often the most difficult patients for the nurse to handle wisely. She must remember that they are passing through a difficult stage in their development, while they are struggling to assert themselves and to 'find their feet'. Much can be done by example; these patients are quick to take their cue from others and soon learn with whom they may take liberties. Mili-tary discipline is useless, but a lax attitude is equally fatal. A firm yet kindly approach combined with suitable occupation and amenities such as those mentioned in previous paragraphs, will usually establish good relations. Companionship is particu-larly important to these patients; ideally, they should be nursed neither with adults nor with younger children, but should be segregated in groups appropriate not only to their physical age but to their stage of development. If their formal education is at an end, every effort should be made to find them interesting occupations and if their stay in hospital is likely to be prolonged, a useful craft should be taught. Some may even further their education through correspondence courses or by private tuition.

Children are our greatest responsibility, because they are dependent on us not only for physical care, but for that love and sense of security which is the essential soil for the healthy growth of the personality. This is particularly important because orthopaedic treatment often requires either a pro-longed stay in hospital or oft-repeated visits.

Each age group presents its own problems; young children should not be separated from their mothers; whenever possible the mother is admitted with the child. In any event, visiting in a children's ward should be 'free', the parents being encour-aged to visit daily by arrangement with the ward sister and even to participate in the care of the child. Indeed this is essential because early discharge home is an important aim of treatment (Chs 11 and 12). Toddlers are no longer deprived of their beloved old 'teddy' or doll or whatever object they always take to bed with them, but are asked to bring it with them. The mode of reception of child and parents is important; both may be bewildered and frightened at the unknown, and the parents needs in this connection are as important as those of the child (Glen, 1982). Parents are asked to co-operate by visiting *at the time promised* and to be truthful in their dealings with the child. If they can-not visit daily, they should keep in close touch with the hospital and with the child, if only by telephone and by letter. The arrival of a picture post-card for the child who cannot be visited will make his day.

During a child's stay in hospital the most impor-tant things are undoubtedly (apart from his treat-ment) attention and activity in an atmosphere of what can only be described as loving-kindness. The nurse in a children's ward must be sure at all times that no child is left sitting in his cot without toys, with nobody to play with or without ocupation of any kind (Fig. 3.12A and B); such inactivity and boredom will inevitably result in temper-tantrums and naughtiness. Children from unsatisfactory homes or who for some reason have been deprived of love may need special consideration, and may present behaviour problems, though these often disappear in a warm, friendly, cheerful atmos-phere. Though iron discipline has no place where children are concerned, it must be remembered that proper 'bringing up' is essential, and training in good behaviour and good manners is as impor-tant in the hospital ward as in the home.

The nurse will be prepared to give her patient

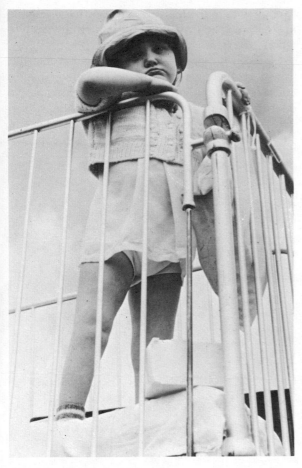

Fig. 3.12A The lonely child.

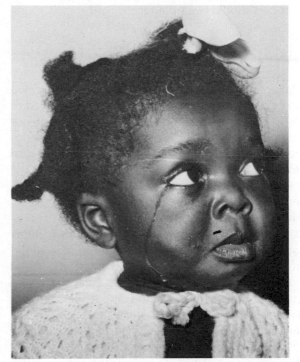

Fig. 3.12B The homesick child.

and his relatives special support at times when this is needed—for example, when an operation is to be performed. Very young children to whom procedures cannot be explained need very careful handling and adequate sedation. Older children are usually very courageous provided they are never told untruths, and learning to face ordeals can be a valuable experience provided proper support is given.

In the case of older children (and even very young children can join in singing games and other suitable pastimes) *education* is of primary importance from the point of view of formal schooling as well as a means of providing interesting occupation. Indeed, nurses should be closely associated with educational programmes devised for individual handicapped children and this reflects the need for inter-professional training between nurses and teachers (Slack, 1978).

It has been said that 'the education offered in hospital should be better in certain ways than that the child would normally receive and not be merely a sophisticated form of child-minding' (Lee, 1982).

During the past two decades there has been a new awareness of the emotional needs of children in hospital and this is illustrated by the wealth of writing on the subject, some of which is listed in the Bibliography (MacCarthy, 1981; Swannick, 1983; Hopkins, 1983; King, 1984) The last-named writer records her 'change of heart' and acceptance of play therapists.

Older children often present problems out of school hours, particularly boys in the 8 to 15 years age group. Normally this is a period of intense activity when the boy is discovering the world around him. Again, *plenty to do* is the answer, and the aid of parents, friends, Scouts, etc., should be enlisted to help the time to pass quickly, and amenities such as radio, television and other entertainments are desirable. Reading, interesting crafts and hobbies should be encouraged.

SENSORY DEPRIVATION

Patients in hospital, and especially those confined to bed for any length of time become deprived of sensory stimuli to a greater or lesser degree depending on their condition, with corresponding deterioration of intellectual processes. Most people can tolerate monotonous conditions provided that the normal flow of sensory stimulation from the environment does not fall below a certain minimum level. In extreme cases however drastic curtailment of stimuli as practised in some institutions or prisons can cause a person to 'go stir simple' (Goffman, 1961); McGhie (1969) gives an interesting account of the reaction of people exposed to 'the dreadful *sameness* of the environment and the persistent monotony of being exposed to an unchanging pattern of stimuli for a length of time; he describes the reactions of patients being nursed in a tank-type of respirator and those of a patient suffering from an eye-injury who, having lost normal visual contract with his environment, might be 'hungry' for stimuli and contact with the outside world. The same author concludes that 'our very hold on reality is basically dependent upon us receiving a continual and uninterrupted flow of sensory stimulation from our environment' and points out that *enforced immobility* of the subject, such as we see in many of our patients, causes reduction in external stimulation; further, it is recommended that such detrimental effects of immobility should be kept in mind when we consider the case of the hospital patient who is forced by his illness to lie in bed for considerable periods of time.

These remarks may help us to understand why some of our patients, notably those whose condition and/or treatment enforces immobility and isolation from external stimuli show signs of intellectual deterioration and consequent inability

to cope with individual problems and to co-operate in treatment and nursing care aimed at rehabilitation for a return to home life and work.

Children require special consideration and this aspect of their care is discussed in later pages, because children are particularly vulnerable to deprivation from lack of sensory stimulus (Fig. 3.13); further reference to this will be found in Chs 11, 12 and 14.

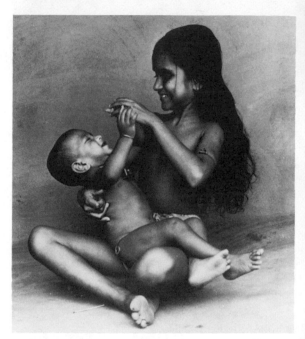

Fig. 3.13 Children all over the world and of all ages need sensory stimulus, particularly if handicapped in any way. This girl is playing with her little brother. (Photo WHO/UNICEF by A. Heyman).

Physiotherapy has much to offer in this connection (Fig. 3.14B) and so has *occupational therapy*; the latter has a role in devising aids which permit disabled patients to make use of sources of stimuli, for example, page-turning devices, aids to using a pen, paintbrush or typewriter; any outlet for self-expression is valuable mental stimulus; some centres employ an Art Therapist and arrangements are made for activities such as cookery, flower arrangement, beauty treatment etc. Handicrafts of all kinds, sports, games and hobbies are also valuable and in some centres special arrangements are made for disabled patients to practice gardening (Fig. 3.14A).

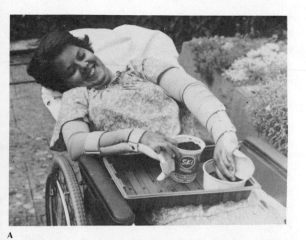

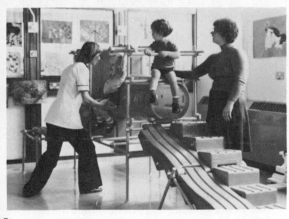

Fig. 3.14 **A.** Gardening can be enjoyed despite disability. (From Mary Marlborough Lodge, Oxford.) **B.** Physiotherapy has much to offer in deprivation of sensory stimulus.

Television and radio are valuable sources of stimuli; but it must be stressed once more that in hospital *individual earphones are essential* so that the noise from these sources does not distress those who do not wish to hear it.

Newspapers, magazines and books are available in most hospitals and the newspaper vendor and hospital librarian give valuable service in this connection. Indeed to some patients in hospital the arrival of the 'library trolley' may mark a red-letter day.

Letters are essential links with home, family and friends and are much prized and looked forward to: *the telephone*, likewise, is an essential part of modern life and must be made available to hospital patients able to make use of it.

Compatible neighbours in the ward situation are a rich source of companionship; it is surprising how often patients from different walks of life find each other's company acceptable, although the converse also holds true, and it is obviously poor nursing management to force patients who do not get along together to remain in each others close proximity.

Visitors are the most valuable source of stimulus and contact with the outside world, and are usually a source of emotional satisfaction as well. All visitors, therefore, unless there is some good reason to the contrary, should be welcomed and given every possible encouragement (Fig. 3.15).

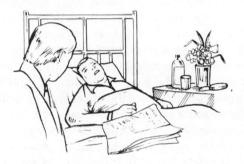

Fig. 3.15 Visitors are a valuable stimulus to the patient in hospital.

Unrestricted visiting has great advantages though nurses sometimes complain that it interrupts ward routine; it is mandatory for children and except during toileting, treatment or examination by the doctor there seems no valid reason for excluding any patient's visitor and indeed, unrestricted visiting allows people to 'pop in' for relatively short periods at the convenience of both visitor, patient and staff; this is often more acceptable to the patient than large numbers of visitors for longer fixed hours, when they feel obliged to stay to the last minute of the time available. It is important to note that a patient can sometimes be visited too often and for too long at one time for his comfort and well-being; conversely there is the lonely patient who is perhaps many miles from home, or who has no close relatives or friends willing or able to visit him; the social worker can give help in this connection and the fact that visitors spend time and money travelling to the hospital and moreover, seldom come empty-handed is often forgotten;

further the demands of other members of a family may prevent individuals from visiting a patient or there may be transport difficulties.

Visitors are not only important to the patient but to the therapeutic team, because the relatives of a disabled person must be taught how to care for him at home; moreover, we acknowledge the concept of comprehensive care which includes the patient's family, so that at the earliest possible moment we must establish lines of communication and good relations with them in the interests of the patient. Learning to take care of a patient might mean that the relatives spend long periods in the hospital at different times of the day or night; relatives of any patient too young, too old or too disabled to feed himself should be requested to visit at meal-times and help to feed the patient.

This deliberate involvement in the care of the patient is not only helpful to him but is also helpful to the visitor, who may experience difficulties in communication, fear of the unknown world of the hospital, and a sense of inadequacy and helplessness caused by the feeling that the hospital has 'taken over' and that their relative is now beyond their care (Speck, 1973). If these factors are present we may falsely assume from the behaviour of the visitor that he lacks interest in and concern for the patient, so that we may unwittingly increase his

feelings of fear, inadequacy and alienation from the situation; early establishment of lines of communication and of good relations are imperative to secure the co-operation of relatives and friends who will continue the care of the patient at home.

In some centres, children under a certain age are not allowed to visit patients; this can cause great distress both to the patient and to a child, especially in the case of a young child separated from a parent; moreover, there are occasions when a child must accompany a hospital visitor because he cannot be left alone at home; a sensible compromise between hospital rules and the well-being of both the patient and the child can usually be reached. Indeed, in at least one hospital, this has been achieved (Goodall, 1982).

SENSORY OVERLOAD

This is discussed briefly here because it is the direct opposite of sensory deprivation. It can be defined as a marked increase in the intensity of stimuli over normal level, leading to disruption of cerebral processes, so that there is decreased reasoning power and disturbance of thought processes which may even lead to hallucinations.

Sensory overload usually occurs only in intensive

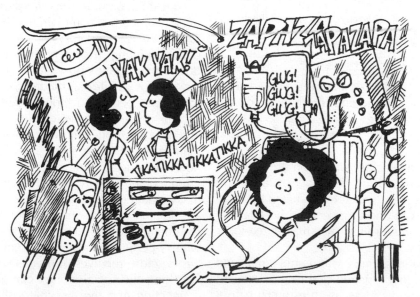

Fig. 3.16 Sensory overload. Copyright, the American Journal of Nursing Company. Adapted with permission from the *American Journal of Nursing*/John Huehnergarth. August. Vol. 80. No. 8.

care units. An interesting experiment was conducted by three American nurses (Lindenmuth et al, 1980) who became experimental 'patients' in a CCU at the busiest time of day. Describing their findings, they mention 'bothersome' noise over which they had no control, especially from telephones and also from toilets flushing, from conversations and from equipment such as respirators and infusion pumps (Fig. 3.16). The nurses noted that time seemed to have slowed down and that they became restless, agitated and lonely, with feelings of isolation, resentment and rejection. They also reported a strong sense of loss of control over their environment, and to anxiety regarding esposure of their bodies and to loss of personal possessions.

Discomfort, with early development of 'pressure areas' was also mentioned, as was discomfort from equipment such as a board for immobilisation of a limb for an intravenous infusion.

As a result of this experiment, the nurses involved developed the patient-care plan seen in Fig. 3.17. A significant statement in this publication is that 'there is a tendency for intensive care nurses to become desensitised to the potential sensory overload factor in their units'.

We do not all work in intensive care units which present the special problems outlined here; but sensitivity to a patient's needs is surely the crux and lynch-pin of professional nursing responsibility in every area of nursing practice. This is also discussed in the *Nursing Times* (Smith, 1982) in an article which describes 'insensitivity to the needs of elderly patients'. Another important article appears in the same journal emphasising the importance of communication between nurse and patient (Börsig et al, 1982).

OUT-PATIENT AND AFTER-CARE SERVICES

The out-patient department is usually situated within the hospital itself or in premises adjacent to it, and large numbers of patients are seen here who receive the appropriate treatment on the spot, which is less expensive than in-patient treatment. The out-patient department is the hospital's 'shop window' (Rayner, 1967) and the nurse has an important role as 'hostess' and as liaison officer between the hospital and the community it serves.

Moreover the hospital will be judged by the behaviour of the staff. Efficient management of an out-patient department requires knowledge of local geography and conditions, for example, availability of public transport.

Communication with patients and relatives is a vital nursing responsibility. Apart from carrying out treatment ordered on the spot, the nurse is responsible for teaching the patient simple active exercises, and giving instructions regarding the administration of drugs or the care of splints and plasters. In many instances, she must interpret and explain the doctor's orders and ensure that the patient and/or his relatives understand them. It is also important for the nurse to remember that she is the guardian of the patient's modesty.

Further, the out-patient requires the same consideration in relation to his social problems as does the one in the ward. Where a social worker is readily available it is easy enough to refer patients to the appropriate department, but this is not always the immediate answer so that this role is often assumed by the nurse, particularly out of 'office hours'.

Out-patients are usually seen by appointment, as opposed to casualties which are dealt with immediately on arrival. *A new patient*, usually referred by his family doctor, has often had no previous experience of hospitals and accordingly his *mode of reception* is important; the patient may be nervous, confused and apprehensive, so that every effort is made to help him to feel welcome. Elderly patients and young children require special consideration; where possible, waiting time should be kept to a minimum. Wilson-Barnett (1981) reports 'Patients are particularly concerned about the long waiting lists for appointments, transport arrangements involving long delays, and overcrowded, drab waiting rooms'.

Extended waiting time is all too common in orthopaedic practice because of the nature of the work. For example, a patient wearing a plaster cast is seen by the doctor, proceeds to X-ray, is seen again by the doctor and finally has the cast repaired, renewed or removed. This process may occupy several hours.

When a new patient is referred to an out-patient department with a suspected orthopaedic condition, it is important to bear in mind that a thorough

Patient Care Plan

Patient problems	Short-term goals (expected outcomes)	Nursing interventions
Potential disorientation due to sensory overload and confinement in an open ward bed.	The patient will maintain reality orientation to person, place, time and purpose.	Orient patient to all spheres as frequently as needed. Arrange time to focus on the psychosocial interaction with patient. Contract with patient for specific rest periods. Thoroughly explain equipment sounds, especially monitor and alarms. Ask patient to feed information back. When possible, keep the lights to the level requested by the patient. Encourage all staff to decrease noise level by talking softly, using sinks away from area of open beds, keeping utility and fire doors closed, as well as doors to other patients' rooms when TVs and radios are in use. Encourage appropriate visiting by family and friends. Provide continuity of nursing care.

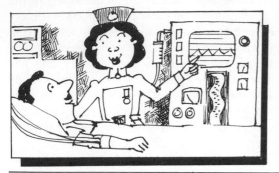

Potential for physical discomfort due to the activity limitations of bedrest.	The patient will state he or she can rest comfortably.	Demonstrate to the patient the extent of limb and joint mobility allowed within equipment restrictions. Do frequent limited passive ROM to limbs, where indicated. Frequently massage pressure points. Maintain adequate fluid and nutritional intake. Use special mattress where indicated. Turn patient at least every 2 hours. Solicit information on patient's comfort level.

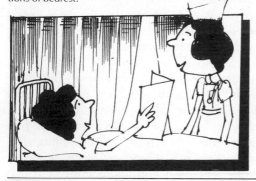

Potential for loss of privacy.	The patient will state that specific privacy needs are being met.	Assure complete privacy during procedures. Ask patients how they would like curtains at all other times, especially when resting, eating, or with visitors. Solicit information from patient about personal privacy needs; ask patients' permission prior to invading their "personal space". Allow patient control over arrangement of objects in his bedside area.

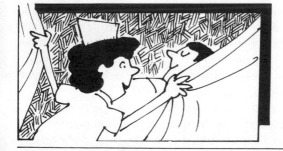

Fig. 3.17 Patient care plan adapted from *Sensory Overload* by Jane E. Lindemuth, Christine S. Breu and Jean A. Malooley in the August 1980 issue of the *American Journal of Nursing* (see text). Copyright, the American Journal of Nursing Company. Adapted with permission from the *American Journal of Nursing*/John Huehnergarth. August. Vol. 80. No. 8

examination of all the systems of the body is usually required and to anticipate the surgeon's wishes in this respect. Not only must the patient be completely unclothed, but apparatus for examination must be readily to hand. Some of these requirements are listed below:

1. Stethoscope.
2. Sphygmomanometer.
3. Ophthalmoscope.
4. Auroscope.
5. Apparatus for urinalysis and for examination of the blood.
6. Tray for neurological examination.
7. Tray for rectal examination.
8. Tray for vaginal examination.
9. Torch.
10. Tongue spatula.
11. Angle measure.
12. Tape measure.
13. Skin pencil.
14. Plumb line.
15. Raising blocks.
16. Apparatus for measuring patient's height.
17. Weighing machine.
18. Tray for injections.
19. Tray for aspiration.
20. The relevant documents and X-ray plates, if any, are placed in readiness.
21. The patient may need help with undressing and while waiting, is kept warmly covered; the bladder should be emptied before examination takes place. Any splint or appliance worn by the patient is presented for inspection.

Notes on preparation for examination of different parts of the body

As already stated, new patients are seen completely unclothed, particularly in the case of children; on the other hand, a patient on a return visit whose lesion is known to be confined to a particular limb may be prepared for examination as described in the appropriate paragraph.

The spine

The patient is completely unclothed, except for underpants or panties or a garment which covers the genital regions and which may be called a 'splash', 'tidy', 'waders', 'bathers' or 'trunks'. The design of this garment varies in different hospitals but a simple one consists of a short strip of cotton material which is placed between the legs and fastened over the pelvis by means of tapes. Women patients may retain their bra or wear a cotton garment to cover the breasts (see Fig. 3.18). A dressing-gown is then put on and the patient made

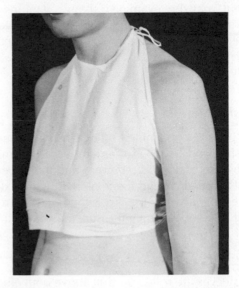

Fig. 3.18 Cotton garment worn by female patient for examination of the spine.

comfortable on a couch and covered with blankets. He is usually examined first in the lying position, and in suitable cases may be asked to stand and walk.

Trays for neurological, rectal or vaginal examination may be required. A tape-measure, skin-pencil, plumb-line, and raising blocks should also be held in readiness.

The hip

The patient is unclothed except for a dressing/gown and modesty garment, and is examined lying. Suitable cases are asked to stand and walk. a tape-measure, skin-pencil, raising blocks and an angle-measure may be required.

The knee

As both knees must be exposed, male patients are asked to remove their trousers; in female patients, a short, tight skirt should be removed. Both shoes and stockings are removed; the patient is examined lying and may be asked to stand and walk. An angle-measure may be required.

The feet

Both shoes and stockings are removed, and the patient may be examined sitting, standing and walking. *The shoes* are presented for the surgeon's inspection; they should not be new ones, and the patient may be asked to bring those which he habitually wears.

The shoulder

The patient is examined sitting. In male patients, the shirt and undervest are removed. In females, the blouse or dress is removed, and the undergarments pinned around the trunk below the axillae. A dressing-gown or blanket is then placed around the shoulders. An angle-measure may be required.

The elbow

The sleeves are rolled up well above both elbows. A dress or shirt with tight sleeves should be removed. An angle-measure is often required.

The wrist and hand

The sleeves are rolled up to the elbow. Wrist-watches or other articles of jewellery should be removed. An angle-measure may be required.

It is important to remember that in cases of injury to the wrist, hand or fingers in which swelling of the extremities is expected (as for example in a Colles fracture) any rings worn by the patient should be removed forthwith, if necessary by means of a ring-cutter. Failure to remove a ring may result in gangrene of a finger.

AFTER-CARE CLINICS

Note The original draft for this section was written by the late Mona Williams when After-care Superintendent, Robert Jones and Agnes Hunt Orthopaedic Hospital, Oswestry.

After-care

The word 'after' means 'behind in place' or 'later in time', and when allied to 'care', i.e. of a patient, it implies continuation of treatment already begun; and indeed, this was the object in view when after-care clinics were first established at the periphery of the area served by an orthopaedic hospital, at a time when large numbers of patients, particularly children suffering from skeletal tuberculosis and poliomyelitis required prolonged supervision, and whose treatment often included wearing a splint or appliance over a long period of time or even permanently. Moreover after-care clinics were first established before the era of modern transportation, so that the peripheral clinic was designed to meet not only physical but social needs, in that 'follow-up' of hospital treatment could be carried out practically on the patient's own door-step.

The social and economic advances, the virtual eradication of some of the crippling diseases of the past, and the improvement in medical care referred to in Chapter 1 are reflected in the diminution in the number of patients now seen at clinics who require months or even years of follow-up treatment. Though there are still many patients discharged from the parent hospital who are referred to their local clinic for continuation of treatment, it now also serves as an extension of the out-patient service and new patients are referred to the consultant orthopaedic surgeon by general practioners in the area.

Clinic premises

Sometimes after-care clinics are held in a peripheral hospital or failing this, in a public building such as a parish hall, and preferably on the ground floor. The chief essentials are—a large waiting room, with lavatory accommodation; cubicles in which the patients can be undressed and examined; facilities for walking; diagnostic X-ray equipment together with viewing boxes; and a plaster room with an impervious floor in which there should be a long wooden table with a deep ledge to take a hip-prop. There should be an ample supply of hot and cold water, storage accommodation for surplus splints and appliances, and a shelter capable of taking prams, invalid chairs etc. Speaking generally, the lay-out and equipment of these orthopaedic clinic premises approximate to an out-patients department in an orthopaedic unit.

Staff

The team consists of an orthopaedic surgeon, an after-care sister, a clinical stenographer, and some-times, a social worker and an orthotist/prosthetist.

Voluntary helpers consist of members of the British Red Cross Society and the Order of St John of Jerusalem, the Women's Voluntary Service, and members of the local Voluntary Orthopaedic Asso-ciation. They help to prepare patients for examina-tion, serve light refreshments and give valuable assistance in a general way.

Transport for patients. In cases where patients are not able to travel to the clinics by public trans-port, the Sister gives details of the case and the type of conveyance required to the transport clerk at the hospital, who makes the necessary arrange-ments.

TYPE OF WORK DONE AT THE CLINICS

New patients

No new patient is admitted to a clinic unless referred either by a local doctor or by the county health authorities. All new patients, particularly those under the age of five years are completely undressed for examination. This is very important, as any assymetry in the lower limbs might be over-looked.

Preventive treatment

Large numbers of school-children are referred to our clinics suffering from postural defects of the spine, feet and knees. In some cases the parents say that they themselves have not noticed anything wrong with the child, others state that they have noticed that the child is round shouldered, or that he 'walks over' on his shoes. Although many of these defects are minor it is important not to ignore them for they may be the beginning of some more serious trouble.

Postural defects of the spine. These patients must be completely undressed for examination. The most common is thoracic kyphosis. Corrective exercises are taught and where room permits the children are treated in classes. They are much keener and more interested than when treated indi-vidually. An attempt should be made to find out the cause of these defects, for example, eyesight might require attention. There may be a history of a chest complaint. The nervous timid child tends to stand badly, or he may be a mouth-breather. There may be some psychological reason due to home influences. In addition to the corrective exer-cises which must be carried out daily at home, it must be emphasised that the child should sleep on a firm mattress.

Postural defects of feet and knees. When children are referred with these deformities it is most impor-tant to examine the footwear as well as the feet and knees. In many cases, the defect is minimal but sometimes the beginning of a more serious deformity is discovered so that every patient must be examined thoroughly. Usually, the necessary shoe alterations and special exercises are sufficient if carried out properly in the home.

Large numbers of infants are referred to us from the child welfare clinics. Many of these children are at the toddling stage and the complaint often is that 'baby turns her feet in when walking'. This of course might mean anything so that the child must be completely undressed and examined thoroughly. As often as not, the defect may be neg-ligible, on the other hand a dislocated hip might be discovered, so that it does not do to disregard these complaints.

Patients discharged from hospital

All patients living within the area served by the hospital may attend their local orthopaedic clinic and are the responsibility of the after-care sister. This means that she is responsible for the continua-tion of the patient's treatment, which might be maintenance of plaster fixation, splintage, re-education of weak muscles, mobilisation of stiff joints, strengthening and corrective exercises, re-education in walking, etc.

Advantages of early discharge from hospital

Children. Parents should not be deprived of their

children longer than is necessary. Furthermore, the parents are expected to take responsibility for the child, and to take an active interest in the treatment. All stages of treatment should be explained to them. Children should mix with other children at school who are physically normal, as far as possible. It has occasionally been noted that if a child has been in hospital for a long period, he has lost his place at home with the rest of the family, and is sometimes unwanted and even treated as an intruder. On the other hand, there is the type of child who, if too long in hospital, receives too much attention on returning home and *demands* constant service, almost to the point of ruling other members of the family. This should be discouraged.

Adults. They, too, can become too hospitalised. Some are quite content to lie in bed and be waited upon. When it is time for their discharge, they just do not want to go. This type of patient is particularly difficult to deal with at a clinic. They will not make the necessary effort to rehabilitate themselves and are horrified when 'returning to work' is mentioned. This type of case requires tactful handling. With the type who is over-anxious about his condition, much persuasion and patience is required. Another type is the one who will not carry out instructions. The surgeon's advice is ignored, and then the patient complains that he is not improving.

Maintenance of plaster fixation

In the case of children, parents are told to take the child to the local clinic on the first possible occasion after discharge. This is very important because they have to be taught to look after splints and plasters, e.g. children sent home in hip-spica plasters need careful nursing to ensure that the plaster does not become wet and sodden.

All patients are encouraged to be as active as possible within reason and without doing anything detrimental to treatment. For example, children in frog plasters are allowed to be placed on the floor, where they move about, in a room or on a lawn, with amazing rapidity. Many find their feet and walk in a fashion. These activities keep the muscles and joints which are free of plaster in good form.

Patients discharged in plasters, particularly walking plasters, need constant supervision; for example, a child admitted to hospital for a foot operation

is discharged home as soon as the plaster is hard. This means that the plaster must be kept in good condition for some months. Boots are worn, but as may be imagined these plasters have to stand a lot of wear and tear. The child goes to school, plays games and in fact leads a practically normal life. If care is not taken, grit, coins, beads, and other miscellaneous articles find their way inside the plasters. These articles invariably cause skin irritation and if this is not investigated at an early date produce a sore. These children, too, seem to have a passion for paddling through every puddle they come across. This, of course, softens the plaster which then becomes quite useless. These plasters therefore have to be renewed quite often. The next problem is the drying. Often parents find it most difficult to keep the child off his feet for the necessary drying period so that the plaster crumbles and cracks and has to be renewed once again.

Hip spicas have to be renewed occasionally but with reasonable care last some months.

Babies in plaster spicas need careful nursing and attention. When these plasters do require renewal the child is admitted to hospital so that a check X-ray can be taken after the new plaster is applied. They are, however, discharged as soon as the plaster is thoroughly dry.

Gradual correction of deformities by repeated plasters

This is done by the Sister at the clinics, for example, relapsing club-feet. The plasters are changed at fortnightly intervals and increased correction is obtained at each change. This procedure sometimes has to be repeated at intervals during the course of treatment because in spite of good correction being obtained and the necessary shoe alterations and splintage worn afterwards, these deformities often recur. It is important, however, to keep the feet in as good shape as possible until the child is old enough for operative correction.

Treatment of congenital deformities

Treatment of congenital deformities such as congenital dislocation of the hip, talipes equino-varus and calcaneo-valgus, Erb's palsy and congenital torticollis is carried out by the Sister at the clinics as soon as possible after the birth of the baby. These babies attend the clinics weekly for manipulations, stretchings, splintage, etc. The mothers are instructed how to look after splints and plasters and to report any complication such as swelling or discoloration of toes.

Other patients treated at a clinic

Apart from continuation of treatment of patients discharged from hospital some patients are treated in plaster wholly at the clinics. These might include plaster cylinders for Osgood–Schlatter's disease, immobilisation of painful joints due to osteoarthritis, rheumatoid arthritis, injuries, sprains, plaster spicas for prolapsed intervertebral disc lesions, plaster corsets for low backache, etc. A large number of out-patients are adults. Besides those who have received treatment in hospital there are those who are referred by local doctors and can be treated by conservative methods at the clinics; for example those who suffer from metatarsalgia or other foot defects. These are usually treated by exercises and special insoles.

Splints

At some clinics the Sister is responsible for measuring, ordering and fitting all splints, for example, a Goldthwait belt, unless the orthotist is in attendance. She is responsible, however, for ensuring that the splint fits well without causing undue pressure, and that it is comfortable. It is sometimes desirable (especially in the case of a child) to have a second splint in case of emergency. If a splint breaks and another is not available, the Sister has to use her ingenuity to hold the correct position by some other means. Usually, she makes a temporary plaster splint. Block-leather splints are always made to a plaster cast which is taken at the clinic.

Boots and shoes

Boots and shoes belonging to patients are brought back to the hospital by the Sister. She writes the necessary instructions for surgical alterations on a label, and attaches it to each individual pair. These are sent to the workshop, and when the work is completed the boots are taken back to the clinic. It should be pointed out here that each patient should have at least two pairs of boots or shoes.

Home visiting

In cases in which a patient is unable to attend the clinic, the after-care sister is expected to visit him in his home. For instance where domestic conditions are good a patient is sometimes nursed entirely at home, although this means regular domiciliary visits by the Sister to ensure that splintage, etc., is satisfactory. Alternatively, the Sister will act as a liaison officer between the hospital and the community nursing service.

Visits to other hospitals

During the course of her work the Sister sometimes visits other hospitals situated within the area served by the clinic, because occasionally patients receiving treatment at our hospital develop some complaint which necessitates treatment in another hospital. They are therefore transferred to the necessary institution and the after-care sister might be responsible for the supervision of their splints or plasters until their return.

Conclusion

Management of an after-care clinic entails liaison between all workers inside the parent hospital and those outside, e.g. general practitioners, community health authorities and community nurses; this liaison is facilitated by the reorganisation of the National Health Service. The after-care sister is able to develop a variety of skills not only in her rôle as a worker in the sphere of orthopaedic treatment, but as health teacher, guide, philosopher and friend to her patient to whom she is a vital link between the hospital and his own 'home ground'.

BIBLIOGRAPHY

Anstice E 1973 Who'll be mother? Nursing Times, 31 May, 714
Ashworth P et al 1978 Rediscovering the patient. Nursing Times booklet, November
Billing A 1982 Central to Care. Nursing Mirror, 11 August

Börsig A et al 1982 Communication with the patient in the intensive care unit. Nursing Times, 24 March

Bowley A H, Gardner L 1972 The Handicapped Child. Edinburgh: Churchill Livingstone

Bromley D D 1966 The Psychology of Human Ageing. London: Penguin

Burrows J, Hughes P 1980 Acute ward planning: an alternative approach. Nursing Times, 24 July

Cavill C A, Johnson J M 1981 Steps towards the process. Nursing Times, December

Chilman A M, Thomas M (eds) 1986 Understanding Nursing Care, 3rd edn. Edinburgh: Churchill Livingstone

Clarke M 1980 Who's afraid of the nursing process? Nursing Times Community Outlook, 12 June

Cohen G L 1964 What's Wrong with Hospitals? London: Penguin

Crow J 1977 The Nursing Process. Nursing Times Publication

Chapman C M 1977 Sociology for Nurses. London: Balliene Tindall

Cruise V J, Wright W B 1978 Better geriatric care—making it happen. Nursing Times, 21 September, 1563

Dickinson S 1982 The Nursing Process and the professional status of nursing. Nursing Times, 2 June

Fanshawe E et al 1978 Disability without handicap. Nursing Times Supplement, 17 August, 3–20

Faulkner A 1981 Aye, there's the rub. Nursing Times, 19 February

Forrest D, Farrow R 1974 The Surgery of Childhood for Nurses. Edinburgh: Churchill Livingstone

Gibbs J R 1977 Net suspension beds for managing threatened and established pressure sores. The Lancet 1: 174

Gilchrist M I, and Blockley N J 1971 Paediatric Orthopaedics. London: Heinemann

Glen S A 1982 Hospital admission through the parents eyes. Nursing Times, 4 August

Goffman E 1961 Asylums. London: Penguin

Gooch J 1981 Change for the better. Nursing Times, 12 February

Goodall J 1982 Children are allowed to visit these wards. Nursing Times, 11 Arpil

Grant P M 1976 Hospitalisation and the elderly patient. Nursing Care Study. Nursing Times, March, 379

Harvey S, Hales-Tooke A 1972 Play in Hospital. London: Faber & Faber

Hector W 1970 Modern Nursing—Theory and Practice. London: Heinemann

Henderson V 1969 Basic Principles of Nursing Care. Published for International Council for Nurses. Basel: Karger

Hopkins J 1983 Spotlight on Children. Nursing Times, 19 October

King S 1984 The story of a convert. Nursing Times, 4 January

Johnson J M 1981 Primary nursing: making a professional commitment. Nursing Times, December

Jolly H 1968 Play and the sick child. The Lancet 2: 1286

Leading article 1981 Doctors and nurses. British Medical Journal 283, No 6293

Lee D H 1982 The education of children in hospital. Nursing Times, 28 July

Lindenmuth J E, Breu S, Malooley A 1980 Sensory overload. American Journal of Nursing 80, No 8, August. University of California, Los Angeles Hospital and Clinics

Lobo E de H 1978 Children of Immigrants to Britain. Their Health and Social Problems. London: Hodder & Stoughton

London P S 1966 Severe injuries that include the head. Nursing Mirror Symposium, 12 August, 1–11

MacCarthy D 1981 The under fives in hospital. Nursing Times Supplement, 22 July

McGhie A 1969 Psychology Applied to Nursing. Edinburgh: Churchill Livingstone

Metcalf C 1978 Owed to the Nightingale but what about the future? Nursing Times, 7 September, 1476

Miller A F 1984 Nursing process and patient care. Nursing Times, 27 June

Nightingale F 1860 Notes on Nursing. London: Duckworth

Noble A, Dixon R 1978 Ward evaluation: St Thomas' Hospital. 'Owed to the Nightingale'. Nursing Times, 3 August, leader and 1273–1284

Norton D 1970 By Accident or Design? Edinburgh: Churchill Livingstone

Norton D 1976 Hospitals of the Longstay Patient. London: Pergamon Press

Norton D et al 1981 The Nursing Process in action 1 and 2. Nursing Times, 17 June, 24

Getting to grips with a problem 1979 Nursing Times, 7 September, 1477

Ogilvie A J 1980 Sources and levels of noise on the ward at night. Nursing Times, 31 July

O'Hare E 1980 The gingerbread man. Nursing Times, 21 February

Robb B 1967 Sans Everything. London: Nelson

Roper N 1982 Principles of Nursing, 3rd edn. Edinburgh: Churchill Livingstone

Roper N, Logan W, Tierney A J 1981 Learning to Use the Process of Nursing. Edinburgh: Churchill Livingstone

Roper N, Logan W, Tierney A J 1983 A nursing model. Nursing Times, 25 May, 1 June, 8 June, 15 June, 29 June

Roper N, Logan W, Tierney A J 1985 The Elements of Nursing, 2nd edn. Edinburgh: Churchill Livingstone

Ross J S, Wilson K J W 1974 Foundations of Nursing and First Aid, Edinburgh: Churchill Livingstone

Rowe J W, Dyer L (eds) 1977 Care of the Orthopaedic Patient. London: Blackwell Scientific

Sancicle L 1982 A double-edged weapon. Nursing Mirror, 4 August

Scales J T et al 1974 The prevention and treatment of pressure sores, using air-support systems. Paraplegia 12, No. 2, 118

Scott D 1977 Net beds in general practice. British Medical Journal (letter) 2: 1156

Scott D 1982 A conflict of interests. Nursing Mirror, 6 January

Skeet M 1970 Home from Hospital. London: Dan Mason Research Committee

Slack P A 1978 Handicap at school. Nursing Times Community Outlook, 12 October, 298

Smith D 1982 Nursing—the caring profession? Nursing Times, 20 October

Smith J P 1982 Graveyards are full of indispensable people. Nursing Times, 6 January

Speck P W 1973 The hospital visitor. Nursing Times, 5 July, 878

Stewart M C 1970 My Brother's Keeper? London: Health Horizon

Swanwick M 1983 Platt in perspective. Nursing Times Occasional Papers 79, No 2, 19 January

Taylor S 1973 Principles of Surgery and Surgical Nursing. London: English Language Book Society

Taylor S (ed.) 1975 Harlow's Modern Surgery for Nurses. London: Heinemann

Wainwright P 1984 Not the nursing process. Nursing Mirror, 23 May

Williamson N 1983 A ward with a view. Nursing Mirror, 27 April

Wilson-Barnett J 1978 In hospital: patients' feelings and opinions. Nursing Times Occasional Papers 16: 3, 29

Wilson-Barnett J 1981 Patients first. Nursing Mirror, 29 July

Younger N R 1978 Children in hospital. Nursing Times, 16 March, Paediatric News, 5

4

Investigations in orthopaedics

INTRODUCTION

X-ray examination of musculo-skeletal disease has now become quite complex. It is important for nurses to have an understanding of the procedures to which their patients are being subjected, together with some knowledge of the necessary preparation and post-examination care when the patient returns from the X-ray department.

The purpose of this section is to describe the types of X-rays available, give an explanation of some radiological terms, describe the preparation of patients for special procedures, the complications which may arise and particular aspects of post-investigational care.

PURPOSE OF X-RAY EXAMINATION

This is fourfold:

1. To confirm a diagnosis, for example, pneumonia.
2. To exclude disease or injury, for example a fracture.
3. To establish the extent of disease, for example metastatic invasion.
4. To assess the progress of disease or its response to treatment, for example healing of osteomyelitis.

TYPES OF X-RAYS AVAILABLE

The examinations described relate mainly to orthopaedic practice but certain patients may also require investigations for a medical condition, e.g. a barium meal.

1. Standard X-rays

In general, no preparation is required for these views. In patients who are restless, sedation may rarely be necessary.

2. Tomograms

By moving the tube and the film, thus blurring out tissues above and below an area of interest, a radiographic section of a bony lesion may be obtained. This produces greater detail and is particularly useful in spinal lesions, bone tumours and in the demonstration of sequestra in chronic osteomyelitis.

3. Xerogram

An image is produced by the action of X-rays on a charged plate rather than on a film. It is especially valuable for demonstrating soft tissues (Fig. 4.1).

4. Computed tomography

A cross-sectional image of the body is created by a computer which collects the information from multiple tiny beams of X-ray as the tube rotates around the body. Many slices are used to cover the part of the body being X-rayed. This allows both bone and soft tissues to be imaged, and is particularly useful in the skull and spine when both the bone and the nervous tissue can be seen at the same time.

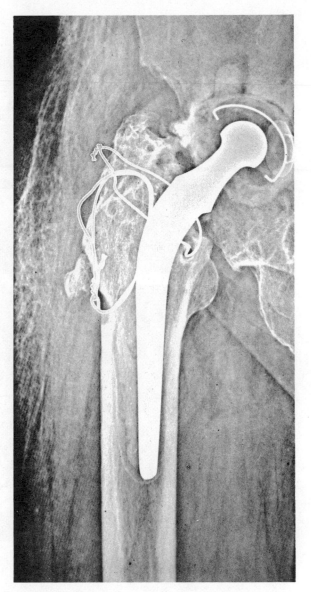

Fig. 4.1 Xerogram of Charnley arthroplasty of the hip.

5. Contrast medium examinations

For this, an injection of radio-opaque substance is used to demonstrate individual organs on X-ray, for example, an intravenous pyelogram (I.V.P.) will outline the kidney structure.

 This type of examination includes the following:

1. Arthrography—in which an injection of air and contrast medium outlines the internal structures of the joint (Fig. 4.2A).
2. Arteriography—demonstrates blood supply to selected organs by direct injection of contrast medium through a catheter in the feeding vessel.
3. Cystogram—is examination of the bladder by injection of contrast medium via a urethral catheter.
4. Myelogram (radiculogram) demonstrates the theca and spinal cord by lumbar puncture.
5. Lymphogram outlines lymphatic vessels and lymph nodes.

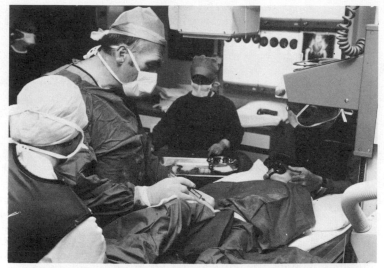

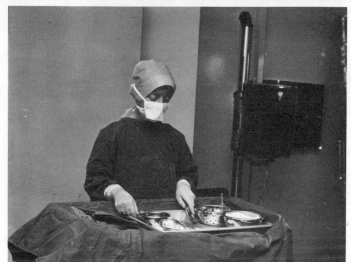

Fig. 4.2 **A.** An arthrogram of the hip in progress. **B.** The X-ray Department nurse assists.

6. Sinogram outlines abscess tracks or fistulae by insertion of a fine catheter into the wound.
7. Venogram shows the venous drainage by means of percutaneous puncture, commonly used to investigate deep vein thrombosis in the leg.
8. Discography—delineates the anatomy of the nucleus of the intervertebral disc.

6. Radio-isotope scan

Substances called radio-isotopes emit radiation, usually in the form of gamma rays. This emission can be detected by special apparatus called a gamma camera. Technetium is such a substance. When joined chemically with diphosphonate and injected intravenously, it is taken up by bone. The amount of uptake reflects both the activity of the bone and the blood supply to the bone. Thus bone death in infarction, bone repair in fractures and tumour invasion of bone can be monitored by this means. It is particularly sensitive and lesions not visible on X-ray may be demonstrated on the scan.

7. Ultrasound

This investigation uses a principle similar to radar to produce echo images of the body. There is no radiation hazard to the patient and the procedure is non-invasive. It is mainly used in obstetrics and in studying the abdominal organs. The applications in orthopaedics are limited but it has been shown to be of value in demonstrating congenital hip dislocation in very young infants.

PREPARATION OF THE PATIENT

It is important that the nurse is acquainted with all aspects of the preparation of the patient for radiological examination and, in particular, is able to offer understanding and reassurance to a patient who is probably nervous and frightened of the unknown.

The introduction of contrast medium into a patient is tantamount to an operative procedure and the patient's informed consent must be sought by the referring clinician. The nurse can often help, by giving an explanation of a complicated procedure and its possible consequences, for example, post-myelogram headache.

It is also important to *check the identity of the patient* before he is sent to the X-ray department.

Bowel preparation is required for certain special X-ray procedures in the abdominal region, for example, intravenous pyelograms.

Skin preparation is the same as for any other surgical procedure, for example, the groin area before femoral arteriography. This procedure also requires a pubic shave.

Premedication—one or two types may be ordered:

1. For examination under sedation, for example, diazepam (valium) before arteriography.
2. General anaesthesia, for example, hip arthrography in infants. Most X-ray departments issue specific written instructions for individual procedures. Examples of such instructions are shown in Tables 4.1–4.5.

POST-INVESTIGATIONAL NURSING CARE

This obviously depends on whether the patient is conscious or unconscious. The majority of examinations are conducted on the conscious patient; this does not mean that on return to the ward, the patient requires no nursing care. On the contrary, he may be thirsty, cold or uncomfortable, with a full bladder and an empty stomach. Wilson-Barnett (1979) recommends that nurses should have time to visit specialised diagnostic departments to learn about the tests.

Table 4.1   Procedure: Hip arthrogram

Name	Ward ....
Registration Number.................................	Patient's Age..
Diagnosis	Date/Time ....

THE EXAMINATION WILL BE HELD IN THE X-RAY DEPARTMENT AT ....

on ....

| General Anaesthetic .... | Local Anaesthetic .... |

1. Please shave pubic area.
2. Give NOTHING TO EAT or DRINK for 4 hours before examination.
3. Give 1 DULCOLAX suppository the night before.
4. Ask the patient to empty his/her bladder IMMEDIATELY before coming down to the X-ray Department.
5. Give ....   as pre-medication at ....
6. Clean bed-linen.
7. Identi-Band.
8. Consent form—SIGNED.
9. Anaesthetic form—COMPLETED.
10. The patient will come to the X-ray Department straight from the ward, but after the procedure will be transferred to the Recovery Ward.

Table 4.2 Procedure: Lumbar venogram

Name	Ward ....
Registration Number..........................	Patient's Age............................
Diagnosis	Date/Time ....

THE EXAMINATION WILL BE AT................................ on ....
in the X-ray Department

General Anaesthetic .... Local Anaesthetic ....

1. Please shave the pubic area.
2. Give NOTHING TO EAT OR DRINK for 4 hours before the examination.
3. Give 1 DUCOLAX suppository the night before.
4. Ask the patient to empty his/her bladder IMMEDIATELY before coming to the X-ray Department.

5. Give .... as pre-medication at ....
6. Clean bed-linen.
7. Identi-Band.
8. Consent form—SIGNED.
9. Anaesthetic form—COMPLETED.
10. The patient will come straight from the ward to the X-ray Department, but following the procedure will be transferred to the Recovery Ward.

AFTER-CARE.

1. Patient may get up and walk around as soon as possible, to assist venous circulation.
2. Quarter-hourly pulse and blood pressure for 4 hours and 4-hourly temperature, pulse and respiration recordings.
3. Half-hourly inspection around the dressing site, to ensure that there is no haematoma formation.
4. Remove dressing (adhesive plaster) after 24 hours.

Invasive investigations

If the patient has had an arterial puncture, the needle puncture site should be carefully examined on return to the ward and at regular intervals thereafter, so that any subsequent haematoma or oozing of blood can be recognised and promptly reported. It is important to remember that in certain investigations where local anaesthetic is introduced, the part will become numb; for this reason, patients who undergo knee arthrography are not permitted to drive a motor car within four hours of the procedure.

Myelography (radiculogram) investigations

The investigation of the subarachnoid space is carried out using water soluble contrast medium. These substances mix readily with the cerebrospinal fluid and provide a clear radiographic detail of the spinal cord, nerve roots and nerve root sheaths.

Great strides have been made in the development of these chemicals and now only non-ionic substances are used. These are isotonic with the cerebrospinal fluid and have a very low neurotoxicity. They can, therefore, be used to examine the

Table 4.3 Water soluble myelography

Name	Ward ....
Registration number	Patient's Age...............................
Diagnosis	Date/Time ....

1. Clean bed linen.
2. Identi-Band.
3. Consent form—SIGNED.
4. Patient MUST be 'clerked' by a doctor.
5. Clean gown.
6. Light breakfast.
7. Patient to remain in bed for eight hours with head elevated.
8. To remain in hospital under observation for 24 hours.

Table 4.4 Treatment of severe reactions following injection of contrast media

There are predominantly four types:	*In any severe reaction:*
1. ANAPHYLACTIC 2. GENERALISED CONVULSIONS 3. HYPOTENSION 4. CARDIAC ARREST	a. Relase abdominal compression (In IVP Patients). b. Administer 100% oxygen by face mask and bag. (Anaesthetic Trolley—Room 1). c. Fetch crash box from X-ray corridor. d. Telephone for assistance (Number for 'cardiac arrest' given). e. Set up an IV Infusion.

Type	Reactions	Treatment
1	ANAPHYLACTIC Mild cases have urticaria. Severe cases have bronchospasm, oedema of glottis and possibly pulmonary oedema.	'Piriton' 10 mg IV and Hydrocortisone 300 mg IV ('Efcortesol'). a. 'Phenergan' 50 mg IV. b. Hydrocortisone 500 mg IV ('Efcortesol'). c. Await response. d. Aminophylline 125 mg IV. e. If necessary Isoprenaline 0.5 mg IM.
2	GENERALISED CONVULSIONS	a. Oxygen 100%. b. Diazepam 100 mg IV. Diluted in Saline to 10 mg.
3	SEVERE HYPOTENSION	a. Hold up all 4 limbs vertically. b. Hydrocortisone 500 mg IV. ('Efcortesol'). c. Rapid IV fluid transfusion of the order of 1 litre in 5 minutes
4	CARDIAC ARREST	a. Clear the airway. b. Ventilate the patient. Mouth-to-mouth or bellows from the crash box. c. Circulation. Cardiac massage.

whole spinal cord. For examination of the lumbar and thoracic regions, the contrast medium is inserted via a lumbar puncture. The cervical cord and nerve roots are best demonstrated by injection of contrast via the lateral C1/2 dural puncture. High concentrations of the contrast medium may still be irritating to the cerebral cortex and slow resorption from the CSF is achieved by the maintenance of the sitting or semi-recumbent position for 4–6 hours after the examination. The patient usually remains in bed for 24 hours following the investigation. Twenty per cent of patients may experience headache and some patients feel nauseated in the 24 hour period following the examination. Increased fluid intake prior to the investigation, may reduce this complication, and mild analgesia is usually sufficient to relieve the symptoms.

The side-effects may be delayed for 48 to 72

Table 4.5 Department of Radiology—contents of emergency trays

DRUGS:	'Piriton' Chlorpheniramine: 10 mg in 1 ml × 5. 'Phenergan' Promethazine Hydrochlor: 50 mg in 2 ml × 10. 'Efcortesol' Hydrocortisone: 500 mg in 5 ml × 3. Aminophylline: 250 mg in 10 ml × 10. Sodium Chloride Inj. 0.9% 10 ml × 10.	
ACCESSORIES:	Syringes (Disposable)	2 ml × 3 5 ml × 3 10 ml × 3
	Needles (Disposable)	19 swg × 10 21 swg × 10
	Butterfly Needles Intermittent type	19 swg × 3 21 swg × 3
	Ampoule Files × 5 'Sleek' 1 Roll.	

DO NOT CLUTTER YOUR EMERGENCY TRAY WITH UNNECESSARY ITEMS

hours. Water soluble contrast medium investigations of the subarachnoid space is contra-indicated in patients who have a history of epilepsy.

INVESTIGATIONS UNDER GENERAL ANAESTHETIC

These require the usual nursing procedures before recovery of consciousness (Fig. 4.3). Note again that puncture wounds should be monitored at regular intervals.

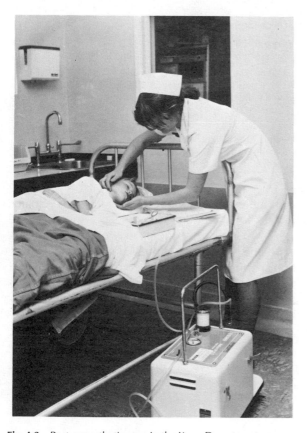

Fig. 4.3   Post-anaesthetic care in the X-ray Department.

THE ROLE OF THE X-RAY DEPARTMENT NURSE

When the patient is given an appointment to attend the department for a spinal procedure the X-ray department nurse should ensure that the necessary instructions are given to the ward staff and to the patient, and that any medical problems are recorded and brought to the notice of the radiologist, e.g. hypertension, diabetes, steroid therapy. The nurse acts as co-ordinator of the patient's care and welfare between the X-ray department, the hospital ward or the community. Preparation and aftercare of the out-patient attending direct from home for examination is the responsibility of the X-ray nurse.

The nurse receives the patient in the department and offers quiet understanding and reassurance, in order to promote a satisfactory level of relaxation. In some patients, sedation may be required in the form of an intramuscular injection which should only be given at the request of the radiologist.

At the conclusion of the examination the nurse will ensure that the patient is transferred to his bed and is made as comfortable as possible. A final check is made of the puncture site and patient's general condition before handing the patient over to the ward staff. Out-patients rest quietly in the X-ray department until fit to leave for home.

Preparation for sterile procedures follow the same general principles as apply to those followed in the operating theatre, and the nurse is responsible for assisting with the procedure (Fig. 4.2B), for the maintenance of sterility standards, for ordering disposable items, and for the general care of instruments.

Emergencies in the X-ray department. Following the injection of contrast medium the patient may suffer a reaction of either minor or severe type. Minor reactions consist of transient hot flushing, nausea, vomiting and headache. These are of short duration and respond to simple symptomatic measures.

Severe reactions are life threatening and an emergency procedure should be established in the X-ray department. An example of the routine is given in Table 4.4. An emergency tray should be set up in each X-ray room where contrast medium is used; the contents are itemised in Table 4.5.

RADIATION PROTECTION

All members of the X-ray staff are required to wear badges which monitor the amount of radiation received by each individual. No member of staff should ever place any part of their body in the primary beam of radiation for any reason whatsoever. A lead-lined apron should always be worn by members of the X-ray staff who are present during Fluoroscopy or television screening.

CONCLUSION

This brief outline is given to indicate in general terms what happens to patients in the X-ray department and to emphasise the supporting role of the nurse. A patient can easily become confused and upset in the 'no man's land' between investigation and management. It is the particular responsibility of the nurse by continuing contact, care and compassion, to ensure that this is minimised as much as possible.

LABORATORY INVESTIGATIONS IN THE ORTHOPAEDIC HOSPITAL

In a short section it is not possible to enumerate all the possible investigations in a pathological laboratory, but simply those pathological tests which are of particular value in the diagnosis of bone and joint disease.

Possible investigations may be classified as:

1. *Simple Haematology*: ordinary 'blood counts' and sedimentation rates.
2. *Biochemical*: e.g. Serum proteins, calcium, inorganic phosphate and alkaline phosphatase, uric acid.
3. *Bacteriological*: the culture of pus, synovial fluid or blood for pathogenic organisms. The same department usually carries out *serological* tests for the antibodies of typhoid, brucellosis, and gonorrhoea.
4. *Histological*: direct microscopical examination of surgical specimens or biopsies removed at operation.

HAEMATOLOGY

The haemoglobin level is the simplest blood test and will be carried out on practically every patient at least once. A low value, less than 10 g in females and 11 g in males, demands further investigation for the type of anaemia. Briefly a low Hb level may be due to

lack of haemopoietic factors;—iron, Vitamin B12;

blood loss whether acute or long standing;

chronic illness; infections, renal disease, or malignancy.

The full investigation of anaemia is outside the scope of this section, but except in emergency as a life saving measure, blood transfusion should not be used as a 'short cut' before the real cause of the patient's anaemia has been found.

The white cell count; the commonest cause of an increased white cell count (leucocytosis) over the normal upper limit of 10 000 is some form of acute infection. *Pyogenic infections* usually by staphylococci or streptococci, cause an increase in the polymorphs (neutrophils) and this is the most likely cause in a patient with postoperative pyrexia and sepsis. Noninfective conditions; a coronary thrombosis or a pulmonary embolus, for example, can also cause a leucocytosis. A raised white cell count therefore, while a useful indication is not completely reliable without bacteriological confirmation.

Erythrocyte sedimentation rate (ESR)

When citrated blood is left standing in a tall narrow tube, the red cells will slowly settle, leaving a clear zone of straw-coloured plasma at the top. In blood from a healthy subject, the rate of fall is very slow, not much more than 5 mm in males or 7 mm in females during the first hour. The rate at which the red cells settle seems to depend on their stickiness, their tendency to collect in piles or rouleaux and it is accelerated in changes in the albumen-globulin ratio. An increase in the ESR is found generally in inflammatory conditions and in orthopaedics the test helps to differentiate rheumatoid disease or bone tuberculosis from osteoarthritis. The test is nonspecific and therefore of limited value. In obvious acute infections there is little point in having the ESR done and the trauma of an operation will also tend to increase it. ESRs taken within ten days post-operatively are therefore futile. Certain malignant conditions also give a raised ESR and the most important orthopaedically, is multiple myeloma, in which it may be over 100 mm in the first hour.

Plasma viscosity

A new test for the measurement of the viscosity or stickiness of the plasma has been devised in the past ten years, comparing it with that of water. Like the erythrocyte sedimentation rate, the viscosity of plasma is raised by increased amounts of the higher plasma proteins, particularly fibrinogen and decreased by low albumin levels. Unlike the ESR which is more rapid in anaemia, the plasma viscosity is not affected by the mass of red cells, since it is carried out on the separated plasma.

The normal values in both sexes are 1.50–1.72 cP (centrepoises) as compared with a value of 1.00 for distilled water.

Platelet count

The blood platelets are concerned with the formation of thrombi and the normal process of blood coagulation. A fall below the normal (lower limit $150\,000 \times 10^9/1$) does not produce the clinical effects of subcutaneous and submucosal haemorrhages (purpura) until the count is about 50 000 or less. A patient with purpura would not normally be admitted to an orthopaedic hospital. Most platelet counts in the author's department are on patients with rheumatoid arthritis. This is because treatment with powerful anti-rheumatoid drugs (e.g. gold, penicillamine) may depress the bone marrow and so reduce the platelet count.

BIOCHEMICAL INVESTIGATIONS

Biochemical tests have doubled or trebled in number and apparatus for their estimation has become much more sophisticated in the past thirty years. Here it is only possible to mention a few investigations which are commonly carried out for the diagnosis of bone and joint conditions.

Plasma and serum proteins

Normal plasma contains 60–80 g/l divided into three important groups, albumin, 35–60 g, globulin, 18–32 g, and fibrinogen, 2–4 g. In practice, orthopaedic surgeons rarely require to know the fibrinogen content; if they do, a heparinised specimen of blood will be sent. During the normal process of clotting, fibrinogen is converted into fibrin which forms the basis of the blood clot. The clotted specimen of blood usually sent to the laboratory will exude serum, containing only the albumen and globulin, but these form the great bulk of the blood proteins. The name 'globulin' in fact comprises a number of different proteins with different properties and molecular weights. These are separated by their different rate of movement in solution when a weak electric current is passed (electrophoresis). Generally globulins are more complex than albumin, and it is from these that the various antibodies are formed. Antibodies are detected by their behaviour towards various antigens, usually living or dead bacterial suspensions and their investigation comes under the heading of *serology*, in the bacteriological laboratory.

One disease, *multiple myeloma*, is of importance in the orthopaedic hospital, since it is usually manifested clinically by bone pain and pathological fractures. In this condition, there is a very marked increase in the serum or plasma globulin with values of total protein up to 200 g/l, most of this being globulin. As was seen this also produces a high ESR (from 80 to 100 mm in 1 hour). The abnormal globulin is produced by the myeloma cells in the bone marrow; these are large neoplastic plasma cells. In about 50 per cent of cases of myeloma, Bence-Jones protein is excreted in the urine. This is only one of the light chains of the myeloma globulin, with a molecular weight of 20–40 000, less than half that of normal serum alubumin. The old test of boiling the urine (when the Bence-Jones substance appeared at about 60°C and dissolved again as the urine approached boiling point), had the advantage of being simple and within the capacity of the nurse on the ward or the general practitioner without laboratory facilities at hand. However, it is now known that B-J protein is missed in about half the cases in which it is present, if the simple heating test is used. Electrophoresis of concentrated urine is more reliable.

Bone metabolism

In an orthopaedic hospital, the three most important estimations for the diagnosis of bone disorders

Table 4.6

Disorder	Mechanism	Se calcium 2.12–2.62 mmol	Inorg. phosphate 0.8–1.4	Alkaline phosphate 3–13 KA u	Faeces Ca up to 560 mg/24 h	Urine Ca 100–300 mg/24 h
Rickets	Deficiency of dietary calcium in infancy and/or failure to form sufficient Vitamin D in skin due to lack of sunshine.	R	R	++	R	R
Osteomalaica	Deficiency of calcium in later life, particularly in old people living alone on inadequate diet and in pregnant women with increased needs for the foetus.	R	R	++	R	R
Hyper-para-thyroidism	(i) Primary due to hyperplasia or more often tumour of parathyroids with excess parathormone production	+	R	++	N	+
	(ii) Secondary; renal disease with loss of calcium in urine and compensatory parathyroid hyperplasia.	N or R	R	N or +	N	Phosphate
Fanconi syndrome	A congenital deficiency of the renal tubules with failure to conserve phosphate. Disease may present in infancy as pseudorickets.	N	R	N	N	Ca N Phosphate +
Myeloma and secondary carcinoma of bone	Destruction of bone with multiple tumours, lead to pathological fractures and secondary attempts at healing.	+	N	++	N	N to +
Paget's disease (osteitis deformans)	Cause unknown. A rarefying osteitis; initial softening and deformity followed by excessive new bone formation.	N	N	+++	N	N
Malabsorption	Defect in intestinal mucosa.	R	R	N	Ca & Phosp +	N

N = normal values.   R = reduced.   + = slightly increased.   ++ = moderately increased.   +++ = greatly increased.

are the serum or plasma calcium, inorganic phosphate and alkaline phosphatase. Here it is only possible to summarise the factors which influence these three substances and then to give in table form, the changes occurring in some of the more important bone disorders (see Table 4.6).

Calcium

Calcium is absorbed from the gastro-intestinal tract by the action of calciferol (Vitamin D) which is itself partly obtained from the diet and partly synthesised in the skin by the action of sunlight. Vitamin D also promotes the utilisation of calcium in the formation of bone. The opposite effect, the withdrawal of calcium from the bones and increase in the blood plasma level is brought about by para-thormone, a hormone secreted by the parathyroids, the four tiny glands behind the thyroid. Therefore in cases of overactivity of these, there will be a progressive rarefaction of the bones with increased plasma calcium and raised excretion in the stools and urine.

Inorganic phosphate

Calcium is deposited in the bones in the form of hydroxyapatite (three molecules of calcium phosphate to one of calcium hydroxide) and therefore the metabolism of phosphate is linked to that of calcium. The red cells contain large amounts of phosphate; therefore to give reliable results specimens of blood for phosphate estimation must be fresh and unhaemolysed.

Alkaline phosphatase

Alkaline phosphatase is an enzyme which acts upon organic phosphate compounds in the body to liberate phosphate at the sites of new bone formation. Alkaline phosphatase levels will be increased in any condition in which bone is being formed but also in bone destructive diseases since these are almost always accompanied by reactive attempts at regeneration. The normal adult values are 3–13 units/100 ml but in small children up to three years old, in whom a lot of bone growth is going on, the normal values are 10–20 units.

Uric acid (normal value, SI units, 0–0.45 mmol/l)

In gout, a disease in which there is an inborn error of purine metabolism, particularly in the acute stage, the plasma uric acid will be raised. It is also increased during treatment by drugs which promote urinary excretion of urates. Impaired renal function will tend to cause a raised uric acid level and therefore the blood urea is usually determined at the same time.

BACTERIOLOGICAL (MICROBIOLOGICAL) INVESTIGATIONS

Specimens of pus, blood, synovial fluid and material removed at operation may all be sent for culture and if organisms are grown, for sensitivity to various antibiotics. There are two things nurses need to bear in mind about specimens for the Bacteriology Department. Firstly *do not* put any operation specimen for culture in formol saline or other strong fixative solution. These will kill any organisms and render the investigation futile. Secondly, however 'urgent' a test may be, culture must take at least 24 hours with a further 24 hours for sensitivity tests. Culture for Mycobacterium tuberculosis will take from two to three weeks. Apparent delay is not due to slackness by the lab staff; it is simply that culturing organisms takes time.

Serology

Serological tests may be performed for many diseases, but the two which most commonly produce arthritis or bone disease are the enteric (typhoid-paratyphoid) group and brucellosis. In the earlier stages of the enteric fevers, blood culture and a little later urine or stool culture, are the best means of diagnosis. Unfortunately arthritis is usually a late complication and one has to employ the Widal test for antibodies. Today, when so many people have had TAB inoculations in the forces or for holidays abroad, the test is difficult to interpret and normally surgeons will consult the microbiologist on the significance of the results.

In brucellosis, a raised titre against Brucella melitensis, abortus or suis will be suggestive in obscure bone or joint disease. Titres of 1/100 to 1/200 would be considered diagnostic in urban areas but in a rural county such as Shropshire, many healthy farm workers and veterinary surgeons will have antibodies and a higher level, say 1/1000 may be found.

HISTOLOGICAL INVESTIGATIONS

Specimens of bone or soft tissue removed at operation are usually sent for microscopical examination by the pathologist:

1. To confirm a fairly obvious diagnosis—e.g. osteoarthritis in a femoral head removed in a Charnley operation.
2. To diagnose a condition not obvious to the naked eye, e.g. a swelling which may be a malignant tumour of some kind.
3. For research purposes.

Specimens for histology only should be preserved in a fixative solution (to arrest the normal process of decay), the most usual being 10 per cent formol saline. Difficulties for the theatre staff arise when the surgeon wants culture and histology on the same small specimen. In cases of doubt nurses should put the specimen in a dry sterile container and let the lab staff deal with it. At night or the weekend when the laboratory is closed, a specimen may be placed in a sterile container and covered with *sterile* normal saline. This will not spoil it for bacteriological examination but at the same time, if refrigerated, will preserve it fairly well for later histology.

BIBLIOGRAPHY

Chesney D N, Chesney M O 1978 Care of the patient in diagnostistic radiography. 5th edn Oxford: Blackwell

Goldman M 1978 A guide to the X-ray department. Bristol: Wright

Parker M J 1978 Microbiology for nurses. 5th edn. London: Baillière Tindall (Nurses' aid series)

Hare R, Cook E M 1984 Bacteriology and immunity for nurses. 6th edn. Edinburgh: Churchill Livingstone

Wilson-Barnett J 1979 Stress in hospital. Edinburgh: Churchill Livingstone

Winner H I 1978 Microbiology in Patient care. London: Hodder & Stoughton (Modern nursing series)

5

Basic principles of nursing care applied to orthopaedic patients

INTRODUCTION

The unique function of the nurse has been defined as 'assisting the individual sick or well, in the performance of those activities contributing to health or its recovery (or to a peaceful death) that he would perform unaided if he had the necessary strength, will or knowledge, and to do this in such a way as to help him gain independence as quickly as possible' (Henderson, 1969). This definition is developed further in 'the Nursing Process' in which Crow (1977) points out that the words 'strength', 'will' and 'knowledge' cover the nurse's triple role of physical helper, emotional supporter and teacher.

In order to fulfil this role, it follows that the basis of effective nursing care is understanding of the patient's physical, psychological, pathological and socio-economic state; this leads us to consider nursing histories, nursing assessment, and nursing care plans.

NURSING ASSESSMENT

Baldwin (1976) discussing 'made-to-measure' care in the *Nursing Times* points out the importance of the assessment stage of the nursing process and states that 'there is much to be said for the nurse taking a comprehensive nursing history', pointing out that the task of taking a new patient's history is frequently given to the junior nurse, ward clerk or receptionist, who merely checks the details on the admission slip. This author further points out that this does not equate with taking a full nursing history which should include the patient's previous experience of hospital and illness, his occupation, social, economic and family status, housing, religion, dietary habits etc. It is also pointed out that a nursing history should be aimed at discovering social problems and as an example, says 'checking that the patient's next-of-kin is his wife does not bring forth the information that she is crippled with arthritis, unable to leave the house and that there is no-one who could readily visit the patient'. The same author points out that taking a nursing history enables one to assess the patient's personality and intelligence as well as his needs so that the objectives of his treatment can be defined, and the concept of comprehensive care applied to his particular requirements. This view is further endorsed in *The Nursing Process* (Crow, 1977), which explains how and why to take a nursing history and states that the aims are to:

1. Establish what is a normal life pattern for that individual.
2. Gather facts and identify specific needs.
3. Allow a care plan to be made that meets individual needs.
4. Establish an early nurse/patient rapport.
5. Save time, as a written history taken by one nurse is then available for others.

Another author, Boylan (1982), suggests that 'the physical assessment undertaken on admission should be total, unless the patient is in crisis'.

Nursing assessment therefore is a valuable tool for ensuring care for all patients but notably for those *at risk*; for example, the elderly patient admitted with a fracture of the neck of the femur requires *immediate* steps to prevent him from developing pressure sores (see Ch. 21) and/or chest complications. Nursing assessment is therefore essential for prompt intervention and initiation of nursing measures aimed at the *prevention* of complications which may hinder the patient's early discharge and return to independence.

NURSING CARE PLANS

All effective nursing care is planned to some extent,

and a written plan *forces* those who make it to give some thought to fit the individual's needs (Henderson, 1969). This is as true in orthopaedics as in every other area of nursing. A written plan is a guide to all those involved in delivering nursing care; periodic revisions and modifications of the plan depend on the patient's condition; drastic changes (e.g. surgery) mean that the plan must be re-written, for example, a patient may be up and about on a pre-operative day and confined to bed in a plaster hip spica on the day of operation and for some weeks or months thereafter. But when the patient has recovered from the effects of surgery, a weekly review of his nursing care plan may suffice. Further reference to nursing care plans will be found in *The Nursing Process* (Crow, 1977). It is interesting to note that nursing care plans recorded in this publication relate to patients with a very common orthopaedic condition— fracture of the upper end of the femur. The Nursing Process has already been discussed in Ch. 3.

We will now discuss some aspects of the nursing care of orthopaedic patients, using Henderson's *Basic Principles of Nursing Care* as set out in Table 5.1. Note that each of these principles is prefaced by the words '*assisting* the patient' and these words imply nursing judgement to preserve a nice balance between that which must be done for the patient and that which he can be helped to do for himself in order to retain or regain independence. This is of particular importance in orthopaedics since our patients have a physical disablement which reduces them, either temporarily or permanently, to varying degrees of helplessness, ranging from the healthy young person forced to lie in bed continuously because of a leg injury, to one who is unconscious from head injury or paralysed from spinal cord damage. Most of our patients however, fall somewhere between these two extremes, and it is the wide variations in the different and constantly changing needs of our patients which makes meeting them an exciting challenge, not forgetting that some of them may suffer from some concomitant medical/surgical condition, and further, that since we deal with all age-groups, the field of our work can range from 'paediatrics' on the one hand to 'geriatrics' on the other.

RESPIRATION

Assisting the patient to breathe normally

This quite naturally takes first place, since cessation of respiration for more than 3–5 minutes results in death. Obvious causes of respiratory failure which require immediate medical and nursing measures are serious injuries to the air-passages or to the chest, or paralysis of the muscles of respiration; similarly, cardiac arrest or pulmonary embolism are medical emergencies. Medical treatment is also needed for established chest conditions such as pneumonia or asthma. Obstruction of the airway by a foreign body or by the position of the tongue in an unconscious patient are obvious causes of respiratory embarrassment; respiratory failure which cannot be treated by simply clearing the airway might require intubation, suction, oxygen therapy, or even tracheostomy.

Assisted respiration is usually given by means of an intermittent positive pressure pump.

Apart from the emergencies outlined above, observation of the respiratory state is particularly important in patients 'at risk', notably those with established chest disease, the very young and the very old, the weak and debilitated, the obese patient and the heavy smoker. The unconscious or paralysed patient has already been mentioned.

Other factors affecting respiration

The environment

Respiration can be inhibited by a hot, stuffy atmosphere or conversely by one that is cold, or by abrupt change from one extreme of temperature to another; the nurse must be aware of these factors in an environment which the patient cannot mani-

Table 5.1 Needs of all patients usually met by the nurse and how modified by conditions always present and sometimes present (Henderson: Basic Principles of Nursing Care, Basel: Karger 1969 by kind permission of the author and publishers.)

Components of basic nursing	Conditions always present that affect basic needs	Pathological states (as contrasted with specific diseases) that modify basic needs
Assisting the patient with these functions or providing conditions that will enable him to: 1. Breathe normally 2. Eat and drink adequately 3. Eliminate by all avenues of elimination 4. Move and maintain desirable posture (walking, sitting, lying and changing from one to the other) 5. Sleep and rest 6. Select suitable clothing dress and undress 7. Maintain body temperature within normal range by adjusting clothing and modifying the environment 8. Keep the body clean and well groomed and protect the integument 9. Avoid dangers in the environment and avoid injuring others 10. Communicate with others in expressing emotions, needs, fears, etc. 11. Worship according to his faith 12. Work at something that provides a sense of accomplishment 13. Play, or participate in various forms of recreation 14. Learn, discover, or satisfy the curiosity that leads to 'normal' development and health.	1. Age: newborn, child, youth, adult, middle-aged and dying 2. Temperament, emotional state, or passing mood: (a) 'normal' or (b) euphoric and hyperactive (c) anxious, fearful, agitated or hysterical or (d) depressed and hyperactive 3. Social or cultural status: A member of a family unit with friends and status, or a person relatively alone and/or maladjusted, destitute 4. Physical and intellectual capacity: (a) normal weight (b) underweight (c) overweight (d) normal mentality (e) sub-normal mentality (f) gifted mentality (g) normal sense of hearing, sight, equilibrium and touch (h) loss of special sense (i) normal motor power (j) loss of motor power	1. Marked disturbances of fluid and electrolyte balance, starvation states, pernicious vomiting, and diarrhoea 2. Acute oxygen want 3. Shock (including 'collapse' and haemorrhage) 4. Disturbances of consciousness, fainting, coma, delirium 5. Exposure to cold and heat causing markedly abnormal body temperatures 6. Acute febrile states (all causes) 7. A local injury, wound and/or infection 8. A communicable condition 9. Pre-operative state 10. Post-operative state 11. Immobilisation from disease or prescribed as treatment 12. Persistent or intractable pain.

pulate himself. Dust, pollen or tobacco smoke in the atmosphere can be very distressing and bed-clothes tucked in tightly over chest and abdomen might inhibit respiration in the weak, debilitated, helpless patient. Chest infection is a hazard in patients with low respiratory reserve; those most vulnerable have already been mentioned and should be protected as far as is humanly possible by constant monitoring of the environment, and by the exclusion of known sources of infection, including carriers of the common cold.

Posture influences the respiratory excursion and consequent interchange of gases in the lungs. This interchange is easiest when the trunk is in the upright or semi-recumbent position with the arms and shoulders in a normal physiological position. Anything which interferes with this position can inhibit respiration. The side-lying position favours the upper-most lung at the expense of the other, and the prone-lying position is not well tolerated for any length of time where there is respiratory difficulty.

Deformity of the spine and thorax for example gross kyphosis, scoliosis, and the deformity seen in ankylosing spondylitis limit lung expansion and may lead to serious pulmonary insufficiency.

Pain is a potent cause of respiratory problems if it prevents the patient from breathing deeply or from coughing, leading to accumulation of bron-chial secretions and atalectasis. Respiration may be inhibited not only by pain in the chest itself from infection, injury or operation but from wounds elsewhere for example, in the abdomen; sufferers from low back pain are only too well aware that coughing exacerbates their pain; spinal surgery has a similar effect.

Analgesics are given with caution since some of them, e.g. Morphine, depress the respiratory centre.

Surgery may contribute to loss of respiratory function, especially if prolonged anaesthesia was required; post-operative shock and pain from a sur-gical wound may inhibit respiration, especially in a debilitated patient.

Immobility, especially associated with uncon-sciousness or paralysis or with some form of splint-age, such as a tight heavy plaster jacket, limits the respiratory excursion and prevents full expansion of the lungs.

Summary of nursing assistance

1. *Observation* of the patient; especially those 'at risk' described in preceding paragraphs; note respiratory rate and skin colour, body temperature; note flaring of nostrils, tension of the accessory muscles of respiration, movements of the chest and abdomen. Note noisy respirations; nasal discharge, 'snuffling'; the cough, whether dry, 'hacking' or productive; sputum—amount, colour, odour, tena-city; collect appropriate specimens.

2. *Monitoring of the environment* to provide the most effective setting for the maintenance of normal respiration.

3. *Seek prompt medical treatment* where indi-cated; e.g. antibiotic therapy.

4. *Posture should be modified* at regular inter-vals (where possible) to favour respiratory excur-sion, and to encourage the patient to cough. *Change of position* no matter how little, is essential not only for the prevention of chest complications but for others, e.g. pressure sores. For example, a patient nursed in the sitting posture as part of the treatment of chest injury may be tilted slightly from one side to the other, by means of a pillow or pad under the raised buttock. If the patient is able to lift the buttocks on alternate sides he is taught and encouraged to do so at two-hourly inter-vals. This does not interfere with the correct pos-ture.

5. *Deformity* which produces respiratory com-plications requires treatment described elsewhere, but it is appropriate to stress here that an important aim in orthopaedic nursing is *prevention* of defor-mity e.g. in ankylosing spondylitis.

6. *Pain* requires treatment by appropriate anal-gesics but those which depress respiration are best avoided. In this connection, attention to all aspects of the general comfort of the patient is axiomatic; if there is a wound, support it firmly yet gently with the hand when encouraging the patient to cough. In this connection, excellent advice is given in the book *Lifting, Handling and Helping Patients* (Dow-nie & Kennedy, 1981).

7. *Immobility* is a common cause of chest com-plications in orthopaedic patients. *Change of posi-tion in bed* is essential; sometimes a patient in a heavy plaster jacket or spica has claustrophobic manifestations and 'cannot breathe'. Medical

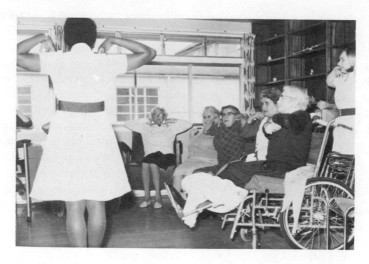

Fig. 5.1 Let's get moving! Exercises are very important for elderly patients.

advice might be required, with administration of a tranquiliser. In the meantime, *change of position* e.g. from the supine to the side-lying or semi-recumbent position, a supply of 'fresh air' from an open window or supplied by a fan, together with relief of pressure on the chest from the edge of a heavy plaster by placing pillows beneath the lumbar spine or even sitting the patient up in a chair or on a stool, for example, the patient in a plaster jacket; the patient in a hip spica may be allowed to stand if the plaster is dry and the doctor gives permission.

Breathing exercises are often the key to the prevention of respiratory complications. For obvious reasons, they cannot be given to unconscious patients and very young children; very old patients may be unable to co-operate; these patients, and those with inadequate respiratory function because of paralysis of the intercostal and/or abdominal muscles require special exercises and chest manipulations to ensure adequate ventilation of the lungs.

Similarly patients with deformity of the thorax may require specialised exercises taught by a physiotherapist; those with established chest conditions such as asthma and emphysema are also helped by specialised physiotherapeutic techniques.

Surgery requires thorough pre-operative investigation of the respiratory state, especially for those patients 'at risk', as already mentioned. Breathing exercises are learned more easily pre-operatively rather than in the presence of a painful surgical wound.

Breathing exercises are aimed at expansion of the whole lung. Unless encouraged, some of our patients use only the uppermost parts of the chest. To encourage deep breathing, place the hands on either side of the ribs and instruct the patient— 'breathe in and push my hands away . . . breathe out . . . and relax.' After each deep breath, taken slowly in and out, there should be complete relaxation; repeat 3–4 times, observing the patient carefully meantime. Then place a hand below the sternum and repeat the instruction—'breath in, push my hand away . . . breathe out and relax'— These exercises ensure maximum excursion of the diaphragm and maximum aeration of the lungs. It should be noted that in some cases abdominal distention may interfere with diaphragmatic excursion and increase respiratory embarrassment; if not relieved by change of position, the use of a flatus tube may be required. Finally in connection with immobility, it should be noted that talking, singing, laughing and crying help to ventilate the lungs. The lesson to be learned is that patients at risk should not be left unattended for long periods and may need to be 'roused up' at intervals to prevent consolidation of the lungs as well as other complications associated with immobility. It should be noted here that breathing exercises not only expand the lungs but assist in venous return to the heart, so helping to prevent deep vein thrombosis.

NUTRITION

Assisting patient with eating and drinking

In this connection we see once more the variations in our patients' needs according to age, pathological state and degree of dependence; nutrition is of equal importance to them all, whether they are fed by the intravenous or intragastric route or by natural means. Yet it has been said that 'there is ample evidence to suggest that nurses do not give high priority to the nutritional aspect of nursing care' (Jones, 1980). The same author states that 'ward sisters are more concerned about special diets and take no account of patients' normal needs'. Furthermore it has been stated that 'Nurse education devotes little time to the nutritional requirements of patients who do not require a therapeutic diet'. Consequently, 'nurses may be less aware of the need to ensure that their patients receive an adequate diet' (Coates, 1984). Concern for this aspect of patient care is reflected in the number of articles on this topic listed in the Bibliography. The majority of our patients with feeding problems have some physical disability, either temporary or permanent which prevents them from taking food and drink in the normal manner.

A meal-time should be an enjoyable event in the hospital ward as well as in the home. This is especially important to the long-stay patient so that treatment and other interruptions should be prevented as far as possible from interfering with patients' meal-times. The patient who is allowed up, whether afoot or in a wheelchair should take the main meal of the day in a dining room rather than from a tray placed at the bedside.

Many of our patients have no specific medical ailments and are blessed with normal healthy appetites; there is a danger however in an era of 'plated meals', often distributed by non-nursing staff, that the nutritional needs of a patient are overlooked; a 'full diet' ordered for a patient will not benefit him if he does not eat it; on the other hand, obesity, diabetes or some other condition may require special dietary measures, and some of our patients may be immigrants with dietary problems associated with different customs and religious beliefs which must be respected. Beck (1978) discusses the composition of a routine hospital diet for different age-groups and points out that menus should provide sufficient choice to enable the nurse to meet the needs of each patient, giving as examples the old and feeble without teeth, and those at varying stages of recovery from illness or injury. The importance of good simple cooking and of the attractive appearance of food is also stressed by this author; co-operation between nurses, nutritionist and Catering Manager is axiomatic.

Feeding the helpless patient

Feeding problems in certain groups of patients, for example, children, and the paralysed and the aged will be referred to again in later chapters.

In regard to children, Winkler (1977) poses a question in the *Nursing Times*—'How well fed are our children?'—and goes on to discuss some of today's problems in this connection, and to point out that affluence does not automatically ensure a correct diet for a child; despite the efforts of health educationists it has been reported that obesity is a big problem among school children (Wells, 1978). More recently Sturt (1984), has expressed concern regarding the nutritional state and future eating habits of school children consuming mainly 'junk' food especially 'chips with everything', or without anything else. In this report, the passing of the traditional school dinner is deplored (The Guardian, July 24th, 1984).

Elderly disabled people present special problems and nursing staff need to decide which patients can feed themselves and which need assistance, such as correct positioning and provision of special feeding utensils (Wainwright, 1978) (see Figs 5.2 A–F). Early training in the ability to feed oneself is also aided by special feeding utensils (see Fig. 5.3).

In some cases feeding by the nurse or by some other person is the only solution, though far from ideal, because an adult dislikes being fed by another and it does not improve the appetite. Some patients take insufficient food because of the effort required to eat it; this may do little harm in the short term but permanent weakness or disablement can lead to malnutrition, for example in the tetraplegic patient (Ch. 23). Then there is the patient whose handicap causes him to eat so slowly that the meal is cold and unappetising long before it is finished, so that the patient loses interest in food. In such cases the *occupational therapist* has an

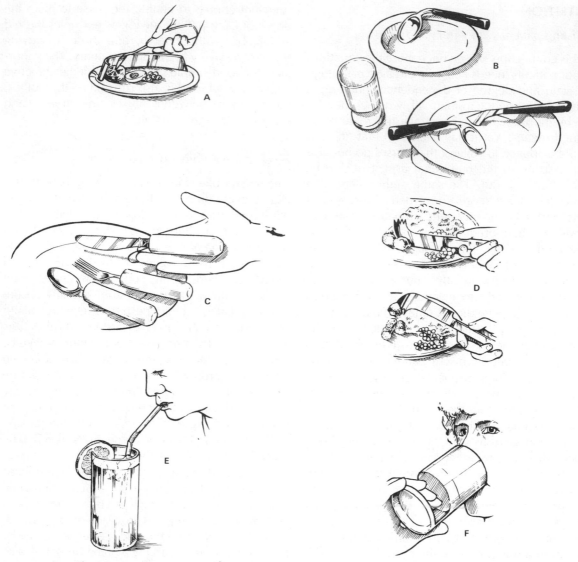

Fig. 5.2 A–F. Special feeding utensils for the disabled.

important contribution to make in devising aids to eating and drinking aimed at the restoration of this essential independence.

Many of our patients can feed themselves with imaginative help, such as changing the posture of the patient, where possible; placing the plate in an accessible position, and cutting up food where necessary. It is important however that the patient sees the complete meal (for example meat and vegetables) neatly arranged on a plate before it is prepared for eating. The recumbent patient may be assisted to eat by using a tilting mirror to reflect a plate of food placed on the chest (Roaf and Hodkinson, 1975).

Some of our patients face problems of tissue repair following major injuries or major surgery; moreover patients treated in prolonged recumbency lose calcium from the skeleton which is not replaced by dietary means; nevertheless once appetite is regained a well-balanced, high-energy, high-protein diet with added vitamins and minerals helps the body to re-establish its equilibrium and to use its natural powers of healing. Beck (1978) gives valuable advice on the dietary needs of the

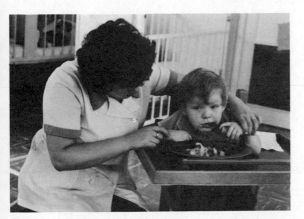

Fig. 5.3 A child being taught to use special feeding utensils.

injured patient, and also discusses artificial feeding.

Artificial feeding is also described by other authors. Hector (1974) gives dietary advice over a wide field; Roper (1971) gives a survey of means of helping the patient in eating and drinking, including advice on the needs of the disabled patient, who is our main concern in these pages; this author, as we do, favours encouraging a member of the helpless patient's family to visit at meal times to help with feeding.

Insufficient fluid intake may arise in connection with bed-fast patients who impose a fluid restriction upon themselves because of fear of using a bedpan, or of not being supplied with one immediately it is required. This must be corrected because immobilised and recumbent patients need extra fluids to maintain renal function and prevent the formation of calculi, and also to prevent constipation. As in the case of food, imaginative nursing help is required to enable the patient to drink, and the use of a straw is required for recumbent patients. In cases where a full fluid intake is essential, as for example, in the paralysed patient (Ch. 23), a fluid balance chart is mandatory.

Patients being fed by artificial means present special problems. Taylor (1973) discusses fluid balance, dehydration and fluid replacement in surgical operations and trauma, and at the same time warns against the dangers of over-hydration. In this connection, the importance of the fluid balance chart must be stressed, especially in post-operative patients, the recently injured, the paralysed and

the unconscious patient where an accurate record of fluid intake and output is essential.

ELIMINATION FROM BLADDER AND BOWEL

The nurse must know the 'normal' ranges of all avenues of elimination, including that from the skin, the lungs and by menstruation, so as to be able to recognise the abnormal, institute appropriate nursing measures, and seek medical intervention when required (Henderson, 1969). In this connection we will briefly discuss only elimination from bladder and bowel.

Assisting the patient with elimination

This nursing duty is often relegated to relatively untrained members of the staff; yet to the patient it is one of the most important, because in the normal course of events elimination is an intensely private function, and many people fear and dread this aspect of helplessness more than any other. It is bad enough to be unable to feed oneself; how much worse to be dependent upon others for the means to eliminate body excreta; at best it is embarrassing (Broad, 1982); at worst, humiliating and degrading. It will be obvious that certain patients have special requirements in this respect, notably the unconscious and the paralysed; we shall discuss them in later chapters.

In many of our patients the main problem is that they are wholly confined to bed; those able to sit upright and use a conventional urinal and bedpan are relatively easy to deal with, though only he who has himself maintained his precarious balance upon a bedpan and struggled to cleanse himself after its use is really in a position to understand the patients' difficulties, not least of which is the fear of upsetting the bedpan, and the embarrassment of producing eructating noises and disagreeable smells (Anderson, 1978). If this is true of the able-bodied how much more it is of the patient disabled by loss of normal function or by means of splints, plasters or traction.

Then there is the immigrant patient no longer able to assume his normal squatting position for defaecation, and who, moreover, is usually extremely modest.

In some patients the use of a conventional bedpan is contra-indicated, for example, following spinal surgery; in these circumstances, intravenous therapy is often ordered until bowel sounds are normal, abdominal complications less likely to occur, and post-operative pain is controlled; similarly an indwelling catheter may be *in situ* in the bladder so that elimination in the immediate post-operative period is not a pressing nursing problem.

Later, however, normal bladder and bowel action must be established and if the patient is not allowed out of bed to use a commode or lavatory he may be faced with serious problems of elimination, especially if immobilised in some form of splintage. Patients able to lift the buttocks from the bed by grasping a trapeze are relatively easy to manage and can use a conventional bedpan provided this does not lead to contamination of a surgical dressing, a splint or a plaster cast.

The recumbent patient unable to sit up is particularly vulnerable to elimination problems and it is well-nigh impossible to empty the bladder or bowel completely in this position, especially in patients who cannot 'strain' because of muscle weakness or pain. Smith and Wright (1984) conducted a research project on constipation in hospital patients and found that those most at risk were patients on traction (i.e. immobilised in bed) for several weeks. The most potent cause however was embarrassment when using a bedpan, with change in the normal bowel habit. These authors recommend encouraging patients to increase their fibre and fluid intake, encouraging mobility, and, in addition, nurses should try to make it as easy as possible for the patient to use normal toilet facilities. Enforcement of the recumbent position leads to the retention of intestinal gas, and many of our patients complain bitterly of indigestion and flatulence; in the normal seated or squatting position excess gas is expelled at the time of defaecation; sometimes the patient, even if semi-recumbent, must retain a limb in a certain position, for example, following hip surgery. In such cases, the use of a urinal is advocated for female patients as well as for males especially where movement causes pain. If a female urinal is not available one must be improvised from a receiver or other receptacle such as a small bowl or dish. An ordinary male urinal is often found to be satisfactory. In the home, the use of discarded domestic dishes, jugs, jars or cans will often solve the problem. In addition to preventing pain from unwanted movement, the use of a urinal prevents soiling of a plaster, splint or surgical dressing.

Technique of use. The urinal (Fig. 5.4A and B) of whatever design is pressed against the vulva while the patient makes a *conscious effort* to initiate and sustain micturition; this skill improves with practice and is well worth the time, effort and perse-

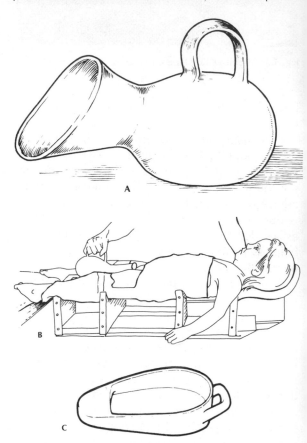

Fig. 5.4 A. Contamination of dressings, splints and plaster is prevented by the use of a urinal for both male and female patients. This urinal is especially designed for female patients. **B.** It is essential that a urinal is used by patients of both sexes to prevent contamination of splintage. This illustration shows a urinal being given to a patient on a plaster bed, which is very readily soiled by excreta. This little girl became expert at holding a urinal herself. Note that in this illustration the feet are in the equinus position. Except when being exercised they should be supported at a right angle to the leg. **C.** A shallow bedpan is recommended for recumbent patients to prevent contamination of wound dressings, splints and plasters. (From Chilman, A. and Thomas, N. 1978 *Understanding Nursing Care.* Edinburgh, London and New York: Churchill Livingstone.)

verance involved both on the part of the patient and of the nurse.

The bedpan. Broad (1982) describes a personal experience in using a bedpan after spinal surgery and developed her own technique. In reply to this article Tostevin (1982) suggests an alternative technique in a letter to the *Nursing Times* and this account is now quoted and the rolling technique is shown in Fig. 5.5.

> Putting a patient onto a bedpan following spinal surgery should not be difficult or painful for her. A simple and comfortable method is to use two pillows as support, bearing in mind the patient should have adequate analgesia to allow her to relax.
>
> Two nurses are required, and after explaining to the patient what will happen, she should be rolled onto her side keeping her spine straight (Fig. 5.5 A, B). A pillow is placed longways along her back.
>
> Two disposable bedpan inserts may be used without the carrier and put in the appropriate place at the edge of the pillow. The patient is rolled back on top of the pillow and bedpans, then the second pillow is placed longways under the other half of the patient.
>
> The patient is, therefore, supported fully along the length of her spine with the bedpan below the edge of the pillow. The problems of bedpans tipping or pressure on the suture line are eliminated.
>
> To remove the bedpan, the procedure is reversed. Care should be taken to hold the pan as the patient rolls off so that its contents do not spill.

Importance of an adequate diet and fluid intake. We have already referred to the importance of an adequate fluid intake in the immobilised patient in order to ensure drainage of the urinary tract and prevention of renal complications; fluids are also necessary to prevent constipation and the diet must be adequate in bulk and roughage. The patient is questioned about his bowel habits; many people worry quite unnecessarily about their bowels and overdose themselves with laxatives; others pin their faith to some special food or medicine. In general however, and in the absence of any relevant pathological state, all that is required is a regular habit

and an adequate intake of food and liquid, including roughage. There are occasions however, in extreme cases, where retention of urine requires administration of drugs or catheterisation, and where impacted faeces require manual removal. Some of these will be discussed in later pages. Further discussion of bowel management in the immobilised patient will be found in Ch. 9.

Patients allowed out of bed, even if not fully weight-bearing and for only a limited period of time, e.g. in a wheelchair, might require the use of a bedside commode or of a sani-chair which can be wheeled over a lavatory. Except in cases where it is either impossible or categorically denied by the doctor patients should be allowed this privilege. Even for the seriously ill, the strain of emptying the rectum while in a semi-recumbent position may be far greater than that required to get out on a commode for a bowel action (Henderson, 1969). This author also mentions the necessity for toilets designed for the use of weak and handicapped patients and various items of equipment in this connection are seen throughout this book. The publications of the Consumer's Association (1974) and of the Chartered Society of Physiotherapy (1975) also give valuable advice on the design of sanitary aids and of helping disabled patients to use them.

In conclusion, Anderson (1977) describing a personal experience, tells of the 'private ecstasy' of a patient able to use a normal lavatory after a period in hospital using 'the bedpan and the commode'. She mentions 'the bliss of a flushable pan, a locked door; privacy'. We who take these privileges for granted must be very well aware of the problems of the patients to whom they are denied.

MOVEMENT AND THE MAINTENANCE OF DESIRABLE POSTURE (assistance with walking, sitting, lying and moving from one to the other)

Orthopaedic treatment often means holding the body or part of the body in a certain position for healing. Good body and limb alignment is essential to prevent deformity. Whilst desirable posture of the body or limb can be maintained by splints or plasters, movement from this posture is not so easy for the patient. Nevertheless it is essential to prevent

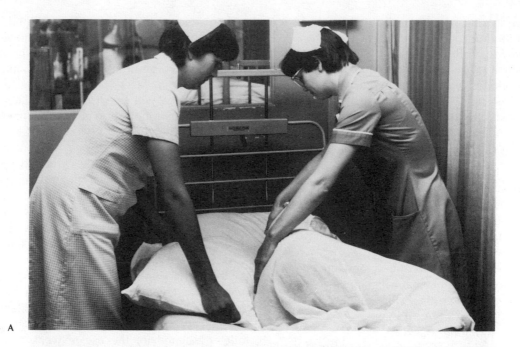

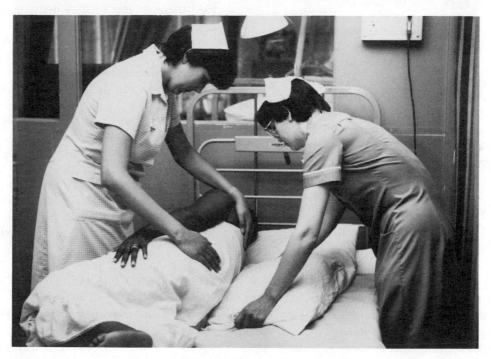

Fig. 5.5   A, B, C. These illustrations show the method of rolling the patient onto the bedpan (from the Royal Orthopaedic Hospital, Birmingham, by courtesy of Miss Patience Reed).

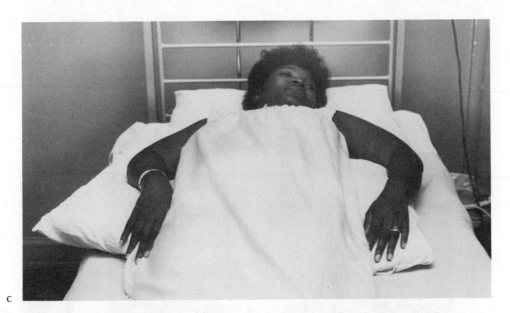

c

pressure sores, joint stiffness and contractures and also to prevent the complications of rest in bed shown in Fig. 2.7. All patients are taught and encouraged to change their position regularly; a *patient who cannot change position himself must have it changed by the nurse.* Sometimes the patient's position can be changed only very slightly, but even minimal change of position will help to prevent the complications already described. This is particularly important in the case of patients requiring special care, i.e. the very ill, the old, the young, the helpless, the unconscious, the paralysed and the mentally confused.

Importance of the prone position

Some illustrations of positions in which patients are nursed together with remarks regarding posture are seen in Ch. 2. But we would make special mention here of the importance of the prone position, especially for patients confined to bed for long periods. Many patients dislike the prone position because it limits their view of the environment. This can be avoided by the use of a hand-held mirror (Fig. 3.8) or by reversing the position of the bed so that the patient does not face a blank wall. Other patients who cannot tolerate the prone position are the obese and those with respiratory problems. Most patients, however, benefit by spending at

least a short time daily lying face down, with a pillow beneath the chest and the toes held clear of the mattress (Fig. 3.4).

Advantages are as follows:

—The act of turning helps to drain the urinary tract and aids the respiratory tract by encouraging coughing.
—Intra-abdominal pressure is increased helping expulsion of intestinal gas and also helping to prevent constipation.
—The spinal and gluteal muscles and unimmobilised knees can be exercised.
—Pressure sores on the sacrum, the heels and other vulnerable areas on the posterior aspect of the body are prevented.

Once accustomed to the position many patients welcome the change.

We have already referred to the 'orthopaedic eye' which is ever alert and to recognise and correct defects of posture in our patient with particular reference to the *prevention* of deformity. The classical example is of a patient's foot which is allowed to assume the 'drop foot' position, unsupported and unexercised, until the tendo-Achilles becomes contracted; and in time the deformity becomes fixed (i.e. structural) so that the patient is thereafter unable to place the foot in the plantar-grade position, i.e. flat on the ground for walking. Moreover,

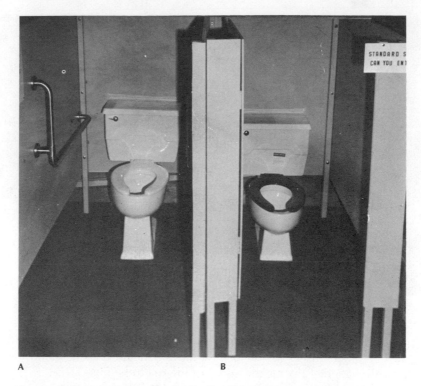

Fig. 5.6 A, B. Patients with orthopaedic disabilities require spacious toilet accommodation with readily accessible fixtures. Similar adaptations may be required in the home. This illustration compares adapted (A) with (B) standard toilet accommodation. (Courtesy Disabled Living Foundation.)

correction of the deformity might require surgery and a prolonged period of treatment which in turn delays rehabilitation for home life and work.

It must be recognised that effective handling, positioning and maintenance of muscle power and joint motion is not only a matter of theoretical knowledge but of practical experience; good movement and handling techniques cannot be learned only from a book; as in all practical skills, *practice in the clinical area* is essential, as is the teaching role of the physiotherapist. Darwin, Markham and Brysson Whyte (1967) illustrate the right and wrong way of handling a patient's limb, which is always lifted in its entirety, never by grasping only fingers or toes. Nurses should study 'Lifting, *Handling and Helping Patients*' (Downie and Kennedy, 1981). Special care is required in handling the limbs of young children, the aged, the paralysed and the unconscious or drugged patient; fragile bones are easily fractured, weak muscles and liga-

ments are easily stretched and lax unprotected joints easily dislocated (Fig. 5.7).

ASSISTING THE PATIENT TO REST AND SLEEP

When nurses discuss the means of helping a patient rest and sleep, the first thing that appears to spring to mind is to give the patient medication. Because it is an easy and quick way to obtain relief from pain and sleeplessness, patients (and nurses) are often tempted to use drugs unwisely (Henderson, 1969). These remarks indicate firstly the heavy reliance on sleeping pills and other medications among the general public, and secondly, the regrettable fact that nurses also regard them as the only means of securing rest and sleep. Moreover, in hospital the nurse is often in a dilemma, for even if she practises her nursing arts in an attempt to ensure his relaxation and comfort, the patient will often demand 'my sleeping pill'.

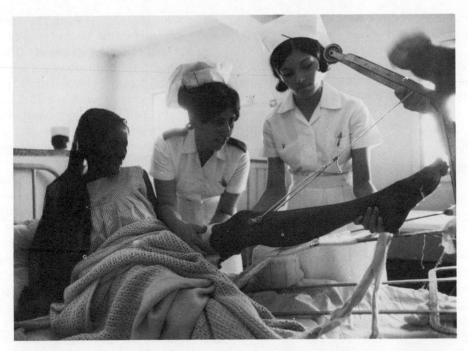

Fig. 5.7 The original caption to this photograph reads as follows: 'Ouch! Nurses at a hospital in Democratic Yemen delicately adjust the traction on a patient's injured leg'. It illustrates *careful handling* of a patient's limb. (Courtesy of WHO. Photo by N. Wheeler).

Relief of pain

Condon (1980) discussing the nurses' role in pain relief says 'So we see the nurse as observer, advocate and administrator of analgesia. But the nurse has one supremely important role. It is at the patient's bedside that the nurse can relieve pain and discomfort in a way uniquely her own. Regular turning and pressure area care, so often seen as a chore, not only relieves but often prevents pain'. This author also states 'in addition to this there are all the other aspects of basic nursing care which help the patient feel clean, comfortable and cared for'.

Armitage (1983) also discusses pain relief and quoting Roqas says 'the best approach is to demonstrate warmth, empathy and genuine regard for the patient'.

The orthopaedic patient who normally sleeps well may have great difficulty in doing so because he cannot adopt his normal posture on account of splintage, traction or following surgery, and it may be a day or two before he becomes accustomed to rest and sleep in a new position. We have already considered some other factors which interfere with rest and sleep and eradication of them, as far as possible, is an essential nursing duty.

Cunningham (1971) discusses deprivation of rest and sleep in a hospital ward and describes disturbances at night such as emergency admissions and 'well-meaning night nurses and sisters with squeaky shoes and flashlights'; while the squeaky shoes are deplored it must be pointed out here that the wearer of the shoes and wielder of the flashlight represents *nursing observation* which may not be vital to one particular patient, but to another, perhaps the difference between life and death. Moreover there may well be patients to whom the squeaky shoes and the flashlight are comforting and reassuring if not actually therapeutic—those, perhaps not ill in the medical sense or in need of specific nursing attention, but who are anxious, lonely, homesick and frightened.

Cunningham further qualifies his remarks by stating that 'a couple of nights of lost or disturbed sleep do little harm to healthy individuals' and goes on to suggest that 'part of the problem arises from having large wards of patients in various stages of recovery'. In an earlier chapter we touched briefly on systems of organisation of nursing care and mentioned *progressive patient care*, a system which entails separation of the 'convalescent' who need minimal supervision from those for whom constant and continuous nursing observation is essential.

CLOTHING

Assisting patients to dress and undress

In this section we will consider our patients under two headings:

1. Those who may be temporarily disabled because of their treatment in hospital e.g. surgery, and:
2. the permanently disabled who might require help with dressing and undressing on return to the community.

PATIENTS IN HOSPITAL

It is still the practice in some centres to deprive patients of their own clothing and among the excuses given are lack of storage space or lack of time to act as custodian of garments which might get lost, for example, in the laundry, and it is true to say that garments do occasionally get lost and irate relatives pursue the staff for 'Grannie's vest'. Yet there is nothing more lowering to morale than sitting around all day wearing a dressing-gown and bedroom slippers and often—in the case of ladies—uncovered hair-rollers as well. There is no reason why ambulant patients should not wear their own clothes, provided they are clean, because they are not merely a covering but are part of the personality of the wearer. One patient, describing his loss of independence in hospital (Macmillan, 1980) said 'Make no mistake about it, you're not free any more. They take your clothes away. You can only walk around when they say.' Unless there is some definite contra-indication, patients should also wear their own *footwear*, avoiding bedroom slippers (Swaffield, 1981). On the other hand Gabell and Nayak (1982) defend 'those Christmas slippers'. Their research suggests that sensible, well-cared-for slippers are actually beneficial for some

old people. This view is shared by Turnbull (1982) who recommends the bootee type of slipper with a zip or lace fastening. There is no reason, other than tradition, for compelling patients to shiver in pyjamas and dressing gowns if dress does not interfere in the slightest with nursing needs (Cunningham, 1971). On the other hand, many patients obviously believe that the very fact that they are in hospital permits them to wear only night clothes; they are sometimes reluctant to wear normal day dress and even more reluctant to discard bedroom slippers. This is perhaps because this mode of dress is associated in the mind with rest and relaxation; whilst we do not deny the patient rest and relaxation, we resist the attitude of mind that prevents him from wearing normal clothing appropriate to the time of day, to his treatment and activities and, moreover, encourages him in self-care and self-respect. The interruption of normal habits of dressing should be reduced to a minimum if we wish to prevent the patient's withdrawal from life (Henderson, 1969). The very minimum allowance of clothing ought to be slacks and shirts for men and the equivalent for women (Cunningham, 1971), and present day fashions and materials help us to advise patients in this connection; simple 'separates' made of easy-care drip-dry materials, and trousers for both men and women are both sensible and becoming, though one cannot always say the same of fashionable footwear. Clothing for patients, whether in bed or afoot, should not interfere with essential treatment and activities, for instance, passive joint movements or active exercises; nor should it interfere with inspection of a splint or plaster; it is often necessary to 'arrange' articles of clothing to accommodate a splint or plaster cast. It should be noted here that wearing a splint or plaster cast produces abnormal wear and tear of clothing.

It goes without saying that clothing should be sufficient to prevent chills but not so heavy as to produce over-heating; helpless patients unable to change their own clothes are very vulnerable in this respect. In cases where there is loss of normal skin sensation, as for example, in spinal cord injuries, the patient is nursed without clothes, but it should be noted that it is *cruel* to expose patients unnecessarily and the innate modesty of the individual must be respected.

Relatives or friends may ensure a regular supply of clean clothes and in this connection it is helpful if patients admitted from a waiting list are asked to mark their garments with the owner's name when they are less likely to be lost. In the case of a helpless patient, a relative may come to an arrangement with the nursing staff so that soiled clothing belonging to the patient is placed in a plastic bag to await regular collection for laundering at home. The helpless (and perhaps indigent) patient without this resource is entirely dependent on the nurse to choose his clothing from what is available; in cases of hardship in this connection the social worker should be informed.

THE PERMANENTLY DISABLED PATIENT

The Consumers' Association publication *Coping with Disablement* (1974) opens with this statement when discussing clothes: 'Most able-bodied people dress every day without giving a thought to how they do it. But dressing is a process calling for balance, reach, strength, nimbleness of fingers and some stamina'. The book goes on to describe suitable clothes and to give advice on the management of dressing and undressing for various types of physical disablement; this advice is particularly valuable to patients with a permanent disability living at home.

In hospital, the occupational therapist who is concerned with teaching activities of daily living is usually available to help patients likely to have permanent difficulties in dressing and undressing; but it is essential that nurses are aware of these difficulties and are prepared to meet them on the lines discussed in the publication named above and in others which will be referred to in Chs 34 and 35.

ASSISTING THE PATIENT WITH
MAINTENANCE OF BODY TEMPERATURE
WITHIN NORMAL RANGE BY ADJUSTING
CLOTHING AND MODIFYING THE
ENVIRONMENT

This note is included here as a reminder of the nurses responsibility only in connection with modi-fication of clothing and of the environment; pathological states which cause variations in body temperature will not be discussed here and this subject is well covered by Roper (1973).

We have already given a brief resumé of the helpless, immobilised patient's dependence on nursing aid in the matter of clothing. The environment of the orthopaedic patient has also been discussed briefly in Ch. 3 but it must be noted that the patient often has little or no control of it. The temperature of the environment may be acceptable to staff members busy about their work, but not necessarily to the patient who is immobile and helpless.

One can well imagine the misery of waking in the night feeling over-hot or cold and being so helpless and disabled as to be unable to adjust one's clothing, bedclothes or the temperature of one's room; however, patients able to communicate can at least make their needs known, but special vigilance and monitoring is required where communication is deficient or impossible, for example, in very young children, the drugged, the unconscious and the very old.

ASSISTING THE PATIENT WITH AVOIDANCE
OF DANGER

The environment of the orthopaedic patient has already been discussed briefly, including the danger of infection, with special mention of the role of the nurse in this connection. It must be noted however that control of the environment is never completely in the hands of the nurse. Ralph (1982) sums this up by saying 'charged with responsibility for achieving a suitable environment in which patients are nursed, she has no direct control over cleaning, catering and ward clerk services'. The nurse must rely heavily upon the hospital administrator, the hospital maintenance engineer, the housekeeping and catering services, and in particular on the integrity of those who carry out sterilising techniques, e.g. in a Central Sterile Supplies Department. On the other hand, she is often responsible for the supervision of cleansing and sterilising activities, for example, the operating theatre technician may operate the autoclave but it is the theatre nurse manager or her delegate who checks the contents.

Other sources of infection include animal or insect pests such as mice, mosquitoes, cockroaches and flies.

The nurse also has responsibilities in protecting patients not only from infection but as far as possible from the effects of administration of potent drugs and application of lotions (Roper, 1973). *Fire hazards* are also discussed by this author, who lays stress on the essential instruction of all hospital personnel in this connection.

Physical dangers in the environment include falls, and highly polished floors are forbidden; wet flooring is also dangerous and spillage of fluid, food or any other substance which might cause a fall is removed immediately; slipping on a banana-skin is a traditional music-hall joke but it is anything but a joke in the patient's environment. Burns and scalds may occur from sources of heat, including hot-water bottles; patients with loss of skin sensation require special protection, and it will be obvious that patients who are confused, mentally ill, or under the influence of alcohol or drugs also require special consideration.

A discussion on the *control of the violent or potentially violent patient* is outside the scope of this book, and advice in this connection is given in the DHSS Health Circular HC(76)11, commented on in leading articles in the *Nursing Times* and *Nursing Mirror* listed in the bibliography.

Castledine (1981) and Cardwell (1984) discuss this topic; in this connection the latter mentions the need for training and guidance of staff.

ASSISTING THE PATIENT WITH COMMUNICATION

'It is as easy to formulate some original thoughts on the subject of communication as it is to write a fresh poem on daffodils or skylarks' (Chisholm, 1976); but we must try to formulate some thoughts here, because nursing cannot be accomplished without communication between nurse and patient (Roper, 1973). Communication with the patient's relatives is also essential. A parent who is also a teacher and an educational psychologist (Dean, 1982) makes a passionate plea for better communication between professionals and the parents of a handicapped child, saying 'But most of all, training

should enable staff to make themselves known as friends and people who are basically interested in people—not just cases'. It goes without saying that in order to assist a patient with communication the nurse must him/herself possess communication skills.

Man has tried to communicate with his fellows from time immemorial, if only by means of the smoke signal and the tom-tom. It could be said that communication is both an art and a science which is never completely mastered, and this is much in evidence at the present time. Despite the advance of modern civilisation, effective communication between man and man, especially in large organisations such as the National Health Service, has paradoxically never been so difficult to sustain as it is today, because of the complexity of the system in which we work, the vast number of people with whom we have to deal and the speed and stress of modern developments and of our way of life, so that the eternal plaintive cry of today is that there is lack of communication (Goodwin, 1973). Yet in health care in any situation, communication is of vital importance; in this connection, the nurse is inescapably an interpreter (Henderson, 1969) as for example, between the doctor, the patient and his relatives; it will be obvious that this communication fails immediately unless it is first established between doctor and nurse. McGhie (1969) refers to *traditional* barriers to communication between medical and nursing staffs, suggest that they are due to faults on both sides and that they can be overcome by free discussion. Nurses cannot give patients correct information and advice unless the doctor's plan of treatment is clearly understood, and in wards where several doctors are involved it is sometimes difficult for nurses to explain variations in treatment, for example, why Mr X's patients are kept in bed for fourteen days following meniscectomy when Mr Y's are allowed out of bed in two days. Moreover, communication must include all those team-members who are in a position to talk with the patient because, to quote McGhie (1969) again, 'a lack of staff co-ordination in communication may also result in the patient being given conflicting information from different staff members'. The most common complaint from patients however, is of lack of information. The present author has been told by patients that they are convinced that there is 'a conspiracy of silence' regarding their conditions; another said that she obtained more information regarding her prognosis from the ward domestic assistant than from any other source. In this connection it did not matter that the information came from the domestic assistant because it happened to be correct; but it is all too easy for incorrect, garbled, and sometimes frightening information to be gleaned by the patient from various sources. On one occasion a patient was examined preoperatively by a doctor who gave him no explanation and who happened to be the District Coroner; the patient asked his neighbour in the ward to identify the doctor and explain the examination, and was told 'he's the coroner who examines you before operation so as to save time afterwards'. The patient was momentarily terrified and being a new admission, was not to know that his informant was, temporarily, the ward comedian.

Cartwright (1964) gives examples of patients stating their views on communication, including one who said 'I would like to be told after the operation what they had done, like. All the staff were the type you couldn't speak to a lot really. When I did once they just said "scrape". I don't know what that was except hearing old wives' tales from other patients'. This example indicates a serious breakdown in communication and one which we should make every effort to avoid; it has been shown that patients who are well-informed about their condition, for example, the nature of an operation, tolerate post-operative pain better than those not so well-informed (Hayward, 1975). It sometimes happens that even intelligent patients, well able to understand their condition, are often 'left in the dark' and staff may assume that such a patient will automatically know what is happening and what is expected of him when in fact this may not be the situation (Chapman, 1977). This author suggests that communication between patient and nurse depends not only upon the nurse's appropriate areas of knowledge but upon development of empathy, and goes on to define and discuss this quality, which, it is suggested, can be described as an attitude of receptiveness and availability, leading to the ability to 'step into the other man's shoes'. It also implies a 'caring' attitude and a sensitivity to the patient's needs. This desirable atti-

tude is highlighted by a letter published in the *Nursing Times* (1978) in which an experience is described by a lady who 'spent eleven dreadful weeks in hospital undergoing corrective orthopaedic surgery'. And who goes on to say 'Life was made bearable by two nurses—the day sister and an auxiliary who worked on nights. They cared. They cared about my pain, my fear, my depression, my inability to sleep, and did something about it.'

Communication between nurse and patient can be influenced by the fact that the nurse may find it easier to relate to some than to others; it can also be influenced by bias and by pre-supposed ideas; for example, in approaching a patient with a reputation as being 'difficult' (Stockwell, 1972).

The following has been described as a source of suffering in a hospital patient:

'Failure to communicate to the patient, immediately upon admittance, a simple timetable of events that lay ahead within the next 24 crucial hours. Patients desperately needed to know when they would be operated upon, when they would be given pre-medication and what this would involve. Surely it is not asking too much to suggest that every patient should be greeted upon arrival by the ward sister or a staff nurse, put at ease and given this information' (Cunningham, 1971).

Visual signals may be as important as verbal ones, such as those conveyed by facial expressions, eye contact, gestures and touch (Roper, 1973); the process of communication is three-fold—firstly, the sensory input of the message sent by sight, sound, touch, smell or taste; secondly the interpretation of the message and thirdly the response or 'feedback' which indicates that the message has been understood. Needless to say, the patient who is deaf or who has a speech handicap requires special consideration—for example the patient with a tracheostomy, with a head injury or with aphasia following stroke.

Stewart (1963) states that good communication is useless without *co-operation*, because it is essentially a two-way process. The same writer points out that barriers to communication exist where people have different backgrounds and experiences and that even those of similar education and background may make different assumptions and misinterpret messages.

Means of communication

The most effective means of communication is usually considered to be by word of mouth in a face-to-face situation. But this is not always sufficient; the message may be inadequately delivered or the recipient inattentive; or there may be difference in language, inadequate command of the language or of the terms used; it is easy to believe that people have understood what one has said; yet we have only to play the parlour game in which a message is whispered along a line of people, to know the garbled version which emerges at the end; often people hear only what they wish to hear; effective communication entails not only delivering a message but ensuring that it is understood.

But defective as it might be, face-to-face communication is irreplaceable, for example we would all rather hear bad news from another person, especially a sympathetic one, rather than from a telegram or some other medium. Communication by word of mouth is often effectively strengthened by written follow-up; an example is seen where a plaster cast is applied to a patient's limb and verbal instructions are given as to its care and the complications which may occur; in addition to verbal instructions, the patient is also given a printed leaflet which repeats them. Note that this *strengthens* verbal instructions, *never* replaces them (Ch. 6). Printed leaflets are improved by the additions of simple illustrations of the instructions to be followed; this is particularly useful where there is a language difficulty. *The Medical Phrase Book* (1978) published by the Health Education Council is very helpful, using several languages, with illustrations to 'tell us what's wrong in pictures', and in one centre, instructions to patients are given by means of a tape-recorder (Welford, 1975).

Where inadequate grasp of a language is a barrier to communication the patient's relatives may have a vital part to play, for example, an immigrant to this country with inadequate grasp of the English language may well have a son, daughter or grandchild able to act as an interpreter. Increasingly, nurses must learn to understand and communicate with people from other cultures (Dobson, 1983). Advice in connection with Asian patients is given in *Chat Sheet* (1982). Hughes (1982) in an interesting and thought-provoking article in the *Nursing*

Times makes a plea for inclusion of relatives in the care of the patient and describes their 'helpless frustration' if this is denied them.

Other patients can also be very helpful; hospital patients never tire of discussing their ailments with their fellows, although as we have seen earlier, they do not always obtain correct information by this means; in most instances however they have much to learn from each other.

It has been stated that 'the ward sister is a key person in the hospital communication network, the main link between medical and nursing staff, between senior administrative staff and nurses, and often between doctors and patients' (Cartwright, 1964). In this connection, we have acknowledged the fact that the doctor is often the co-ordinator of the therapeutic team and therefore, the manner and extent of his communication with nursing staff, with other workers, and with patients sets the tone and the standard of the level of communication between the patients and the team members.

ASSISTING THE PATIENT TO KEEP THE BODY CLEAN AND WELL-GROOMED

'One of the hallmarks of nursing since its inception has included assisting patients to meet hygienic needs when they are unable to do so on their own. *Nursing has changed, but this important aspect of care should still command the nurse's attention and concern*' (Wolff et al, 1978).

Inability to keep the body clean and well groomed because of physical disability can be very damaging to the self-esteem; in common with elimination, once childhood has passed, one's personal toilet is a private affair; physical disablement however, reveals the details of our toilet to others and we must often forego familiar routines and settle for the essential basic item . . . bodily cleanliness; and even this may be impossible to attain without the help of others.

Every nurse should be able to keep a patient clean regardless of his size, position, physical or emotional state (Henderson, 1969). These remarks are particularly relevant to orthopaedic practice, because a nurse trained in conventional methods may have difficulty in modifying them in relation to patients in splints, plasters and traction devices;

it is essential that what the patient can do for himself he must be expected, encouraged and helped to do; for example it is a waste of nursing time to bed-bath a healthy young adult whose only disability is that he is confined to bed with his leg fixed in balanced traction; on the other hand he needs privacy, a supply of essential toilet accessories and, perhaps, help in reaching inaccessible parts, for example the foot and toes of the immobilised leg. An ill, elderly or very obese patient, on the other hand, has different needs; the first-named may be too feeble even to wash her own face unless the wash-cloth is placed in her hand; the second may be quite unable to wash areas which can be reached by the more athletic, for example, the back, buttocks, foot and toes. Whenever possible, the patient himself should wash his own external genitalia, but if this is impossible it is an essential daily nursing duty. In female patients, the labia should be separated and the area gently swabbed with a damp, soapy cotton wool pad. Similarly in the uncircumcised male the foreskin must be retracted for cleansing purposes. Where possible the nurse should wear gloves but if they are not available the penis is handled in a towel or similar piece of cloth. Nursing situations where a complete daily bed-bath cannot be given must be accepted, but the axillae and in particular, *the external genitalia must be washed daily*, if only for aesthetic reasons. It does not matter if the feet are not washed for a day or two, but even one day's neglect of the areas mentioned is a failure in nursing care. Female patients immobilised by some means—for example, in a hip spica—can often reach the genitalia by using a long-handled domestic dish-mop rather than a bath sponge or wash-cloth, which in any event must be kept for this specific purpose.

The hair and nails require regular grooming, and in some centres the attendance of a chiropodist and of a barber/hairdresser for men and a hairdresser/beautician for women is a great help to the nursing staff and a morale booster for the patients; there is danger of infestation by lice in patients whose treatment includes immobilisation of the head (Roaf and Hodkinson, 1975).

The mouth, teeth and nose deserve special mention; there can be few things more demoralising to the helpless than a dirty mouth which one cannot cleanse oneself, or one more indicative of nursing neglect. The mouth toilet of the recumbent patient is described in Ch. 9; the use of an electric toothbrush may be indicated and the care of dentures is also outlined in Ch. 9. There are patients who cannot remove crusts that form in the nose by blowing into a handkerchief; these must be gently dislodged by the nurse, using moistened cotton-wool-tipped applicators.

For the patient who can leave his bed, by whatever means, in wheelchair, sani-chair or with the aid of crutches or some other walking aid, special adaptations to bathroom and lavatory may be required, as shown in Fig. 5.6.

PREVENTION OF PRESSURE SORES (BED SORES, DECUBITUS ULCERS)

A pressure sore is a localised area of tissue necrosis, due to interruption of blood supply which in turn leads to interruption of nutrition to the part. A review of the literature describes the prevention of pressure sores as one of the oldest nursing problems known to man, since they have been discovered in Egyptian mummies (Pinel, 1976). This author also quotes an estimation that about 25 000 people in Great Britain suffer from pressure sores.

Despite the antiquity of this problem it still exercises the minds of very many nurses, as evidenced by the vast amount of writing on the subject. This is listed in the Bibliography, and includes a series of six articles in the *Nursing Times* (1981) 'The perennial pressure sore', and 'Tissue breakdown' a Clinical Forum feature in the *Nursing Mirror*. Treatment of pressure sores in the community is also discussed in these journals (Hibbert, 1980; Bendle (interviewed by Swaffield, 1980). A pressure sore survey (O'Reilly et al, 1981) appeared in the *Nursing Times Theatre Nursing Supplement*. In nursing practice, they are a highly emotive subject because their occurrence implies nursing neglect and engenders feelings of guilt and inadequacy; even doctors, patients' relatives and patients themselves tend to regard pressure sores as failure of nursing, and the reputation of many hospitals and of particular wards within them has been damaged because a patient developed a pressure sore, whether or not it was actually due to nursing neglect. This is particularly noticeable when a patient nursed at home or in some other institution where pressure sores are avoided develops one soon after transfer to a different situation; the fact that the sore may not be directly due to nursing neglect and that there may be other contributory factors is often overlooked. On the other hand, this highlights the necessity for *prompt nursing assessment of patients at risk and immediate institution of preventive measures* (Fig. 5.8).

a patient with an infected pressure sore is a danger to others in a surgical ward. Then there are *socio-economic sequelae*; the annual cost to the nation for the treatment of pressure sores is quoted by Torrance (1983) as being in the region of £100 million per annum; the patient with a pressure sore cannot be discharged home so that the bed he occupies at public expense cannot be used for other patients awaiting treatment. Further, a long period

A		B		C		D		E	
PHYSICAL CONDITION		MENTAL CONDITION		ACTIVITY		MOBILITY		INCONTINENT	
Good	4	Alert	4	Ambulant	4	Full	4	Not	4
Fair	3	Apathetic	3	Walk/Help	3	Sl. Limited	3	Occasionally	3
Poor	2	Confused	2	Chairbound	2	V. Limited	2	Usually/Ur.	2
V. Bad	1	Stuporous	1	Bedfast	1	Immobile	1	Doubly	1

Key: total score of 14 or below='at risk'. (Report: An Investigation of Geriatric Nursing Problems in Hospital. Norton *et al.*)

Fig. 5.8 Pressure sore risk assessment form.

Ross and Wilson (1970) list the pressure areas and predisposing causes and point out that pressure sores occur not only over bony prominences but where two moist surfaces are in contact, for example, beneath the breasts and between the buttocks. These authors give warning of patients particularly at risk, notably helpless, unconscious or paralysed patients; those with general debility or with disease or injury of the central nervous system; those who are incontinent, obese, emaciated or oedematous or have poor circulation or metabolic disease; immobilised patients; and those in which convulsive movements cause friction.

A pressure sore is a calamity for various reasons; feelings of guilt and inadequacy experienced by conscientious nurses is only one of them. Other reasons include the following: the *comfort* of the patient is affected; there may be pain at the site of the sore and it may cause limitation of movement; then there is the discomfort of treatment of the sore, and the clothing or bed-linen may become soiled by discharge which is aesthetically displeasing to the patient and his relatives. The patient's *health* cannot but be affected adversely, since a pressure sore inevitably becomes infected. Further, large chronic discharging sores cause loss of body protein, which is seriously debilitating and which may even lead to amyloidosis and death; again,

of treatment may be required entailing prolonged separation from home, family and a job of work; a pressure sore might interfere with the rehabilitation of a patient and it may also preclude surgery; for example, the patient admitted with a fracture of neck of femur cannot be operated upon because of a pressure sore on the sacrum or the heel; or one who has had a successful operation cannot be rehabilitated for early discharge home for the same reason. On the other hand, it is all too easy to blame pressure sores on nursing neglect when there are other powerful factors which are not entirely in the hands of the nurse, for example, fever, serious malnutrition, vitamin deficiency, anaemia, cardiovascular disease, diabetes etc. Again, the patient may be so immobilised by apparatus used for orthopaedic treatment that prevention of pressure sores by nursing measures alone becomes well-nigh impossible, especially if the patient is also unconscious, paralysed, grossly obese or emaciated and/or has some concomitant medical condition as outlined above. Other contributory factors as already outlined are incontinence of urine and faeces, oedema, friction and mental derangement. There is no doubt however that the main cause is *prolonged pressure* on a vulnerable part of the body, notably the sacrum, the heels, the greater trochanters and in certain patients (notably the unconscious and the paralysed) the malleoli and the condyles of the femur.

PREVENTION OF PRESSURE SORES

We have already seen that the first nursing measure in prevention is *prompt recognition of patients at risk, and immediate institution of preventive measures*. For example, an elderly patient with a fracture of the neck of the femur is admitted during the evening shift; no active treatment is ordered by the doctor and if there is failure of nursing intervention the patient may be left to lie in bed, in pain, immobile, perhaps dehydrated, incontinent of urine and confused in mind, until the next morning; it may well be that the patient has sustained her injury several days before admission and may have lain for some hours on a hard surface; further she may well suffer from some concomitant medical condition. To delay preventive nursing measures until morning comes and active treatment is ordered will probably be TOO LATE, and a pressure sore on the sacrum or heel will be present or imminent. We shall discuss this nursing problem again in Ch. 21, but it is mentioned here in order to indicate the necessity for *immediate* preventive nursing intervention.

The main principles of preventive measures are summarised briefly below.

1. *The relief of pain.* Patients in pain will not move themselves and will resist being moved by the nurse. Simple splintage or traction which makes it possible to change the patient's position (even if only very little) should be applied forthwith; analgesics may be required and *attention* to the *general comfort is axiomatic*, including attention to the bladder and bowel and to the mouth.

2. *Change of position* (again, if only very little) at *regular intervals* is imperative; patients who cannot change their position themselves must be lifted, tilted or turned by the nurse. *Continuous pressure on vulnerable parts of the body, notably the sacrum and heels must be prevented.*

3. *The skin must be kept immaculately clean and dry at all times.* Moisture predisposes to pressure sores; incontinence of urine and faeces requires positive treatment to avoid contamination of the skin.

4. *The use of nursing equipment.* A clean, dry smooth bed with a firm base is the first essential item; other equipment is valuable in the prevention and treatment of pressure sores, including mechanical devices such as tilting and turning beds (Ch. 23) alternating pressure mattresses, sheepskin pads, ripple beds, water beds and air beds. It is imperative, however, to bear in mind that nursing equipment is only an *aid* and cannot replace the primary medical and nursing measures outlined above.

5. *Treatment of concomitant medical conditions*, for example, correction of anaemia, dehydration, vitamin deficiency, malnutrition; treatment of metabolic or cardio-vascular disease.

6. *Peace of mind* for the patient; those who are worried and frightened may be tense and restless, especially in old age.

N.B. Prevention of pressure sores in patients wearing splints and plasters is discussed in Chs 6 and 7.

Treatment of pressure areas by the traditional method of rubbing the part with soap and water followed by the application of alcohol and/or talcum powder now appears to be open to question and indeed, it seems illogical to wet the skin when moisture is recognised as a contributory cause of pressure sores; on the other hand accumulation of skin secretions or soiling by excreta are also contributory factors and the skin must be kept *clean* and *dry*.

Dyson (1978) reports a research project involving 200 aged patients when tissues over the sacrum were found to be actually damaged by rubbing, in contrast with a control group not so treated. This author says 'we now stress that change of position is the most valid of all the treatments with washing of the area if incontinence or sweating occurs'. It follows therefore that the chief benefit of the traditional routine 'back round' is that *the patient's position is changed, his bed is smoothed, his skin cleansed and his pressure areas inspected for premonitary signs so that further prolonged pressure is prevented.*

TREATMENT OF ESTABLISHED PRESSURE SORES

It has been pointed out that many ward sisters and doctors have their own methods which they have found to be successful in the past (Ross and Wilson, 1970).

Crow et al (1981) suggest 'an overall plan' and state that 'Although we are still a long way from full understanding of pressure sores, we know enough to say that every nursing unit should make it their business

—to know what factors make each patient potentially vulnerable to pressure sores

—to know the dangers of the furniture that is in use

—to understand the different methods of prevention as they relate to the different causes

—to ensure that equipment sitting in cupboards is both complete and in working order.'

Finally the situation is summed up in the statement 'it does not matter what you put on a pressure sore provided you do not put the patient on it' (Pratt, 1971).

ASSISTING THE PATIENT TO WORSHIP ACCORDING TO HIS FAITH

Patients wishing to attend religious services should be given every facility to do so, and should also be allowed visits from ministers of their own faith, if possible in privacy. Some patients in hospital who do not normally practice their religion overtly find a renewal of their faith and seek spiritual help in the face of illness, adversity and helplessness; conversely, others either have no faith or they turn away from it in bitterness and will not seek or accept its help. In the ward, it is our duty to show tolerance ourselves and perhaps to help our patient to tolerate a religious belief different from his own and to respect its laws and taboos. Richards (1977) in a series of articles in the *Nursing Mirror* describes the different religions we might encounter among our patients.

In some cases, a minister of religion can give not only spiritual guidance but practical help in family affairs and in solving social problems.

ASSISTING THE PATIENT TO WORK AT SOMETHING THAT PROVIDES A SENSE OF ACCOMPLISHMENT

Despite modern evidence to the contrary, some people regard work as a necessary (and perhaps even enjoyable) part of their lives. People raised in this idiom find that inability to work causes a deep sense of deprivation, frustration and futility, so that we feel that we 'are no good to anyone'. To some of us work is a habit, but both in ourselves and in our patients, idleness all too readily also becomes a habit. It will be obvious that the management of a patient in relation to work requires *nursing judgement*; it is wrong to expect the ill patient, perhaps in pain or with a serious disability, to 'work' until such time as his activities can safely be directed towards his rehabilitation for physical and socio-economic independence. On the other hand unless the patient is seriously ill in a medical sense, the habit of idleness must not become so established as to prevent the attainment of such independence.

In the rehabilitation of the orthopaedic patient, his most important 'work' is directed towards his own recovery, so far as this is possible. Medical, nursing, physiotherapy and occupational therapy resources are directed towards encouraging and maintaining old physical and mental skills and in learning new ones, and, eventually and where necessary, retraining the patient in activities of daily living and in work which will bring the maximum physical and socio-economic independence commensurate with his disability (Fig. 5.9). Further discussion of this topic will be found in Chs 34 and 35.

ASSISTING THE PATIENT TO PARTICIPATE IN VARIOUS FORMS OF RECREATION

In a previous paragraph, we discussed helping a patient work, and this is often closely allied to recreation. For example, a patient may enjoy some creative handicraft which at the same time is of therapeutic value. It is important to find something the patient likes to do; some, apparently, are quite happy to do *nothing*, but this must be discouraged. It has been pointed out that even aged patients benefit from 'meaningful and creative activity' (Brocklehurst, 1975). How much more, therefore, does the child, or the adult who is father or mother of a family. Physiotherapy and occupational therapy is valuable; it is the nurse's duty to encourage the patient to take advantage of such recreational

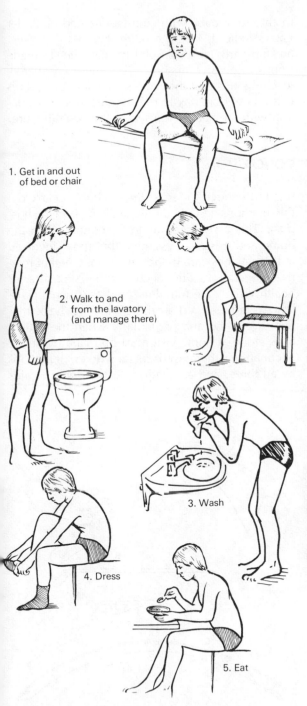

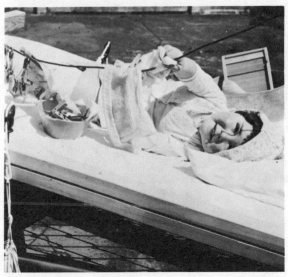

activities as are offered and in their absence, to arrange them herself. In hospital, these may be limited, but radio and television are valuable stimuli and library books and periodicals can usually be borrowed. Daily newspapers and other items are offered for sale in most wards. Patients can also play cards, chess or checkers or work at some handicraft under the supervision of an occupational therapist. We have already seen that patients confined to bed for long periods may suffer from sensory deprivation so that the introduction of any sensory stimulus is to be encouraged. *Visitors* provide valuable stimulus and contact with the outside world. Children require special consideration because play is essential to their normal development and also allows them to 'work out' frustration, anxiety and fear (Fig. 5.10).

Fig. 5.10 Traction and immobilisation must not rule out play, which is essential to normal development.

ASSISTING THE PATIENT WITH LEARNING

Life, even as a patient in a hospital ward, is (or should be) one long process of learning. Children in hospital for long periods must, in ideal circumstances, continue their education (Ch. 12); adults of good intelligence continue to learn from books and other media. But each patient should learn, if nothing else, the nature of his own condition and the aim of his treatment, and how to assist

1. Get in and out of bed or chair

2. Walk to and from the lavatory (and manage there)

3. Wash

4. Dress

5. Eat

Fig. 5.9 *Basic personal independence* is illustrated here. It is the ability to perform these acts *unaided*: 1. Get in and out of bed or chair; 2. Walk to and from the lavatory (and manage there); 3. Wash; 4. Dress; 5. Eat. (Adapted from *My Brother's Keeper* by Monnica Stewart, with the permission of the author and the Chest, Heart and Stroke Association.)

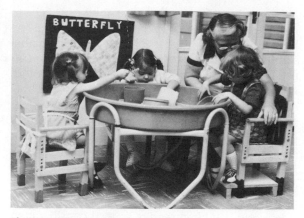

Fig. 5.11 Play-school.

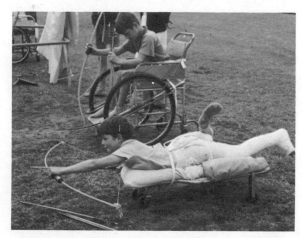

Fig. 5.12 Confinement to a wheelchair or wearing a plaster spica for some weeks/months need not prevent patients from enjoying sporting events.

in his rehabilitation for a return to normal life and work.

Each member of the therapeutic team has something to teach the patient and/or his relatives, particularly where there is likely to be permanent physical disability. Sometimes a nurse maintains that she 'cannot teach', because she visualises the teaching function as one which takes place in a schoolroom; in fact, she teaches continuously, if only by example. It is self-evident that no teaching, and therefore no learning will take place without *communication* between the teacher and the learner. Teaching methods are worked out according to the situation and the use of a slide-projector or tape recorder is very helpful; tape recordings have been used, for example, to teach a mother

to care for a baby with club-feet treated in plaster casts (Welford, 1975). Models (Fig. 5.14), posters and flip-cards are also useful and can often be made from inexpensive materials, but these are merely teaching *aids* and the most successful teaching is carried out from day-to-day in a face-to-face situation with the patient himself as the central figure.

CONCLUSION

It is not enough to '*assist the patient*' to carry out the functions described only while he is in the hospital. This assistance has to be continued in the home and it is most essential that those involved in the patient's care in that situation, whether relative, general practitioner, district nursing sister or health visitor, are fully informed as to what assistance is required. Where there is likely to be permanent disability, and particularly when the patient lives alone, a home visit must be made by nurse, occupational therapist or social worker, or perhaps by all three, and adaptations to the home or aids

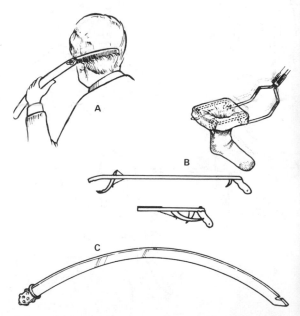

Fig. 5.13 Aids to dressing and grooming. **A.** A long-handled comb (Homecraft). **B.** A stocking-aid and 'helping hands' reachers for grasping objects (Mecanaid). **C.** A coathanger with the hook removed, fitted with a stationers thimble at one end and a notch at the other is useful for 'hooking' clothes over the shoulders and for dealing with shoulder straps (Nuffield Orthopaedic Centre).

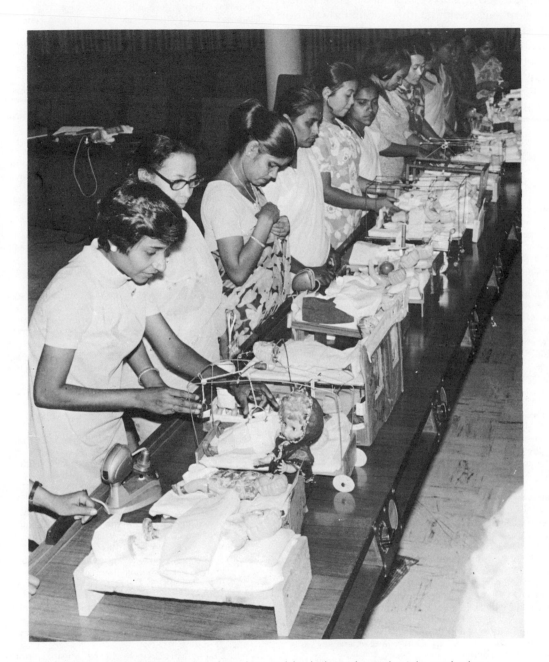

Fig. 5.14 Nurses in South-East Asia learn by making models which are afterwards used to teach other nurses, patients and their relatives. (Photo: WHO.)

on the lines discussed in Ch. 34, might be required. It should be stressed once more however, the aids are not advised until it is established that the patient cannot manage without them. Similarly liaison with employers might be required to enable the patient to return to work. In the case of children, continued education, companionship and opportunities for play are mandatory (see Chs 11 and 12). Further reference to resettlement at home and at work will be found in Chs 34 and 35.

BIBLIOGRAPHY

Anderson E 1978 The bedpan and commode. Nursing Times, 20 April, 684

Anthony D, Barnes E, Smith I, Wade W 1984 Pressure sores 1, 2 and 3. Nursing Times, 5 September

Armitage P 1938 Strategies for dealing with discomfort. Nursing Mirror, 30 March

Ascher R A J 1947 The dangers of going to bed. British Medical Journal 2: 967

Asian Diet Fact Sheet 1978 Nursing Times Community Outlook, 13 April

Autton N 1969a Pastoral Care in Hospitals. London: Society for Promoting Christian Knowledge

Autton N 1969b Pastoral Care of the Mentally Ill. London: Society for Promoting Christian Knowledge (SPCK)

Autton N 1970 A Manual of Prayers and Readings to the sick. London: Society for Promoting Christian Knowledge

Baldwin S M 1976 Made-to-measure care. Nursing Times, 25 March, 460

Beck M E 1975 Nutrition and Dietetics for Nurses. Edinburgh: Churchill Livingstone

Bendle (interviewed by Swaffield) 1981 Pinpointing the problem. Nursing Times Community Outlook, 14 May

Bleakley R (ed.) 1974 Despite Disability. Reading. Educational Explorers

BMJ 1978 Treating pressure sores. British Medical Journal 1: 1232

Börsig A et al 1982 Communication with the patient in the intensive care unit. London: Nursing Times, 24 March

Bowen M 1983 Fighting Fire. London Nursing Mirror, 29 June

Boylan A 1982 Assessment of the patient's physical condition. Nursing Times, 1 September

Broad J 1982 How to use a bedpan after spinal surgery. London: Nursing Times, 7 April

Capper W M Questions Colleagues have Asked me. London: Christian Medical Fellowship

Cartwright A M 1964 Human Relations and Hospital Care. London: Routledge and Kegan Paul

Cardwell S 1984 Violence in accident and emergency departments. London. Nursing Times, 4 April

Castledine G 1981 Encounters of the violent kind. London. Nursing Mirror, 16 September

Chartered Society of Physiotherapy 1975 Handling the Handicapped. London: Woodhead-Falkner

Chat Sheet 1981 reprinted from Asian patients in hospital and at home (Alex Henley (1981) Kings Fund) London Nursing Times Community Outlook, 17 June

Chilman A M, Thomas M (eds) 1986 Understanding Nursing Care, 3rd edn. Edinburgh: Churchill Livingstone

Chisholm M 1976 Communications—choke or channel? Nursing Mirror, 18 March, 70

Clark M O et al 1978 Pressure sores. Nursing Times 2, 3: 363

Coady T J, Bennett A 1978 Respiratory failure. Nursing Times, 25 May, Scan 17

Coates V 1984 Inadequate intake in hospital. London. Nursing Mirror, 1 February

Condon P 1980 Pain relief—the nurse's role. London. Nursing Times, 12 June

Consumer Publications 1974 Coping with Disablement. London: Consumer's Association

Crow J 1977 The Nursing process. Nursing Times, Publication

Crow R et al 1981 Pressure sores and their prevention. Nursing 26. Oxford: Medical Educational (International) Ltd

Cunningham C 1971 Traditional nursing—a harsh regime? Nursing Mirror, 4 June, 38

Darwin J, Markham J, Brysson W 1967 Bedside Nursing—An Introduction. London: Heinemann Medical Books Ltd

David J, Wells R 1984 Tissue breakdown. Nursing Mirror Clinical Forum, 7 March

Davies E M 1975 Let's Get Moving. Mitcham, Surrey: Age Concern

Deakin H G, Rann S E 1969 Artificial ventilation. Nursing Times Occasional papers, 27 March, 49

Dean J E 1982 Communication between professionals and parents of handicapped children. London. Nursing Times, 11 August

DHSS 1976 The Management of the Violent, or Potentially Violent Patient. London: DHSS Health Circular HC (76) 11

Dobson S 1983 Bringing culture into care. London. Nursing Times, 9 February

Dooley T P 1981 Fire! The nursing response. London. Nursing Times, 21 October

Downie P, Kennedy P 1981 Lifting, handling and helping patients. London: Faber and Faber

Dyson R 1978 Bedsores—the injuries hospital staff inflict on patients. Nursing Mirror, 15 June, 30

Fanshawe E et al 1978 Disability without handicap. Nursing Times Supplement, 17 August, 3-20

Gabell A, Nayak U S L 1982 Those Christmas slippers. London. Nursing Times Community Outlook, 12 January

Gent A, Sanderson P, Speechley V 1984 Intravenous nutrition. Nursing Mirror, 30 May

Gibbons C 1980 Religion as a way of life. Nursing, 16. Oxford: Medical Educational International Ltd

Glidden P, Powell M 1952 Called to Serve. London: Hodder and Stoughton

Goff M 1982 Speak to me, Nurse! London. Nursing Mirror Education Forum, 6 January

Goodwin P 1973 People with all the needs . . . Nursing Times, 9 August, 1039

Gore I 1976 Physical activity in old age. Nursing Mirror, 19 February, 48

Gould D 1983 A perennial problem. Nursing Mirror, 27 July

Grant P M 1976 Hospitalisation—and the elderly patient. Nursing Care Study. Nursing Times, 11 March, 379

Guilbert J J 1977 Educational Handbook for Health Personnel. Geneva: WHO Offset Publication No. 35

Guild of St Barnabas for Anglican Nurses 1969 To the Anglican Nurse. Foreword by S Reeve, Bishop of Lichfield. Revised edn. London: Church Information Office

Harvey S, Hales-Tooke A 1972 Play in Hospital. London: Faber and Faber

Hawker M 1976 Keep-fit exercises for geriatric patients. Nursing Mirror, 19 February, 50

Hayward J 1975 Information—A Prescription Against Pain. London: Royal College of Nursing

The Health Educational Council 1978 The Medical Phrase Book, 78 New Oxford St, London, WC1A 1AH

Hector W 1970 Modern Nursing—Theory and Practice. London: Heinemann

Henderson V 1969 Basic Principles of Nursing Care. Published for International Council of Nurses. Basel: Karger

Henkey A Practical Care of Asian Patients. London: Nursing 16

Hewitt F S 1981 Rôle and the presentation of self. Nursing Times, 28 May

Hibbert D L 1980 A sore point at home. Nursing Mirror, 7 August

Hibbs P 1982 Pressure sores: a system of prevention. Nursing Mirror, 4 August

Hughes Jill 1982 Helplessness and frustration! The relatives dilemma. London. Nursing Times, 9 June

Hunt P (ed.) 1966 Stigma—the Experience of Disability. London: Geoffrey Chapman

Johnstone V L 1959 A Hospital Prayer Book. Oxford: Oxford University Press, for the Nuffield Orthopaedic Centre

Jolly, H 1968 Play and the sick child. The Lancet 2: 1286

Jones D 1980 Careful Diet. London. Nursing Mirror, 24 July

Leaves A 1982 A question of fibre. Nursing Mirror, 6 January

Lelean S 1976 Ready for Report, Nurse? London: Royal College of Nursing

Lobo E de H 1978 Children of Immigrants to Britain. London: Hodder and Stoughton

Lowthian P 1982 A review of pressure sore pathogenesis. London. Nursing Times, 20 January

McGhie A 1969 Psychology Applied to Nursing. Edinburgh: Churchill Livingstone

Mirror leading article 1976 Management of the violent patient. Nursing Mirror, 18 March, 33

Moghissi K et al Reprint of 1977 The pleural cavity and injuries of the chest. Nursing Times, Publication

Morrew S 1982 Clinical Nurse Specialist in the nutritional therapy team. Nursing Times, 4 August

Macmillan P 1980 Strange encounter. Nursing Times, 6 November

Norton D, Maclaren R, Exton-Smith A N 1975 An Investigation of Geriatric Problems in Hospital. Edinburgh: Churchill Livingstone

Nursing Mirror Clinical Forum 1983 Pressure sores, 8 June

Nursing Times Community Outlook 1983 Vitamins and People, 8 June

Nursing Times leading article 1976 Common sense made official. Nursing Times 18: 393

O'Reilly M et al 1981 A pressure sore survey, Theatre Nursing Supplement, Nursing Times, 30 September

Pinel C 1976 Pressure sores. Nursing Times, 5 February, 172

Pratt R 1971 Nursing care of paraplegic patients. Nursing Times Publication

Procedures for nasogastric feeding 1984 Nursing Mirror Clinical Forum, 16 May

Ralph C 1982 Angels by any other name. London. Nursing Mirror 1982

Richards R 1977 What they believe and why—Parts I, II and III. London. Nursing Mirror, 14, 21, 28 April

Roaf R, Hodkinson L J 1976 Textbook of Orthopaedic Nursing, London: BIScientific

Roper, N 1982 Principles of Nursing, 3rd edn. Edinburgh: Churchill Livingstone

Roper N, Logan W W, Tierney A 1985 The Elements of Nursing, 2nd edn. Edinburgh: Churchill Livingstone

Roper N, Logan W W, Tierney A 1981 Learning to Use the Process of Nursing. Edinburgh: Churchill Livingstone

Ross J S, Wilson K J W 1970 Foundations of Nursing and First-Aid. Edinburgh: Churchill Livingstone

Rowe J, Dyer L (ed.) 1971 Care of the Orthopaedic Patient. Oxford: Blackwell Scientific

Rudinger E (ed.) 1974 Coping with Disablement. London: Consumers' Association

Smith B 1983 Danger: Points under pressure. Nursing Mirror, 20 April

Smith E M 1981 total parenteral nutrition—a team concept. Nursing Times, 19 August

Smith S, Wright D 1984 Constipation 1 & 2. London. Nursing Times, 30 May

Stanton B R 1971 Meals for the Elderly. London: King Edward's Hospital Fund for London

Stewart R 1963 The Reality of Management. London: Pan

Stockwell F 1972 the Unpopular Patient. London: Royal College of Nursing

Sturt J 1984 Eating themselves to death. Education Guardian, 24 July

Swaffield L 1981 Foot care—with older people in mind. London. Nursing Times Community Outlook, 9 September

Swaffield L 1982 Pressure for progress. Nursing Times Community Outlook, 10 March

Taylor S 1973 Harlow's Modern Surgery for Nurses. London: Heinemann

Thomson W 1978 Health Education. London. Nursing Times, 14 September; 21 September; 28 September; 5 October; 12 October; 19 October

Torrance C 1981 the perennial pressure sore. Nursing Times, 12 February—18 June

Torrance C 1982 Pressure sores; Aetiology, Treatment and Prevention. London: Groom Helm

Tostevin, Marlene 1982 Bedpans and spinal injuries. London. Letter in Nursing Times, 9 June

Turnbull P 1982 Slippers. London. Nursing Times letter

Wainwright H 1978 Feeding problems in elderly disabled patient. Nursing Times, 30 March, 543

Welford W 1975 Closing the communications gap. Nursing Times, 16 January 114

Wells D 1978 Nitty Nora—the reality. Nursing Times Community Outlook, 12 October, 293

Winckler I 1978 How well fed are our children? Nursing Times Supplement, 30 March, 3

Wolff L, Weitzel M H, Fuerst E V 1978 Fundamentals of Nursing. New York: J B Lippincott Co

Wright H 1982 Swallow it whole. New Statesman, 7 May

Wright L 1974 Bowel Function in Hospital Patients. London: Royal College of Nursing

Yearwood-Grazette, H S 1978 An anatomy of communication. Nursing Times 12: 1672

6

Plaster of Paris technique

Plaster of Paris technique is easy to write about but not so easy to execute; in fact it can be learned only by experience. On the other hand, every orthopaedic nurse must understand its basic principles and should be able to apply an effective plaster cast in an uncomplicated case. If practical experience under skilled supervision is not available, much can be learned from watching *practical demonstrations* given by an acknowledged expert in this field.

It is important to remember that expertise is not acquired overnight, either from a textbook or in the classroom, but in the process of the actual day-to-day application of every variety of plaster cast.

But even if expertise in the application of plasters cannot be acquired overnight, the nurse caring for patients wearing plasters must acquire, *from the first*, a sound knowledge of their needs with particular reference to recognition of and reporting on the complications which are discussed later in these pages.

Plaster of Paris consists of calcium sulphate, which is obtained as gypsum and rendered anhydrous by calcination; when mixed with water, it swells and sets rapidly, to form a hard cement.

Plaster bandages are made by rubbing prepared plaster into strips of crinoline. *Home-made plaster bandages* have now been abandoned in favour of proprietary brands (Gypsona or Velroc). Roaf and Hodkinson give a description of the function of plaster of Paris in modern orthopaedics, and Kennedy in her book *Orthopaedic Splints and Appliances* gives a comprehensive study of plaster technique (see Bibliography).

PLASTER SLABS

These are of two kinds:

1. *Dry slabs* are supplied by manufacturers in ready-to-use dispensers of 20 m lengths. They are six layers thick and 15 cm or 20 cm wide. Narrower slabs can be made by folding a bandage backwards and forwards on itself to the required length and thickness.
2. *Wet slabs* are made as required and applied at once. A plaster bandage is soaked, then folded over and over on itself on a glass or enamelled surface, and applied to the limb. There are various methods of preparing slabs (Kennedy, 1974).

REQUIREMENTS FOR APPLICATION OF PLASTER

1. *Bandages and slabs* of the correct size.
2. *Deep bowls or buckets of water* in which to soak the bandages. The water should be comfortably warm to the hand. Tests have shown that the ideal temperature is 24°C. This gives the best lamination of layers and therefore results in the strongest cast. This factor is sometimes outweighed by the need for a slower or faster setting time, and colder or hotter water is used accordingly. The water should be changed frequently, or the bandages will be slow in soaking and the centres will tend to fall out. When emptying buckets, drain off the water and empty the sediment into a dustbin, otherwise it will set in the drains. Most plaster-rooms are fitted with a specially built sink to prevent this.

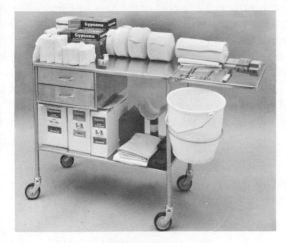

Fig. 6.1   Trolley set for application of plaster.

3. *Padding* under plasters is used in recent injuries or after operations, in anticipation of reactionary swelling. Unpadded plasters provide better immobilisation and are used when swelling is not expected. Too much padding can be as detrimental as no padding at all. Plaster is applied over stockinette, which is supplied in rolls of various sizes.

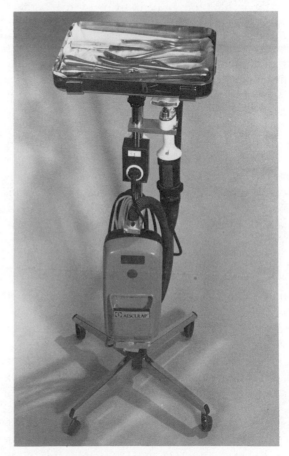

Fig. 6.2   Plaster room equipment: shears, openers, benders, knives, electric cast-cutter and vacuum extractor.

Bony prominences may be protected by grey felt, white adhesive felt, double-faced wool rolls or synthetic cast padding. These newer synthetic materials do not retain water and therefore do not become flattened and wet as does wool.

4. *Protective boots and aprons* are worn by the operators; gloves are required for all modern casting materials. Cotton or polythene sheets are used to protect bedclothes, and pillows covered with waterproof material and then with towelling are placed beneath wet plasters.

5. *Plaster knives* are required for trimming. A plaster knife should have a large handle which is easily grasped, so that it is not liable to slip. It must be very sharp. Linoleum or cobblers' knives are satisfactory; it is dangerous to use discarded scalpels.

6. *Any special apparatus*, such as an orthopaedic table, hip prop, or head-suspension apparatus, should be placed in readiness.

To soak a plaster bandage. Immediately before it is required, immerse the bandage in water until air bubbles cease to rise; lift the bandage from the water, using both hands, and squeeze it very gently towards the middle. Free the end and hand it to the operator. As the bandage is lifted from the bucket, a fresh one replaces it, lifted with a *dry hand*, or small lumps will collect on the bandage. *Do not splash* the bandages which are put out ready for use; a splashed bandage will contain hard lumps which will cause pressure sores and should be discarded.

Application of a plaster cast

In suitable cases, vesting or padding is applied beforehand; otherwise it is applied when the patient has been placed in position. *The surgeon will hold the limb in the correct position throughout the procedure, while the nurse applies the plaster.* It is most essential that the correct position is maintained continuously. A plaster cast will not benefit a patient unless it is correctly applied in a correct position. NEVER ATTEMPT TO CORRECT POSITION BY PULLING ON A PLASTER BANDAGE OR BY CHANGING THE POSITION OF THE LIMB WHEN THE PLASTER IS PARTLY APPLIED. Such attempts will be met only by disaster. Creases or ridges will form at the point where the bandage is pulled or where movement takes place, and pressure sores and/or interference with circulation are certain to occur. Routine changes of plaster are frequently delegated to the nursing staff, when a responsible person will hold the limb while the cast is applied.

To apply a plaster bandage. The bandage is *rolled* round the limb, and contact between it and the part to which it is being applied must always be maintained. *Do not pull the bandage away from*

the limb, or the edge may form a tight strand. The edge of a bandage should never coincide with the line of a joint. When changing direction so as to follow the contour of the limb, take a tuck at the upper or lower edge of the bandage. Always cover two-thirds of the previous turn, and smooth the plaster continuously with the free hand. A cast which is perfectly smooth is not likely to cause pressure sores, and the smoothing will cause each layer of plaster to adhere to the previous one. Air spaces weaken a plaster, and indeed, a complete cast should not be a series of layers, but one homogeneous mass.

Slabs. These are applied wet and sloppy. In limb casts it is usual to begin with a smoothly applied bandage and then with a smoothly moulded slab; otherwise they are applied at strategic points where added strength is required, for example, behind and in front of the hip joint in a hip spica. Cover the slab at once with a bandage, otherwise it will not merge with the rest of the cast.

Moulding. The plaster is very carefully moulded round bony prominences, using the thenar and hypothenar eminences of the hand rather than the fingers. Speed is essential when applying plasters, but the comfort of the patient is the first consideration. It is wicked to apply a plaster roughly and then polish the outside. *The patient feels the inside.* Aim for neatness and smoothness first, and speed will come with practice. Only experience can teach the number of bandages required for a particular cast; it should be as light as possible; a heavy plaster is not necessarily an efficient one.

Trimming. The edges of the cast are trimmed with a sharp knife. Edges should be smooth and rounded. Sharply-angled edges—for example, at the groin in a hip-spica—make the plaster more liable to crack. If stockinette is used, it can be turned over the edges and secured either with a strip of Gypsona or with flour-paste. Alternatively, it can be secured with adhesive strapping when the plaster is dry.

NURSING CARE IMMEDIATELY AFTER APPLICATION OF PLASTER

Handling

A wet plaster must be handled with the greatest

care. *The cast must be supported in its entirety;* for instance, never lift a hip spica by the leg only, or it will be certain to crack at the hip or the knee. Do not dig the fingers into a wet plaster; use the thenar and hypothenar eminences of a relaxed hand. Do not attempt to move the patient until the plaster has 'set'. Plasters set more slowly in a hot, humid atmosphere or if applied over a great deal of padding. Before the patient returns to the ward, excess plaster is cleaned from the skin with warm water, using no soap.

Drying

The appearance of a plaster sore is always blamed on the plaster-room staff. Though it may indeed be the result of a badly applied plaster, it may also be due to mismanagement during the drying period. A fracture board is placed beneath the mattress to prevent sagging of the plaster. The patient is received on to pillows, arranged so that while the plaster is supported in its entirety, bony prominences such as the heels, the sacrum or the iliac spines are not receiving direct pressure (Fig. 6.3). *In no circumstances must these prominences rest on a hard surface.* When possible, patients in jackets and spicas should commence the drying period lying on the face; four-hourly turning is essential for even drying. Drying of plasters is best done in the open air, or if this is not possible, in a warm room. *A wet plaster must not be covered*; it dries by the evaporation of moisture, and covering the

plaster delays the process. Areas not enclosed in plaster can be covered with a shawl or a blanket. A newly applied plaster feels very hot and later becomes intensely cold. A dry plaster is the same temperature as the patient's body and is resonant on percussion. The patient must be kept away from any direct heat source until the cast is perfectly dry as heating of the retained water can cause scalds. A plaster cast should be dried as it is applied, that is, as one homogeneous mass. *Heat-cradles are not used unless rapid drying is a dire necessity*, because casts dried in this manner are very brittle. Great care must be taken to prevent burns and overheating. The patient must not be left unattended whilst under the heat-cradle.

Turning

Patients in large casts such as jackets and spicas should be turned four or six-hourly to ensure even drying. Two nurses are required to turn a patient in a spica, and more may be needed. Lift the patient from the side of the leg which is enclosed in plaster, and roll him over on the free one. If turned on to the enclosed leg, the spica will crack. A double or one-and-a-half spica must be turned in the air. Sitting cases—for example, shoulder spicas—can sit in a warm room. All plasters should be allowed a minimum of 48 hours to dry, and large casts may require a longer period. Walking in a newly applied leg plaster is not permitted for at least three days,

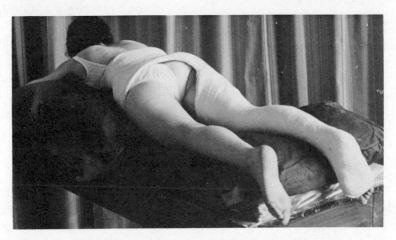

Fig. 6.3 Single hip spica supported on pillows. Note that the pillows should be covered with turkish towels to absorb the moisture from the plaster.

and in large casts it is better to defer weight-bearing for five days.

Inspection of the extremities

This is *essential*, especially after operations or recent injuries. Note the temperature and colour of the fingers or toes and whether there is pallor, cyanosis, swelling or loss of movement. *Report any of these findings at once.* The fingers or toes must be *warm* and *rosy* and must flush quick with blood on release of digital pressure. *Special note.* In dark-skinned patients test the finger or toe-nails rather than the surrounding skin. *Nail varnish must be removed.* If there is any doubt as to the circulation, it may be necessary to split the plaster; this must be done *from top to bottom* down one or both sides, and if there is no improvement *any padding beneath it is divided down to the skin.* Alternatively, the cast is bivalved and the top half removed. Some surgeons insist that casts applied post-operatively are split before the patient leaves the theatre. In this connection, or after recent injury, remember that intractable pain may indicate incipient ischaemia or even gangrene of the extremities (Ch. 19).

DAILY NURSING CARE OF PATIENTS WEARING PLASTER

The patient

Examine the patient himself; note the general appearance, question him as to the comfort. *Never ignore a complaint*, even if the patient seems unduly fussy. This is particularly important in every patient wearing a body cast. It has been said that 'many patients have suffered serious and irreversible complications because no one listened and responded appropriately to their complaints' (Luckman & Sorenson, 1980). In particular, any complaint of abdominal pain or discomfort should be reported to the doctor because of the danger of the so-called 'cast syndrome'. This is thought to be due to mechanical compression of part of the duodenum by the superior mesenteric artery, causing bowel obstruction.

Body casts may also be invaded by insects, e.g. fleas or bed-bugs, and can be extremely uncomfortable in hot weather. A little alcohol on a soft cloth may be rubbed gently on the skin at the edges of a cast and an electric or hand-held fan may be used for cooling purposes.

Sometimes severe skin irritation requires the administration of anti-histamine preparations.

Be certain that full movement of joints not immobilised is being preserved; if ambulant, note the gait; be on guard against deformity of other parts.

Stains on a plaster cast can be removed by gentle rubbing with a damp cloth and a little cleansing powder, e.g. Vim. Damp patches can be dried by means of the cautious use of a hand-held hair-drier.

The plaster

Examine the plaster for cracks or limpness; report these at once. A cracked or limp plaster is not functioning as a splint. A metal back-splint may be bandaged on to a cracked plaster as a temporary measure. The cast is then either renewed, or repaired with a plaster slab and bandage. Ambulant patients must be kept in bed pending repair or renewal of broken plasters.

PLASTER SORES

These occur from the following causes;

1. *Pressure*, due to carelessness in moulding, handling or drying, or to insufficient protection of bony prominences. Sores at the edge of a plaster may be due to roughness or tightness.
2. *Friction*, as when a loose plaster rubs against a bony prominence.
3. *Foreign bodies* inside the plaster, such as food crumbs, beads or coins.
4. *Delay in repairing cracks*, so that the rough edges chafe the skin.

INDICATIONS OF A PLASTER SORE

These include the following;

1. Itching beneath the plaster.
2. A burning pain; this is characterised and must on no account be ignored. If pressure continues, the tissues become anaesthetic and the pain disappears, because a deep sore has developed.

It should be remembered that a loose plaster is as likely to cause sores as one which is too tight.

3. Rise of temperature.
4. Disturbed sleep; the night nurse must report restlessness or night-cries.
5. Fretfulness, especially in children.
6. An area of local heat on the plaster.
7. Swelling of the fingers or toes, once reactionary swelling has subsided.
8. An offensive smell. Sometimes the first warning of a plaster sore is a faint but unmistakable smell noticed when the bedclothes are first disturbed in the morning, as when stripping the bed.
9. The appearance of a discharge.

TREATMENT OF A PLASTER SORE

Cut a window in the plaster by sawing out a small square over the suspected area. Lift the cut-out section away and gently remove the padding until the skin is exposed. Sloughing wounds require a moist dressing until the slough separate, then a dry dressing which is changed once weekly. The window is then packed with felt or wool, and the piece of plaster which has been removed is reapplied and secured with adhesive tape or a plaster bandage. This is to prevent swelling through the window. A sore due to the edge of a plaster should not be treated by cutting the offending edge horizontally. This will only produce another sore higher up. Split the edge longitudinally and insert a piece of adhesive felt, sticky side towards the plaster. Bind firmly with adhesive tape; this will relieve the pressure.

Dermatitis occasionally occurs during plaster fixation in patients whose skins are delicate. Treatment consists of talcum powder blown through a window in the plaster.

Blisters may appear over an unprotected area after an injury. Treatment consists of aspiration of the blisters and the application of talcum powder.

NOTES ON THE APPLICATION AND CARE OF SPECIAL PLASTERS

Wrist plasters. These extend from the head of the radius to the knuckles; if they are carried only half-way up the hand, the fingers will swell. Unless otherwise ordered, the plaster extends only to the transverse creases in the palm, so as to allow full flexion of the metacarpo-phalangeal joints and approximation of the thumb and little finger (Fig. 6.4).

Above-elbow plasters extend from just below the axilla to the knuckles, and unless otherwise ordered, are supported in a sling or collar-and-cuff.

Shoulder spicas. Unless the patient is under anaesthesia, a shoulder spica can be applied as he stands or sits on a stool. Otherwise it is applied on a shoulder prop; alternatively, the patient lies on a thin narrow plank of smooth polished wood which is placed so that it projects over the end of the table. The plank is then pulled out at the bottom of the completed spica. A supporting strut is frequently required as the weight of the arm piece tends to crack the cast, except when using the modern materials. It should be avoided whenever possible because it prevents the patient from wearing normal clothing. The internal epicondyle of the humerus may require protection by a felt ring. Where possible, drying is best commenced with the patient in the sitting position.

The spica includes the whole of the upper limb

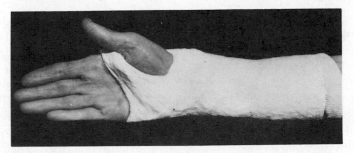

Fig. 6.4 Wrist plaster.

and must extend below the iliac crests (Fig. 6.5). The wrist and hand may or may not be included.

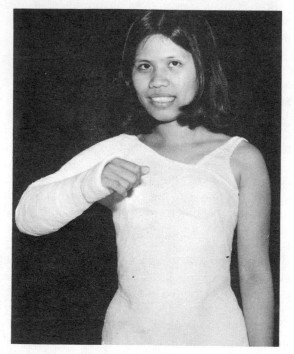

Fig. 6.5 Plaster shoulder spica.

The position of the shoulder is decided by the surgeon and is governed by the clinical and X-ray signs and the patient's age and occupation. The most usual position for an adult is abduction 70 degrees, flexion 40 degrees and enough external rotation to allow the mouth to be reached by the fingers when the elbow is flexed. In all cases, the elbow is flexed to the right angle, the forearm is held in mid-rotation and the wrist is dorsiflexed. Children are as a rule fixed in a greater degree of abduction than adults on account of the greater mobility of the scapula.

If the patient is confined to bed, he may be propped up with a back-rest and plenty of pillows, which are usually removed at night. The arm must be supported and the extremities watched for circulatory interference.

Knee-guarding or cylinder plasters. These extend from the groin to just above the malleoli. The plaster is applied over stockinette and the minimum of padding. A strip of felt is placed just above the malleoli and the plaster rolled on as snugly as possible. This must be a well-moulded cast to prevent

slipping down onto the malleoli and Achilles' tendon. Unless otherwise ordered, the knee is held a few degrees short of full extension.

Above-knee plasters. These extend from the groin to the web of the toes. The plaster is carefully moulded round the knee, the malleoli, and the arches of the foot, and must not prevent full flexion of the metatarso-phalangeal joints. The knee must have 5 degrees to 10 degrees of flexion and the ankle joint held at 90 degrees whenever possible.

Below-knee plasters. These are trimmed sufficiently at the top to allow full flexion of the knee. The head of the fibula and the malleoli may require protection. For walking plasters, the sole is reinforced and a plaster boot supplied. Alternatively a rubber sole, which covers the whole of the bottom of the plaster, can be incorporated into the cast. Rocker rubbers are not used because the concentration of pressure in one area of the foot leads to the softening and denting of the plaster. If a rubber sole is used, a raise may be needed on the shoe of the unaffected leg.

Plaster slippers are shaped as the name suggests and the toes are covered completely except for the tips.

FUNCTIONAL BRACES

The introduction and uses of functional braces are described in Ch. 19. This method of treating fractures enables the unaffected joints to be kept fully mobilised, while the pressure of the soft tissue splints the fracture. It is therefore very important for the Plaster Room staff to understand the principle and put it into practice.

Method of application

Femoral cast-brace. A doctor should always be present to remove the skeletal traction and maintain the position of the limb. A full length cast sock is applied to the limb. Felt or synthetic foam strips are positioned around the groin, above and below the knee, and above the malleoli (unless the foot is included). The cast is rolled on in two sections; the thigh section and the below-knee section. The thigh section must extend to the greater trochanter. A mould is applied externally to give the quadrilateral thigh shape and then removed. The centre of the patella is marked. Knee hinges are inserted into the alignment jig and this is positioned over the mark. The hinges are held in position by large Jubilee clips until incorporated into the cast, when the jig can be removed. A heel cup with ankle hinge is added and the patient cleansed of any plaster on his skin. The patient will then have a check X-ray before returning to the ward. See Fig. 6.6.

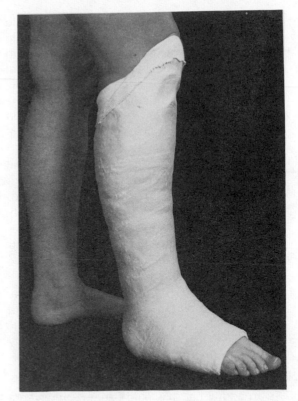

Fig. 6.7   Tibial cast brace.

Both these casts are usually made from the newer materials as the weight to strength ratio is better than plaster of Paris and mobility is improved.

INSTRUCTIONS TO OUT-PATIENTS WEARING PLASTER

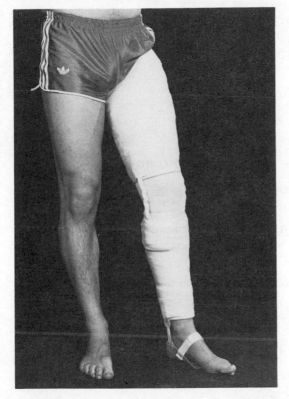

Fig. 6.6   Femoral cast brace.

Tibial cast-brace (Sarmiento). A cast sock is applied from the toes to above the knee. Extra padding may be applied to the head of fibula, spine of tibia, ankle and foot. The cast is then rolled on firmly but without tension from above the patella to the toes, leaving room at the back of the knee for full flexion. Moulding is done around the patella, into the patella tendon and around the malleoli. The top of the cast is moulded into a triangular shape in cross section, which compresses the gastrocnemius-soleus muscle mass, which in turn splints the fracture. A check X-ray is performed before the patient returns to the ward. See Fig. 6.7.

The patient is not allowed to leave the hospital or clinic unless it is certain that the circulation in the extremities is unimpeded. He is given the following verbal instructions:

1. The date of his next attendance at the hospital or clinic.
2. If there is swelling of the extremities, the patient may be instructed to remain recumbent with the limb elevated. Swelling of the extremities is not a contra-indication to exercises; on the contrary, their performance is then imperative because muscle activity increases the venous return. Even if there is no swelling, the patient is instructed not to allow the limb to hang down

whilst sitting about the house. It is useless to instruct the patient 'keep your foot up'. Explain that a foot in plaster must be raised at least to the height of a chair seat, and in the case of the hand, the wrist is raised above the elbow and the elbow to a higher level than the shoulder. If the fingers or toes become cold and blue the patient should report to the hospital immediately.

3. The fingers and toes are actively exercised at regular intervals, but never passively stretched; other joints not immobilised are also exercised. Patients in newly applied plasters generally attend the hospital or clinic daily for exercises until it is certain that full movement of all joints not immobilised is being preserved, and active use of the limb is encouraged.
4. The patient should report to the hospital or clinic *at once* if the plaster cracks, but he should not interfere with the plaster himself.
5. He is told to report anything which may indicate a plaster sore.
6. The plaster must be kept dry.

As an additional safeguard patients are given a written summary reminding them of the possible complications that can occur (Fig. 6.8).

REMOVAL OF PLASTER

Requirements

The following are required: electric cast-cutter with vacuum extractor (to comply with Health and Safety at Work Act), plaster shears, openers, knives, aprons and covers to protect operator and patient.

Procedure

A plaster cast is *bivalved*, that is, it is deliberately cut in half, not merely hacked off the body or limb. The patient lies comfortably on a table or couch of convenient height. Approach the patient quietly, especially if he is a child. Avoid noise, fuss and flourishing of implements. Explain to the patient what is about to be done, and reassure him. Place a mackintosh or cotton cover beneath the plaster. Mark in pencil the line you wish to follow. Insert the cutter blade beneath the plaster, keeping it flat

You have been given instructions in the care of your plaster. If you do not understand, please ask now.

Patient's Name:

Hospital No.:

Signature:

Date:

Checked by:

ORTHOPAEDIC HOSPITAL CLINIC

Do not wet, cut, heat or otherwise interfere with your plaster.

REPORT AT ONCE:

(1) If there is PAIN.

(2) If the fingers or toes become
    (a) SWOLLEN.
    (b) BLUE.
    (c) NUMB OR DIFFICULT TO MOVE.

(3) If the plaster cracks, becomes loose or otherwise uncomfortable.

Fig. 6.8 Written instructions for patients in plaster of Paris casts.

on the limb; do not dig the point into the patient. With the cutters at a right angle to the plaster, cut or nibble a millimetre at a time. Be deliberate; it is better to remove a plaster slowly than to cut the patient. *Exercise special care when passing over joints, in young children, in cases where there is loss of skin sensation, and in patients under anaesthesia.* In foot plasters, cut behind the internal malleolus and in front of the external malleolus. This exerts the minimum of pressure on bony points. Large heavy casts may require to be sawn, rather than cut with the shears. An electric cast-cutter is used in most hospitals and is particularly suitable for bivalving large heavy casts. A great disadvantage of its use is the noise of the motor, which often terrifies the patient, although there are now much quieter direct current models available. The problem of dust has necessitated the use of vacuum extractors, which makes this a very cumbersome tool to use (see Fig. 6.2). When both sides of the plaster have been cut, secure it with strips of bandage tied round it at intervals. Then encase the whole cast in a firm bandage. A bivalved plaster may be retained as a splint. The surgeon may remove only the top half of the case for inspection, or the limb may be lifted out altogether after pressing out the sides of the cast with the openers. *Never remove a plaster altogether without permission from the surgeon.*

CARE OF THE SKIN ON REMOVAL OF PLASTER

When plaster is worn for any length of time, the top layer of the skin cannot flake off normally and so collects beneath it. This dead skin should not be forcibly removed; it is better to wash the limb frequently with soap and water in the normal way, or soaking the limb in a warm bath may be allowed. Scrubbing the skin with strong cleansing agents should be avoided. If it is imperative that dead skin should be removed immediately (e.g. for an operation), then the area should first be soaked in warm olive oil, washed with soap and water and finally cleansed with Savlon.

PLASTER JACKETS, HIP SPICAS

Plaster jackets

These may be applied with the patient in one of the following positions:

> Standing between two upright supports. Sitting.
> Suspended by head traction (Fig. 6.9).
> Lying on a hip prop, orthopaedic table or Abbot's frame.
> Drying is preferably commenced either sitting or in the prone position.

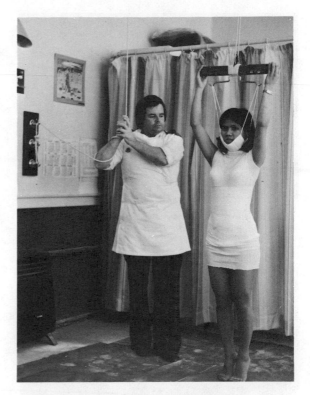

Fig. 6.9 Application of a plaster jacket in head-suspension. The patient is suspended so that only the toes touch the floor.

A layer of stockinette is applied and felt or synthetic foam is placed over the iliac crests and the spinous processes. This is then covered with a thin layer of cast padding. In female patients the breasts are either enclosed completely in the plaster or left out altogether; in most cases the patient is more comfortable if they are enclosed.

If the jacket extends over the shoulders, it is very important for the shoulders to be held down, to prevent 'winging' of the straps.

Abdominal windows. A window or 'blow-hole' may be cut over the abdomen in jackets and spicas; this is not a routine procedure but is necessary in emphysematous patients or to relieve abdominal distension. Except in an emergency, a window is not cut until the plaster is dry.

Hip spicas

These are applied on an orthopaedic table or on a hip prop screwed to an ordinary table (Figs 6.10 and 6.11): the shoulders are then supported on a

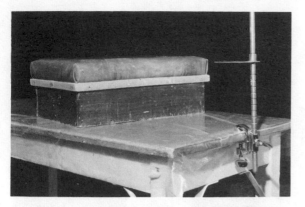

Fig. 6.10 The hip prop. The pelvis is supported by the prop and the shoulders rest on the box as shown in Fig. 6.11.

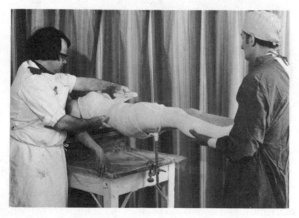

Fig. 6.11 Application of a plaster hip spica. The hip prop, and the box which supports the shoulders is shown in Fig. 6.10.

box of suitable height. The spica extends from the nipple line to either above or below the knee on the affected side; the foot may or may not be included. Double spicas enclose both legs, and both legs may be joined by a strut. One-and-one half spicas enclose the sound leg to just above the knee, the position of the limb will be decided by the surgeon. Unless otherwise ordered, the hip is held in extension and neutral rotation. The degree of abduction depends upon the condition; in the absence of specific orders, the limb is placed in the neutral position. The knee is held in 5 degrees or 10 degrees flexion, and the foot, if included, is held at a right angle and in neutral rotation. *The anterior superior iliac spine, the inner border of the patella and the inner border of the great toe*

must be in the same straight line. The spica is trimmed at the groin sufficiently to allow for nursing. It is trimmed round the buttocks at the level of the tip of the coccyx, and in a single spica enough to cut away in front to allow right-angled flexion of the sound hip.

A *Minerva jacket* (Fig. 6.12) or *doll's collar* (Ch. 22) is applied either in the sitting position, or the

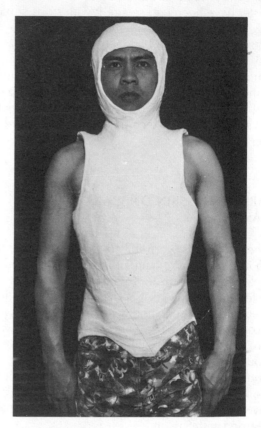

Fig. 6.12 Minerva jacket.

patient lies on a table with the shoulders supported by a smooth piece of wood which in turn is supported by a stand. The head projects over the end of the stand and the surgeon will hold it in the position he desires. Drying is best commenced sitting if possible, or, if not possible, in the prone position, and regular turning is carried out as already described. When the plaster is dry the patient may be allowed up, or better still, he will be more comfortable if it can be dried while he is ambulant rather than confined to bed. For further points in nursing please see the following pages.

Protection and reinforcement of a plaster cast

In some cases, particularly in children who are not toilet-trained or in those wearing leg plasters which are liable to wear out quickly, protection and reinforcement can be achieved by using one of the new synthetic materials described later in this chapter.

Care must be taken in the post-operative cases because many of the new materials are water resistant and will therefore mask any leakage from the wound.

NURSING CARE OF PATIENTS IN PLASTER JACKETS AND SPICAS

Patients in large heavy body casts require special care, and the reader is referred to Chs 3, 5 and 10, because the observations made therein apply with equal force to the patient being nursed in plaster jackets and spicas, and especially to patients confined strictly to bed. A plaster jacket, in particular, is widely used in various conditions: in infective lesions (Chs 16 and 17), in injuries to the spine (Chs 22 and 23) and in the treatment of low back pain (Ch. 28). In the early stages, before the patient is accustomed to it and particularly during the drying process, it is quite extraordinarily uncomfortable; the patient is rendered helpless by the plaster and until it is dry is quite unable to move so that he feels like 'a beetle on its back', impotent, frustrated and confined, and indeed, some patients develop claustrophobic symptoms and a few are quite unable to tolerate the situation. Most patients however suffer their discomfort with fortitude, especially if adequately prepared both mentally and physically, and those whose jacket or spica is applied in preparation for 'getting up' will welcome the change.

Patients needing special consideration are those recovering from operation, the very young, the elderly, the heavy and those confined to bed for long periods.

Preparation of the patient

The surgeon will explain the necessity for fixation, particularly if the plaster is to be applied post-operatively. If the patient has never been immobilised before, he will be more comfortable if an aperient or suppository is given so that the bowels are evacuated before the plaster is applied. This is advisable even in routine changes of large plasters, because an adequate bowel movement before the plaster is applied ensures that in most cases the patient need not be lifted on to a bedpan during the most important part of the drying period, i.e. the first 12 hours.

Position in bed

When the plaster is first applied, the patient is received on to firm pillows covered with turkish towelling as already described (Fig. 6.13). In children, the pillows are removed in 48 hours when

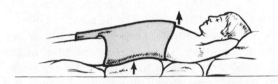

Fig. 6.13 Jacket spica. Note position of pillows so that it does not press on chest and abdomen.

the plaster is dry, but adults generally prefer to retain them. They are arranged so that one or two support the lumbar spine, one is placed beneath the shoulders, one beneath the knees and as many beneath the head as the patient finds comfortable. In the case of a hip spica, one or two pillows between the legs, one under the lumbar spine and two or three under the shoulders and head will enable the patient to lie on the side of the leg which is enclosed in plaster. *This manoeuvre is never attempted until the plaster is thoroughly dry*. Children, and such adults as can tolerate the position, should spend part of the day lying on the face (Fig. 6.3). Helpless patients in heavy plasters must be turned from front to back or from side to side four-hourly throughout the day, and at night are fixed up in the position they find most comfortable.

In very heavy patients wearing plaster spicas, suspension by means of weights and pulleys attached to an overhead beam may be ordered. This enables the patient to raise himself for nursing purposes and helps to prevent the complications of prolonged recumbency.

Exercises

Movement in bed is encouraged once the plaster is thoroughly dry; exercises given for joints not immobilised, and breathing exercises are practised regularly. The complications of rest in bed and of immobilisation are discussed in Chs 2, 3 and 5.

The daily toilet

This is carried out in much the same manner as that described later (Ch. 9) for a patient in a plaster bed, except that the patient can be turned on to the side of the immobilised leg (in the case of a spica) for washing and attention to the buttocks. The edges of the plaster are kept clean, smooth and dry and talcum powder is dusted along all plaster edges and between all skin-folds. Beware of overusing talcum powder. Excess powder will mix with perspiration forming beads which will irritate under the plaster. A pulley over the head of the bed enables the patient to lift himself for bedpans to be given. *Female patients must be taught to use a urinal.* It is imperative that the plaster is not soiled by urine and faeces; the head and shoulders are raised on pillows so that excreta does not flow upwards under the cast and plastic material (such as that used for food wrapping) is placed around the edge of the cast to prevent soiling. Soiled spots on a cast can be cleaned by means of a little Vim or other cleansing powder applied on a damp cloth. A localised wet patch can be dried by the cautious use of a hand-held hair-dryer, followed by the application of a sprinkling of talcum powder or a little white shoe-polish. Plaster 'crumbs' at the edge of the cast which may irritate the skin can be removed by the cautious use of a hand-held vacuum cleaner such as that used to clean the inside of a motor-car.

Complications

If the patient is confined to bed, be on guard against the following complications:

1. Bronchitis, especially in the very young, the aged, the corpulent and the alcoholic.
2. Renal calculi, from prolonged recumbency.
3. Abdominal conditions, such as acute dilation of the stomach or paralytic ileus. Abdominal

distension, pain, vomiting or constipation is a matter for concern and must be reported at once.

Further nursing details will be found in Ch. 10 and a useful booklet on the care of a child in a hip spica cast is published by the National Association for the welfare of children in hospital (Greenwood, 1980).

PLASTER BEDS AND TURNING CASES

A plaster bed extends from the seventh cervical vertebra to the tip of the coccyx. From this level two leg pieces extend to just above the malleoli, or, in some cases, to just above the knees. A head-piece may be ordered. The patient lies prone with his arms to his sides and his scapulae level. Be sure the head is central, the spine straight, and hips in extension, neutral rotation, and sufficient abduction to allow for nursing purposes (Fig. 6.14). The

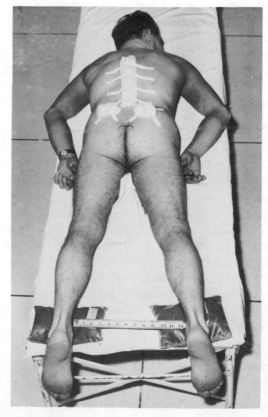

Fig. 6.14 Patient in position for making a plaster bed.

knees are slightly flexed and the feet hang over the end of the table. If the feet require to be supported, separate plaster shells are made when the patient is lying on his back. Footpieces should not be incorporated in a plaster bed; not only is it practically impossible to make them in a correct position, but the patient levers himself up the plaster bed by pressing against them. Moreover, foot exercises cannot be carried out and there is the possibility of increased risk of deep vein thrombosis.

Plaster bed method

Smear the patients back and legs with olive oil or liquid paraffin. Protect the hair with a piece of stockinette. The nurses stand on either side of the patient. Using the 90 cm roll, make a three or four layer slab covering the length of the patient's body. Soak this, and lay it smoothly over the whole body, making sure there are no creases next to the skin. Split between the legs and fold back. Continue with plaster bandages rolled smoothly to and fro over the back and legs. Be sure that there is a good overlap at the hips, between the back and legs. This procedure can be carried out by two people but is easier and quicker with four operators.

Finishing the bed

The bed remains on the patient's body until it has set. A plaster bar unites the legs. The bed is marked and cut out opposite the tip of the coccyx for nursing purposes, and lifted off *en masse*. It is then trimmed, dried and lined, either with felt gamgee tissue or with three layers of splint wool, and covered with stockinette secured with flour paste. It is most essential that there are *no wrinkles* in the padding; a smoothly made bed should in fact require no padding at all. When finished, it is mounted on wooden blocks made by the hospital carpenter (Ch. 9). In an emergency, it may be supported on firm pillows arranged to fit the curves of the bed.

To make a turning-case for use with a plaster bed or straight frame

Remove the clothing and protect the pubic hair with a thin piece of wool. Protect the posterior shell and the bed with plastic sheeting and proceed as for making a plaster bed. When completed, wash the patient, replace clothing and leave the patient comfortable.

Plaster shells

These are used to support the limbs and to prevent deformity. They are not suitable for *correction* of deformity; a complete plaster is always necessary. Plaster shells are best made over stockinette and a smoothly applied wool bandage. Enclose the limb with bandages as if making a complete cast, using a slab for strengthening if necessary. Mould the plaster very carefully round bony prominences. When set, mark the edges of the shell, and cut out with a sharp knife. When the shell is dry, turn the edges of the stockinette over neatly. The shell is either bandaged on to the limb, or canvas bands and buckles are incorporated in it. Velcro fastenings are very useful.

The newer casting materials make very good, light and strong shells as described further on.

THE USE OF SYNTHETIC CASTING MATERIALS

There are several new synthetic materials available as alternatives to plaster. Each major manufacturer today is striving to find the perfect synthetic cast material to replace plaster of Paris.

Advantages

1. A cast which is a third or less of the weight of plaster, whilst being three times stronger.
2. Weight-bearing in up to thirty minutes as compared to 48 to 72 hours.
3. Resistant to water when used with polypropylene stockinette and padding, therefore useful with incontinent patients. They can frequently be used for bathing and hydrotherapy.
4. Increased radiolucency for checking fractures without removing cast.
5. Greater durability for long-term immobilisation.
6. Less bulk (except Hexalite) so that the patient can wear ordinary clothes.
7. Clean to apply and wear.

Disadvantages

1. Not as easy to mould except for the plaster associated group such as Zoroc, Orthoflex and Crystona; therefore cannot safely be used with newly reduced fractures.
2. Cost of material. It is inadvisable to use them in a patient requiring early or frequent change of cast, because all these materials are very much more expensive than plaster.
3. There is an increased cost of accessory equipment such as specialised shears and electric cast-cutter blades.
4. Wastage due to premature opening of packets or short shelf life.
5. Sharp edges and rough surfaces can cause damage to clothes and furniture as well as the patient's skin.
6. Minor burns can arise when using Hexalite (from the water it is heated in), and from the exothermic reaction in some materials.
7. Skin reactions can occur from contact with the polymers in most modern materials and from formaldehyde in Zoroc.

Methods of application

Plaster affiliated materials (Zoroc, Crystona and Orthoflex)

These are immersed in tepid water and applied by the same technique as plaster. Orthoflex is plaster on an elasticated bandage which gives a closer fitting cast. This can be used on its own or with Zoroc (see Figs. 6.6 and 6.7) or Crystona which are resin based plasters. They take longer to set than plaster but allow weight bearing within half an hour.

Polyurethane impregnated fibreglass (Scotchcast, Scotchflex, Delta-lite and Dynacast)

In these materials the polymer is water-activated and sets within six to eight minutes of immersion. These need a little more expertise in application because they do not mould as easily and tucks often have to be held until bandaged over. Either a wet crepe bandage or hand cream is applied to smooth the final cast and quicken setting. These casts are all weight bearing in thirty minutes. An example of Scotchflex is shown in Fig. 6.15.

Resin-impregnated cotton bandage (Baycast)

Again the polymer is water activated. Do not open the packets until ready to use them. The water should be tepid. The hotter the water the greater is the exothermic reaction which can lead to burns. This produces a very light cast but does need more layers than the previous group. It is usually finished by applying a wet bandage until it has set and is weight bearing in thirty minutes.

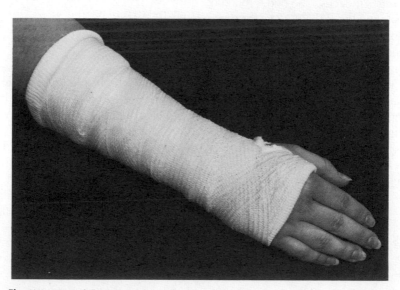

Fig. 6.15 Scotchflex.

Thermo-plastic materials (Orthoplast and Hexalite)

Both these materials are light but rather more bulky than the previous groups. These is a slight danger of scalding the operator or the patient as the water has to be so hot for malleability. These are commonly used for splinting (Fig. 6.16) rather than complete casts. The edges frequently have to be covered by protective tape to prevent chafing.

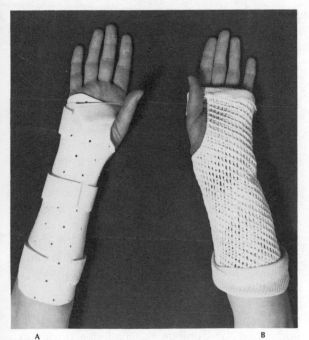

A   **B**

Fig. 6.16   **A.** Hexalite. **B.** Orthoplast.

Conclusion

Every plaster room operator will find reasons for and against using one or more of these materials.

The list of advantages shows the sort of patient for whom the cast outweighs the disadvantages.

Pre-fabricated braces

A short note is made about these because until recently the plaster room staff made Orthoplast braces to measure, for the patients with fractured humerus, ulna, femur or tibia. There are now available ready-made braces for this purpose which the plaster room staff or the orthotists can apply.

BIBLIOGRAPHY

Bradley D 1974 Checking a plaster—how and why. Nursing Times, 1 August, 710: 1190
Douglas R 1982 Baycast moulding Nursing Mirror, 21 July
Farrell J 1977 Illustrated Guide to Orthopaedic Nursing. Oxford: Blackwell Scientific
Greenwood A 1980 Your child in an immobilising plaster. London. National Association for the Welfare of Children in Hospital
Kennedy J M 1974 Orthopaedic Splints and Appliances. London: Ballière Tindall
Lane P 1982 New synthetic casts: what nurses need to know. United States of America. Orthopaedic Nursing 1(6): 13–20
Lavalette R 1982 Setting temperatures of plaster casts. London. Journal of Bone and Joint Surgery 64A: 907–911
Luckman J, Sorenson K C 1980 Medical-Surgical nursing: a psychophysical approach. New York. W B Saunders
Massie S 1981 Cast bracing of femoral shaft fractures. London. Nursing Times
Reid H 1984 Plastering in the 80s. Nursing Mirror Clinical Forum, 29 August
Roaf R, Hodkinson L J 1975 A Textbook of Orthopaedic Nursing. Oxford: Blackwell Scientific
Rowe J W, Dyer L (eds) 1977 Care of the Orthopaedic Patient. London: Blackwell Scientific
Stone E, Pinney E 1978 Orthopaedics for Nurses. London: Ballière Tindall

7

Splints and appliances (orthotics)

ORTHOTICS AND PROSTHETICS

Orthotics is the science of fabrication and fitting of a splint to an existing part of the body. 'An orthosis is a device applied directly and externally to the patient's body with the object of supporting, correcting, or compensating for an anatomical deformity or weakness however caused. It may be applied with the additional object of assisting, allowing, or restricting movement of any part of the body.' This definition is taken from *Classification of Orthoses*, published by the Department of Health and Social Security.

Prosthetics is the science of fabrication and fitting of an appliance to replace a missing part of the body, and the appliance is called a *prosthesis*, which may be, for example, a glass eye, a set of false teeth, an artificial leg or heart valve, or a joint replacement device (Chs 25 and 27). Artificial limbs will not be discussed in this book and are referred to briefly in connection with amputations (Ch. 33).

Persons trained in the skills required for this special work are called *orthotists* and *prosthetists* respectively; sometimes both types of skill are acquired by the same person when he is called an orthotist/prosthetist, and is supported by technicians trained to work in materials used in the fabrication of orthoses–prostheses, namely, wood, leather, metal, canvas, and plastics of various kinds.

Definition of orthotist. This again is taken from the publication referred to above. 'An orthotist is one who is qualified to measure fit and supply all types of orthoses.'

Plaster of Paris is used not only by itself in the form of a cast, but in combination with other materials as in a temporary prosthesis following amputation of a limb (Fig. 33.3) or in cast-bracing (Fig. 19.24). It is also used to make a solid mould or a cast of a part of the body on which a splint or appliance is fabricated to obtain a perfect fit (Fig. 7.14).

Home-made splints such as plaster shells for the foot or a cock-up splint for the wrist are usually made in the outpatient department or the plaster room. Physiotherapists and occupational therapists are adept at this work. Plaster spinal jackets and other spinal supports also come into this category. Cervical collars are frequently ordered and if required immediately, might be made of sorbo rubber or some other soft material or from other materials such as plastics (Kennedy, 1974).

ORTHOTICS

The splints and appliances (orthoses) described in this book are capable of many variations and improvements but the principles underlying their application and care remain the same. Moreover, there are numerous devices which are not described in detail but which can be found in excellent modern publications devoted entirely to this subject (see Bibliography).

Measurements are included here for interest's sake. They must be accurate, and in many cases a plaster cast of the part is required, especially if deformity is present. The measurements given in this book are not arbitrary, and will vary with different orthotists.

In general, nurses are not expected to measure patients for splints except for those taken from hospital stock, notably the Thomas bed-splint, Braun splint and perhaps a metal cock-up wrist splint (Fig. 7.1).

THE USE OF SPLINTS AND APPLIANCES

Splints and appliances are used for the following purposes, as already described in Ch. 2. We will however, repeat this information here.

1. To provide immobilisation and local rest by limiting movement of a part.

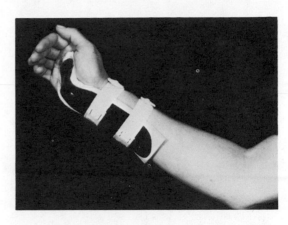

Fig. 7.1 Metal cock-up wrist splint secured by Velcro straps.

2. To provide fixed traction (e.g. the Thomas bed-splint) (Fig. 7.2D).
3. To provide a cradle for the limb in the application of balanced traction (Thomas splint, Braun splint etc.) (Figs 7.2 and 7.3A and B).
4. To prevent deformity, or to correct *mild* deformity, or, to retain correction when this has been achieved; for example, an inside iron outside T strap (short leg brace) is used for an inverted foot in hemiplegia (Fig. 7.7). Corrective/retentive splintage is also applied in club-foot. A Milwaukee brace is used in the treatment of scoliosis (Fig. 15.4A, B, C, D) and maintains continuous extension of the spine so that further deformity is prevented and may even correct itself as the child grows.
5. To relieve weight, as in a weight-relieving caliper (brace with ischial seat) (Fig. 7.2A) or Thomas patten-ended caliper (Fig. 7.2C).
6. To stabilise joints and to protect weak muscles, as in poliomyelitis or muscle weakness from some other cause, for example, spinal cord injury.
7. To maintain extension of the spine/or hips and knees for maintenance of the erect position with weight-bearing, as in the examples given above or in allied conditions; for example, spina bifida.

THE ROLE OF THE NURSE IN RELATION TO ORTHOTICS AND PROSTHETICS

As stated above, fitting of orthoses and prostheses has now become the province of specially

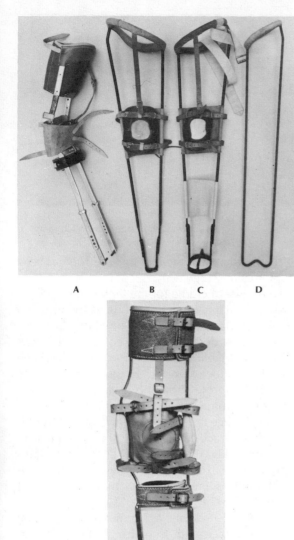

A   B   C   D

E

Fig. 7.2 A–E. Lower limb splints. **A.** Jointed bucket-top caliper. **B.** Walking caliper. **C.** Thomas patten ended caliper. **D.** Thomas bed splint. **E.** Band-top caliper (Taylor).

trained personnel. But the care of the patient is still in the hands of the nurse and it is an essential part of her duties to see that unsatisfactory orthoses/prostheses are not accepted. She will work closely with the doctor and the orthotist/prosthetist not only in the fitting of the splint or appliance and the care of the patient, but in teaching him to manage it. Where appropriate, this instruction must include the patient's family; the general practitioner and community nurse will be informed of any special problems relating to the patient's home-care.

General notes on splints, with related nursing management have already been given in Ch. 2 in connection with the provision of local rest for some part of the body.

The principles of the application and care of splints and appliances will now be described in broad outline. The management of particular splints is described in subsequent chapters dealing with the conditions for which they are used.

PREVENTION OF SPLINT SORES

This is an important nursing responsibility. Splint sores occur from the following causes:

1. An ill-fitting splint. One which is too small will cause sores from pressure; one which is too large will cause sores from friction.
2. Neglect of the skin or of the splint itself.

Care of the skin. Three essential points must be observed:

1. The *circulation* in areas subjected to pressure must be maintained. Where possible, the skin and soft tissues should be moved beneath the splint (for example under the ring of a Thomas bed-splint) so that slightly different areas receive the pressure of the splint. Patients should be taught to do this, but in very young, elderly, unconscious or unco-operative patients it must be carried out regularly by the nurse.
2. The skin must be kept scrupulously *clean* in this way.
3. It must be kept *dry*.

In general, when the splint is first applied, the areas of skin beneath it which are subjected to pressure must be treated every two hours by movement of the skin. Once the skin has hardened and become accustomed to pressure, treatment is carried out once or twice daily.

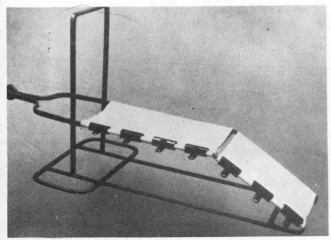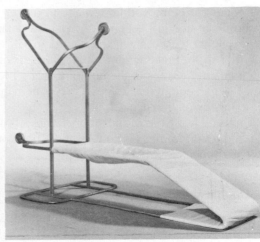

B

Fig. 7.3 A, B. Braun splint.

Dampness is a contributory cause of pressure sores. Large quantities of dusting powder should not be used, and spirit should never be used in conjunction with leather splints as it hardens, and cracks them. Grease is not used except in the case of young children or incontinent patients.

Care of the splint. This is inspected daily for signs of wear and tear. Any necessary repairs are executed promptly. Avoid careless handling which may damage the splint. *Cleanliness of the splint is as important as cleanliness of the skin.* Leather splints should be cleaned and rubbed daily with saddle soap to keep them soft and smooth. In children, splintage must not become outgrown.

TREATMENT OF A SPLINT SORE

If this calamity should occur, first consider the *cause* of the sore. Make every effort to remove it, whether it be a fault in fitting or cleanliness. The commonest cause is undoubtedly pressure, and this must be removed at all costs, the aim being to relieve local pressure by distributing it over a larger area. It is therefore quite useless to place pieces of gauze, wool or other material over a sore or an impending one. Rather, place protective material on either side or all around the area. Once the skin has broken, the sore must be treated with sterile dressings, and the surrounding areas only treated in the usual way. Again, movement of the

skin and soft tissues beneath the splint is most important.

The patient and his splint

It is important that whenever possible, the patient, his relatives and the community nurse should be taught the management of his splintage before being discharged from the hospital. The patient should understand the purpose for which it is worn, so that his co-operation is assured.

THOMAS STRAIGHT FRAME

This splint was originally designed by Hugh Owen Thomas as a means of transporting patients suffering from tuberculosis of the spine. It was once used in that condition to provide 'rest—enforced, uninterrupted and prolonged' (H. O. Thomas). It is no longer used and is mentioned here *en passant* for historical reasons, and because the abduction frame (still used occasionally) was developed from it (Ch. 14).

JONES ABDUCTION FRAME

This splint is still used occasionally in some centres in any condition in which traction and counter-traction to the hip joint are required; it is an excellent method of maintaining traction whilst allowing the patient to be moved from place to place, and it permits of free inspection of the part. A detailed description of its use will be found in Ch. 10, whether in the treatment of tuberculosis or other inflammatory lesions of the hip joints (Chs 14, 15 and 17) or in epiphyseal lesions (Ch. 16) or in injuries to the lower limb (Ch. 21).

There are two types of abduction frames: (1) double abduction frame; (2) double abduction frame with C-shaped cross-bar.

1. Double abduction frame

This presents two longitudinal bars, nipple bars, pelvic bars and knock-knee bars as in the straight frame. The cross-bar is pierced by a series of holes and the lower longitudinal bars are jointed at their union with the upper ones, as shown in Fig. 7.4.

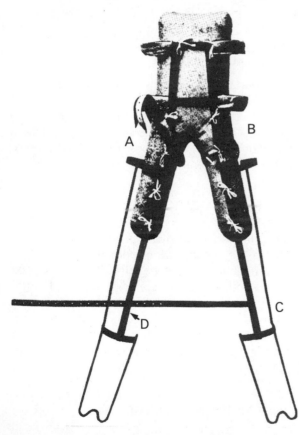

Fig. 7.4 Jones double abduction frame (posterior view). The screws are removed from the joints marked C and D. The degree of abduction is then adjusted at the joints marked A and B.

A further joint between the longitudinal and cross-bar permits of abduction of both legs to about 90 degrees. When adjusting the degree of abduction, the screws are removed from the joints marked C and D in Fig. 7.4. The lower bars can then be adjusted to the required degree of abduction at joints A and B. The bars terminate in W-shaped extension bows, to which skin extensions are fastened (Fig. 7.5).

The guards are made from tubular leather.

The saddle is made of high-quality leather and stuffed with lamb's wool.

The groin strap. This strap is placed on the sound side to provide counter-traction against the pull of skin extensions tied to the extension bows. It is made of boiler-felt covered with leather and is fastened by means of eyelets to metal studs at the back and front of the pelvic bar (Fig. 7.4).

Measurements
1. Nipple line to gluteal fold.
2. Gluteal fold to 4 cm above lateral malleolus.
3. Round fully expanded chest at nipple line.

In addition, state whether 25 cm or 30 cm extension bows are required, according to the size of the patient.

2. Double abduction frame with C-shaped cross-bar

This is used for gradual reduction of a congenital dislocation of the hip (Ch. 14) and permits of abduction of both hips to 180 degrees. It is similar in construction to the double abduction frame, except that the C-shaped cross-bar is pierced with holes along its entire length and is moveable at both ends as shown in Fig. 7.5.

Two saddles are required. One is made as for an ordinary double abduction frame, and is used until 50–60 degrees abduction is reached. The second saddle is made with the legs abducted 180 degrees (Fig. 7.5).

Measurements. These are the same as for double abduction frame and saddle.

THE THOMAS BED-SPLINT

The Thomas bed-splint is widely used to provide immobilisation and traction in injuries, e.g. frac-

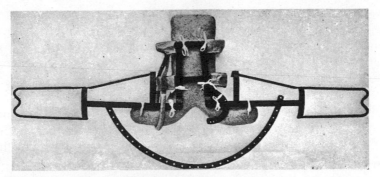

Fig. 7.5 Posterior view of double abduction frame with C-shaped cross-bar, allowing abduction of both hips to 180°.

ture of shaft of femur (Ch. 21). It can also be used in inflammatory lesions, e.g. septic arthritis of knee. Details of its application and care in this connection will be found in Ch. 16. It can be used to correct flexion contracture of the knee, as in rheumatoid arthritis (Ch. 25).

It consists of a metal ring padded with boiler-felt and covered with leather, from which two parallel bars terminate in W-shaped extension bows (Fig. 7.2D). Skin extensions are fastened to the bows to provide traction, which is countered by the pressure of the ring against the ischial tuberosity (Fig. 10.21). The splint is specially made for the right or left leg. The ring is not circular, but is so shaped that the larger half is at the back. The outer side of the ring is at a higher level than the inside. When choosing a splint from stock, place a tape-measure or piece of string across the ring between the parallel bars; whether it is a right or left splint will then be determined by the fact that the larger half of the ring should encircle the back of the thigh. The slings are made of leather, and support the thigh, the knee and the calf. They are secured to the splint by means of paper clips or safety pins.

Measurements. The patient lies comfortably on a couch.

Measure:

1. Round the thigh at the level of the adductor tendon. In obese patients, the tape-measure should be pulled tightly.
2. From the adductor tendon in the groin to the heel, plus 20–30 cm to allow for the extension bows.

State whether a right or left bed-splint is required.

WALKING CALIPER (LONG-LEG-BRACE)

A walking caliper or long-leg-brace (Fig. 7.2B) is similar in construction to a Thomas bed-splint except that instead of terminating in extension bows, the parallel metal bars are fitted with prolongations which slot into a tubing placed in the heel of the boot. The knee is supported posteriorly by a leather sling and anteriorly by a knee-shield, which is attached to the ring by means of a strap. A heel strap prevents the lower prolongations from slipping out of the tubing, and extension pieces allow of alteration in the length of the caliper. It is used for the following purposes:

1. To prevent direct weight-bearing on the lower limb.
2. To maintain extension of the knee.

The essential difference in the application of the splint for either of these two purposes lies in its length. If the caliper is applied to relieve weight, it must be of such a length as to allow the ring to be pressed firmly against the ischial tuberosity whilst the under surface of the heel is clear of the inside of the boot; the limb is then suspended in the splint and the body weight is transmitted to the ground by means of the ring and parallel bars. This is known as the 'long' or 'weight-relieving' caliper, and is used in the late treatment of tuberculosis or other inflammatory lesion of the knee joint (Chs 16 and 17), after fracture of the femur (Ch. 21) or in any other condition in which it is necessary to prevent direct weight-bearing through the knee joint.

The 'short' or 'non-weight-relieving' caliper is ordered in cases of poliomyelitis affecting the quadriceps (Ch. 18), in spastic paralysis (Ch. 14) or in any other condition in which it is desirable to protect the knee and hold it in extension whilst at the same time permitting weight-bearing. it should be of such a length as to allow the ring to fit comfortably in the groin, while the under surface of the heel is in contact with the inside of the boot.

Measurements

1. Round the thigh at the level of the adductor tendon.
2. From the adductor tendon in the groin to the heel, with the foot held in right-angled dorsiflexion.

If the caliper is to be weight-relieving, add 1–2 cm according to the size of the patient.

State whether a right or left caliper is required; the boot is tubed in readiness.

BUCKET-TOP CALIPER (BRACE WITH ISCHIAL SEAT)

The construction of this splint is similar to that of an ordinary caliper, except that a leather bucket encases the top of the limb instead of the ring. The leather bucket has a turned-over lip posteriorly to support the ischial tuberosity (Fig. 7.2A). It is used for conditions already mentioned in connection with an ordinary caliper, but this type is chosen for aged or obese patients in whom an ordinary ring would be uncomfortable.

Measurements. These are as before. In addition, a plaster cast is taken of the patient's thigh. In some centres, an aluminium mould is used instead of a plaster cast.

JOINTED CALIPER

This may be of the ordinary or bucket-top variety, and presents a knee-joint which can be manipulated by the patient (Fig. 7.2A). The degree of flexion allowed is decided by the surgeon. It is used in cases where a certain degree of movement with protection is desired, for example, in poliomyelitis affecting the quadriceps (Ch. 18) or in cases of osteo-arthritis of the knee-joint (Ch. 27).

Measurements. These are as already described.

A paper tracing of the limb is essential, and in most cases a cast is necessary, especially if deformity is present.

THE THOMAS PATTEN-END CALIPER

This consists of a padded ring and longitudinal bars as in an ordinary caliper, but the bars terminate in a circular plate covered with rubber on which the weight is taken (Fig. 7.2C). A patten is applied to the boot on the sound side, and the affected limb hangs free in the caliper. A leather sling supports the back of the knee and a knee-shield is provided. In addition, a webbing strap fastens the caliper ring over the shoulder of the opposite side. It is used in tuberculosis or other inflammatory conditions of the ankle joint (Ch. 17), after amputation of the lower limb (Ch. 33) or, occasionally, in Perthes' disease (Ch. 15).

Measurements

1. Round thigh as for a caliper.
2. From the adductor tendon in the groin to the heel, plus sufficient to allow for the patten. If the caliper is to be worn after an amputation, it is made the same length as the sound limb.

KNEE-CAGE

This splint is used in any condition in which it is necessary to protect the knee whilst at the same time allowing weight-bearing and a certain degree of movement, for example, in osteo-arthritis of the knee (Ch. 27).

It consists of longitudinal bars, jointed at the knee according to the degree of flexion allowed, and joined by leather straps which encircle the thigh at two levels, the calf just below the knee, and the ankle (Fig. 7.6). The outer bar may be prolonged and inserted into tubing in the boot.

Measurements. A cast of the leg is necessary. State the degree of knee-flexion required. If a prolongation to the heel is required, the boot must be tubed in readiness.

THE GIRDLESTONE MERMAID SPLINT

This is a simple yet effective night splint for use in the treatment of knock-knee deformity. It consists

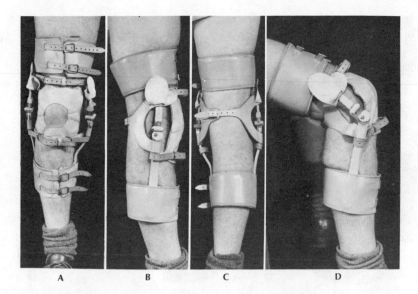

Fig. 7.6 A–D. A knee cage is occasionally useful in instability of the knee following severe ligamentous damage, or in painful rheumatoid arthritis or osteo-arthritis.

of two metal gutter-splints riveted back to back. The upper end of the splint is wider than the lower, and it must be of such a length as to extend from the groin to the inner side of the heel (Kennedy, 1974).

Measurements
1. Round the leg at mid thigh.
2. From this point to the knee joint.
3. From the knee joint to the heel.

BRAUN SPLINT

This splint is used as a means of support in injuries to the lower limb, particularly where skeletal traction is employed. It consists of a metal framework, shaped as shown in Fig. 7.3. A flannel bandage is placed across the upper bars of the splint to support the limb, and a cord carrying weights runs over the pulley placed at the end of the splint (Ch. 21).

DOUBLE BELOW-KNEE IRON (SHORT-LEG-BRACE)

This splint is used for the following purposes:

1. To prevent movement of the ankle joint whilst at the same time permitting weight-bearing, as

in the late treatment of tuberculosis of the ankle joint (Ch. 17). *If all movement is to be prevented, the iron is either fixed in the heel of the boot or the boot is fitted with contrary stops,* i.e. one behind the iron on one side of the boot and one in front of the iron on the other.

2. To prevent plantar-flexion of the ankle joint beyond the right-angled position, as in poliomyelitis affecting the anterior tibial muscles (Ch. 18), in spastic paralysis (Ch. 14) or in drop-foot deformity from any other cause. In these cases the stops are placed behind the iron. They are referred to as *posterior or drop-foot stops* [Fig. 7.7B(A)].

3. To prevent dorsiflexion of the ankle joint beyond the right-angled position, as in poliomyelitis affecting the calf-muscles (Ch. 18). In this condition, the stops are placed in front of the iron—*anterior stops.*

The double iron consists of a semi-circle of metal, covered by a circular leather strap which encircles the leg just below the knee and buckles on the outer side. Two longitudinal metal bars are attached and fit into tubing in the heel of the boot.

Measurements
1. Round the leg just below the knee joint.
2. From head of fibula to heel.

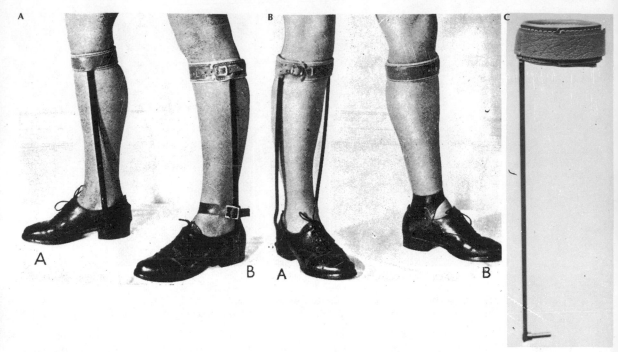

Fig. 7.7 **A.** (A) Lateral view of double iron, drop-foot stops. (B) Lateral view of double iron, outside T-strap. **B.** (A) Anterior view of double iron, drop-foot stops. (B) Medial view of outside iron showing attachment of inside T-strap. **C.** Single leg-iron.

State whether a right or left double iron is required. The boot is sent to the orthotist for tubing and fitting of stops.

SINGLE BELOW-KNEE IRON

This splint is similar in construction to the double iron, but there is a single longitudinal bar which fits into tubing in the heel of the boot. It is combined with a T-strap, i.e. a T-shaped piece of leather sewn on to the opposite side of the boot to which the iron is placed; the arms of the T pass over the iron and are fastened by means of a buckle [Fig. 7.7B(B)].

A single iron is used to correct varus or valgus deformity of the foot. *It is placed on the side to which the foot is turned*, so that the corrective force is applied on this side and increased by the pull of the T-strap fixed on the opposite side.

An inside iron. This is therefore used to correct a varus deformity of the foot.

An outside iron. This is used to correct a valgus deformity (Ch. 15).

A T-strap. In addition a T-strap may be used in combination with a double iron or a caliper, in cases in which a single iron would not provide sufficient support. It is placed on the opposite side to which the foot is turned, and passes over the longitudinal bar of the double iron or caliper on the opposite side.

Measurements. For a single iron the measurements are exactly as for a double one. State whether right or left, inside or outside, and send the boot to the splintmaker for tubing and application of the T-strap.

METAL GUTTER-SPLINTS (BACK-SPLINTS)

These splints are made of malleable metal covered with felt. They are used for the following purposes:

1. *As temporary splintage in disease or injury of the lower limb.* The back-splint must be long enough to extend well above and below the site of disease or injury. For example, if it is used as temporary immobilisation in injuries of

the leg, it must extend from the upper thigh to the lower calf.

2. *As an adjunct to other splintage.* Metal gutter-splints may be used in combination with a Thomas bed-splint in inflammatory lesions of the knee (Chs 16 and 17) and in fracture of the femur (Ch. 21).

3. *As a knee-splint in injuries to the knee or after removal of a cartilage* (Ch. 21).

DENIS BROWNE CLUB-FOOT SPLINT

This splint is used in the correction of congenital talipes equinovarus (Ch. 14). It consists of two aluminium plates bolted to a transverse bar of the same metal. The sole of the foot rests on one plate, whilst the other is in contact with the outer side of the ankle (Fig. 7.8). After padding with felt, the foot pieces are strapped on and bolted to the transverse bar as shown in Ch. 14.

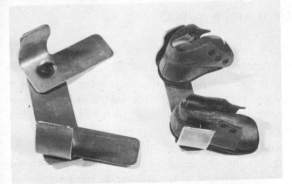

Fig. 7.8   Denis Browne club-foot splints and boots.

Measurements. The length of the foot from the toes to the heel.

Denis Browne boots are used as night splints in the later treatment of the same condition. They are bolted on to a transverse bar as shown in Fig. 7.8. The toes of the boots are left open to accommodate the growing foot, so that the boots do not require renewal throughout the course of treatment.

Measurements are as for Denis Browne splints.

LITTLER-JONES ABDUCTION ARM-SPLINT

This is an abduction arm-splint made of a framework of tubular metal. Leather slings support the limb and the splint is fastened round the pelvis by means of a webbing band.

It is a difficult splint to fit and an uncomfortable one to wear, other than over the clothing. it is used in injuries to the shoulder joint (Ch. 20), in late treatment of tuberculosis of the shoulder (Ch. 17), in poliomyelitis affecting the deltoid (Ch. 18) or in axillary (circumflex) nerve palsy (Ch. 22).

Measurements. If possible, the arm should be held in the desired position while the metal is moulded to the body and limb by the splintmaker. If this is impossible, the limb is held in the correct position by an assistant and measurements are taken as follows:

1. Round the pelvis, halfway between crest of ilium and great trochanter.
2. From a point in this line above the symphysis pubis to the supra-sternal notch.
3. From supra-sternal notch to shoulder joint anteriorly.
4. From shoulder to elbow joint.
5. From the elbow to the transverse skin creases in the palm of the hand.
6. Round the chest at the nipple line.

When ordering, *state the position in which the arm is to be held*, and whether a right or left splint is required.

ELBOW-CAGE

This splint may be ordered in any condition in which a degree of protected movement of the elbow is required. it is similar in construction to a knee-cage.

Measurements. A cast of the limb is required. State the range of movement to be permitted.

COCK-UP SPLINTS

Metal long and short cock-up splints are used as purely temporary splintage in injuries to the wrist, hand or fingers (see Fig. 7.10).

Measurements: Long cock-up. From the fingertips to the middle of the forearm (see Fig. 7.9).

Short cock-up. From the transverse creases in the palm of the hand to mid-forearm (Fig. 7.10). (See

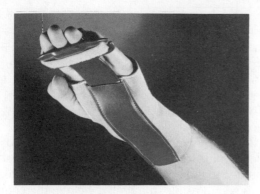

Fig. 7.9 Long cock-up splint.

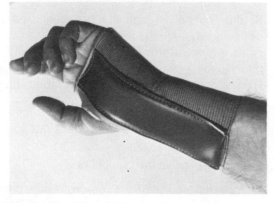

Fig. 7.10 Short cock-up splint.

also Kennedy: *Orthopaedic Splints and Appliances*.)

CRAMER WIRE

Cramer wire is used for making abduction splints to support the shoulder and arm, as for example in Erb's palsy (Ch. 14). The wire is bent to fit the part and is padded with wool covered by a gauze bandage.

MOULDED BLOCK-LEATHER SPLINTS

Block-leather splints are made on a plaster cast of the part of the body or limb to be supported. The method of making the cast is described later. The leather is soaked in water, and then stretched tightly over the cast, so that it is moulded closely to its contours. Figure 7.14 shows a block-leather hip spica cast in process of construction. After the block-leather has dried on the cast, it is removed and sent for fitting. The edges to be trimmed off are also marked at this time. On return to the orthotist, the block-leather is reinforced with metal strips and treated with varnish (Fig. 7.11). Block-leather hip spicas are mentioned in Ch. 10.

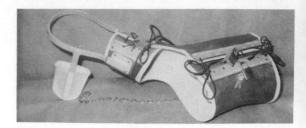

Fig. 7.11 Birmingham splint. An example of a moulded block-leather (Taylor).

SHOE ALTERATIONS

The nurse may be asked to advise patients as to the type of shoe suitable for alterations ordered by the surgeon. In general, a shoe which the patient knows to be comfortable is preferable to a new one, provided that it is in good repair and is otherwise suitable. A shoe presented for alteration should be a perfect fit, and have a strong leather upper which is deep enough to embrace the foot firmly, a straight inner border, a rounded toe and a wide flat heel. Women patients who are unused to wearing flat-heeled shoes may be adverse to this, but they should 'be persuaded to adopt this type of shoe except on 'dressy' occasions. In general, slip-on shoes or those fastened by means other than lacing are not suitable, and crêpe soles are definitely contra-indicated. Children are often best served by the 'Start-Rite' type of shoe; it is essential that they do not become outgrown and that they are kept in good repair.

Inside raising to the heel (crooked heel). This may be ordered in any condition in which inversion of the foot is desired, notably in flat-foot and in knock-knee (Ch. 15). It consists of a piece of leather, of a thickness decided upon by the surgeon, *placed between the upper and the sole on the inner side of the heel of the shoe*. The shoe

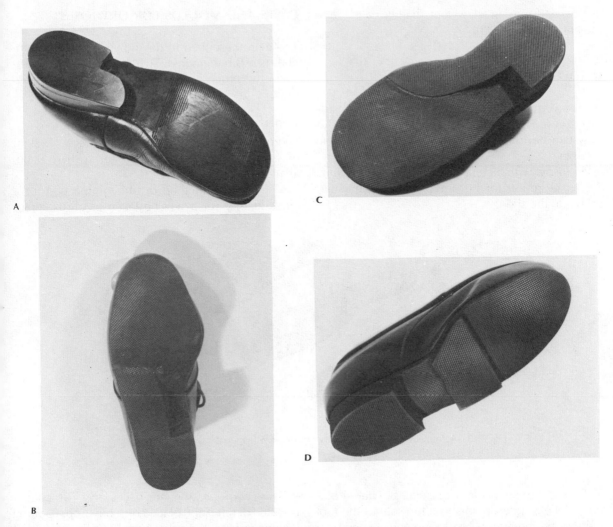

Fig. 7.12 Shoe alterations. **A.** Crooked and enlongated heel (Single Thomas heel). **B.** Double Thomas heel. **C.** Outside raising to heel and sole of shoe. **D.** Metatarsal bar.

can then be repaired in the normal way without interfering with the raising (Fig. 7.12A and B). More rarely, inside raising is also applied to the sole of the shoe.

Single Thomas heel (inside raising and elongated heel—crooked heel and elongated heel). This is ordered in the same conditions when a greater degree of inversion of the foot is desired (Fig. 7.12A).

Double Thomas heel. The crooked elongated heel is prolonged until it merges with the sole. It is ordered when still greater inversion of the foot is desired (Fig. 7.12B).

Outside raising to the heel of the shoe (Fig. 7.12C). This is applied in the same way as inside raising. It is ordered only in the late treatment of congenital talipes-equino-varus (Ch. 14) and occasionally in the treatment of strain or rupture of the external collateral ligament of the ankle joint (Ch. 21).

Metatarsal bar. This consists of a strip of leather nailed to the sole of the shoe behind the metatarsal heads. It is placed obliquely so as to conform with the arrangements of the metatarsal bones (Fig. 7.12D). It is ordered in any condition in which it is desirable to relieve weight-bearing on the metatarsal heads, as in claw foot, hallux valgus and metatarsalgia (Ch. 15).

INSOLES

Insoles are made of leather and are worn inside the shoes. They are convenient for the patient as they can be transferred from one pair of shoes to another.

An insole with metatarsal button or bar. This (Fig. 7.13A) is ordered for the same purpose as a metatarsal bar to the shoe.

CASTS AND MOULDS FOR ORTHOSES

These are described in detail by Gleave and Kennedy (see Bibliography). To help the nurse to understand the process, a brief description is included here.

To make a cast for a splint

Requirements. Vesting or oil to protect the skin; plaster bandages, buckets of water, a sharp knife; an indelible pencil.

Method. The method of obtaining a cast for a block-leather spica will be taken as an example.

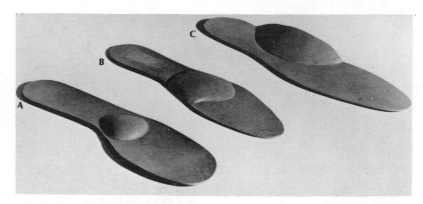

Fig. 7.13   **A.** Insole with metatarsal button. **B.** Insole with metatarsal bar. **C.** Insole with inside raising to heel.

To trace for an insole with metatarsal bar or button. Place a little ointment on the sole of the foot behind the metatarsal heads; previous experiment with felt pads and strapping should have determined its exact situation; the patient then stands and places the foot on a piece of paper, and a tracing is taken by holding a pencil upright and outlining the foot. An impression is left by the ointment which indicates the situation of the button. It is necessary to outline this, or the ointment may soak into the paper and cover too large an area.

Insoles with inside raising to heel and/or sole. This may be ordered in cases of flat-foot. A tracing of the foot is required.

Moulded leather insoles. These are made on a cast taken with the foot held in the desired position. They are ordered in conditions in which support for the foot is required, as in permanent flat-foot (Ch. 15).

At least two operators are necessary. The patient is vested or oiled and placed on a hip prop. Padding is unnecessary; the splint should fit like a second skin. Proceed as for applying a plaster spica; *be certain that the first layer of the bandage is absolutely smooth*; any creases, ridges or lumps will be reproduced in the splint, with disastrous results. The spica extends from the nipple line to above or below the knee. When sufficient plaster has been applied (about five layers of bandage should be sufficient), mark the sides in transverse lines with an indelible pencil. The lines are approximated when the cast is cut, to secure accurate apposition of the cut edges. When nearly set, cut the case down one side with a sharp knife. Remove it, and while an assistant holds the edges together, enclose the cast with a circular plaster bandage. The 'hole' left by the sound leg is also covered over. Figure 7.14 shows the negative cast.

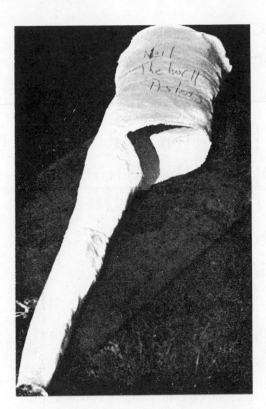

Fig. 7.14 The negative cast.

To make a positive cast

Requirements. One or two operators; a piece of metal or wood, buckets of water, an enamel jug, petroleum jelly or olive oil, and either dry white plaster or the coarse pink casting variety.

Method. Place the cast on a mackintosh with the leg piece upwards and grease the inside. Insert the strip of metal or wood. This is to facilitate handling of the cast. Prepare a sufficient quantity of sloppy plaster cream, pour it rapidly down the leg piece, until the whole cast is filled. When firmly set, cut away the negative cast. The positive cast is then smoothed over with a sharp knife, thoroughly dried, marked with the patient's name and sent to the orthotist.

BIBLIOGRAPHY

Adams J C 1971 Outline of Orthopaedics. Edinburgh and London: Churchill Livingstone
Apley A G 1977 A System of Orthopaedics and Fractures. London: Butterworths
Day B 1972 Orthopaedic Appliances. London: Faber and Faber.
Department of Health and Social Security 1980 Classification of Orthoses. London: Her Majesty's Stationery Office
Gleave J A E 1972 Moulds and Casts for Orthopaedic and Prosthetic Appliances. Springfield, Illinois: Thomas
Kennedy J M 1974 Orthopaedic Splints and Appliances. London: Ballière Tindall.
Roaf R, Hodkinson L J 1976 Textbook of Orthopaedic Nursing. London: Blackwell Scientific.
Rose G K 1977 Orthotics. Physiotherapy 63: 78.
Rowe J, Dyer L (ed.) 1977 Care of the Orthopaedic Patient. Oxford: Blackwell Scientific.

8

The orthopaedic operating theatre and care of the patient undergoing surgery

The term 'operating theatre' originates from the days when the surgeon conducted his operations on a table watched by crowds of apprentice surgeons sitting on tiers of benches around him.

The acceptance of aseptic techniques pioneered by Joseph Lister and the introduction of steam sterilisation to render instruments, dressings and drapes germ free were important developments.

Simultaneously, anaesthetics were being developed—initially, using liquid ether dropped on to a cloth placed over the patient's nose and mouth, then via a face mask. Progress to endotracheal anaesthesia soon followed to give complete control of breathing during operations.

Thus, by the turn of this century the origins of our modern operating theatre were already in existence. The combination of improved techniques and equipment led to the development of today's surgical suite.

THE SURGICAL SUITE

This is an area specially designed and constructed to provide an environment that is convenient and safe for both patients and staff where surgery is performed.

Commonly, the suite comprises a number of operating rooms and all the rooms with services

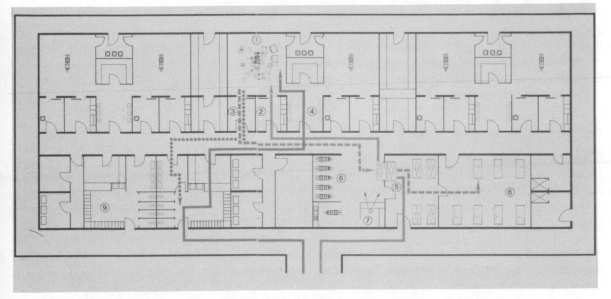

Fig. 8.1A. Layout of operating suite 1. Operating room 2. Induction room 3. Exit room 4. Scrub 5. Transfer area 6. Table parking 7. Table cleaning 8. Recovery 9. Staff changing

necessary to its function. It is a self-contained unit and may take up a whole floor of a hospital. Usually, it is set off from the main flow of the hospital traffic and is separated by an 'unclean' corridor.

Reception and transfer area

Patients are received into the department and transferred from their ward bed to a theatre trolley or bed before entering the clean zone.

Pre-operative holding area

The patient waits in this area until the staff in the theatre are ready for him.

Post-operative recovery

This area is staffed and equipped for the immediate safe recovery of the patient from his anaesthetic. He remains in this area for observation until his condition is stable and he is fit to return to his own unit. Patients who need specialised care would be transferred to Intensive Care.

Theatre sterile supply unit

Here, instruments and equipment are prepared, sterilised and stored for use. Some supplies may be provided by the hospital Central Sterile Supplies Department.

Storage rooms

Adequate storage is essential for all supplies and equipment necessary to the unit function.

X-ray facilities

X-ray machines and image intensifiers are mandatory for use intra-operatively in orthopaedic theatres. A room must be provided for developing films within the clean area and for storage of films and accessories.

Plaster room

This is essential for patients requiring plaster casts at the completion of their surgery. Additionally, traction may be set up in this area and plaster casts changed.

Office accommodation

Offices are required for the nursing and medical staff with their secretaries so that administrative duties can be carried out.

Communication

An area should be assigned for control of communication within the unit. Often an intercom from room to room is included. Telephones are manned from this area to communicate within and with other departments external to the unit.

Teaching and demonstration rooms

These are essential for training of new staff. Demonstration of new equipment is a 'must' so staff can handle the equipment efficiently.

Rest rooms and kitchen

Minimal kitchen facilities are necessary for beverages and light refreshments to be taken during hours of duty. Comfortable seating should be provided.

Staff changing rooms

Changing rooms are necessary for all grades of staff with facilities for personnel to change from outdoor clothing to theatre wear. Lockers must be provided for safe storage of personal property. Toilets and showers are installed in the changing area.

Each operating room has its own:

Anaesthetic room

For the induction of anaesthesia and positioning of the patient ready for surgery.

Preparation area

Storage and supplies of sterile stock and equipment for use during surgery may include a 'laying up area' for preparation of sterile trolleys.

Scrub up area

For hand washing, gowning and gloving of the surgical team.

Disposal area

For the disposal and cleaning of used instruments and equipment.

Exit area

Preferably a room where patient has immediate post-operative care before proceeding to recovery area.

FABRIC AND CONSTRUCTION WALLS, FLOORS AND CEILINGS

Walls and ceilings

These should be covered by a material which is easily cleaned. Tiles and stainless steel are a popular finish in modern suites; they are durable and require little maintenance.

Colour is important—it should be restful. In areas where assessment of the patient's colour is important, blues and greens should be avoided.

Floors

Hard wearing properties are essential in floors so that the heavy wheeled equipment which is in daily use in the unit can be supported.

Quiet flooring is also important, especially in patient areas. Terrazo tiling is ideal but the cost is high and often heavy duty vinyls are used.

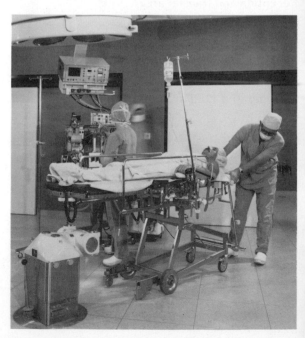

Fig. 8.1B. General view of operating theatre showing fabric.

Lighting

Natural lighting is the most pleasant to work in and windows should be incorporated in the suite wherever possible. Double glazing eliminates noise. Opaque windows on operating theatres ensure privacy.

Artificial light is usually provided by fluorescent lighting. Operating lights should move easily. It is important that they are shadowless, that the light can be focused and that they do not give out unnecessary heat.

CLEANING THEATRES

At the end of each operating list, the theatre is completely cleaned. Theatre walls, all furniture and equipment are washed and dried with great care. Floors are scrubbed, using machines, and dried. Clear instructions should be written for daily or weekly cleaning which should be carried out in all areas of the theatre unit. This also gives the opportunity for all the equipment to be checked and tested.

MAINTENANCE OF UNIT

Regular maintenance should be carried out on a weekly basis. At this time, engineers check the fabric of the unit. Particular attention is paid to autoclaves, ventilation systems and electrical equipment.

The theatre staff are responsible for routine maintenance on suckers, tables, instruments and equipment in daily use.

The electro-bio-mechanical engineers are responsible for maintaining sophisticated equipment such as tourniquets, monitoring devices, anaesthetic machines. They also arrange servicing (by companies) of equipment as necessary.

The following section includes extracts from Howorth's leaflets on 'Prevention of air-borne infection during surgery with the exflow clean zone' by kind permission of F. H. Howorth OBE FRSA FIIC FIPI PPI HospE.

ENVIRONMENTAL CONTROLS

Air conditioning is essential throughout the operating suite.

In an operating theatre equipped with a conventional air conditioning system, air is supplied at controlled temperature and relative humidity through integral or terminal bacterial filters and is introduced into the operating rooms by diffusers situated in either the walls or the ceiling. It is well-established that the main source of infection in an operating theatre is people who are constantly emitting contaminants on their body convecting current and on their exhaled breath. From tests, it was found that the clean incoming air was contaminated by entrapped ambient air almost at once (see Figs 8.2 and 8.3). Because of the general pattern of the incoming air, this mixture of clean and grossly contaminated air is circulated around the operating room and therefore, inevitably, into the wound.

In some specialised procedures, such as total joint replacement, where prevention of infection is of extremely high importance, special systems of controlled air distribution have been devised to minimise the risk of air borne contamination.

The first surgeon to conceive this idea was Sir John Charnley who, in 1961, invited engineers to design an air system which would prevent air borne infection of the wound during surgery.

Thus, in 1963, the first 'clean air enclosure' in the world was installed. By 1970, clinical results had established the effectiveness of clean air in eradicating air borne infection. At the same time, the necessity for a total body exhaust system preventing contamination of this clean air by members of the surgical team was established beyond all reasonable doubt.

The Charnley Howorth Exflow Clean Zone System eliminates perimeter entrainment and contaminants and provides total protection against air borne contamination.

The Charnley Total Body Exhaust System consists of a lightweight face mask which has a removable visor, together with a one-piece hooded gown made of 'ventile' material. A specially-designed

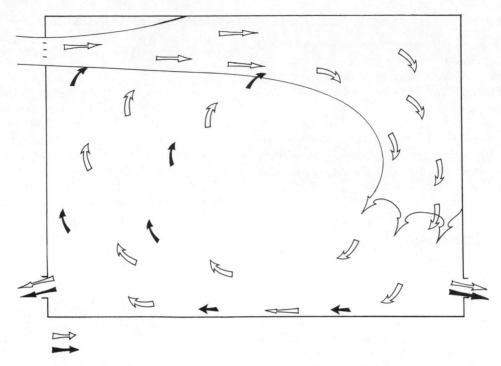

Fig. 8.2 Entrainment of contaminants with conventional side wall diffuser.

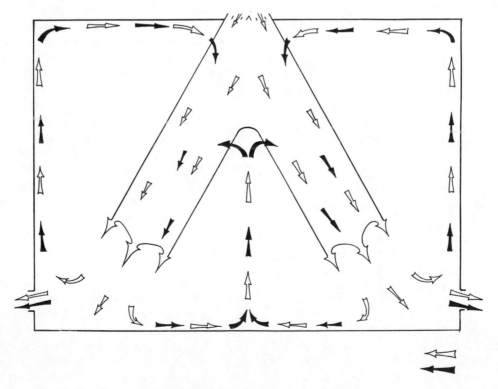

Fig. 8.3 Entrainment of contaminants with conventional ceiling diffuser.

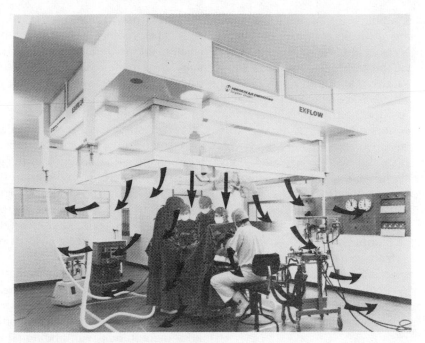

Fig. 8.4   Charnley/Howorth Exflow System.

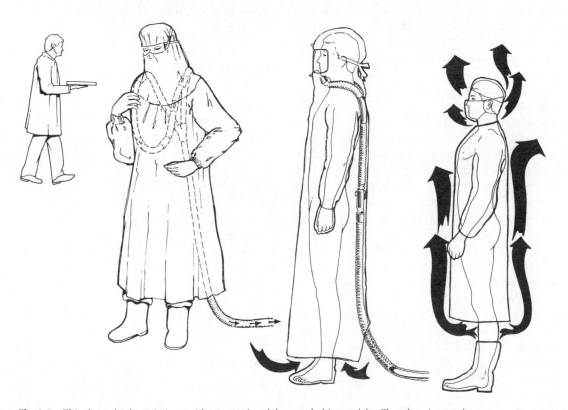

Fig. 8.5   This shows body emissions with conventional theatre clothing and the Charnley visor and gown.

exhaust fan unit is supplied for installation outside the theatre, discharging to atmosphere. Lightweight flexible tubes are connected to the face masks via suction points in the theatre, so that the area underneath the wearer's gown is at negative pressure and the bacteria-carrying particles which are constantly emitted cannot escape into the ambient air. Because of the continuous flow of air upwards under the gown and over the wearer's body, he is cooled, refreshed and well-oxygenated, thus reducing fatigue. A full audio system is available enabling clear communication to be made between the operating team, the anaesthetist and service team.

Extensive investigations have proved beyond doubt that 'Ultra clean air systems' dramatically reduce post-operative infection in major joint replacement surgery. With the increase of revision surgery for joint replacement, they may become the accepted standard design for all future orthopaedic theatres.

In recent years, concern has been expressed about the possible harmful effects of waste anaesthetic gases, namely halothane and nitrous oxide, being exhausted into the theatre atmosphere. 'Scavenging systems' are now mandatory to remove waste gases from the air.

SAFETY IN THE OPERATING DEPARTMENT

Regular checking and maintenance of all equipment used in the suite is essential. All new equipment should be tested prior to use and instruction given to the staff using it, to ensure it is used correctly. Any equipment not working properly should be removed from use and arrangements made for its early repair by the appropriate department or supplier.

It is essential that the operating suite has a generator which can take over if there is a failure in the power supply as this could have disastrous effects, particularly during surgical operations.

Fire drill policies should be laid down and all staff using the unit should be instructed in the procedure to follow in case of a fire.

Static electricity can be a hazard in the operating department, particularly where sparks may occur in the presence of explosive anaesthetic gases. This is particularly likely when plastic and nylon materials are in use. To lessen the risk, clothing used in theatre should be made of cotton or non-inflammable materials. Shoes are fitted with anti-static strips in their soles. All wheeled furniture and equipment is fitted with anti-static rubber wheels; anaesthetic tubing and face masks are made from anti-static rubber.

Every hospital has an operating department committee made up of surgical, anaesthetic and nursing representatives to ensure theatre procedures are reviewed regularly with regard to staff and patient safety. The Medical Defence Union and Royal College of Nursing issue memorandums with recommendations of procedures which should be followed to safeguard against patients having the wrong operation.

Similarly, there are recommendations to safeguard against failure to remove swabs and instruments from patients. A 'Theatre procedure' booklet incorporating the advice and recommendations of these memoranda with additional and alternative details approved by the committee, is issued to all medical and nursing staff using the department who should follow the procedures laid down in the interests of safety.

THE OPERATING LIST

Specialisation in surgery has evolved from the development of more sophisticated equipment and instrumentation, which, in turn, has led to the introduction of more advanced and complex surgical procedures. Nowhere is this more evident than in the orthopaedic theatre. Today's operating list may consist of:

1. Cold orthopaedic cases
2. Traumatic cases
3. External fixators
4. Non union of fractures
5. Microsurgery
6. Spinal surgery
7. Total joint replacement

COLD ORTHOPAEDIC CASES

Foot surgery

The foot is prone to numerous disorders due to

trauma, disease or congenital deformity. Many of these conditions can be treated by surgery, e.g. hallux valgus, foot instability, congenital talipes equino varus.

Hand and wrist surgery

Surgical treatment may be undertaken to correct problems such as: carpal tunnel syndrome, Dupuytren's contracture, ganglions, syndactyly, replacement of joints.

Shoulder surgery

Instability of the shoulder joint caused by lax ligaments and capsule resulting in recurrent dislocation of shoulder can be surgically treated. Two common operations are the Bankart and Putti Platt procedures, Arthroplasty of shoulder.

Growth disorders

Growth disorders (e.g. limb inequality) can be operated on by either lengthening the short limb or shortening the good limb. Staple fixation can be used to restrict epiphyseal growth in conditions such as knock knees. Slipped upper femoral epiphysis can be pinned surgically to maintain correct position until growth is completed.

Congenital deformities

Open reduction and osteotomies with or without internal fixation may be performed to correct deformity. Now, with improved conditions for surgery, the necessary operations may be carried out simultaneously, e.g. in congenital dislocation of the hip, it is possible to do an open reduction and pelvic osteotomy at the same operation.

Arthroscopy

Surgery under endoscopic control has improved enormously. Diagnostic arthroscopy to detect pathology in the knee is now commonplace. From this, the concept of dealing with lesions seen through the scope became a challenge and instrumentation has been developed to do this. Menisectomy, synovectomy and removal of loose bodies are just some of the conditions treated by this method.

TRAUMATIC CASES

Soft tissue operations

These range from simple toilet and suture of wounds, skin grafting and tendon repairs to reconstructive procedures such as cruciate ligament repairs.

Fractures

Many fractures are treated by open reduction and internal fixation. Rigid fixation and accurate anatomical reduction allow direct bony union. Improved implants control the fracture without additional external support, thus allowing early mobilisation and recovery.

X-ray image intensification at surgery shortens the operating time as reduction and fixation can be carried out under direct vision.

EXTERNAL FIXATORS

These are a method of immobilising fractures using percutaneous transfixing pins in bone attached to a rigid external metal frame. The frame can be adjusted so that distraction or compression can be maintained according to the fracture. Initially, the system was devised for tibial and femoral fractures but frames can be made to control pelvic fractures and those of the upper limb and shoulder.

The external fixator is particularly useful in the treatment of open fractures; as well as the fracture being stabilised, the wounds can be observed and treated as required (often mobilisation can be commenced earlier). The same apparatus can be used to control the limbs during reconstructive plastic surgery procedures such as a cross leg flap graft.

External fixation is also used for arthrodesis and as a fixation in non-union fracture cases where it may be used following bone grafting procedures.

NON-UNION OF FRACTURES

Delayed union and non union of fractures may require further surgical procedures. As previously mentioned, external fixators can be applied to control the position of the fracture. Bone grafting may be necessary. Frequently, the bone ends at the fracture site need re-fashioning so that the fracture can be fixed internally.

Bone grafting

Bone can be transferred for grafting from one area of the body to another. Some procedures commonly using bone grafts are anterior and posterior spinal fusions, additional fixation in fracture repair following internal fixation, secondary grafting to non union of fractures and arthrodesis of joints. The sites bone can be obtained from are:

1. *The ilium.* This may be done via an anterior or posterior approach.
2. *The greater trochanter; head of tibia.* These supply good source of cancellous bone.
3. *Ribs.* In anterior approaches to the thoracic spine, one or two ribs are removed to provide good exposure of the spine. These can be used for bone grafting.
4. *Fibula.* Useful as a strut graft in spinal procedures where height restoration and stabilisation is necessary, for example, following removal of diseased vertebrae either infective or tumour ridden.

Bone can be stored in sterile containers and frozen up to twelve months before use. It can be stored from a donor and used on a different patient without any harmful effect.

MICROSURGERY

The use of the microscope in surgery has made possible not only repairs of nerves but replantation of digits and limbs. This type of surgery is usually only carried out in specialised centres.

SPINAL SURGERY

Spinal surgery may be contemplated for three types of disorder:

1. Spinal injury
2. Back pain
3. Spinal deformity

Since the 1960s, instrumentation for spinal deformity has provided a solution to stabilise as well as correct deformity, allowing the patient to be mobilised in a plaster jacket a mere two weeks after surgery. In the late 1970s, a segmental spinal fixation was devised originally for use in paralytic curves. This does away with the use of plaster jackets entirely. In correction of severe deformity, the patient may require staged operations from anterior and posterior approaches, sometimes with a period of skeletal traction in between operations.

Similar instrumentation can be used to stabilise the spine in spinal fracture patients with unstable fractures. Instability following cervical spine fractures may necessitate fusion of the damaged area.

Operations for back pain include laminectomy, spinal decompressions, anterior and posterior spinal fusions.

TOTAL JOINT REPLACEMENT

Although the hip and knee are the most common joints being replaced, it is not uncommon to replace shoulders, finger joints, elbows, wrists and ankles.

Even though thousands of successful hip and knee replacements are carried out annually, the problems which can arise post-operatively may lead to the need for further surgery. A great deal of progress has been made over the last decade on the part of surgeons and engineers so that 'revision joint replacement' can now be successfully achieved.

ANAESTHESIA

In a chapter such as this, it is impossible to describe anaesthetic techniques. However, the reader should be aware that without the armamentarium of equipment necessary for giving the anaesthetic and the excellent monitoring equipment available, much of the major orthopaedic surgery today could not be contemplated.

The anaesthetist does not only provide general anaesthesia but also regional local anaesthetics for patients undergoing limb surgery and spinal or epidural anaesthesia when general anaesthesia is considered unsuitable. 'Pain clinics' are now being set up for patients with chronic pain and the anaesthetist may have his own session to deal with these cases.

INSTRUMENTATION

When the new nurse commences orthopaedic theatre, the maze of instruments required for bone and joint surgery may seem bewildering.

A basic knowledge of requirements for surgical operations lays the groundwork on which to build. Regardless of what type of surgery is performed, be it general, orthopaedic, ophthalmic or whatever, the same basic tools are required. Firstly, the patient's skin is prepared, using sponges on *sponge-holders*. Next, the patient is draped to occlude all but the area around the incision. The towels are held in place with *towel clips*. A *knife* is required then to make the incision—with a knife, one uses a fork. The surgeon's fork is his *dissecting forceps*. Usually, these are toothed to grasp tissue. *Retractors* are used to hold tissue apart so that the operation can be performed. In addition, *tissue forceps* may be used to aid exposure. *Scissors* may be used to divide tissues and a *blunt dissector* to probe or identify layers of tissue. In all operations, blood

vessels may be divided. *Artery forceps* are used to control bleeding. Having controlled the bleeding with the forceps, the vessels may be ligated or coagulated using diathermy. Having completed the operation, the wound must be closed. *Needle-holders* are used to carry the needles of the suture material and special *suture holding forceps* to pull through the suture material.

These basic soft tissue dissecting instruments come in a wide variety of sizes for various parts of the body, for example:
1. *Minor surgery* can be used for small operations such as carpal tunnel syndrome, tendon repairs or suturing of lacerations.
2. *Medium soft tissue.* Basic instructions include those for surgery on knees, shoulders or an infants hip.
3. *Large set.* Basic requirements for operations on the adult hip.

Thoracotomy instruments are required for operations where it is necessary to open the chest cavity.

In orthopaedic surgery, it is essential that the nurse understands the anatomy of the area to be operated on. Thus, if a knee joint is to be replaced, instrumentation can be based on this knowledge. In addition to a basic medium soft tissue set, instru-

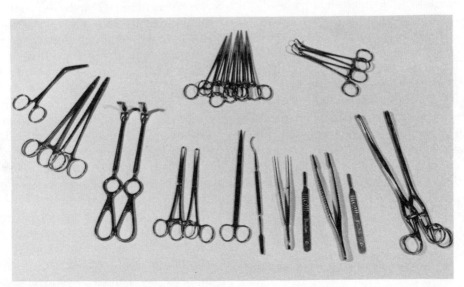

Fig. 8.6A. *Medium soft tissue set* (reading right to left)
Front row Sponge holder, B.P. handles, Bonneys dissecting forceps, Gillies dissecting forceps, McDonald dissector, McIndoe scissors, Vulsellum tissue forceps, Langenbeck retractors, Mayo needleholders, Galabin forceps
Back row Artery forceps, Towel clips

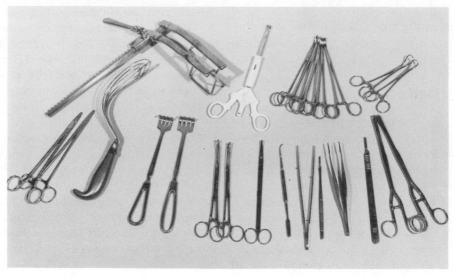

Fig. 8.6B. *Thoracotomy set* (reading right to left)
Front row Sponge holders, Long B.P. handle, Ramsay dissecting forceps, Waugh dissecting forceps, McDonald dissector, Duval lung tissue forceps, Volkmann retractors, Lung retractor, Mayo needle holders
Back row Finichietto retaining retractor, Autosuture vessel clip dispenser, Sawtell artery forceps, Towel clips

ments are required to strip periosteum which covers the bone (a *periosteal elevator*). *Bone levers* are used to retract soft tissue and support the bone surfaces which require cutting and shaping to accept the prostheses. *Power saws, osteotomes* and *chisels* are used to cut the bony surfaces. *Bone holders* may be necessary to align bone ends. *Curettes* can be utilised to curette out bone cysts, *bone files* to further smooth rough edges.

Each type of prosthesis has its own set of precision instruments designed so it can be fitted exactly to restore function of the joint it is replacing. Often it is necessary to have different sized components so that an accurate fit can be obtained for the individual. In the knee, separate components are made for the femur and tibia; often a replacement patellar component is included.

IMPLANTS

Implants are used to repair or replace parts of the body. Orthopaedically, they are used to relieve pain, increase stability and improve mobility.

It is really only this century that implants have been used with any degree of success. Historically, various materials were tried for making implants such as ivory, Pyrex, silver, nickel and Teflon. Smith Peterson in 1937 used a chrome cobalt alloy cup. During the 1950s a lot of progress was made. Stainless steel, vitallium and titanium were used to produce implants of good quality which were implanted without any rejection from the body as long as the metals were used in isolation; for example, if a vitallium plate was used to fix a fracture, the screws had also to be made from vitallium.

Orthopaedic surgeons also enlisted the help of engineers in designing prostheses which were biomechanically sound. Additionally, they were able to produce instrumentation necessary for the accurate fixation of the implant.

The use of a high density polyethylene component when reconstructing a total joint replacement by Sir John Charnley was a major advance and it is commonplace in this decade that total joints comprise a metal and a polyethylene component.

In the 1960s, the introduction of bone cement (methylmerthracrolate) to stabilise prostheses furthered the success for joint replacement surgery.

Silastic, which is a silicone elastomer, has been

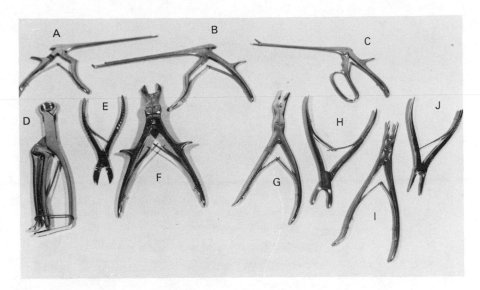

Fig. 8.7A. *Bone nibblers and cutters*
A. Kerrison rongeur. **B.** Cloward rongeur. **C.** Ferris Smith ronguer. **D.** Vehmehron rib shears.
E. Single action Liston bone cutter. **F.** Keys laminectomy shears. **G.** Leksell rongeur. **H.** Rat tooth
rongeur. **I.** Smith Peterson rongeur. **J.** Heanley rongeur

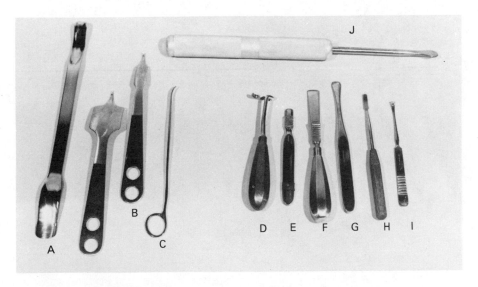

Fig. 8.7B. *Bone levers and periosteal elevators*
Front row **A.** Murphy skid. **B.** Hohmann levers. **C.** Trethowan bone lever. **D.** Doyen rib raspatory.
E. Farabeuf rugine. **F.** Mitchell periosteal elevator. **G.** Dewar periosteal elevator. **H.** A/O periosteal
elevator. **I.** Pennybacker periosteal elevator
Back row **J.** Cobb elevator

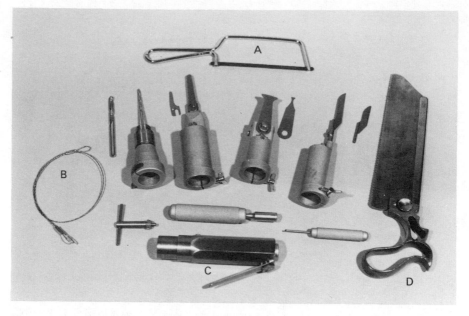

Fig. 8.8A. *Drills and saws*
A. Hack saw. **B.** Gigli saw. **C.** Chirodrill i/c drill attachments, Tuke saw, Oscillating saw, Reciprocating saw. **D.** Amputation saw

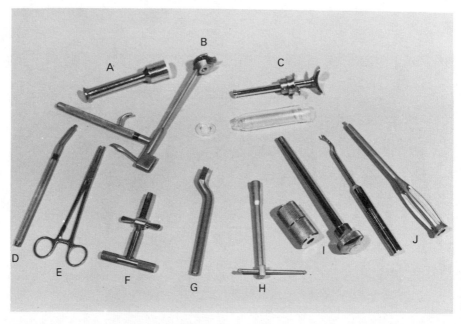

Fig. 8.8B. *Assorted introducers and punches*
A. Charnley femoral prosthesis punch. **B.** Charnley acetabular cup holder. **C.** Cement syringe i/c disposable insert. **D.** Harrington hook introducer. **E.** Harrington hook holder. **F.** Guide wire introducer. **G.** Angled bone punch. **H.** McLaughlin spanner. **I.** McLaughlin introducer and extractor. **J.** Kuntscher nail extractor and introducer

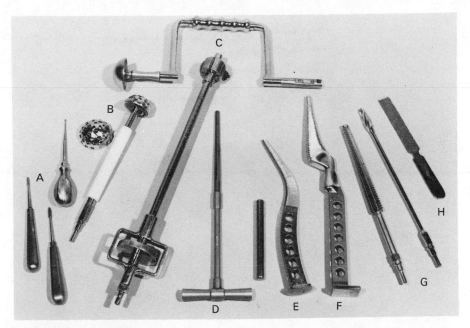

Fig. 8.9A. *Variety of reamers*
A. Bone awl and paton burr. **B.** I.C.L.H. acetabular reamers. **C.** Charnley expanding acetabular reamer i/c brace. **D.** Femoral taper reamer. **E.** Charley femoral reamer i/c tommy bar. **F.** Iso-elastic femoral reamer. **G.** Iso-elastic reamer for use i/c hand or power, Iso-elastic drill for use i/c hand or power. **H.** Bone file

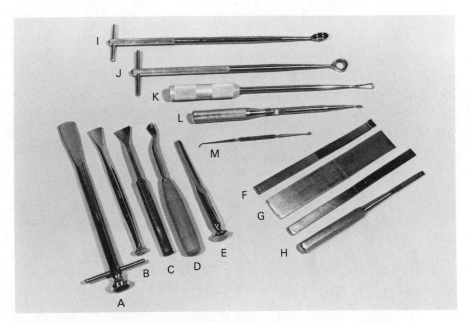

Fig. 8.9B. *Assorted gouges, osteotomes, chisels, curettes*
A. Watson Jones gouge. **B.** Buck's gouge. **C.** Putti gouge. **D.** Capener gouge. **E.** Robert Jones gouge. **F.** Curved Lambotte osteotome. **G.** Straight Lambotte osteotome. **H.** Chisel
Back row **I.** Charnley spoon. **J.** Charnley ring curette. **K.** Oswestry spinal currette. **L.** Chou curette.
M. Mastoid curette

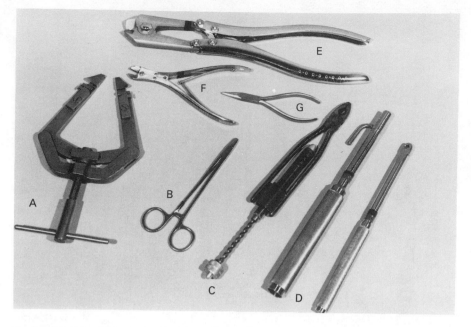

Fig. 8.10A. *Wire tighteners, rod benders, pliers and cutters*
A. Charnley wire tightener. **B.** Charnley wire holding forceps. **C.** Robinson wire twister. **D.** Luque rod benders
Back row **E.** Berbecker wire cutters. **F.** Double action wire cutter. **G.** Small pointed pliers

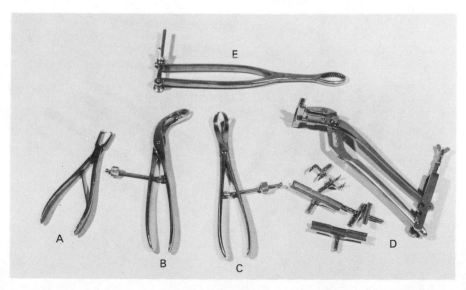

Fig. 8.10B. *Bone holders*
A. Frosch bone holder. **B.** A/O Bone holder. **C.** A/O Reduction forceps. **D.** Charnley bone holding forceps i/c attachments
Back row **E.** Hey Groves bone holder

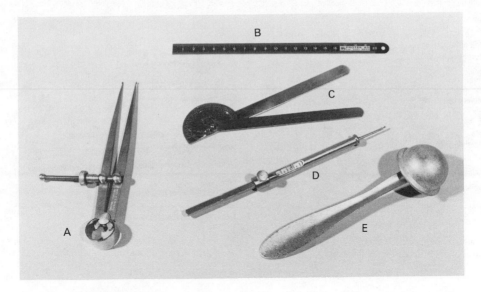

Fig. 8.10C. *Bone measuring devices*
A. Bone graft measuring caliper. **B.** Rule. **C.** Goniometer. **D.** Depth gauge. **E.** Acetabular gauge

successfully developed as an implant material for small prostheses to replace such joints as metacarpals, radial heads and lunate bones.

Damaged ligaments can now be repaired using carbon fibre implants. Initially, the implant acts as a simple prosthesis but research has proved that new ligamentous material forms within and around the carbon fibre. Synthetic Terylene ligaments are now being developed. These also act as scaffolding to support new fibrous tissue.

Iso-elastic is a new material which is being used in joint replacement. It is made from a polyacetyl plastic. The idea was conceived by Robert Matthys in 1967. He made an iso-elastic prosthesis which could be anchored into the bone without using cement. After extensive experimentation in 1973, the first cementless hip was inserted.

CLEANING, CARE AND STERILISATION OF INSTRUMENTS AND IMPLANTS

Nowadays, surgical instruments are almost always made from high grade surgical steel.

Proper care of instruments, especially ensuring that they are only used for the purpose of which they are designed, is essential. The many sets of instruments used in orthopaedic surgery take care

of a large share of the operating theatre budget. For instance, a basic set of instruments on a minor orthopaedic set costs £400—a special set for hip replacement may cost nearer £2000. Well cared-for instruments will last for many years.

DISINFECTION

After the instruments have been used, they should be sent to the area where they are to be processed. This may be part of the operating department or at the CSSD elsewhere in the hospital. Ideally, the instruments should be returned in closed containers, thus avoiding the danger of contamination. If cleaning cannot be guaranteed within a short time, they should be immersed in a disinfecting solution.

CLEANING

By hand

The instruments are scrubbed with a nylon scrubbing brush in a detergent solution. This may have added ingredients which dissolve blood. Instruments which consist of several parts such as introducers and acetabular reamers should be disassembled so all parts are thoroughly cleaned.

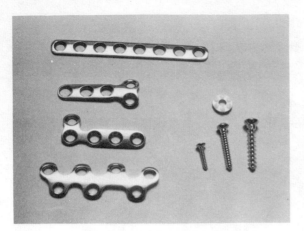

Fig. 8.11A. A/O Mini fragment plates
i/c Cortical and cancellous screws and washer

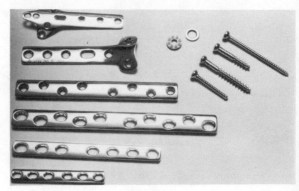

Fig. 8.11B. A/O Plates
i/c Cortical cancellous and malleolar screws

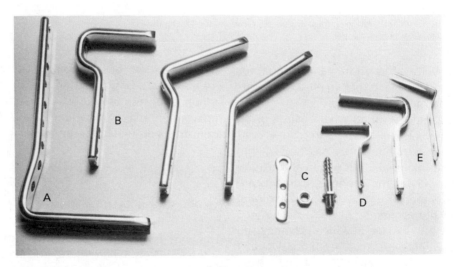

Fig. 8.11C. A. A/O Condylar plate. **B.** A/O Osteotomy plates.
C. Coventry lag screw and plate. **D.** A/O Children's. **E.** Wagner infant plate

Hollow instruments and suction tubes require a suitable range of bottle type brushes so they can be cleaned internally. Special pressurised water jets are useful for removing impacted bone from instruments.

Particular care must be exercised when cleaning sharp instruments such as gouges and osteotomes to ensure the cutting edges are not knocked as this may blunt them.

By machine

Special washing machines are now available which disinfect, wash, rinse and even dry instruments. Ultrasonic cleaners are especially useful for cleaning orthopaedic instruments; ultrasonic waves pass through the water and remove the debris. After thorough cleaning, they are then passed into a rinsing tank.

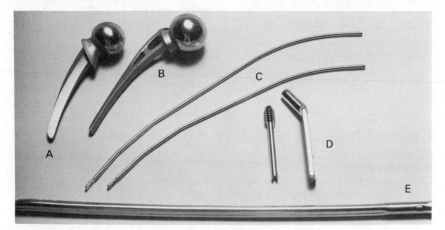

Fig. 8.11D. **A.** Thompson & **B.** Moore's prosthesis
C. Enders nails
D. Dynamic hip screw and plate
E. A/O Intermedullary nail

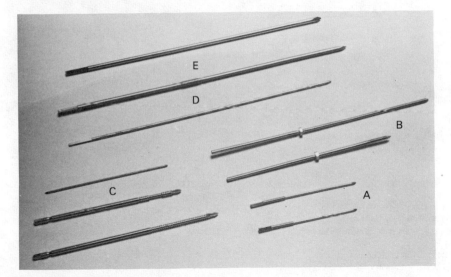

Fig. 8.11E. **A.** Crawford Adams pins
B. Knowles pins
C. Threaded pins and half pins for use i/c Hoffman apparatus Kirschner wire
D. Graduated guide wire
E. Steinmann's pin

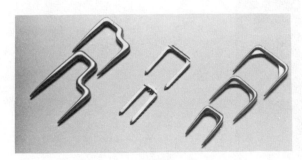

Fig. 8.11F. Coventry stepped staples
Richards staples
Vitallium staples

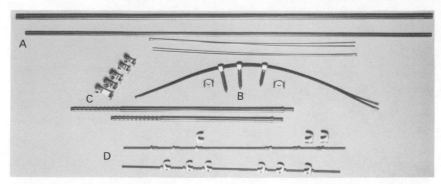

Fig. 8.12A. **A.** Luque rods and wires
B. Dwyer cable screws and staples
C. Harrington hooks and distraction rods
D. Harrington compression rods

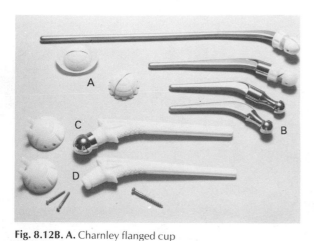

Fig. 8.12B. A. Charnley flanged cup
Charnley L.P.W. cup
B. A selection of Charnley femoral prostheses
C. Iso-elastic hip prosthesis femoral component i/c head
D. Iso-elastic hip prosthesis femoral component without head
  Acetabular cups
  Small screws for fixation of acetabulum
  Cancellous screws for fixation of femoral component

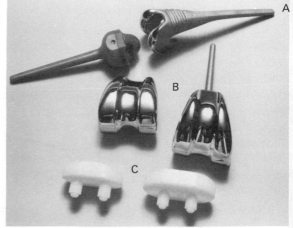

Fig. 8.12C. **A.** Sheehan knee showing femoral and tibial component
B. Freeman Samuelson femoral and revision femoral component
C. Freeman Samuelson tibial components

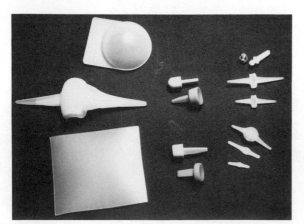

Fig. 8.12D. Varian shoulder prosthesis (silastic)
Silastic elbow prosthesis
Silastic sheeting
Ulnar head
Radial head
Trapezium
Great toe
Iso-elastic M.C.P. joint
Silastic M.C.P. prosthesis
Calnan Nichol M.C.P. prosthesis
Nicholl I.P. joint prosthesis

Drying

After cleaning, instruments should be thoroughly dried either by hand, at which stage they can be inspected to be sure they are in good working order, or alternatively, they may be dried in heated cabinets.

Lubrication

Instruments with working parts should be lubricated before they are re-assembled, either using a spray or immersing the instruments in a special solution.

Checking and packaging

Instruments are checked and set out in trays for sterilisation. Sets may be autoclaved in special filter casks or double linen or paper wrap. Individual instruments can be packed in double sterilisation bags, preferably see-through so the instrument can be seen. All types of package should have sterility indicators. These usually change colour during sterilisation indicating that the pack is ready for use. Every package is dated with the day of sterilisation. All items should be used within a given period. This varies with type of package and the storage area. Three months is a reasonable shelf life for paper packages.

METHODS OF STERILISATION

Autoclaving

Sterilisation is achieved by steam at a temperature of 134°C and pressure at 32 lb per square inch for a period of three and a half minutes.

Autoclaves vary in pattern and cycle. Most departments use high vacuum autoclaves for sterilising soft goods, linen and instrument packs in everyday use.

Daily testing of autoclaves is mandatory to ensure their effective functioning.

Hot air sterilisation

This is used as a method of sterilising glass syringes, needles and drills where the motor is not enclosed and would be damaged by steam autoclaving. The items are packed in metal or glass containers. These are placed in a hot air oven. The air is heated to 160°C and circulated by a fan. This temperature is maintained for one hour to effect sterilisation.

Ethylene oxide sterilisation

Ethylene oxide gas is used commercially for sterilising items that would be affected by heat. These include plastic, rubber and bone. Some hospitals utilise this process. Special instructions must be followed to protect the operators and make sure the products are aerated adequately to remove the gas, which is highly explosive. Toxic effects and irritation to skin and mucous membranes are side effects produced by the gas.

Gamma radiation

This is a widely used commercial process for sterilisation of single use items like syringes, needles, blades and sutures as well as implants and bone cement. The items are packaged and exposed in a special plant to gamma rays. Chemical changes can occur in some items rendering them unsuitable for re-sterilisation.

Disinfection by chemical solutions

Re-usable items that cannot be readily sterilised by heat may be disinfected by soaking in fluid. This process will destroy all micro-organisms if the manufacturer's instructions are followed carefully. No test can be performed to show that the item is sterile and there is always risk of contamination in delivering the item to the sterile field. Additionally, these chemicals are toxic and equipment has to be rinsed prior to use.

IMPLANTS

Sterilisation of implants depends on the type of implant and of the material of which it is made. Sets of nail plates and screws are packed in sets as the exact size cannot be determined until the actual operation. Individual trays, often compartmental, are available so that the implants are kept separate to prevent surface damage. Special screw racks provide storage for different sizes of screw. Some companies supply implants with autoclavable caps or bags to further lessen risk of damage. These are packaged in a similar way to the instruments. During surgery, the sets should be set aside from the main instrument table, so they do not become contaminated with blood. Any implant that does need cleaning should be washed by hand using a soft brush. Any implant such as a nail which has been implanted, must never be re-used.

Prostheses for joint replacement are often bought sterile. Many of these components are made of high density polyethylene and cannot be autoclaved. Usually, they are sterilised by gamma radiation which individual hospitals do not have a facility for. Once items are opened, they cannot be resterilised. It is essential the correct size is determined before the package is opened. To aid this, most prostheses have autoclavable trial components.

The molecular structure of iso-elastic prostheses is altered by autoclaving and it must not be sterilised more than three times. Additionally, it is recommended that it should be left twenty hours after autoclaving before it is implanted.

Silastic prostheses are supplied sterile but can be resterilised by autoclaving. Special care must be taken. The implant must be cleaned using a non oily soap such as Lux flakes, and rinsed in distilled water. It should be handled using gloves, and dried on a lint-free cloth. Initially, problems were met when oil-based soaps were used for cleaning. These were absorbed by the prosthesis and leaked out after implantation.

STAFFING THE OPERATIVE DEPARTMENT

The staff of the operating theatre is led locally by a nursing officer; she is responsible for the daily management and welfare of staff and patients in the unit. She is accountable to a senior nursing officer.

A permanent team of trained sisters, staff nurses, operating department assistants, State Enrolled nurses and auxiliary nurses work under the direction of the nursing officer. Theatre clerks and domestic assistants are also part of the permanent team.

Additional staffing is provided by student, pupil and post-registration nurses, to further their training needs on a rotational programme.

The surgical team is headed by a consultant surgeon. He may operate, assisted by senior registrars, registrars or house surgeons. Alternatively, when the registrars are competent to operate, they may perform operations delegated by him and under his control.

A consultant anaesthetist is responsible for anaesthesia. He may delegate operating lists also under supervision, to the junior medical staff in the anaesthetic department.

The number of beds in the hospital and number of operating theatres governs the number of staff employed in the department.

The staff of the operating theatre are a closely knit team. Each member, regardless of his role, has an important part to play, from the domestic assistant to the senior surgeon. Everyone involved shares the responsibility to do his best to achieve the patients' restoration to full bodily health. Once the patient has signed an operative consent form, he is completely dependent upon the skills and care of the team.

Often, operations are the results of weeks of careful planning and evaluation involving many other departments in the hospital.

CARE OF THE PATIENT

'Total patient care' cannot be related solely to the operating theatre. The patient's care can be divided up into three phases: pre-operative, intra-operative, post-operative. The first two phases are described below.

THE PRE-OPERATIVE PHASE

The patient's admission to hospital commences this phase. The ward sister is responsible for familiarising him with ward routines and facilities.

An identification bracelet is applied to the patient's wrist; this should be referred to when any treatments or medications are given. This is especially important when the patient comes for his operation; when he is anaesthetised he cannot identify himself.

A medical history and physical examination must be completed to ensure the patient is fit for surgery. Routine tests such as X-rays, blood work, urine testing and ECG are completed at this stage: likewise any special tests which may assist in confirming a diagnosis.

An accurate record should be made giving relevant details of the medical history and physical status of the patient, so that these can be used as a basis for comparison throughout all stages of treatment; for instance blood pressure and pulse recordings post-operatively mean little unless the pre-operative recordings are available. Results of all investigations carried out must be included in the notes. Any treatment required pre-operatively is instigated, e.g. special medications.

The psychological state of the patient is of prime importance, and everything possible should be done to set his mind at ease with regard to his surgery and hospitalisation.

He may have family problems arising from his stay in hospital and these can be sorted out with the aid of the social worker. Similarly, thought should be given as to how he will cope with convalescence.

A consent form for operation must be completed by the patient and surgeon. To be valid the surgeon must explain the nature of the operation and the patient should sign to give permission and to confirm he clearly understands what procedure is to be carried out. Where the patient is unfit to sign either through physical disabilities or mental incompetency, consent must be signed by a relative, also in the case of a child under 16. When investigations are complete, the date for surgery is decided and the surgeon hands in his operating list.

This indicates the name, unit no., age and ward of the patient. The diagnosis, type of anaesthesia and operation to be performed are included. The surgeon and his assistants are named as is the anaesthetist. Information is listed as to the site of the operation; this is especially important where left or right is applicable or if the operation is on a digit. Details of blood available and any investigations required during surgery must be listed.

The operating list provides the basis around which the operative care is planned. The procedure the surgeon plans indicates what equipment may be required. Most theatres have 'FAD' cards for each surgeon. These determine the requirements for a given case, skin preparation, instruments, sutures, dressings, splintage, position to be used and table accessories. These details, with a knowledge of anatomy and surgical techniques, help the theatre team with their preparations. The anaesthetist bases his requirements on the type of surgery to be performed, and similar information to that of the surgeons is used to prepare his needs.

The sister-in-charge of a theatre is responsible for planning the care of her patients through the intra-operative phase. She will be assisted by other nurses and ancillary personnel and must be assured that these staff are competent to carry out their delegated tasks.

Effective performance is best assured when assignments are made in advance and adequate preparation can be made to ensure that the necessary supplies, equipment and information are to hand. This allows the operation to be accomplished with safety and efficiency. Poor organisation can result in diminished care and slow down the operative procedure. In these times when hospital costs are soaring, efficient use of time, equipment and staff is essential.

Ideally, the theatre nurse who is making the care plan should visit the patient on his ward. A pre-operative assessment helps plan the intra-operative care. Not only does this individualise patient care but helps the nurse foresee special problems. The patient is deaf; often this information is not charted, and how distressing this can be for the patient arriving in theatre when no-one knows. The age of the patient she knows, but this in no way relates to size, and the latter information is very relevant to the size of instruments required. Having assessed the size of the patient the correct instrumentation can be processed. The consent form can be checked and all relevant reports which may be needed for referral at operation. Allergies may be noted; it is surprising how many patients do not recall these until questioned. Limitations of mobility are important when patient transfer has to be considered—from bed to stretcher, stretcher to table. Disability, such as a stiff shoulder, should be borne in mind, so overstretching whilst the patient is anaesthetised can be avoided and this in turn reduces post-operative discomfort.

In the assessment the theatre nurse establishes a rapport with the patient; he is grateful to be able to know and identify the person who will be looking after him during his operation. For the nurse it is gratifying to see the smile of recognition when the patient arrives in theatre.

Often the patient will ask questions which he was reluctant to bother the surgeon with. Where will his incision be? What does the prosthesis look like? The nurse understanding the operation can endorse what the surgeon has already told the patient and help put him at ease. Immediate pre-operative procedures can be explained.

—The reasons for nil by mouth prior to a general anaesthetic
—The purpose of shaving and skin preparation
—Bowel preparations
—Pre-operative medications. When explaining the purpose of pre-medication drugs a patient has often confessed the worry that he won't sleep the night before. Sedation which is not mandatory can be arranged.

He may question what will happen when he is transferred to theatre for instance, how will he be anaesthetised? Similarly, the patient often wonders where he will awake? Will it be very painful? Answers to these questions reduce anxiety and help the patient understand what is expected of him.

The pre-operative phase involves innumerable detailed observations and procedures. Their importance cannot be over-emphasised; everything possible must be done to ensure the patient arrives for his operation in the best physical and psychological condition; this can only increase the likelihood of an uncomplicated return from surgery.

INTRA-OPERATIVE CARE

The patient's pre-operative care is almost complete; special procedures laid down by the surgeon depending on the type of surgery have been completed. All investigations are reported; the consent is signed. Skin preparation is done and the patient is dressed for his operation. The pre-medication drug is given and the patient is left to relax.

Meanwhile the theatre team prepare for his operation. Environmental controls must be checked; scrupulous cleanliness is essential in preparation of the theatre and anaesthetic areas. All electrical equipment is tested to make sure it is in good working order.

The theatre staff are dressed for the occasion; trouser suits are worn. These allow minimal dispersion of skin scales; hair is completely covered with a cap; outdoor shoes are exchanged for theatre shoes, which incorporate a conductive strip to prevent the build up of electrical charges. Face masks are worn in theatre areas.

The sister checks with the theatre team that all the necessary equipment and supplies which may be required for the operation are available and that the staff feel competent to undertake their delegated tasks. She sorts out any problems they may have. She checks in the anaesthetic room that the equipment is working and all relevant supplies are ready for use.

A porter from the theatre is sent to collect the patient; he takes a 'collection slip' which gives details of the patient he is to bring. The ward nurse checks this slip with the name on the patient's bed and his identification bracelet; together they verify the details are correct. The patient is transferred carefully onto a stretcher, made comfortable and covered with a blanket. The ward nurse who is familiar to the patient accompanies him to the theatre transfer area.

When the patient arrives in theatre he is greeted by the nurse who carried out the pre-operative assessment. She checks his identification bracelet with the ward nurse and peruses the notes making sure the consent and relevant reports are present and correct. This done the patient is ready for transfer to the theatre table. The ward nurse leaves the patient indicating she will see him on his return to the ward, and the theatre nurse and assistant wheel him into the anaesthetic room.

Here the anaesthetist is ready to begin; firstly he identifies the patient with the nurse; he verifies what operation is to be performed and that the consent form is valid.

Induction is usually achieved by intravenous injection of pentothal; he explains what he is doing to the patient, and an assistant may apply pressure to help display the vein. The nurse may hold the patient's hand or just stay close to reassure him. Anaesthesia is usually maintained via an endotracheal tube; a short-acting muscle relaxant facilitates passage of the tube, once the patient has lost consciousness. The tube is connected to the anaesthetic machine and a check is made to ensure it is in place. Cuffed tubes are commonly used when the cuff is inflated; this prevents any backflow of secretions into the trachea. It is important to secure the tube so it does not become disconnected when the patient is moved.

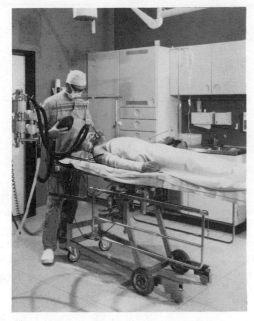

Fig. 8.13A. Patient in anaesthetic room

Depending on the extent of the surgery, monitoring equipment may be applied at this stage. Blood pressure and ECG readings are commonly taken during surgery. In major cases arterial and central venous pressure monitoring is usual. Intravenous transfusions are commonly used to replace fluid loss. Strict aseptic technique must be observed when setting up any intravenous system. All infusion sets should be flushed through to eliminate air from the apparatus before connecting to the cannula. Careful anchoring of cannulae is essential so they are not displaced. When these tests are complete, the patient is positioned for his operation; this should be supervised by the surgeon. Movement should be done carefully to avoid injury to the patient and prevent the displacement of the various tubes. When positioning is satisfactory to the surgeon, a final check must be made to ensure there

is no impediment to respiratory, circulatory or neurological functions. Bony prominences may require extra padding to prevent pressure sores. If diathermy is to be used, the indifferent electrode should be applied in an area of maximum contact, usually on a thigh; at the same time a check should be made to see the patient is not touching metal so he is protected from burns when the diathermy is activated.

Simultaneously the scrub team are preparing in the theatre. Skin disinfection with a suitable antibacterial skin cleanser is performed in the routine manner. A hand scrubbing brush is used; the arms are washed up to the elbow and the hands and nails are scrubbed for five minutes.

The hands are then dried in a prescribed manner and a sterile gown and gloves are donned taking care that the outside of the gown and gloves do not come in contact with the bare hands.

The circulating nurse opens the outer layer of the packs which provide a working base on the instrument trolleys; care must be taken not to contaminate the inner covers. These are opened by the scrub nurse. She then instructs the circulating nurse to open instruments and sterile supplies necessary to the operation. Each package must be examined to ensure its sterility and be dispensed with care to avoid contamination. Preliminary checks of swabs and needles which must be accounted for are carried out between these two and the details recorded on a special board.

When the patient is brought into the theatre, position is finally checked and all equipment is plugged in ready for use. The surgeon prepares the operation site with a suitable skin disinfectant and sterile drapes are placed to cover all but the operative site, care being taken to anchor them in place, usually with an adhesive plastic; diathermy and suction are connected and the surgeon confirms with the anaesthetist that he may begin the operation.

An experienced scrub nurse with a knowledge of surgical techniques is able to hand the surgeon the correct instruments as required. Basically all operations follow a similar pattern. The incision is followed by exposure which involves separation and retraction of tissues, blood vessels being coagulated or ligated. When adequate exposure is achieved the surgeon can carry out the main part

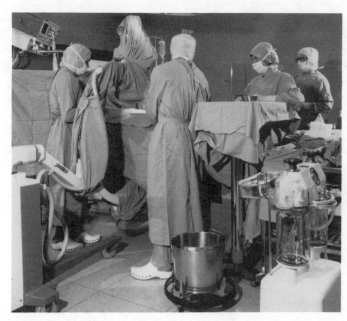

Fig. 8.13B.   Scrub team at operation

of the procedure, removing, repairing or replacing structures.

The nurse in charge is checking that tasks are being performed correctly; she may assist or relieve the circulating nurse. Extra swabs opened must be checked and recorded. All swabs in theatre should be radiopaque, so if any are missing and believed to be still in the wound an X-ray can be taken to confirm this.

Dropped instruments must be shown to the scrub nurse; if she needs the instrument again it must be re-sterilised, otherwise it is kept in theatre till the end of the operation.

During the operation the anaesthetist monitors the patient's condition carefully, replacing fluids and maintaining a satisfactory level of anaesthesia. Maintenance of asepsis throughout the procedure is essential to prevent contamination. Used swabs are placed on a rack in multiples of 5, so they are easily visible for checking; blood loss may be estimated by weighing swabs, similarly blood sucked from the wound may be measured; care must be taken to deduct any amount of irrigation fluid which has been used.

Specimens taken during the operation should be put into appropriate containers and labelled correctly ready for dispatch at the end of the case when the specimen forms have been completed.

When the main part of the procedure is finishing the scrub nurse prepares the sutures for reconstructing the wound. Before any closure is commenced the scrub and circulating nurses check the swabs together; in addition the scrub nurse checks her instruments. If all are correct the surgeon is told; the surgeon confirms his agreement and the wound closure may commence. Wound drains may be used; the type and amount must be recorded in the patient's notes, similarly any packs which may be left in situ.

Needles should always be handed to the surgeon on a one-for-one basis to ensure none are lost. Before the skin is closed a final check of swabs and instruments is made and the information related again to the surgeon. A needle check should be instigated before the wound is cleaned and dressed at the end of the procedure.

Details of the surgery are recorded in the theatre register; these include the details on the operating list. The surgeon is responsible for stating and signing for the operation, swabs and needles used are recorded and nurses involved in their checking must sign to verify they were correct. The total anaesthetic and surgery time is also noted.

Immediately after the procedure the wound is carefully dressed, special attention is paid to the anchoring of drains. Electrode leads etc. are

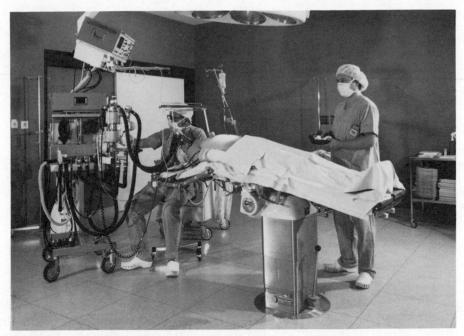

Fig. 8.13C. Patient ready for transfer to bed in recovery.

removed; the nurse checks the skin is clean and intact. A clean gown is put on the patient and he is covered with a warm blanket. Usually the anaesthetist will extubate the patient and 'equipment' should be available in case there are problems in maintaining an airway. As soon as his condition is stable the patient is transferred to his bed and returned to the recovery area. The nurse accompanies him and reports to the recovery staff details of surgery, what drains are in situ and the 'instructions' for immediate post-operative care.

Throughout the patient's treatment nursing care has been continuous; if nursing records are accurately kept, evaluation can be made between ward and theatre nurses. This gives us valuable guidelines for setting standards of basic care and brings to light procedures which need revising to improve care for all patients.

BIBLIOGRAPHY

Howarth F H 1975 Air Technology in Medicine. Building Services Engineer, London
National Association of Theatre Nurse 1978 Codes of Practice. Guide Lines to the Total Care and Safe Practice in Operating Theatres. 2nd edn. London

9

The spine: immobilisation and nursing care

GENERAL NOTES

Before discussing methods of immobilisation of the spine and the nursing care required, some *general principles* on the management of patients immobilised in this way are about to be discussed. Fixation in the lying position is an ordeal for anyone, and the aim of the nurse must be to help her patient over the initial and most difficult period of fixation by the means about to be described. Once the patient accepts the position he soon becomes accustomed to it, and in fact if immobilised for any length of time in a plaster bed he may feel quite bereft when removed from it, though this sensation soon passes. The method of making a plaster bed is described elsewhere (Ch. 6). Preparation of the bed is a simple matter but preparation of the patient himself involves the expenditure of time and trouble not only by the nurse, but by the surgeon and other members of the team. The surgeon will explain to the patient and where indicated, to his relative the reason for his treatment but may allow the ward sister to give further information; in any case this must be given by a responsible person, since the patient can be unduly alarmed if information is gleaned only from his fellow-sufferers or from some other unreliable source. On the other hand, conversation with a cheerful patient already comfortably immobilised can be very helpful to a new one. The nurse may often be questioned by a patient or his relatives and if the patient seems unduly worried, she should refer the matter to the ward sister. The patient's family is brought into the picture at an early stage in the treatment; sometimes difficulties at work or at home are encountered, and it does not require a great deal of imagination to visualise the misery and frustration of lying in bed in hospital while one's professional and domestic affairs deteriorate outside. A patient worried in this way is less likely to settle down to his treatment and make a good recovery than the one whose wife and family is taken care of, whose job is secure and who, at visiting time, is surrounded by friends and well-wishers. Patients who are not in this happy situation may need the help of the medico-social worker, whose services in this connection can be of inestimable value. The family doctor, health visitor and community nurse are also important members of the team caring for the patient.

A patient who is to be immobilised lying on his back requires a tilting mirror fixed to his bed (Fig. 9.2B). Before fixation is started, he should lie on his bed for long periods and learn to focus the mirror, for example, on his food. Roaf and Hodkinson show a recumbent patient eating with the aid of an overhead mirror (see Bibliography). Patients should practise shaving, eating, and making-up in this position, and using a bedpan and urinal. *Female patients must be taught to use a urinal*, so that when fixation is started splintage is not contaminated by urine. A special female urinal is shown in Fig. 9.3, but if one is not available a small kidney-dish or ordinary male urinal often serves the same purpose. Apart from the obvious difficulties of passing urine and faeces while in the lying position, the nurse will again use her imagination in this connection, because the patient is dependent upon her in the performance, in a hospital ward, of acts which are normally an intensely personal and intimate part of his life; this can be embarrassing and even humiliating unless those responsible are careful at all times to preserve the patient's dignity and self-respect. It is also vital that the nurse realises her responsibilities in regard to the toilet of the genital and anal regions of immobilised patients; again, it is humiliating to be unable to perform one's own genital toilet without help and to be quite unable to reach one's anal region for cleansing purposes; routine, daily, matter-of-fact performance of this important nursing duty is imperative.

Although plaster beds are rare now, the nursing problems associated with them must be known.

IMMOBILISATION AND NURSING CARE OF A PATIENT ON A PLASTER BED

Immobilisation of the spine by means of recumbency on a plaster bed may be ordered in any spinal condition, for tuberculosis of the spine, osteomyelitis of the spine, for pain in the back from any cause, e.g. congenital abnormalities or disc lesions, or for fixation following spinal surgery, notably spinal fusion. Briggs & Evans (1982) describe the care and immobilisation of a patient operated on for spondylolisthesis. Other nursing details will be found in Ch. 5.

Preparation of the patient

The surgeon will have explained the necessity for fixation. Except in an emergency, the patient is usually allowed a day or two to 'settle in' before being immobilised, so that he can get to know his fellow patients, his nurses and other members of the ward team, including the physiotherapist, the occupational therapist and if necessary, the medico-social worker. He is admitted to a bed with a sponge-rubber or interior spring mattress, but this can be exchanged for a hair mattress supported by fracture boards as soon as immobilisation commences. Immobilisation is more easily tolerated if the patient remains in bed for a day or two beforehand, lying flat for long periods and practising eating, drinking and using a tilting mirror, bedpan and urinal in that position. Any investigations required, such as radiographic examination, are carried out during this period, especially if surgery is contemplated.

Special clothing is prepared; many hospitals provide large flannel garments but some patients prefer to provide their own pyjama jackets, shirts or nightgowns, split down the back and large enough to tuck in comfortably round the plaster bed. Wool socks, bedjackets and cardigans may be necessary.

Sedatives may be ordered to ensure a good night's sleep and some 'tranquilising' drug may be ordered for nervous, apprehensive individuals.

On the morning of the day of immobilisation, it is essential that the bowels are emptied and it is always advisable to give a small enema or a suppository. This wards off abdominal complications and helps the patient over the initial settling into the bed, if only by relieving his mind about the state of his bowels. Immediately prior to immobilisation, the patient is bathed, either in bed or in the bathroom, and the hair and nails should be scrupulously clean. If a headpiece is ordered, as in a cervical or high thoracic lesion, the hair is best cut short at the back.

Preparation of the plaster bed

The bed is made for the individual patient as already described (Ch. 6). It is of vital importance that it is a *perfect* fit and moulded like a second skin to the contours of the patient's body. Particular attention should be paid to the position of the patient when the bed is made; if it is made with the arms held above the head it cannot be comfortable when the arms are brought to the sides. The legs must be comfortably abducted for nursing purposes, but not so widely that the feet stick out on either side of the mattress; an excessive degree of abduction gives the patient a disagreeable sensation of being 'spread-eagled' and moreover may lead to strain of the inner side of the knee. Unless otherwise ordered, both legs are abducted equally, or the patient may feel that he is 'lying crooked'.

Padding the bed. Unless it is a perfect fit, no amount of padding will make it comfortable. In fact, as already stated, padding should be unnecessary and in some centres patients are nursed successfully in completely unpadded plaster beds

(Fig. 9.1). In most hospitals, however, some form of padding is used and the material does not matter provided it is perfectly smooth and unwrinkled. Sometimes a thin layer of sterilised white or grey felt is cut to fit the contours of the patient's body and the plaster bed made over it; the disadvantage is that the felt tends to ruckle as the wet plaster is moulded over it. When the bed is dry, the felt is covered with a layer of stockinette secured at the edges with plaster cream or adhesive tape. In some centres, splint wood (sheet-wadding) is slit into three thin layers and laid in the bed, then covered with stockinette secured at the edges as described above. This makes a thin, smooth and comfortable lining. In other hospitals, gamgee tissue is used, which looks and feels cosy but is expensive, easily soiled and has a tendency to wrinkle.

When the bed is completed it is sent to the hospital carpenter who mounts it on a wooden support (Fig 9.2B). Some surgeons order suspension of the bed by means of cords and multiple pulleys which the patient can manipulate himself so that he tilts from side to side or from head to foot, the object being to prevent renal complications (Fig. 9.1).

The turning case is made as already described (Ch. 6) as soon as convenient and when the patient is comfortably settled in the bed and able to tolerate the procedure.

Method of immobilisation

The patient's bed should be in a warm room. If

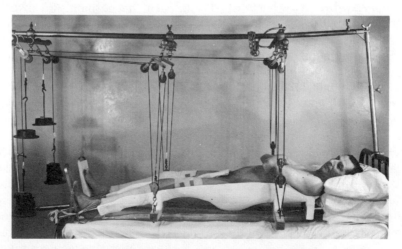

Fig. 9.1 A plaster bed suspended by means of cords and multiple pulleys. Note that this bed is unpadded. (With kind permission from the Insitite of Orthopaedics, Royal National Orthopaedic Hospital.)

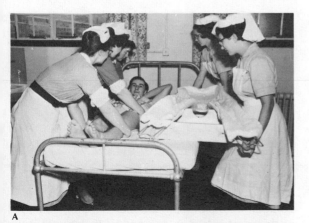

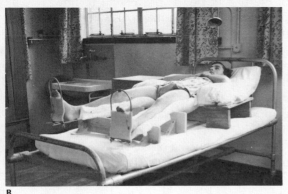

Fig. 9.2 **A.** First stage of immobilisation. A team of nurses lift the patient into the plaster bed as shown. **B.** The patient is now immobilised. Note the firm mattress (fracture boards are not seen in this illustration) the tilting head mirror attached to the bed, and the comfortable supports for the arms and feet. The knee bandages have not yet been applied.

his condition allows, he may sit out of bed while it is stripped, the mattress changed if necessary and supported by fracture boards. Otherwise a completely new bed is prepared and the patient is lifted on to it and laid towards one side of the mattress. Four nurses take up their positions; one grasping the shoulders, one the pelvis and the third the legs just below the knees. The fourth nurse stands on the opposite side of the bed and holds the plaster bed ready in position opposite the patient as shown in Fig. 9.2A. At a command, the patient is lifted while the fourth nurse lifts the plaster-bed into the centre of the mattress and the patient is lowered into it. Unless a headpiece is used, pillows are now placed under the head so that it is comfortably supported. The team leader then satisfies herself that

the patient is lying comfortably, inspecting the shoulders, the trunk and the legs. Run the fingers along the edges of the bed since these sometimes turn in a little during the drying process. If the bed digs into the patient at any point it can be cut or pressed out with shears but 'easing' with the fingers is usually all that is necessary. Be sure that the patient is lying straight with the shoulders and pelvis level and the patellae pointing towards the ceiling; pay special attention to the buttocks; the fork of the bed should be at the level of the tip of the coccyx so that the anal region is free and easily reached for cleansing, but the buttocks should lie evenly in the bed and must not bulge out unsupported or they will become swollen and indurated. Inspect the points where the bed terminates just above the malleoli; a hard edge may cause pressure on the legs and interference with the circulation which may have serious consequences.

Knee bandages. Some surgeons prefer the legs left free, but in general they are bandaged into the bed if strict immobilisation is required. Place a pad of splint-wool over the knee and bandage over the knee and the plaster bed. In some cases the bandages may be removed daily for leg exercises. *The feet* are not allowed to dangle and are either supported by a footboard and pillow or by gallows as shown in Fig. 9.2. These also serve to support the weight of the bedclothes. High footboards and very large bed-cradles should not be used since they cause draughts and obstruct the patient's view over the foot of his bed. *Foot exercises* are given daily. *Arm pillows* are always required since the bed is raised on a platform (Fig. 9.2B).

IMMEDIATE NURSING CARE

When immobilisation is complete, the clothing is put on and the bed is made. A warm, light blanket is usually placed beneath the top sheet and tucked snugly round the plaster bed. *Warmth* is important and a covered hot-water bottle is comforting. Place the locker and personal possessions near at hand, and do not leave the patient unattended for long periods. Though he may not be in actual pain, some discomfort is inevitable, especially in the older, heavier patient and especially towards evening when he becomes tired of his new position. Children and young adults usually suffer no ill effects but they too require attention to their general comfort.

Diet

At first a light diet is offered and help is given in cutting up food. At meal-times a large table-napkin is spread over the chest; the plate is placed on it and the head-mirror is focused on the plate. The majority of patients soon learn to feed themselves and can tolerate a full varied diet within a few days. Refusal of food must be reported to the ward sister.

Fluids

It is vital that adequate fluid intake is ensured from the start, in order to prevent the formation of renal calculi and subsequent infection. Stagnation of urine in the renal pelvis can occur in the early stages of fixation when the patient has difficulty in taking fluids in the new position. At least three pints of fluid should be taken in twenty-four hours and in the early stages it is safest to maintain a fluid intake and output chart. The necessity for a full fluid intake must be explained to the patient and drinks should be made attractive by the addition of fruit juices. Tea and coffee should be freshly made and served to the patient's liking. Some patients like a feeding-cup, but most prefer an ordinary cup or glass, a straw or an angled glass rod which is kept for each patient's exclusive use.

Micturition

Difficulty of micturition is not uncommon in the early stages of fixation. *Inability to pass urine must be reported to the ward sister.* Male patients may need help in placing a urinal in position and if necessary it should be supported on a pillow. In female patients a special urinal (Fig. 9.3) may be used, though an ordinary male urinal is often quite satisfactory. At first, the nurse must hold the urinal in position against the vulva, but most patients soon learn to manage it themselves. Explain to the patient that she must make a definite effort to pass urine. Though more time-consuming in the early stages than simply placing a bedpan in position, it is infinitely more comfortable for the patient since

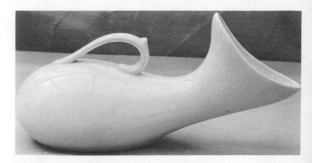

Fig. 9.3 A special urinal for a female patient.

contamination of both the surrounding skin and of the plaster bed is prevented. If, however, the patient finds it impossible to use a urinal, warmed, non-absorbent brown wool is packed round the anal and genital areas to prevent contamination and a tray or bedpan is placed underneath the patient. If difficulty persists, the time-honoured method of running the taps and placing a warm compress over the lower abdomen may prove effective. If the bowels have not been opened for twenty-four hours an enema or Dulcolax suppository may be given and urine may be passed during defaecation. As a last resort, catheterisation may be necessary.

Pain

Many patients complain of aching pain in the lower back and this is due to the 'settling' of the lumbar spine into the bed. There may be abdominal pain and aching of the thighs; this is due to stretching of the abdominal muscles and hip flexors and is usually relieved by a simple analgesic and attention to the general comfort. If it is severe the knees may be flexed for a short period on pillows laid on the leg-pieces of the plaster bed, but this only delays the 'settling' process and the pillows should be removed as soon as possible.

Vomiting

If this occurs it is a danger signal and should be reported to the ward sister immediately; she, in turn, will report it to the medical officer on duty. It must on no account be ignored since it may be the first sign of dilatation of the stomach or paralytic ileus. The knees are flexed on pillows as described above and sips of water only are given. If the bowels have not been opened for twenty-four hours a small enema or suppository is usually ordered, or a flatus tube passed. Persistent vomiting may necessitate removal of the patients from the plaster-bed, administration of fluids by the intravenous route and continuous gastric suction.

General comfort

Attention to the general comfort must not be forgotten in relation to the foregoing observations. The patient often rests quietly throughout the day when there may be distractions in the ward such as visitors, television, etc. but in the evening he becomes tired of his position and will require special attention before settling down for the night. Sponge the hands and face, attend to the hair and the mouth toilet, change the clothing, adjust the pillows and remake the bed. See that the feet are warm, covered and comfortably supported. Refill the hot-water bottle, offer a hot drink, see that fresh drinking water or fruit juice is at hand, and leave the patient comfortable.

DAILY NURSING CARE

A cup of tea is offered on waking and the patient's general condition observed and reported on to the sister in charge. After breakfast, the bed is screened and brown wool is packed round the anal region and a bedpan placed in position. If the bowels are not opened in twenty-four hours a suppository or mild enema is less distressing to the patient than drastic purgatives. Some patients establish regular habits very quickly; others worry about the state of their bowels and many rely on some favourite food or aperient. 'All-bran' cereal with stewed prunes for breakfast is excellent. An adequate fluid intake and plenty of fruit and vegetables are essential during immobilisation to prevent chronic constipation, which may occur although the patient succeeds in passing a small stool each day. Sometimes this state of affairs persists until the rectum becomes full of impacted faeces and manual evacuation is the only remedy. When the bedpan is given, a urinal is also offered and the importance of the use of a urinal in female patients has already

been stressed. When the bedpan has been used, clean the patient with toilet tissue or damp swabs wrapped round the fingers. In female patients, always use a downward motion so that the urethral and vaginal orifices do not become contaminated with faeces; infection of the genital or urinary tract may arise in this way.

The toilet is then commenced. Ideally, the patient is covered by a bath-blanket and all exposed surfaces are washed each day. In the early stages of fixation, or if the patient is too young, too old, too feeble or too ill to wash himself, this must be done by the nurse and in any case the genital region cannot easily be reached by the patient, and the anal region not at all. *Thorough daily cleansing of these parts must on no account be neglected.* Often these patients cannot sit in a bath for some months and are entirely dependent on their nurse for this vital part of their toilet. Most patients prefer to wash the hands and face themselves, and indeed, should undertake as much of their own toilet as they can manage without detriment to their fixation. When the face, neck, arms, axillae and trunk have been washed the nurse must use a separate flannel and towel to wash the genital and anal regions. As already suggested in Ch. 5, the use of a long-handled domestic dish mop may enable patients to wash themselves. Adult male patients can be handed flannel and towel in turn to wash as much of the genital region as can be reached under the bedclothes, but they too require attention to the buttocks and anus. It is important that these areas are thoroughly dried after washing and after using a bedpan, and talcum powder is applied to all skin folds.

During the toilet, see that the buttocks lie evenly in the plaster bed and that there is no swelling or excoriation of the skin. Inspect the shoulders, chest, abdomen and thighs; remove and reapply the knee bandages if necessary; see that the patellae point towards the ceiling; inspect the feet, reporting any swelling or loss of movement to the ward sister. Pressure on the lateral popliteal nerve may cause a drop-foot deformity. Any complaint of pain in the calf should be reported at once; it may indicate a venous thrombosis. The head of the fibula and the malleoli should be inspected since these bony points are subject to pressure.

Attention to the mouth. A tooth-mug filled with

water, and a receiver are required. Place a towel under the chin; patients who are able to clean their own teeth are handed the moistened toothbrush loaded with tooth-paste, and when the teeth have been brushed the tooth-mug is held so that the patient can rinse his mouth into the receiver held to the cheek. Helpless patients must have their teeth cleaned by the nurse; the use of an electric tooth-brush may be indicated; *false teeth* can be soaked in a solution of *hot* water and denture cleansing powder, unless the patient prefers some other cleansing agent. Many endentulous patients allow their dentures to soak overnight, but they must be rinsed in warm water before wearing. False teeth are difficult to clean except under running water and become very uncomfortable if soiled; some patients like to rinse them after each meal.

TURNING

The patient is turned at the discretion of the ward sister, and in general not more often than neces-sary, which may be once a week or once a month, depending on the circumstances. Regular and fre-quent turning helps to prevent renal complications, but in some patients it produces headaches, dizzi-ness and vomiting. Sometimes daily turning is necessary, e.g. if there is a wound or pressure sore on the back.

The use of a mechanical turning device is often urged because hand-turning is said to cause undue strain on the nursing staff, but a well-trained ortho-paedic team who understand the technique of lift-ing and turning can in fact hand-turn a patient in less time, less space and with less disturbance than by mechanical means. The art of hand-turning must be part of every orthopaedic nurse's training since mechanical aid may not always be available or it may break down. Hand-turning with a plaster of Paris turning-case will now be described and since a crane is used in some centres this is also included.

Hand turning with plaster of Paris turning case. The patient should be in a warm room. Place the turning-case and straps at hand. Prepare a trolley with toilet articles, bowl of hot water, clean wool and bandages, nightwear and fresh bedclothes. If a wound is to be dressed a dressing trolley is also prepared.

Strip the bed, remove the knee bandages and the clothing. Line the turning case with wool and lay it in position over the patient's trunk and limbs. Reassure him from time to time: fasten the long turning strap around the trunk and two shorter ones around the legs, keeping the buckles to the outer side. Three nurses stand on one side of the patient and at a command lift him together whilst a fourth removes the wooden platform on which the bed rests. The patient is now lying in his plaster bed with the turning-case strapped on. Two nurses take up their positions on either side of the bed. At a command, the patient is lifted to the end of the bed so that the feet hang over when he is turned, and is thereafter lifted, turned in the air and brought smoothly down on the bed. A pillow is then placed under the head and the patient reassured. In high thoracic or cervical lesions, it is the responsibility of another nurse to steady the head, and the arms are kept out of the way by instructing the patient to clasp his hands behind his neck. Now unfasten the turning-straps and lift the plaster bed off the patient. Inspect the back, noting any swelling red-ness or excoriation of the skin. Wash the back, the buttocks and the backs of the legs, and inspect all pressure areas, the scapulae, the spinous pro-cesses, the sacrum and the posterior iliac spines. The hair may be washed if desired. Cover the patient and leave him comfortable, and inspect the plaster bed. Renew the padding, if required; rough edges may be smoothed off by applying adhesive tape as shown in Fig. 9.4C. When the toilet is com-plete, place the plaster bed carefully on the patient and turn back in the same way. Replace the pil-lows, the knee bandages and the clothing, make the bed and leave the patient comfortable.

Turning with pillows. Where a plaster of Paris turning-case is not available, three or four pillows are placed over the chest, abdomen and legs and fastened in place with the turning straps; the patient is then turned over in the manner already des-cribed.

TURNING WITH THE AID OF A CRANE

Prepare the patient as already described, placing the turning straps in position. Wheel the crane into position over the patient's bed and apply the brake. Place the canvas slings around the patient, bed and

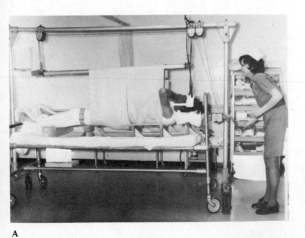
A

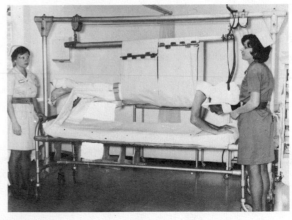
B

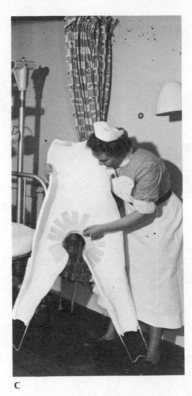
C

Fig. 9.4 **A.** Turning by means of a crane. **B.** The position of the patient is reversed.
C. The edges of the plaster bed are protected as shown.

turning-case as shown in Fig. 9.4A and fasten them securely. Release the brake and wind the patient into the air until he is clear of the wooden platform. The bed is then wheeled away and at a command, the patient is turned in the air while a nurse steadies the head and the patient's hands are clasped behind his neck (Figs 9.4A and B). The bed is replaced under the crane and the patient is lowered on to it for treatment of the back, etc. (Fig. 9.4B) as already described. The same process in reverse is used to return the patient to his plaster bed and he is left comfortable.

TREATMENT OF SORES ON THE BACK

As already stressed, the plaster bed which fits like a second skin should not cause pressure sores, but these sometimes occur if the patient loses weight while lying in the bed. It is quite useless to put thick dressings, pads of wool or other material over sores on the spinous processes, posterior iliac spines or sacrum; this will only increase the pressure and make matters worse. The most satisfactory method of treatment is to make an entirely new plaster bed to fit the patient's altered contours.

THE MARGATE TURNING FRAME (FIG. 9.5)

This was developed at the Royal Sea Bathing Hospital, Margate. The frame has a dual purpose; firstly, it forms a foundation and support for plaster-bed fixation and the accompanying turning-case. Secondly, by joining the two halves together the patient can be rotated from the recumbent to prone position, and vice-versa very easily, quickly, and by one person.

Advantages of the Margate frame

1. Sturdy support for the plaster bed and turning case.
2. The ability to rotate the patient frequently with ease is reassuring and comfortable for the patient and less likely to strain the nurse.

Disadvantages of the Margate frame

1. Because of the depth of the frame when the plaster bed is mounted, a bedstead no higher than 50 cm from the floor should be used to support the frame, otherwise it becomes impossible to attend to the patient. Ideally, a King's Fund bed at its lowest level should be used.
2. For plaster beds with headpiece, special joinery arrangements must be made, otherwise the headpiece remains unsupported.
3. For obese patients there is the occasional difficulty of being unable to oppose the plaster bed and turning case because the connecting pins are too short. This difficulty can be overcome by the joiner constructing four baffles to protect the pins, but in this case, leather turning straps must encircle the patient for security.

These disadvantages can always be overcome and are outweighed by the advantages of a simple and safe piece of apparatus for both patient and nurse.

The nursing care is similar to the classical method of plaster bed fixation as already described. In addition, great care must be taken to support the patient's arms on firm pillows to prevent nerve palsy which could result from pressure against the frame.

NOTES ON NURSING CARE FOR SPINAL SURGERY

Preparation

Major surgery on the spine is not undertaken until the patient is quite at home in his plaster bed. In this connection, adequate preparation for fixation

A
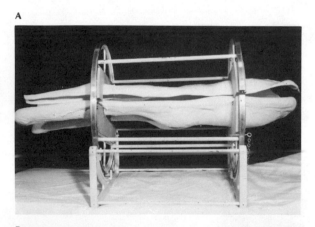

B
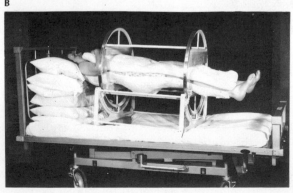

Fig. 9.5   A, B. The Margate turning frame. (See text).

as already described cannot be too heavily stressed, and must include sedation when necessary.

Psychological preparation is very important; the most 'experienced' patient and most phlegmatic individual is afraid of surgery. The first explanation is given by the surgeon but this very often needs to be followed up by other informed people, for example, the Ward Sister. A patient can be helped by talking to another who has had a similar operation, though this too has its dangers because the result of the operation may not be precisely the same in any two people and then one of them believes that he was misinformed.

It has been noted that children sometimes find it amusing to frighten a new patient with horrific tales (Rowe & Dyer, 1977) or a child may have a mistaken but terrifying idea of an operation, such as having his head cut off (*Nursing Times*, 1976). Preparation of the young child is often achieved through play (Ch. 11). Before operation, a thorough physical examination is carried out to exclude chest, urinary or abdominal complications. The patient is visited by the anaesthetist, appropriate drugs are ordered and specimens of blood may be obtained for haemoglobin estimation, grouping and cross-matching in case transfusion is necessary. *Breathing exercises* are usually ordered, and if immobilisation has been prolonged, special exercises may be ordered to regain knee flexion. The day before operation, an enema may be ordered, the patient is bathed and turned for preparation of the skin of the back according to the surgeon's wishes. The plaster bed is relined and clean clothing applied. Pay special attention to the turning-case, in which the patient will lie for the operation; make sure that it is clean and free from cracks or dents. On the morning of operation, the patient is given a light, early breakfast; false teeth and jewellery are removed and urine should be voided immediately before premedication is given. The patient is taken to the operating theatre in his own bed, accompanied by his own nurse, his turning-case and straps, notes, X-rays, receiver, towel and post-anaesthetic instruments.

At the conclusion of the operation, the patient is turned back into his plaster bed, and brought back to the ward by his own nurse who takes over his care from the anaesthetist.

Post-operative care is given as for any other major operation; a clear airway is maintained and the pulse rate, respiration rate and blood-pressure charted half-hourly, or more frequently if indicated. Continuous monitoring of the neurological status is imperative (Chs. 15 and 28). Staining of blood through the plaster bed should be noted and reported to the surgeon. During the first few days following operation, the patient invariably complains of some pain in the back and if this is not relieved by a simple analgesic it should be reported to the surgeon. It is most noticeable that patients who have had bone grafts taken from the iliac crest complain more of pain at this site than at the site of major operation. Sometimes the dressing applied post-operatively becomes soaked with blood which subsequently dries and forms a hard mass over the wound. This causes pressure on the back and it may be necessary to turn the patient to apply a fresh dressing. Otherwise turning is carried out at about the tenth day and the sutures are removed.

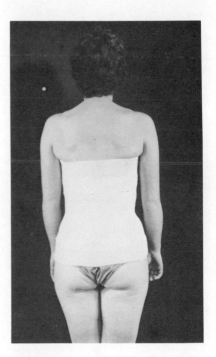

Fig. 9.6 A plaster jacket.

Late treatment of spinal conditions may consist of the wearing of some form of spinal support, such as a plaster jacket (Fig. 9.6) or supporting belt.

BIBLIOGRAPHY

Anderson E 1978 The bedpan and commode. Nursing Times, 20 April, 684

Farrell J 1977 Illustrated Guide to Orthopaedic Nursing. Oxford: Blackwell Scientific

Norton T H, Tait J M 1971 Orthopaedic Surgery. London: Heinemann

Nursing Times 1976 A man without a head. News Feature. Nursing Times, 11 March, 363

Roaf R, Hodkinson L J 1975 A Textbook of Orthopaedic Nursing. Oxford: Blackwell Scientific

Rowe J, Dyer L (eds) 1977 Care of the Orthopaedic Patient. Oxford: Blackwell Scientific

Stone E, Pinney E 1978 Orthopaedics for Nurses. London: Ballière Tindall.

10

The hip and knee: immobilisation and nursing care

THE HIP: IMMOBILISATION AND NURSING CARE

GENERAL NOTES

A variety of conditions relating to the hip joint require treatment quite different from that discussed in this chapter, which is devoted to nursing care in conditions where *immobilisation* and *traction* may be ordered, namely, infective lesions such as septic arthritis (Ch. 16), tuberculosis (Ch. 17) or Perthes' disease (Ch. 15). Such strict immobilisation as that about to be discussed is not nowadays so often ordered as in the past, but every orthopaedic nurse must be familiar with the principles of the techniques described.

In conditions where *movement* of the joint, however limited, is the aim of treatment, as for example after arthroplasty of the hip, splintage which allows controlled movement is ordered, and this is discussed in relation to the particular condition to which it applies, as in Ch. 27. This does not mean to say that a patient immobilised on an abduction frame will necessarily end up with a stiff hip; on the contrary, in infective lesions effectively treated a freely moveable joint is expected, and children treated on abduction frames for Perthes' disease soon recover full movement. It must be borne in mind however that the chief function of the hip joint is that of *weight-bearing*, so that *stability* is of primary importance; a hip joint which, although allowing some movement, is disorganised, unstable and perhaps painful, may be deliberately stiffened by arthrodesis; on the other hand, arthroplasty may be preferred, especially if both hips are affected. The surgeon's advice in this connection will depend on the patient's age, occupation and personal wishes.

The reader is again referred to Chs 2 and 3 on the care of immobilised patients, and also to Chs 5 and 6 which discuss the general care of patients wearing plaster of Paris casts. Some other forms of protective splintage which may be ordered in the late stages of treatment are included at the end of this chapter, together with notes on the correction of flexion deformity of the hip.

TRACTION

The principles of traction are described in Ch. 5. *Skeletal traction* is used mainly in the treatment of fractures and is discussed in Ch. 21. *Skin traction* is supplied by some form of adhesive strapping which is applied lengthwise to the limb and secured by ties either to the foot-end of the bed, which is then elevated to provide counter-traction (Fig. 10.14) or the extensions are attached to weighted cords which run over pulleys fixed to the end of the bed as shown in Fig. 10.15—this is *balanced traction*. Alternatively, as in the method of applying traction about to be discussed, extensions are tied to the end of a splint which exerts counter-traction against another part of the body—this is *fixed traction* as seen in the Thomas bed-splint used in Fig. 10.24.

Application of skin extensions. In the past skin extensions were made by nurses, but have been superseded by commercial packs (Fig. 10.1). The material used is unimportant provided certain rules are followed, now to be described.

1. The limb should be clean and the skin free from blemishes. If there is an abrasion, apply a

Fig. 10.1–10.9 Application of extensions shown in illustrated form (Illustrations by courtesy of Seton Products.)

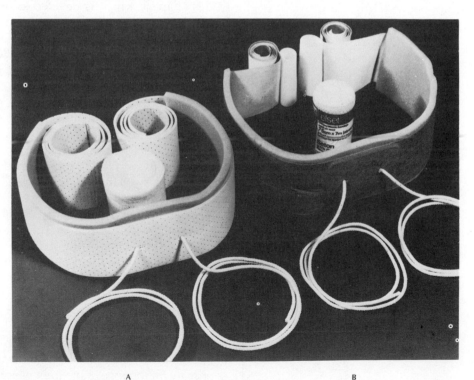

A   B

Fig. 10.1 The pack is chosen according to the size of the patient and the type of traction required. **A.** A non-adhesive pack (page 207). **B.** A two cord adhesive pack suitable for fixed skin traction on a Thomas bedsplint, as seen in Fig. 10.22.

dressing beneath the strapping, or cut a hole in it to accommodate the lesion. *Shaving* the limb is a controversial subject; if it is shaved the skin may be damaged, and in any event new hair will grow in close contact with the strapping; if there is a heavy growth of hair, this may prevent adherence of the strapping. In women and children, shaving is usually unnecessary but it may be required in male patients with excessively hairy legs.* The application of Tinct. Benzoin is favoured in some centres but must not be used with some commercial hypo-allergic strapping. (Seton products).

2. During application, the patient should lie flat in a comfortable position; only the leg involved in the procedure is exposed. An assistant is seated at the foot of the bed or table and exerts gentle steady manual traction on the limb. This keeps the skin 'on the stretch' and helps adherence of the strapping. (Figs 10.2–10.6) (For application of strapping in fracture of the femur see Ch. 21.)

3. The extension strapping must be applied *smoothly*, without creases. Sometimes diagonal cuts in the strapping are required to mould it to the shape of the limb (Fig. 10.6).

4. Apply the strapping so that it lies in the long axis of the limb; i.e. more towards the back of the limb than the front.

5. Bony prominences must be protected, including the malleoli and the head of the fibula.

6. In fixed traction, skin extensions should be tied while an assistant maintains traction on the limb. This prevents the strapping from being stripped off the skin surface.

7. The crest of the tibia and the patella are never covered by the strapping. In above-knee extensions it is best to cover them with two separate bandages, one below the knee and one above.

8. Bandages must be applied firmly but not so tightly as to interfere with the blood or nerve supply to the limb. For the same reason care must be taken to see that they do not crease at the ankle joint.

Skin reactions to extension strapping can be a nuisance both to the patient, who may suffer great discomfort, and to the nurse, who is responsible for keeping up his traction. Treatment of extension sores and of skin reactions is discussed in later

*Patients of the Sikh religion are not permitted to shave body hair.

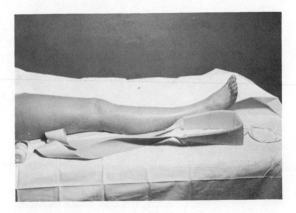

Fig. 10.2 Preparation for application.

pages but sometimes they are so severe that traction has to be discontinued. Since skin extensions are part and parcel of immobilisation by means of a Jones abduction frame, their application and care will be discussed in that connection.

Application will now be shown in illustrated form. (Illustrations by courtesy of Seton Products.)

1. The pack is chosen according to the size of the patient and the type of traction required. Figs 10.1 to 10.7 show a pack with spreader and two cords suitable for fixed skin traction on Thomas splint. Fig. 10.9 shows a one-cord pack suitable for Pugh's or Hamilton Russell traction. *Skin preparation* has already been outlined.

2. Two operators are required; one exerts continuous manual traction on the limb while the other applies the extension. The foot is flexed to a right angle and the spreader plate is placed in position 5–7 cm from the sole of the foot, and at right angles to the leg (Fig. 10.3).

3. After measuring, cut the strapping to the required length (Fig. 10.4).

4. Remove the backing material and smooth the strapping on to the limb eliminating all bubbles and wrinkles. Stretch it in both dimensions so that it conforms to the shape of the limb (Fig. 10.5).

5. Small cuts in the strapping may be required to conform to the shape of the limb (Fig. 10.6).

6. Apply the retaining bandage, starting at half-stretch tension which is decreased as bandaging proceeds up the limb (Fig. 10.7).

7. Always leave the patella free for inspection and practice of quadriceps drill. Most authorities

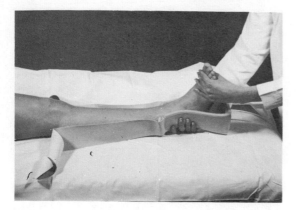

Fig. 10.3 Two operators are required; one exerts continuous traction on the limb while the other applies the extension. The foot is flexed to a right angle and the spreader plate is placed in position 5–7 cm from the sole of the foot and at right angles to the leg.

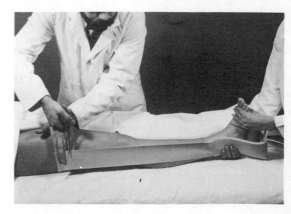

Fig. 10.4 After measuring, cut the strapping to the required length.

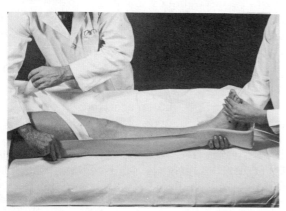

Fig. 10.5 Remove the backing material and smooth the strapping on to the limb eliminating all bubbles and wrinkles. Stretch it in both dimensions so that it conforms to the shape of the limb.

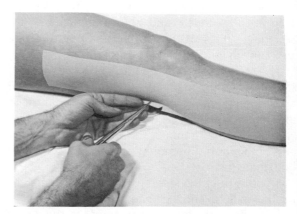

Fig. 10.6 Small cuts in the strapping may be required to conform to the shape of the limb.

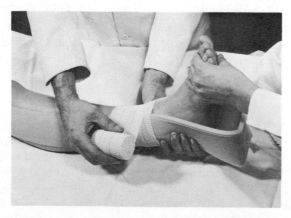

Fig. 10.7 Apply the retaining bandage, starting at half-stretch tension which is decreased as bandaging proceeds up the limb.

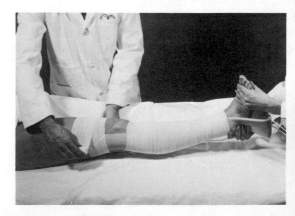

Fig. 10.8 Always leave the patella free for inspection and practice of quadriceps drill. Some authorities suggest the use of two separate bandages—one applied above and one below the knee.

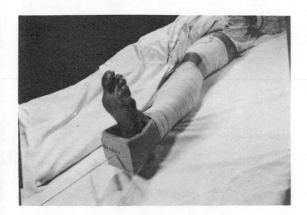

Fig. 10.9 This illustrates the completed extension; in this instance with a single cord attached to the spreader.

suggest the use of two separate bandages—one applied above and one below the knee (Fig. 10.8).

Fig. 10.9 illustrates the completed extension; in this instance, with a single cord attached to the spreader.

Gallows (Bryant's) traction is used for babies and very young children. Skin extensions are applied as already described and are either tied directly to an overhead bar or to weighted cords running over pulleys. The traction force should be sufficient to hold the buttocks just clear of the bed (Fig. 10.10).

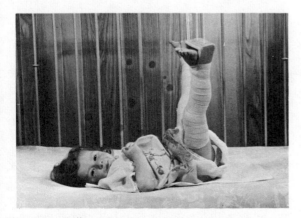

Fig. 10.10 Gallows (Bryant's) traction.

Nursing notes. Feeds are given with caution until the child becomes accustomed to the position, because of the danger of digestive upsets; a napkin is placed beneath the buttocks and the usual care

is given. *Regular inspection of the feet is imperative*; any sign of swelling of the toes is reported to the doctor immediately. Be sure that the encircling bandage is not wrinkled or displaced and that it does not press on the ankle or foot; this might either cause a sore or interfere with the circulation.

Buck's extension hook (Zimmer) is sometimes used in conjunction with skin extension. This extension apparatus may be hooked over the end of any style of bed for the application of traction and it does not need bolts or clamps. It is rubber protected to prevent marring the bed rails. Cord and rod do not interfere with each other. The Carrier Arm is attached to the hook by a ratchet joint which allows the pulley to be securely locked in the desired elevation (Fig. 10.11).

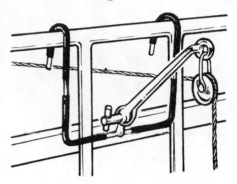

Fig. 10.11 Extension apparatus. Buck's extension hook. (Zimmer.)

Nursing care of patients in traction

Figures 10.12A–D illustrate some of the observations required by the patient in traction:

1. General observations
Is the patient comfortable?
Note the overhead pulley—an essential adjunct to the traction device. To use this the patient grasps the trapeze, bends the sound leg with the foot flat on the bed and lifts the buttocks 'making a bridge'.
2. Is the limb in alignment with the trunk—iliac crest, inner border of patella, inner border of great toe in one straight line?
3. Is the patient practising quadriceps drill at regular intervals?
4. Is the bandage pressing upon the foot?
Is the foot warm, of good colour, and moving freely?
Is there any pain in the calf of the leg?

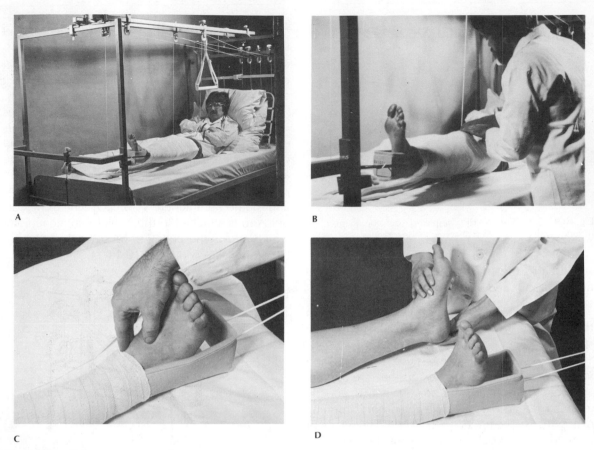

Fig. 10.12 A–D show the observations required by patients on traction. Additional observations required by the patient immobilised in a Thomas Splint (Fig. 10.19–24) will be discussed later in this chapter.

5. Is the heel of the sound foot becoming sore from pressure or friction?

Note that in these illustrations the fixed skin traction applied by means of cords tied to the end of the Thomas splint has been augmented by a cord attached to the splint and running over a pulley placed at the end of the bed—thus adding an additional traction force to the limb.
(Illustrations by courtesy of Seton Products).

IMMOBILISATION AND NURSING CARE OF A PATIENT ON A JONES DOUBLE ABDUCTION FRAME

Preparation of the patient for frame fixation

The patient is prepared as for a plaster bed including psychological preparation (Ch. 9). In addition,

skin-extensions are applied to both legs immediately prior to fixation.

Preparation of the frame

Remove saddle and guards. The degree of abduction is adjusted according to the surgeon's orders by moving the joints of the frame as described in Ch. 7. Bind the frame with strips of gauze. In addition, cover all screws with a little wool and adhesive strapping to prevent them from becoming loose and to protect the bedclothes. Place the frame on a table with the saddle in position, but not tied. With a Lucas wrench, *kink the pelvic-bar on the side of the unaffected hip, and apply the guard and groin-strap.* Apply the shoulder ties.

The degree of abduction is decided by the surgeon and is governed by the clinical and X-ray signs. Wide abduction is sometimes necessary if there is danger of pathological subluxation and in Perthe's disease in order to contain the femoral head in the acetabulum; children as a rule require more abduction than adults. The method of measuring for an abduction frame and saddle is described in Ch. 7.

The patient is generally allowed a day or so in hospital before being fixed on his frame. If, however, the condition is acute and painful, immobilisation may be carried out at once.

The patient lies on a firm couch. Five operators are necessary. Nurse 1 takes up her position at the bed-side, holding the frame with saddle in position level with the patient's body. Nurse 2 stands at the head of the bed and grasps the shoulders. Nurse 3 will lift the pelvis. Nurse 4 steadies the affected limb, one hand beneath the knee and the other around the ankle exerting gentle manual traction against Nurse 1. Great care must be taken in handling the limb and Nurse 4 must concentrate her whole attention upon her particular task. Nurse 5 steadies the unaffected limb in the same way. At the command given by Nurse 1, the patient is lifted *en masse* and the frame slipped beneath him, Nurse 1 satisfies herself that he is correctly placed, with the tip of the coccyx level with the fork of the saddle. Then the already kinked pelvic-bar is pressed into position round the patient's body and the groin-strap is fastened to the studs as shown in Figure 10.13. Nurse 1 then exerts traction *above the knee* in the long axis of the limb, and Nurse 4 ties the extensions. The unaffected limb is dealt with in the same way. This means that traction and counter-traction has been applied and the affected joint immobilised. Other adjustments can then be made without disturbing fixation. The patient is lifted to each side of the bed, the saddle is tied, the remaining bars kinked and the shoulder ties fastened. See that the anterior superior iliac spines are exactly level. Support the knees in slight flexion. Be certain that the knock-knee bars fit closely in the long axis of the limb, and always bandage the whole length of the limb in order to prevent adduction. When bandaging, pay special attention to the position of the limb. Unless otherwise ordered, the patella must point straight forward. It is sometimes difficult to correct rotation and special bandaging or strapping may be necessary.

Figures 10.13A, B and 14 shows patients cor-

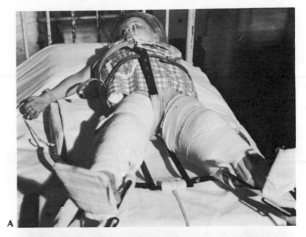

A

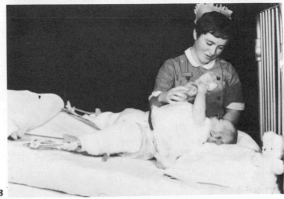

B

Fig. 10.13 **A, B.** Patients immobilised on double abduction frames.

rectly immobilised on double abduction frames. Figure 10.13A shows the moulding of the bars and the position of the groin-strap.

Immediate nursing care

General care. This is as previously described for a plaster bed. The onset of vomiting etc. requires general treatment as already described for a plaster bed. In this connection, the importance of correct preparation of the patient for immobilisation, and of immediate measures to prevent vomiting from becoming established cannot be too heavily stressed. If vomiting commences, the nipple bars may be unfastened and the head and shoulders raised on pillows. In extreme cases, it may be necessary to remove the patient from the frame and apply Pugh's traction until the condition subsides.

Treatment of the groin, by movement of the skin,

must be carried out four-hourly until it has become accustomed to the pressure of the groin-strap. The method of treating the groin is described in the paragraph dealing with the daily toilet.

Daily nursing care

Once traction and counter-traction has been applied, *it is the duty of the nurse to see that it is NEVER relaxed.* The extension ties must be kept taut at all times; they must *never* be loosened unless an assistant is holding the limb above the knee in order to maintain traction. The groin-strap must *never* be unfastened unless counter-traction is provided, this is done either by an assistant exerting traction on the shoulders, or by elevating the foot-end of the bed, so using the patient's own body weight to provide the counter-traction. Flexion contracture, if present, will be reduced by the traction, the lumbar spine will settle on to the saddle and readjustment of the pelvic-bars will be necessary. The extension ties must be inspected frequently as the lampwick may stretch.

The daily toilet is carried out as for a straight frame. After washing the exposed surfaces of the body, pay special attention to the area under the groin-strap.

To treat a groin. Raise the foot-end of the bed on a block or elevator. Remove the groin-strap carefully, so as not to pull on the skin. Inspect the part for signs of pressure (i.e. redness, bruising); if these signs are present the groin-strap must be released for ten minutes (with foot of bed elevated) at two-hourly intervals, day and night. The patient able to co-operate is instructed to use his fingers to ease the skin away from the pressure of the strap at half-hourly intervals; otherwise this should be carried out by the nurse.

When the groin has been inspected, wash the areas beneath the strap, and the external genitalia and powder *lightly*. Any excess will collect in little lumps and cause pressure. Cover the patient and treat the groin-strap. *Do not straighten it*, or the leather will crack and cause sores. Clean the strap with a fairly dry well-soaped flannel. When it is perfectly clean, rub it in the same way as the groin, using plenty of saddle soap. Do not wet it too much. Powder when dry and reapply it, taking care not to damage the skin. A groin-strap which is perfectly clean, soft and smooth will not cause pressure sores, and constant attention to this is as necessary as the treatment of the skin itself. As in the case of any other splint, the patient must be taught to ease the skin and underlying soft tissues away from the strap at regular intervals.

Pressure sores under the groin-strap. The most usual site for a localised sore is the adductor tendon. Once the skin has broken, only the surrounding areas must be rubbed and the sore itself is treated with sterile dressings. Pressure can be relieved in the following manner:

1. By placing a roll of lint on either side of the sore and applying the groin-strap over them. They must be of sufficient thickness to prevent the groin-strap touching the sore.
2. By elevating the foot of the bed and temporarily removing the groin-strap. This must only be done in extreme cases and the frame must be tied to the end of the bed by the cross-bar.

Very young or incontinent patients may require the application of grease instead of powder. Zinc and castor oil ointment, with the addition of sufficient Tinct. Benz. Co, to render it beige-coloured, has been found to be very useful. It should not be used unless absolutely necessary as it quickly ruins the groin-strap, making it black and soggy. If blisters should form beneath a groin-strap, they should be aspirated and treated with sterile dressings. It is always advisable to keep two groin-straps for a child or an incontinent patient.

To give a bedpan to a patient on an abduction frame. This is given as to a patient on a plaster bed; it is not good nursing to elevate the foot of the bed and remove the groin-strap, as urine and faeces may track upwards and ruin the saddle. Female patients should be taught to use a urinal, and cleansing is done in the same way as for a plaster bed.

Maintenance of correct position

The patient is inspected daily to see that the tip of the coccyx approximates to the fork of the saddle and that the ischial tuberosity rests in the gluteal bend of the frame. If incorrect, the patient must be adjusted forthwith.

Procedure

Four nurses are necessary. Remove the bandages and shoulder ties and bend back the nipple bars. Nurse 1 exerts traction under the shoulder-blades as previously described. Nurse 2 steadies the affected limb, Nurse 3 the unaffected one. Nurse 4 then unties the extension tapes, removes the groin-strap and bends back the pelvic-bars. She then grasps the pelvis, and at her command the patient is lifted up or down the frame. The pelvic bar on the unaffected side is then adjusted and the groin-strap applied. Nurse 1 can now release her hold. Nurse 4 then grasps the affected limb above the knee, and exerts smooth gentle traction while nurse 1 ties the extension. Similar traction is exerted on the unaffected limb and the extensions are tied. The extensions should be tight enough to twang like a violin-string. *They must never be tied without traction being exerted on the limb above the knee,* or the strapping will merely be stripped off the skin and no real traction obtained. The pelvic-bar is then adjusted on the affected side. The anterior superior spine of the ilia must be exactly level at all times. Pelvic tilt will result in compensatory deformity of the spine. Place the thumbs on the anterior superior iliac spines and see that they are in the same line. The patient can be taught to do this.

Tilting of the pelvis may be due to one of the following:

1. Extensions being tighter on one side than the other. If so, tighten the extension on the side on which the pelvis is raised.
2. Pressure of the groin-strap. The groin-strap should be tight enough to press against the groin, but not so tight as to produce a deep groove in the skin. The patient may tilt the pelvis down on the unaffected side in an effort to escape the pressure of the strap. In cases where a second groin-strap is necessary to secure immobilisation (e.g. in young and lively children) it must never be so tightly applied as to press on an acutely inflamed hip joint.

The limbs are then examined for swelling or deformity. Special care is needed in supporting the knees. Subluxation is very likely to occur as the traction tends to pull the knee into hyper-extension.

The extensions must be inspected for signs of sores, and no complaint of irritation or pain under them must be ignored. The presence of a sore may be indicated by rise of temperature, by disturbed sleep, and finally by an unpleasant smell or an offensive discharge. Any patient with extensive sores is liable to toxic absorption and albuminuria. The urine must be tested and copious fluids given; the bowels must be kept open. In patients whose skins contain very little pigment, extension sores may become so severe and intractable that a plaster spica is substituted for frame fixation, but this is an admission of failure and is only employed as a last resort.

Treatment of extension sores

A localised sore is easily dealt with by cutting a hole round it in the strapping and applying a sterile dressing. Sloughing sores require a Eusol dressing until the sloughs separate. Thereafter a simple dry dressing is usually adequate. A generalised skin irritation under extensions is more troublesome, and may necessitate removal of the extensions. A temporary extension may be applied (Fig. 10.1A). A generalised skin irritation will often heal quickly if the skin is cleansed with saline and the limb exposed to the air. The application of calamine lotion or of cod-liver oil compresses may prove effective.

Sorbo-rubber temporary extension

A very satisfactory temporary extension can be made by preparing below-knee extensions of Taylor's perforated zinc-oxide strapping and sticking them on to matching strips of 1 cm ($\frac{1}{4}$ inch) sorbo-rubber or by the use of a special pack as shown in Fig. 10.1A. The extensions are then placed, rubber side inwards, on each side of the leg and bandaged on firmly with a crêpe bandage. The extension ties are then fastened to the end of the splint in the usual manner or they may be attached to a spreader, cord and weight as shown in Fig. 10.9.

The ankle must be inspected daily as the extension tends to stand away from the skin after a time and, as traction is applied to it, slips down the limb and may cause pressure behind or in front of the ankle joint.

The feet

When the toilet is complete and splintage adjusted, inspect the feet. Be certain that full movement is present and that they are warm and of good colour, especially if corrective bandaging of any kind is used. Foot exercises are practised regularly.

Deformities

The ones specially to be guarded against are:

1. Tilting of the pelvis.
2. External or internal rotation at the hip.
3. Genu-recurvatum or genu-valgum.
4. Talipes cavovarus. Children must be specially watched for this as they curl their feet inwards under the extension bows.

PUGH'S TRACTION

This may be ordered for any of the conditions mentioned in the opening paragraph, namely, septic arthritis of the hip joint, tuberculosis or Perthe's disease. It is also used in the treatment of low back pain (Ch. 28).

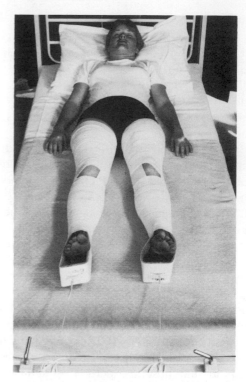

Fig. 10.14 Pugh's traction. The strapping extensions are fastened to the end of the bed, which is raised.

Method of application

After applying the skin extensions, well-padded back-splints may be applied to the legs, extension ties of sufficient length are attached to the extension loops and tied to the end of the bed or to a special wooden cross-bar. The knees must be held in 5 degrees of flexion. In the original Pugh's bed the knees were supported in flexion by a piece of wood inserted beneath the mattress and back-splints were not used. It has been found, however, that the skin-extensions last longer if covered by bandages and splints, and are not easily interfered with by the patient. The foot-end of the bed is then elevated (Fig. 10.14). Never remove the elevator, or all traction on the joint will be lost.

Daily nursing care

After the routine toilet, remove the leg bandages, inspect the extensions, and see that there is sufficient packing under the knee to prevent hyperextension. See that the back-splint, if used, is not pressing into the thigh or the calf, that the extension does not chafe the ankles or feet, and that the feet are warm, of good colour, and moving freely. The heels must not press into the bed, and bedclothes must be supported. Examine the patient for swelling or deformity. Pugh traction exerts no control over pelvic tilt, and is ineffective if the patient sits up. Apart from this it is not an agreeable position for the patient. Copious fluids must be given, and the urine tested regularly as the position prevents proper drainage of the kidneys.

WEIGHT AND PULLEY TRACTION (Modified Pugh's traction)

Weight and pulley traction may follow more stringent immobilisation, or be ordered as a form of treatment in itself.

Method of application

A metal or wooden cross-bar is attached to the end of the bed directly above the mattress and fitted with small pulleys in line with the lower limbs. Strapping extensions are attached to a spreader, and to a cord which runs over the pulley carrying a small weight, as shown in Fig. 10.15. The foot-end of the bed is then elevated to provide counter-traction and the patient may be encouraged to pull the weight over the pulley.

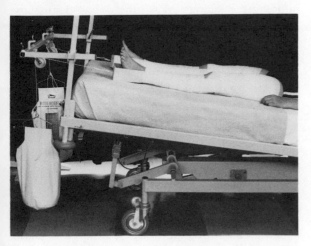

Fig. 10.15 Simple weight and pulley traction (Modified Pugh's traction).

Nursing care

The extensions are inspected daily, and the knees must not become hyperextended. See that the cord does not slip off the pulley and that the weight does not rest on the floor.

PLASTER SPICA, PATTEN AND CRUTCHES

A description of this apparatus is included here because full weight-bearing may not be allowed immediately upon removal from a frame or from other forms of traction. The plaster spica may be single, extending below the knee or including the foot, or it may be double if more fixation is desired. The plaster spica is applied and dried as described in Ch. 6 and the patient is encouraged to roll about in bed. Exercises are given by a physiotherapist to regain flexion of the free knee, and to strengthen the arms preparatory to using crutches. Meantime, crutches are ordered and a patten is applied to the boot of the unaffected side. The height of the patten varies with the size of the patient. For a child, 8 cm at the heel sloping to 6 cm at the toe is usually sufficient, but it must be remembered that though a high patten makes for an unsteady gait, one which is too low will allow the patient to take weight on the toes of the affected side.

To measure for crutches. The patient lies on a firm couch with his arms to his sides. Measure from the axilla to the heel of the boot, and add sufficient to allow for the patten. Crutches must be exactly the right length. If they are too long the patient may develop a crutch-palsy, if they are too short he stoops over them and develops a kyphosis. When the general musculature is good and flexion of the free knee has been regained to at least 90 degrees, weight-bearing is gradually introduced. A physiotherapist will get the patient up for short periods several times a day to avoid fatigue. Exercises, particularly quadriceps drill, are continued, and standing and balancing on the crutches must be taught before actual walking is commenced. If the patient is to be discharged in this apparatus, he must be taught to get on and off his bed unassisted and to negotiate steps. *On discharge*, the nurse must instruct the patient's relatives in the care of the plaster, and the general practitioner and community nurse will be informed of his condition. An appointment should be made for his attendance at the hospital or outside clinic for supervision.

SPLINTAGE WITH WEIGHT-BEARING

Some patients may be allowed to weight-bear in plaster without crutches after frame-fixation (after a preliminary period of kicking about in bed) depending on the individual case, or, direct weight-bearing may be ordered after a period on crutches. The patient may continue to wear a below-knee plaster spica, or, it may terminate above the knee. During the change from a below-knee to an above-knee spica, the patient must regain 90 degrees flexion of the newly freed knee before weight-bearing is introduced. Any patient wearing an above-knee spica must be watched for genu-valgum, and it may be necessary to raise the inner side of the heel of the boot.

COMPENSATION FOR SHORTENING

Real shortening

This is due to destruction or displacement of bone.

Measurements. The patient lies on a firm couch. The anterior superior spines of the ilia must be level. Mark these bony points and the upper border of the medial malleoli. Any difference in measurements between these points constitutes real shortening.

Apparent shortening

This is due to pelvic tilt.

Measurements. The patient lies on a firm couch, with the legs in the position in which they are habitually held. Mark the medial malleoli. Measure from the umbilicus to the points marked. If there is no real shortening, apparent shortening of the limb indicates *adduction*. On the other hand, apparent lengthening indicates *abduction*.

Real shortening of 1.5 cm or less can safely be ignored, but more than this must be compensated for by raising the foot-wear, or deformity will result. To ascertain the amount of raising required, the patient stands upright and graduated wooden blocks (0.5 cm, 1 cm, 2 cm, etc.) are placed under the foot of the affected side until the anterior superior spines of the ilia are level. The amount ordered is generally 1 cm less than the amount of real shortening, and the heel of the boot is usually raised 1 cm more than the sole; for example, a patient with 5 cm real shortening may require 4 cm raising to heel, and 3 cm to sole. The boot is raised by layers of cork placed between its upper and sole (Fig. 10.16B). Fowler (1973) states that if the patient is capable of a normal heel-to-ball gait, the tip of the raised boot should be rounded off to give a toe roll with the same contour as a wooden clog (Fig. 10.16C).

Block-leather spica

After a further period of weight-bearing in plaster, the surgeon may decide to substitute a block-leather spica for the plaster. This is made as described in Ch. 7. It may be made in two halves, or laced down the centre or down one side only, and it may terminate above or below the knee.

Application. The patient is lifted *en masse* into the block-leather.

Daily care of a patient in block-leather spica. Four-hourly treatment of pressure points must be carried out when the splint is first applied; once or twice daily is usually sufficient once the skin has become accustomed to it. After the routine toilet, remove the top half of the block-leather by undoing the lacings. Wash the exposed surfaces, and inspect all pressure points (e.g. the iliac spines). It may be necessary to pad them off with felt, or to hammer out the block-leather a little. Lace the block-leather, turn the patient on to his face and treat the back in the same way. Inspect the spica daily for signs of wear. It is always advisable to keep the bivalved plaster from which the patient has been removed, so that it can be worn should alterations or repairs to the block-leather become necessary.

A caliper

In some cases a caliper may be ordered to afford some protection to the hip joint. This is applied as described later in this chapter and the same care is needed.

Correction of flexion deformity of hip

Correction of flexion deformity of the hip joint may be required in a variety of conditions and the method used will depend upon the cause. In nursing patients suffering from orthopaedic conditions, especially those confined to bed for long periods, it is important to guard against this deformity; for example children with Perthe's disease (Ch. 15) may develop flexion contracture of the hip from constant sitting, and should spend part of each day lying in the prone position. In fact it should be a rule that every patient confined to bed spends at least one hour a day in this position, especially those in whom flexion contracture is likely to occur, for example, in rheumatoid arthritis (Ch. 25), ankylosing spondylitis (Ch. 26), cerebral palsy (Ch. 14) and amputations (Ch. 33). Quite apart from correcting a tendency to hip-flexion deformity, the prone lying position helps to maintain the tone of the erector spinae, the gluteus maximus and the hamstrings; moreover a change of position

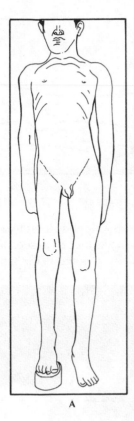

A

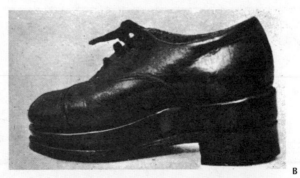

B

Fig. 10.16 A, B. To compensate for shortening of the limb. A layer of cork is placed between the upper and the sole.

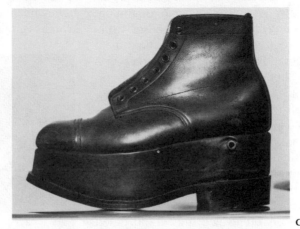

C

Fig. 10.16 C. Patients capable of a normal heel to ball gait should have the tip of a raised boot rounded off. (Courtesy of Mr H. W. Fowler.)

helps to prevent pressure sores, renal and abdominal complications and congestion of the lungs. On the other hand some patients, particularly the elderly, the heavy and the helpless, may find it difficult to tolerate the position and may require special care to prevent the nose being buried in the pillow or the toes being driven into the mattress. The foot hangs over the end of the bed and the upper chest and arms are comfortably supported by pillows; patients who are unable to raise the head should have the forehead supported by a rolled towel or by a sand-bag. During prone-lying it is kinder to reverse the position of the patient's bed, so that he looks into the ward and not at a blank wall. Many patients, especially young subjects, learn to enjoy lying in the prone position and may actually find it most comfortable for meals,

drinks, reading and the pursuit of hobbies or educational projects.

THOMAS TEST FOR FLEXION CONTRACTURE OF THE HIP

The patient lies on a firm couch. The sound limb is flexed on to the abdomen until the lumbar lordosis is obliterated. This position is then held, and if the patient cannot lay the affected leg flat on the couch, flexion contracture is present (Fig. 10.17).

Correction of established deformity

Hip flexion which cannot be corrected or controlled by prone-lying requires treatment according

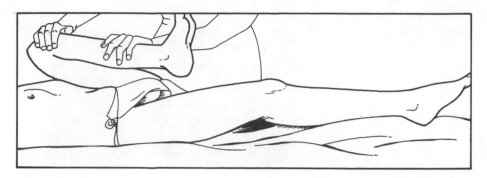

Fig. 10.17 Thomas test for flexion contracture of the hip.

to the cause. Irreversible bony change cannot be corrected by any means other than operation; adaptive shortening of muscles and other soft structures may also require surgical lengthening, as in the Sharrard operation (Ch. 14). Surgical correction is discussed in later chapters relating to the conditions in which it is commonly used.

Correction of flexion contracture of the hip by conservative means is useful where the deformity is due to contracture due to muscle imbalance, as in poliomyelitis, or cerebral palsy, or to muscle spasm as in rheumatoid arthritis. It is important to remember that flexion contracture of the hip joint cannot be corrected unless the pelvis is fixed and the lumbar lordosis obliterated; this is illustrated by Thomas' test (Fig. 10.17).

1. *Correction by means of skin-traction and double-abduction frame* may be ordered in mild cases; application and nursing care has already been described.
2. *Dame Agnes Hunt plaster*. This may be ordered in late cases, where deformity is already established.

Application. A single plaster spica is applied with the sound hip and knee flexed at the right angle and the lumbar lordosis obliterated. The foot may or may not be included. The opposite limb is then fixed in a Thomas bed-splint with skin-extensions in the usual way or immobilised in a plaster cast. At first, the splint or plaster is supported on pillows in the flexed position, then gradually lowered until it rests on the bed. The flexion-contracture of the splinted limb is thus gradually reduced (Fig. 10.18).

In cases where both hips are affected, correction of one will be followed by application of a single

spica. The opposite limb is then fixed in a Thomas bed-splint or in a plaster cast as seen in Figure 10.18 which is gradually lowered in the same way.

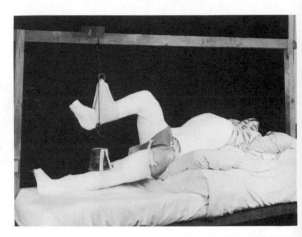

Fig. 10.18 Dame Agnes Hunt plaster for correction of flexion contracture of the left hip. (See text.)

SURGERY

Operations on the hip joint are performed for the following purposes:

1. To correct deformity and promote healing (osteotomy).
2. To fuse the hip joint (arthrodesis).
3. To provide movement at the hip joint (arthroplasty).
4. Operations may be performed to adjust the length of the limbs (leg-shortening or leg-lengthening), especially if there has been interference with growth of the limb.
5. Local excisions may be performed either in an

attempt to eradicate a local focus or to establish a diagnosis.

Preparation for operation proceeds on the same lines as discussed in connection with lesions of the spine. Post-operative care also proceeds on the same lines, and in addition, the splintage applied in the theatre requires attention according to the individual case. The care of plaster of Paris casts has already been discussed and other forms of splintage are dealt with in relation to the conditions for which they may be ordered

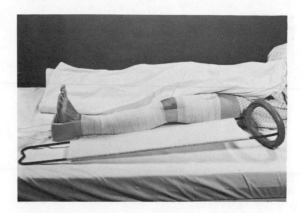

Fig. 10.19   Application of Thomas splint with skin traction.

THE KNEE: IMMOBILISATION AND NURSING CARE

THE THOMAS BED-SPLINT

The Thomas splint is widely used in injuries to the lower limb, in inflammatory lesions of the knee joint such as septic arthritis or tuberculosis of the knee in osteomyelitis of femur or tibia (Chs 16 and 17), or in the correction of flexion contracture of the knee joint as described at the end of this chapter.

Since a *caliper* may be ordered in the late stages to retain extension of the knee or to relieve weight a description of its use is included at the end of this chapter together with notes on the correction of flexion deformity.

Skin-traction is applied by means of commercial extension packs supplied for the purpose. Skin-extensions extend from just below the knee joint to just above the malleoli; *counter-traction* is supplied by the pressure of the bed-splint ring against the ischial tuberosity.

APPLICATION OF THOMAS SPLINT WITH SKIN-TRACTION

Preparation of the patient

Except in an emergency, the patient is usually allowed a day or so to settle into hospital routine before treatment is started, and requires preparation on the same lines as that described for any patient facing immobilisation or rest in bed. Above or below-knee skin extensions are applied as described earlier in this chapter and may be allowed to adhere to the skin for a few hours before being tied.

Preparation of the splint

The method of measuring for a Thomas splint is described in Ch. 7, and the reader should also study Fig. 21.6.

Skin extensions. A commercial pack is generally used.

An assistant steadies the affected limb throughout by grasping the foot.

To apply the bed-splint. Prepare a tray with bed-splint, wool, bandages, and large pins. Two nurses are needed. The patient lies (not sits) on a firm couch, and the affected limb is steadied throughout by an assistant (not shown here). Great care must be taken in handling the limb. While an assistant steadies the limb below the knee, slip the ring of the bed-splint over the patient's foot. The assistant then changes her grasp to the foot and exerts gentle traction. Grasp the splint in the right hand and push it gently up the limb. As the ring reaches the thickest part of the thigh, do not continue to ram it higher in such a manner as to pinch the skin. With the free hand, draw the skin and subcutaneous fat from under the ring, and finally press it firmly into the groin (Figs 10.20 and 10.21). *The bed-splint ring must fit exactly*; one which is too small will cause sores from pressure, one which is too large will cause sores from friction. Adjust the slings with large safety pins, or with paperclips. The slings should be at just sufficient tension to allow two-thirds of the limb to be seen above the splint; if

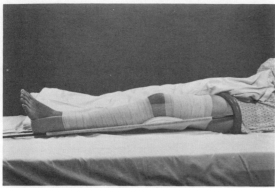

Fig. 10.20   Bed-splint *in situ*.

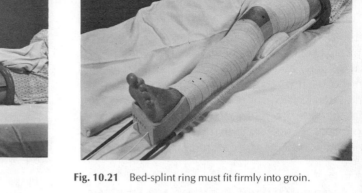

Fig. 10.21   Bed-splint ring must fit firmly into groin.

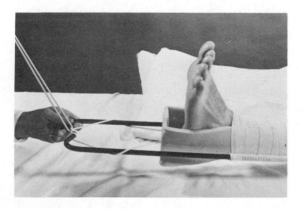

Fig. 10.22   Traction is applied.

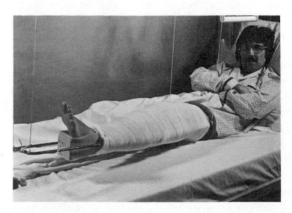

Fig. 10.23   Splint in suspension. An overhead pulley is an essential aid to the patient.

a metal back-splint is used to provide additional support posteriorly, lay it on the slings and pad it with splint-wool; sufficient padding must be placed under the head of the tibia to prevent hyper-extension. The splint must not dig into the thigh or calf. Grasp the ankle above the malleoli and exert smooth gentle traction whilst the assistant ties the extension cord (Fig. 10.22). Traction and counter-traction has now been applied and must NEVER be released. Counter-traction is provided by the pressure of the ring against the tuberosity of the ischium. Now place a thick pad of splint-wool over the knee and bandage securely.

Figure 10.23 shows means by which the splint can be suspended; an overhead pulley or 'monkey-pole' is an invaluable aid to the patient's comfort, since he can then lift himself for bedpans, toilet

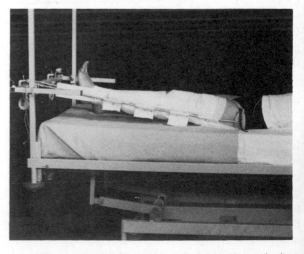

Fig. 10.24   Continuous fixed skin traction on a Thomas bed-splint without suspension.

purposes and for attention to the buttocks and the back of the ring area. If however the patient is unable to raise himself, two nurses stand on either side of the patient and raise him while a third carries out the necessary treatment. In some conditions, the surgeon may give permission for the patient to be turned on his side; in these circumstances the splint is lifted in line with the body while the patient turns on the free leg.

Patients able to sit up are given a back-rest but this is usually removed at night unless there are chest complications.

Care of the skin

The area of skin under the bed-splint ring is very liable to pressure, especially in patients whose general condition is poor and in those suffering from recent injuries or recovering from operations which may cause reactionary swelling of the thigh. It is very difficult to reach the skin under a well-fitting bed-splint and attempts to 'treat' the ring area by conventional washing and rubbing with soap and water are doomed to failure, and in fact may well aggravate the situation by rendering both the surrounding skin and the ring of the splint damp and soggy. *It is vital that the skin and subcutaneous tissue beneath the ring is moved constantly* 'a little this way and a little that way' (Professor McFarland), so that no one area of skin receives constant pressure. At first this treatment should be carried out at *hourly* intervals, especially in an unconscious patient; later the patient is taught to do this himself; a little talcum powder is dusted lightly around the ring area or, if the skin is very dry, a little zinc and castor-oil cream may be applied.

Pressure sores under the bed-splint ring

These should not occur if the splint is a perfect fit and is kept immaculately clean, and if the skin is conscientiously eased away from the ring at regular intervals from the first moment. The most usual sites for localised pressure sores are the adductor tendon in the groin, the front of the hip joint, and the ischial tuberosity. The aim in treating these must always be to relieve the pressure which is the exciting cause, and this can usually be effected by changing the position of the splinted limb. If the sore is on the adductor tendon, abduct the limb, so that pressure in the groin is relieved. If on the front of the hip joint, tie the splint to the end of the bed, elevate the foot of the bed on an elevator, and keep the patient lying so that the body weight falls away from the ring, and pressure is relieved. Pressure sores on the ischial tuberosity may be treated by elevating the end of the splint on a 25 cm wooden block or sand-bag so that the hip is flexed. Generalised skin irritation under the ring is best relieved by tying the splint to the elevated foot-end of the bed, and keeping the patient recumbent.

Daily care of splintage

After the toilet and treatment of the ring area, inspect the extensions and make sure that they are taut.

To tighten extensions. Two nurses are necessary, and the patient must lie down. Remove the bandages. If plaster or metal lateral splints are used, remove them. If anterior and posterior shells are used, the anterior shell only should be removed. Nurse 1 grasps the limb above the malleoli and exerts smooth gentle traction, whilst Nurse 2 secures the extension cord. Inspect the knee for swelling, increased local heat, or increasing deformity. Inspect the extensions. If extension sores form, they may be treated as described in the previous chapter, and extensions are reapplied in the same way, the limb being supported throughout by an assistant. If packing is used under the knee, be certain that it is sufficient in amount to prevent hyperextension. See that the foot is warm, of good colour, and moving freely. Foot exercises are practised regularly. If the surgeon allows, the patient should spend part of every day lying on his face, with the foot over the end of the bed. This preserves the tone of the back muscles and gluteal muscles and prevents the contracture of the hip-flexors which may follow prolonged sitting.

To give a bedpan to a patient in a bed-splint. If the patient is able to raise himself, the bedpan is placed beneath him in the usual way. If, however, the condition is acute, or the patient is old or ill, one or two nurses may be necessary to raise the patient whilst a third places the bedpan in position. Female patients should be encouraged to use a urinal. The patient is either turned on to his side, or lifted as already described for cleansing purposes.

TO APPLY A CALIPER (long leg brace)

A caliper may be ordered to protect the lower limb after disease or injury, and to restrict weight-bearing. The boot must be tubed to receive the caliper. Prepare a tray with gauze bandage, swabs, receiver, a cleansing agent such as ether, roll of Elastoplast or other supporting bandage if ordered, the caliper and a screwdriver. Two nurses are necessary, and the patient must lie down. While an assistant steadies the limb by grasping the foot, the bandage is removed. Slide the bed-splint down the limb, the nurse who is steadying the limb supporting the head of the tibia with one hand whilst maintaining traction with the other. Remove the extensions, and clean the limb with ether or spirit. An Elastoplast or other supporting bandage may be ordered to prevent swelling of the limb; it must be applied smoothly and evenly, leaving no gaps and it must extend from the web of the toes to well up the calf. Slide the caliper up the limb until the ring fits snugly into the groin. Sometimes the caliper ring can be split and fastened with a strap and buckle. Put on the boot and lace it; slip the prolongations into the tubed heel; it may be necessary to shorten or lengthen the caliper by adjusting the screws. Fasten the sling behind the knee with safety pins and see that the knee is completely supported between the slings and knee-shield. A guarding plaster is sometimes used with a caliper to provide additional immobilisation. On removal of the bed-splint, apply the caliper, then the cylinder, and allow it to dry; then proceed as before. To relieve weight efficiently, the ring of the caliper must fit closely against the ischial tuberosity, and the under surface of the heel must be just clear of the boot, so that the limb is suspended in the caliper and weight is borne through the ring and not directly through the knee-joint. Boots are to be preferred to shoes, especially in children, because if the caliper is truly weight-relieving the heel tends to slip out of a shoe. It may be necessary to place the heel tubing at an oblique angle to correct a persistent intoeing gait. Later, the guarding plaster may be discarded and a caliper only be worn. The application of a caliper only is carried out in the same way, but special care must be taken to see that the sling behind the knee is tight enough to prevent hyperextension. The soft portion in the centre of the knee-shield should fit exactly over the patella and the lower straps must be tight enough to hold the knee firmly. The upper straps should not be so tight as to press on the quadriceps.

Nursing care

The caliper must be worn continually unless otherwise ordered. The boot should be wrapped in old linen to protect the bedclothes, and the ring area and the heel must be inspected for signs of pressure. If pressure sores occur under the ring-area, the patient is confined to bed and they are treated as for a bed-splint. For pressure sores on the heel, the boot is reversed, i.e. while an assistant steadies the limb, the boot is removed and the sole covered by a piece of felt. The sole of the boot is then placed against the patient's foot and the caliper ends are replaced in the tubing. Fixation is thereby maintained, but pressure on the heel is removed. When the patient is accustomed to the caliper, he is taught to stand and walk by a physiotherapist. The patient is taught to lift the affected leg straight forwards. He must not be allowed to swing it out sideways.

A *bucket-top caliper* is ordered if it is thought that an ordinary caliper will not be well tolerated, for example in elderly or obese patients. It is made on a cast of the patient's thigh and requires the same care as an ordinary caliper.

CORRECTION OF FLEXION DEFORMITY OF KNEE

Correction of flexion deformity of the knee may be attempted by conservative means in cases where contracture is due to soft-tissue changes rather than to bony ankylosis. The method used may be a plaster or a splint.

1. Corrective plasters

1. *Wedged plaster*. The knee is covered with a thick layer of felt and wool, and the limb is immobilised in a plaster cast. When it has thoroughly

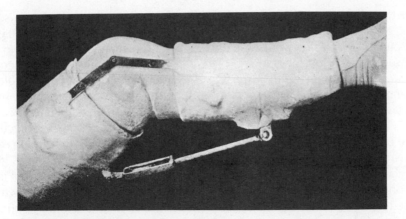

Fig. 10.25 Turnbuckle plaster for correction of flexion contracture of the knee joint (see text).

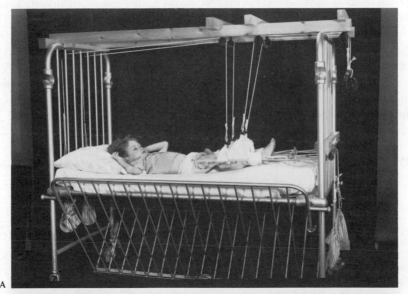

A

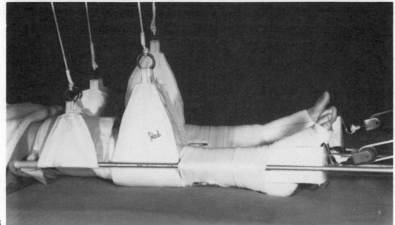

B

Fig. 10.26 **A, B.** Dynamic traction (see text).

set, the back of the plaster is split three-quarters of the way round at the line of the knee joint. The split is opened, pieces of cork are wedged in and gradually increased in size until the desired position has been reached. This method of correction is not without danger because the knee joint is hidden inside the plaster and may easily become dislocated.

2. *Turnbuckle plaster.* The limb is covered with a thick layer of wool-roll, or with felt, and plaster is applied from the top of the thigh to just above the knee joint, and from just below the knee to the malleoli. The two halves are joined by a turnbuckle which is opened a few degrees each day and the knee is gradually brought into the extended position (Fig. 10.25). Again, great care is necessary to prevent subluxation of the knee.

3. *Thomas bed-splint.* A Thomas bed-splint, either bent at the knee or combined with a Pearson flexion attachment.

A. *The Thomas bed-splint is bent* at the level of the knee joint to the same degree of flexion as the knee. It is applied in the usual way, and the extensions tied. The splint is then gradually straightened a few degrees every second or third day until the extended position is reached. *The knee must not be allowed to become subluxated*; adequate support for the head of the tibia must be ensured.

B. *The Thomas splint is applied in the usual way*, with Pearson flexion knee-piece attached at the level of the knee joint. The skin extensions are tied to the flexion piece, and this is gradually straightened until the extended position is reached.

C. *Dynamic traction* is shown in Figs 10.26A, B. It consists of a Thomas splint with weighted slings applied as in B, i.e. one over the knee joint giving downward pressure, countered by a further sling giving pressure under the upper end of the tibia and fibula. This traction can be used to correct flexion deformity of the knee in rheumatoid arthritis and it is also employed to stretch soft tissues before a knee replacement operation (Chs 25 and 27).

Note: This traction must be applied and monitored with the utmost care to avoid subluxation of the knee joint.

BIBLIOGRAPHY

Adams J C 1971 Outline of Orthopaedics. Edinburgh: Churchill Livingstone

Apley A G 1977 A System of Orthopaedics and Fractures. London: Butterworths

Chilman A M, Thomas N (eds) 1978 Understanding Nursing Care. Edinburgh: Churchill Livingstone

Farrell J 1977 Illustrated Guide to Orthopaedic Nursing. Oxford: Blackwell Scientific

Fowler A W 1983 Rigid footwear. Letter in British Medical Journal, 3 March, 553

Kennedy J M Orthopaedic Splints and Appliances. London: Ballière Tindall

Owen R 1972 Indications and contra-indications for limb traction. Physiotherapy, 58, 44

Powell M 1972 Application of limb traction and nursing management. Physiotherapy, 58, 46

Powell M 1973 Limb traction—some aspects of nursing management. Nursing Mirror, 27 July, 26

Roaf R, Hodkinson L J 1976 Textbook of Orthopaedic Nursing. London: Blackwell Scientific

Rowe J, Dyer L (eds) 1977 Care of the Orthopaedic Patient. Oxford: Blackwell Scientific.

Stewart J D M 1975 Traction and Orthopaedic Appliances. Edinburgh: Churchill Livingstone

Stone E, Pinney E 1978 Orthopaedics for Nurses. London: Ballière Tindall

SECTION TWO

Paediatric Orthopaedics

11

Paediatric orthopaedics 1: general considerations

INTRODUCTION

Provision for the care of children is changing in response to shifting disease patterns; diphtheria, poliomyelitis and tuberculosis have almost been eliminated, while road accidents, burns and birth defects have resulted in new attitudes and in new orthopaedic skills in treating these children. Small numbers of children are nursed for long periods in special hospitals, e.g. Orthopaedic or Plastic Surgery Units and those for the mentally handicapped, which are often sited in rural areas where access is difficult. Modern thinking has led to the encouragement of hospital visiting and the provision of 'mother-in' units. This has greatly relieved the anxieties of children and their parents needing these services. Responsibility for child health is jointly shared by the Health, Education and Social Services Departments. Such a system could result in duplication, omission and confusion; but dramatic changes are slowly taking place. A blue-print for the next 20 years has been published by HM Stationery Office, December 1976, entitled *Fit for the Future* in which a visionary approach by Professor Court and the Committee on Child Health offers guide-lines for the integration of all children's services with emphasis on efficiency in the preventive fields.

A new era of multi-disciplinary care has arrived; the aims and objectives shared by paediatric and orthopaedic teams now overlap considerably.

THE CHILD AS AN ORTHOPAEDIC PATIENT

A consistent policy in caring for all children in hospital must:

1. Recognise the special needs of children as children.
2. Have experts in child health (medical, nursing, para-medical, social, etc.) available for all children.
3. Maintain close contacts between the child and his family during the hospital stay.
4. Ensure that the duration in hospital is kept to a minimum, or if possible, avoided altogether.

It is easy to collect data about patients before they leave school, hence it is not surprising that sixteen years is conveniently used by statisticians as the 'age break' between child and adult. In clinical practice judgement must be used by applying the behavioural and emotional developmental status to the various physical signs of puberty, all of which make purely age-related policies unwise. The physical and social maturity of children must influence their medical care, as should their own wishes and those of their parents.

An arbitrary period of 'over three-months in hospital during the previous 12 months' has been generally used to quantify the inmportant group of long-stay patients. Fortunately, as far as Orthopaedic Units are concerned, the numbers of long-stay children are rapidly diminishing. Just a few years ago the average length of stay of a child having spinal surgery was 15 weeks, now it is 21 days. No doubt this is a measure of changing expertise as well as an updated attitude of orthopaedic surgeons who are interested in the total care of children and their families.

Discharging children from hospital between various operative procedures can be commendable but can also create problems. Children sometimes react adversely to repeated changes of environment and the interruption of their educational programmes is also disconcerting. Such requests from parents are therefore best left to the discretion of the ward Sister, who after consultation with team colleagues could then reason with the parent and patient in order to justify the variable decisions which are taken in different cases.

Special needs

All children, whether they be infants, juniors or adolescents have special needs, especially regarding the following:

1. Quality of preventive health service.
2. The environment in which they live.
3. Education.
4. Nutrition.

PREVENTIVE SERVICES

Many paediatricians have developed a keen interest in skeleto-muscular growth problems and some orthopaedic surgeons have shown great concern in *fetal* development; if this were not so, how could defects having medical as well as surgical implications, such as Duchenne dystrophy, haemophilia or multiple birth defects be managed? Babies born with myelomeningocoele have various multi-disciplinary problems both medical and surgical, which demand the team approach by many therapists (Fig. 11.1). For these reasons, orthopaedic surgeons need to acquire experience in examining normal babies before they can become competent in making pronouncements about such conditions as clicking hips, varus feet, tibial bowing, spinal defects, etc. They must be quick to recognise 'funny-faces' and other stigmata suggesting possible chromosomal defects before they embark on major, life-threatening operative procedures. Likewise, paediatricians must be aware of the common orthopaedic problems of childhood, such as congenital dislocation of hips, Perthes' disease and slipped upper femoral epiphyses, so that earlier diagnosis and a shorter stay in hospital can be directed to the child's benefit.

In the nursing field, the RSCN qualification in addition to the orthopaedic certificate should equip the ward Sister admirably for the special needs of children on orthopaedic wards. Unfortunately, these wards are frequently lacking in such skilled manpower. Many also lack the nineteen members of nursing staff which is quoted as being required for a 20-bed childrens' ward. It is certainly helpful for permanent paediatric nursing staff to have their horizons expanded by short periods of practical attachment to physiotherapy, occupational therapy, dental, hairdressing and canteen departments;

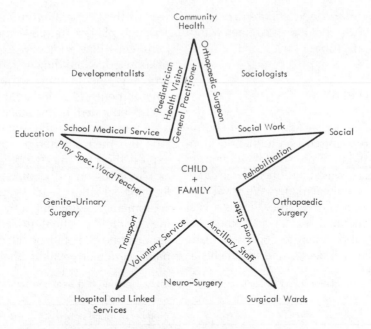

Fig. 11.1 Spina Bifida multidisciplinary service:
1. To reduce social and emotional burden on the child and family.
2. To promote family integration and social adaptation.

while outside the hospital field they might well be attached to pre-school playgroups, schools for physically handicapped children and community adventure playgrounds.

ENVIRONMENT

Four points should be borne in mind:

1. That orthopaedic children are not usually ill, they just happen to be 'relatively fixed' for a spell.
2. Paediatricians have a general concern and responsibility for the welfare of children in whatever department they may be nursed.
3. Provisions should routinely be made for the parents of 10 per cent of children to stay in. This figure could be higher in rural areas.
4. Children's sensory organs need exercising for fun as well as their limbs for locomotion; but excessive noise such as ward radio and TV must be disciplined by the ward Sister who uses tact and reasoned selectivity.

In order to avoid unnecessary ward admissions or to shorten the duration of stay in hospital, clinical investigations and treatment of children should be done on a day basis. Hence facilities for this must be available for all children's departments. Daycare programmes are ideal for radiological investigations, minor dental, orthopaedic and general surgery. Accommodation in the in-patient unit has to be specially planned and staffed for this purpose.

All children attending as orthopaedic outpatients should be seen at a special children's clinic, except where bulky diagnostic equipment is required, which is housed elsewhere and which can only be provided in one area of the hospital. Special attention must be paid to waiting lists, waiting times, courteous reception, patient facilities and departmental management.

In intensive care units which are primarily designed for adults, children should be protected from the sight and as far as possible, from the sound of other patients.

The table shown below was first published with the Hospital Building Act No. 23 for Childrens wards in 1964. It is intended to be a guide for the type, numbers and size of rooms in a children's ward complex. *For orthopaedic children a play and teaching area must be included*, together with a room for plaster work (Table 11.1).

EDUCATION AND PLAY

The therapeutic value of play for children in hospital is now widely recognised as a further development for the well-being of pre-school children. In the past, when play was mentioned to an adult it was interpreted as a trivial matter. We now know that for children the reverse is true. Play is a vital factor in their intellectual, social and emotional development. It enables them to cope with many of the stresses of their illnesses and treatments as well as their separation from homes and families. Through play, a toddler learns; observes and experiments. Play adds new experiences to his store of knowledge, building up language, reasoning out problems and learning to adapt socially to new environments. Play and education in hospital cannot be separated. In hospital it is important to create a secure and interesting setting, as well as to provide the means whereby children can learn to express their feelings (Noble, 1969). What begins as play goes on to become a more conventional learning situation, each stage of the child's development growing out of the previous one. Holding a child's attention and helping him to concentrate can often be difficult to achieve in hospital, particularly with the handicapped child who

Table 11.1 Basic accommodation for a ward unit of 20 beds (12 children in multi-bed areas and eight children in single bed rooms)

Type of room	Number of rooms or beds	Area per room etc. (sq ft)
1. Wards		
(a) and (b) single/mother and child rooms	8 rooms	Min. 120
		Max. 200
(c) Multi-bed rooms or bays	12 beds	100–110 sq ft per bed
2. Day space (play area, dining and schoolroom)	1	30 sq ft per bed
3. Treatment room		
4. Utility rooms		
(a) Clean utility	1	100
(b) Dirty utility	1	100
5. Bathroom	1	200
Shower cubicle	1	
6. Patients' washing facilities	3 cubicles	
7. WCs	7	
WCs area for potting	pot area	
8. Sluice and test room	1	100
9. Sisters' room	1	120
10. Nurses' station	1	80–100
	(possibly 2)	
11. Ward pantry	1	140
12. Linen bay	1	50
13. Stores	3 or 4	300–400 total
14. Cleaners' room	1	50
15. Trolley/wheelchair		
16. Flower room or bay	1	50
17. Staff lavatories and cloakrooms		
(Female WC)	1	
(Female cloakroom)	1	
(Male WC)	1	
18. Doctors' room	1	120
19. Rooms for relatives	1	120
20. Visitors' waiting space	1	
21. Visitors' lavatory accommodation		
(Male)	1	
(Female)	1	
22. Parents' sitting room	1	
23. Mothers' washing facilities		
24. Sundry facilities		
25. Circulation space		

may not be able to concentrate at all. The play specialist has therefore, to find or create situations which make children eager to learn. Children who are restricted—for example by a plaster cast or a traction device—need to use the limbs which are free. Stimulation through musical toys, action songs and nursery rhymes are important to promote these movements. Involvement of parents in planned programmes of play is important, even when the visits are only of short duration. For the babies, such play could be vital. If babies are 'good' they might be left for too long in a calm and peaceful setting; we now realise that if babies are not played with and talked to, their language development can be inhibited.

Hospital staff should help mothers to appreciate the connection between play and learning. Bonding processes which are stimulated in the perinatal period should be reinforced when there is prolonged separation (Jolly, 1978). Remember that in this context, a day in the life of a baby may be equivalent to a month for an older child. Coordination of these ward activities, like many others, involve harmony between nursing, play and teaching staff, and in working with the parents. Play therapy should be available constantly (seven days a week and holidays) because of its catalytic contribution to the child's overall recovery.

NUTRITION

Babies in orthopaedic units are usually hand (bottle) fed. However, breast-feeding should be encouraged wherever possible and suitable accommodation should be offered to the mother. Ward construction must allow designated areas for feed preparation and for bottle and teat sterilisation (using pressure cookers if necessary). Alternatively, ready prepared, humanised milk feeds are satisfactory and time saving, but they are more costly. During the first three months (or until a weight of 15 lb) the well baby thrives on four-hourly feeds of 2.5 fluid ounces per pound body weight per day. Weaning foods are slowly introduced over the next three months to ensure adequate calorie intake— about 1300 calories daily until aged 1–2 years, and 2700 calories daily at age 11–14 years. We must remember that one pint of cow's milk (silver-top) supplies 360 calories and that this volume contains enough calcium to meet all the child's needs. Adequate fluid, calorie and salt intake is reflected in the weight gain and stools. A baby gains an ounce a day in the first three months after birth. He doubles the birth weight at age five months and trebles the birth weight at one year. He is four times the birth weight at two years, and when age seven years he should weigh about $7 \times 7 = 49$ lb.

Hospital meals for older children need joint action between the Catering Department, Dietitian, and the ward Sister (who is consulted about the various likes and dislikes of the children); foods with new flavours must be introduced with care. Food should be attractive in appearance and texture, well-cooked and finely chopped for very young children. Meals must be served punctually at regular times and the utensils for the young child should be coloured and unbreakable. Plastic-wear is probably better than white china; mugs and cups are easier than glasses for small children to hold and drinking straws are useful for children to take fluids post-operatively without spillage.

Obesity is often the sign of parentally mismanaged eating habits at home and at school. In the prevention of overweight, we must aim either to stop weight gain or to reduce weight by a maximum of 2 lb a week. A reduction of weight over a long term must be maintained and dietetic prevention of regained weight should be achieved by careful discipline and a positive attitude to food selection such as taking protein for breakfast and avoiding fried food. A low calorie intake of half to two-thirds of normal requirement and 20 per cent of the total calories through protein, can also be highly effective for children. Adequate vitamins—especially C and D—as well as minerals (phosphate and calcium) must be taken. Avoidance of ketosis is important.

For the under-weight child, attempts should always be made to institute oral rather than parenteral feeding. This can be provided in several ways. Liquid food products can be administered via nasogastric tubes if the usual palatable oral nutritional supplements such as Complan, Calorine and Hycal combinations are not tolerated. These foods can supply most of the calorie, nutritional, mineral and vitamin requirements for a few weeks.

NORMAL GROWTH AND DEVELOPMENT IN RELATION TO ORTHOPAEDIC CONDITIONS

Embryonic development is mostly under the influence of genetic control which governs rapid cell division and determines cell 'layering'. Formation and function of organs is very soon complete within this completely new creation. At three months' gestation, placentation enables the fetus to flourish. The environmental influences *in utero* during all this time are important for the skeletomuscular system. The secret of many postural, metabolic, deficiency and infective disorders can be determined prenatally. Fetal malformations may be environmentally induced or have some hereditary (genetic) basis. The birth process itself has become less significant now that fetal monitoring and elective procedures enable obstetricians to control fetal hypoxia as well as length of gestation.

Amniocentesis, at 4–5 months of pregnancy has offered new opportunities in the field of preventive paediatrics, which together with the availability of abortion poses new ethical and moral problems for doctors, parents and nurses. Genetic counselling and accurate, careful advice about family planning are essential within all systems of management at this time.

Nursing staff are occasionally involved in a special way with the surviving babies or their families. Conflicts can arise from the social, financial and resource allocation which must determine specific strategies for treatment. Judgements about the advisability of intervening to promote the best possible state of survival must therefore be made by co-ordinating medical and nursing policies (see Fig. 11.2 for intra-uterine and postnatal growth).

Normal growth of childhood is in three separate phases. The first is in the first year of postnatal life

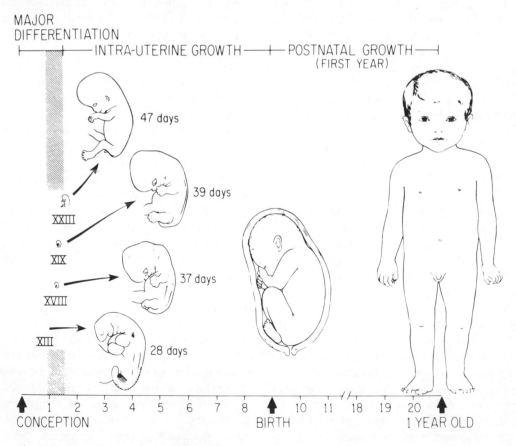

Fig. 11.2 Intra-uterine and postnatal growth.

(babyhood). The second has its peak at the sixth or seventh year (second dentition) and the third is the adolescent spurt (puberty).

Each of the three periods of growth is associated with its own developmental and disease problems. Thus, the first year is concerned with the baby's nutritional problems. In the second, there is increased risk of infection as the environmental contacts increase. When schooling commences in the third period we have the catarrhal and infectious diseases being common, while after the second dentition the period of adolescence is probably the healthiest time of our lives.

The growth of the skeleton after birth—short stature

The growing period of life extends from conception until full skeletal maturity has been reached—at about 25 years of age. During this time, the skeleton of the different regions of the body changes not only in size, but also in shape (Fig. 11.3).

As seen in Fig. 11.3 the head becomes relatively smaller. The limbs, and especially the lower limbs, become relatively longer, so that in adults the level of the pubis divides the body into two equal segments—an upper segment (head to pubis) and a lower segment (pubis to heel). During adolescence, the growth spurt occurs more in the spine than in the legs. This is the time when predisposed girls develop the common type of lateral spinal curvature known as adolescent idiopathic scoliosis. In normal boys, the adolescent growth spurt peaks at about the age of 14 years—two years later than in normal girls.

Growth is a complicated process. First and fore-

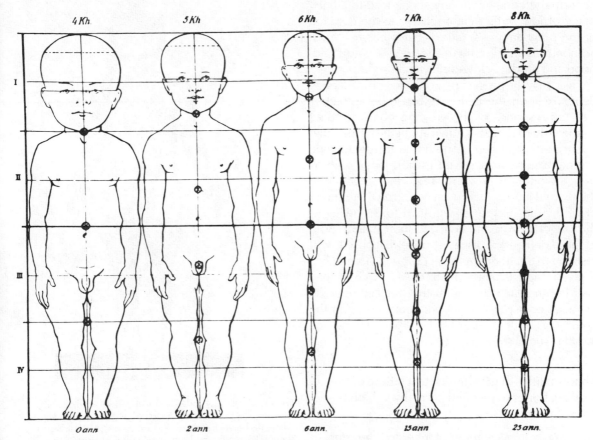

Fig. 11.3 The changing skeletal proportions with increasing age from birth to 25 years. The individuals shown at birth, 2 years, 6 years, 15 years and 25 years have been drawn to the same absolute height. Note that with increasing age the head gets relatively smaller and the pubic level moves upwards to about the midpoint of the body—due to the legs getting longer relative to the spine. (Reproduced by kind permission of Professor V. A. McKusick and C. V. Crosby Company.)

most it depends on the inheritance of the individual—paternal and maternal. Great variations in height and weight must therefore be accepted as normal. If the parents are small, their children are likely to be small. This is known as genetic short stature. The term 'dwarfism' to mean short stature for age is now no longer used.

Maternal inheritance includes not only the genetic characteristics of the mother but also any characteristics determined by the uterine environment during pregnancy. Thus the children of mothers who smoked 10 or more cigarettes a day during pregnancy are about 1 cm shorter at the age of 7 years than the children of mothers who did not smoke and chronically alcoholic mothers are known to produce children with an increased incidence of growth retardation, odd facies, other malformations and psychomotor disturbances. An abnormal uterine environment can lead to a baby being of low birth weight relative to the duration of the pregnancy—'small for dates babies'. Such an abnormality of growth may persist into childhood and produce 'low-birth weight short stature'.

Basically, the process of growth after birth largely depends upon the action of blood-borne factors and the response of the growing bones to these factors. Much more is known about the former than about the latter. The blood-borne factors include essential nutrients, as well as hormones such as from the pituitary (e.g. growth hormone) and from the thyroid gland. A deficiency of growth hormone or of thyroid hormones will lead to a slowing of the rate of growth and hence to short stature. Both of these deficiency diseases, once diagnosed, will respond to treatment by the appropriate hormone(s) if given early in appropriate doses. A child may also fail to reach his full stature for age because of social or psychological problems arising in the home, or trouble at school or with the police (psycho-social short stature).

Abnormalities of growth due to a failure of the growing bones to respond normally to blood-borne factors

There are a large number of inherited disorders of the skeleton which arise from an abnormality within the growing tissues of the bones themselves. The spine may be particularly involved and cause the trunk to be short relative to the limbs (e.g. spondylo-epiphyseal dysplasia). Alternatively, the bones of the limbs may be particularly involved and be short relative to the trunk (e.g. achondroplasia and hypochondroplasia). When the limbs are involved, the shortening may particularly affect the proximal (rhizomelic), middle (mesomelic) or distal (acromelic) segments (Greek, rhiza = root, mesos = middle, akron = extremity, melos = limb). The bones of the limbs on one side of the body may be affected (e.g. Russell-Silver syndrome). These are only a few examples, for there is a wide variety of other inherited disorders of the growing skeleton (see Beighton, 1978).

Two examples are illustrated (Figs 11.4 and 11.5). In Fig. 11.4, the boy's limbs are short relative to his trunk. He has a relatively common disorder

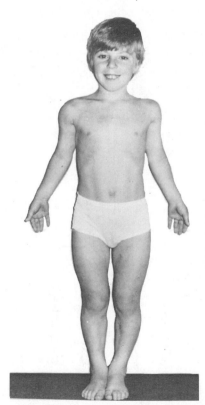

Fig. 11.4 This boy at the age of 11 years 8 months had a standing height of 119 cm. Plot his height for age on Fig. 11.10 where his height lies below the 3rd centile. He has short stature. Moreover, his limbs are disproportionately short relative to his trunk. The diagnosis is hypochondroplasia which is akin to achondroplasia. This boy's hypochondroplasia was caused by a mutation in an autosomal gene of one of his parents.

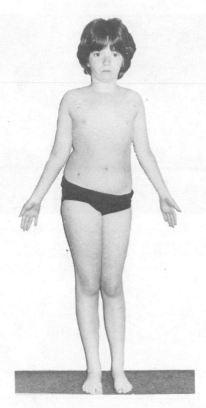

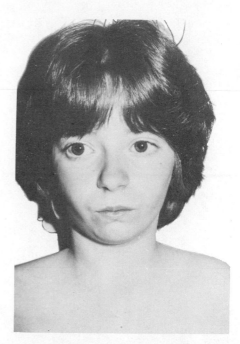

Fig. 11.6 The face of the girl shown in Fig. 11.5. The skull is broad and the chin both small and receding, giving her face a triangular outline.

Fig. 11.5 This girl at the age of 12 years 5 months had a standing height of 131 cm. She has short stature and was a 'small for dates baby'. Note the shorter arms and legs on one side of the body (left). The diagnosis is the Russell-Silver syndrome.

known as hypochondroplasia. In Fig. 11.5, the girl has an inequality of limb length on the two sides of the body. Thus, her left arm and leg are shorter than her right arm and leg. Orthopaedically she presents the problem of leg length inequality. The cause was 'intra-uterine' and she also has low birth-weight short stature. She has the Russell-Silver syndrome with the characteristic triangular face (Fig. 11.6).

Abnormalities of proportionate skeletal growth in children with Perthes' disease and idiopathic scoliosis. Screening for scoliosis

It is generally considered that Perthes' disease of the hip is due to a local vascular obstruction of the blood vessels supplying the head of the femur (femoral capital epiphysis). However, recent research has shown a growth abnormality more

widespread than that of the hip (Burwell et al, 1978). To reveal these changes, the modern techniques for measuring man (anthropometry) have been used (Figs 11.7, 11.8 and 11.9).

Using such anthropometric techniques it has been found that children with Perthes' disease are not only generally small for their chronological (birthday) age, but the various skeletal regions of the body are disproportionate (Figs 11.10, 11.11 and 11.12). The reason for this abnormality of the mechanisms which determine proportionate skeletal growth in the body of the growing child is unknown; but it may be determined by factors acting before birth. Additional support for the view that children with Perthes' disease may have a major congenital defect is the finding of a high incidence of minor congenital anomalies in such children (Hall et al, 1979).

Another possibility is that blood-borne factors may be involved. In this connection, recent work using monkeys has shown that poor nutrition slows growth, not only of the animal as a whole, but particularly of the most peripheral parts of the limbs. Such malnutrition unmasks the presence of ill-understood mechanisms which in health coordi-

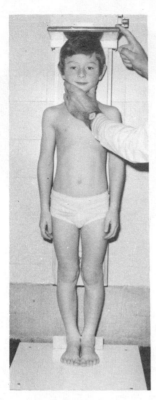

Fig. 11.7 Measuring the standing height using a modern instrument (the Harpenden Stadiometer).

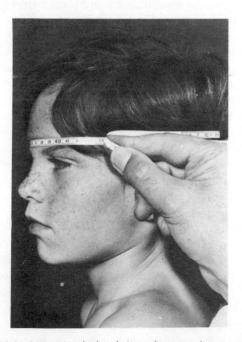

Fig. 11.8 Measuring the head circumference using a steel tape.

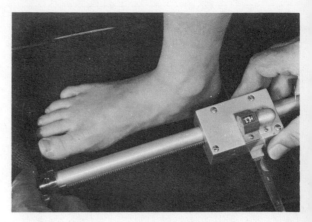

Fig. 11.9 Measuring the length of the foot using a modern instrument (the Harpenden anthropometer). This instrument can also be used to measure the width across the shoulders, across the hips and segments of the upper as well as of the lower limbs.

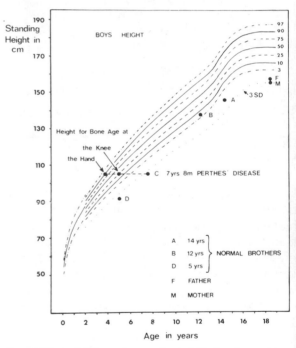

Fig. 11.10 In this figure the standing height of each member of a family is plotted on the centile charts for British children. The boy aged 7 years 8 months has Perthes' disease. He has short stature. All the family are small so that his short stature is probably familial (genetic short stature). However, his *biological age* assessed from radiographs of the bones at the hand and at the knee was retarded—and the hand more so than the knee. When his standing height is plotted against his bone age, his height is normal. (Reproduced from Burwell, Vernon and Dangerfield (1980) and by kind permission of the Editors and William Heinemann Medical Books Ltd., London, England.)

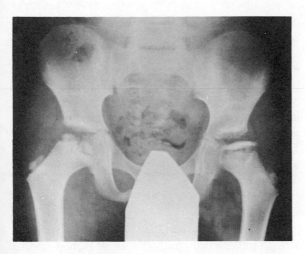

Fig. 11.11 Radiograph of the pelvis of the boy with Perthes' disease whose standing height is plotted in Fig. 11.10. The disease of the hips is bilateral.

nate the growth of individual bones throughout the body and which produce the normally proportioned adult. Factors in blood and bones are likely to be involved.

The pattern of disproportionate growth in the limb bones of malnourished monkeys is strikingly similar to that found in children with Perthes' disease. It begs the question: *'Is there a nutritional deficiency in children with Perthes' disease?'* (Harrison & Burwell, 1981).

In this connection a recent survey of Perthes' disease of the hip in three regions of England showed

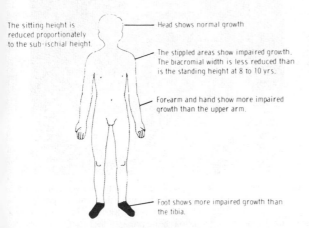

The sitting height is reduced proportionately to the sub-ischial height.

Head shows normal growth

The stippled areas show impaired growth. The biacromial width is less reduced than is the standing height at 8 to 10 yrs.

Forearm and hand show more impaired growth than the upper arm.

Foot shows more impaired growth than the tibia.

Fig. 11.12 A drawing to show the pattern of abnormal growth in boys with Perthes's disease. Note the more normal growth of the upper regions of the body (rostral sparing). (Reproduced from Burwell *et al.*, 1978 and by kind permission of the Editor of the *Journal of Bone and Joint Surgery.*)

a higher incidence in the Mersey region compared with Trent or Wessex. To explore this further a case register was set up in Liverpool. Analysis of all new cases that occurred in Liverpool during 1976–81 showed a steep gradient with social class, ranging from 7.7/100 000 children in the higher classes to 26.3/100 000 in social class V. The inner city of Liverpool, which has been shown to be underprivileged, had the highest yearly incidence of the disease ever reported—21.1 cases/100 000 children aged 14 years and under.

The association with poverty supports the hypothesis that undernutrition is a causative factor in the disease (Hall et al, 1983).

Similarly in children with idiopathic scoliosis, an abnormality of growth has been found in which the upper limb shows asymmetry of length (Dangerfield et al, 1980). The reason for this arm asymmetry is unknown but it is possible that it indicates a disorder of proportionate growth in which the scoliosis is the most obvious feature. Disproportionate growth in another region of the skeleton has been found in girls with adolescent idiopathic scoliosis— they are 4–6 cm taller than average with a disproportionately tall pelvis (Nicolopoulos et al, 1984). These observations on skeletal growth are useful in our attempts to unravel the biological mechanisms which lead to some children getting idiopathic scoliosis. It is not known yet whether the first changes of scoliosis are in bone, intervertebral disc, muscle, nerve or central nervous system. Once a spinal curve has formed, gravity will tend to make it worse until the spine stiffens in its deformed position; or the ribs impinge on the pelvis and stop the spinal curve progressing. Further research, including three-dimensional techniques of body measurement of children with scoliosis, may ultimately aid management and possibly help us to understand how such a deformity can arise in an otherwise apparently normal child (see Burwell, 1978).

The detection of idiopathic scoliosis in adolescents for early brace treatment to stop the curve progressing has now moved to the schools—this is because mothers, brothers, sisters and friends at school usually spot the deformity too late. There is a problem in our attempts to bring children from school to hospital early enough to avoid a surgical operation. The screening test is difficult. In it, the child is asked to bend forwards (forward bending test), and the screener looks for a rib hump on one side of the chest (Fig. 11.13A). The difficulty arises from the fact that about 25 per cent of healthy children have such rib humps (10 right to 1 left) (Burwell et al, 1983). Hence the screener has to decide whether any hump observed is either normal or abnormal and whether or not to send the child to hospital for an orthopaedic opinion. The test is too subjective—relying as it does on the screener's experience.

These and other difficulties led the British Orthopaedic Association and the British Scoliosis Society in 1983 to recommend that it should not be national policy, at present, to screen children for scoliosis routinely throughout the United Kingdom (Report,

1983). One subjective way of aiding the school nurse and school doctor in early diagnosis is the use of a new inclinometer now available commercially and termed the 'scoliometer' (Fig. 11.13B) (Bunnell, 1983). The British Scoliosis Society has a Study Group which is working to make screening for scoliosis more efficient as well as learn more about the natural history of smaller spinal curves. This is necessary because early diagnosis can lead to the unnecessary early treatment of some children—particularly as it is now known that many small lateral spinal curves in adolescents resolve (disappear).

The nervous system has an entirely different growth pattern from the skeleton. It is through this system that an animal is made aware of his immediate dangers and so we find that it is much more fully developed at birth than in other species. Indeed, it is the rapid growth of the brain which causes the remarkable head enlargement in the first eighteen months of life, when the fontanelles and sutures of the separate skull bones allow the brain to expand.

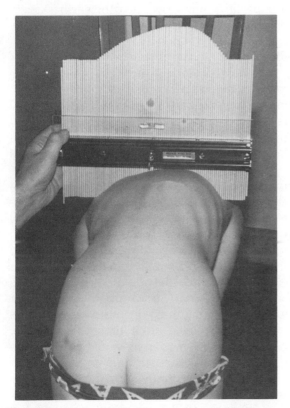

Fig. 11.13A A healthy child in a standing forward bending position with an instrument (Formulator Contour Tracer) taking up the outline of the back. The rods of the instrument move under gravity into positions determined by the contours of the back; using a pencil the contours are then transferred to paper for examination and analysis to give a trunk asymmetry score. This procedure is repeated at least two levels on the back (thoracic and lumbar regions). (From Burwell et al, 1983 with kind permission of the editor, *Journal of Bone and Joint Surgery*).

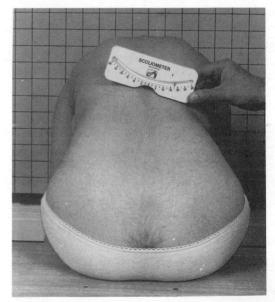

Fig. 11.13B A child with scoliosis in a sitting forward bending position with an instrument (scoliometer) showing the angle across the back. the 'scoliometer' is a commercial inclinometer which gives a direct reading of the angle of inclination across the trunk: in this child 15–20° which is abnormal. A reading is taken on at least two levels on the back (maximum in each of the thoracic and lumbar regions). The instrument is currently being evaluated for the early detection of scoliosis in schoolchildren.

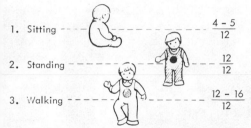

1. Sitting $\dfrac{4-5}{12}$

2. Standing $\dfrac{12}{12}$

3. Walking $\dfrac{12-16}{12}$

4. Urine + Bowel Control – At age for family, 2–4 years.

5. Adolescent Sex Confrontation – Critical time 10–16 years.

6. Life Goal Concepts – in child and in the family – unrealistic before growth complete.

Fig. 11.14 Some normal milestones.

Mental and emotional growth is an even more complicated process, but this too follows a more or less fixed pattern. Certain milestones, both physical and mental must be checked if the child's response is to be assessed.

It must be recognised that in Table 11.2 the figures are average. Their importance lies not only

Table 11.2 Some milestones in development

Age		Ability
4	weeks	Follow bright light
6–8	weeks	Smiles
		Makes noises
8	weeks	Follows moving objects
		Recognises familiar sounds
12	weeks	Lifts head off pillow
3–4	months	Holds head up steadily
		Fixes objects with eyes
5–6	months	Grasps objects firmly in hands
6–9	months	Can sit up unaided
		Moves an object from one hand to the other
9–12	months	Begins to crawl
		Can drink from a cup
12–15	months	Stands up and begins to walk
		Can say a few single words
18	months	Anterior fontanelle should be closed
20–24	months	Says a few simple sentences; rapidly increasing vocabulary
		Urinary control by day.

in the age of their accomplishment but also in their orderly progression.

Any acute illness can arrest skeletal growth. This is shown by the deposition of calcium in the long bones—Harris's lines on X-rays. Chronic illness, such as cystic fibrosis or persistent respiratory infection, as well as malabsorption of food can cause growth retardation. Cyanotic congenital heart dis-

ease results in tissue hypoxia which impedes skeletal growth, while endocrine disorders, especially pituitary and thyroid can lead to either gigantism or stunting. Insulin and Adrenalin also play their part in controlling metabolic systems especially during the rapid growth periods of infancy and puberty.

The new science of auxology has taken paediatricians into greater accuracy with the weighing and measuring of stature, skinfolds etc. in out-patient departments. The bodily transformations of puberty have variable rates of maturity which are measured by different scales. The rising tides of different hormones from early childhood to maturity, each in its own time influence the skeleton, the breasts, gonads, pubic hair, etc. Accuracy in measuring skeletal maturity and bone age needs radiological examination of the bones of the hand, carpus and other selected epiphyses.

When growth is not influenced by some pathological process it is now possible to predict the final height. Such forecasts are particularly necessary for exceptionally tall girls for whom hormonal treatment to arrest growth might be considered. Psychosocial growth suppression, with combined influence of stress and nutritional lack is more commonly seen than the 'hypo-pituitary dwarf'. It must be realised therefore that the various risks of hormone treatment which have to be balanced against the advantages, demand expertise and great care in making a correct diagnosis.

PSYCHOLOGICAL EFFECTS OF ORTHOPAEDIC CONDITIONS ON THE CHILD AND ON THE FAMILY

We should consider four components contributing to the behaviour patterns of children, with the family reactions to them during the stressful period in hospital.

A deformity which mars the perfect body image is a very important factor in the emotional well-being of both child and adult. In general, the child with a birth defect or deformity accepts and adapts to his situation better than one who acquired such defects in later life; on the other hand, severe birth defects, such as spina bifida, achondroplasia and even undescended testes can motivate young

adults into full co-operation with treatment programmes. When the child is of good intelligence,
his determination towards achieving independent
mobility frequently leads to success. With regard
to locomotion, a sensitive adolescent often chooses
wheelchair existence in preference to cumbersome
splintage in order to retain self-esteem. There is
less public attention towards the cosmetically
acceptable and easily manipulated wheelchair
compared with the personal struggle and effort
involved in assisted, slow bipedal gait.

Behaviour problems

Behaviour problems associated with deformity do
not usually become troublesome before school
age, but children of 7–10 years old can be very
unkind to each other when the social and intellectual differences become evident. Children with
minor physical handicaps become more aware of
their differences at this age. They can exhibit emotional and psychosomatic symptoms such as bed-
wetting, nightmares, recurrent abdominal pains,
headaches, all of which need careful unravelling
and different management. In some cases, residential schools for the physically handicapped provide
the best means of training older children to be independent; but compared with being integrated into
normal day schools the cost-effectiveness favours
'shared care' locally. This is especially the case
where the patient's family is eager to participate
in overall education and in treatment programmes.

Effects of prolonged hospitalisation

Long periods of separation from parents can certainly produce symptoms of deprivation and stress,
especially in children aged 2–4 years (Bowlby,
1951) (Fig. 11.15). Three phases of the young
child's altered behaviour are described; these are
protest, despair and detachment (Vernon et al,
1965).

At first, the child shows a warm response to the
new situation; this is soon followed by quiet anxiety
as reflected in the child's face and hands; later he
becomes anxious, crying loudly and often rocking;
finally, his acceptance of the inevitability of his
loneliness is shown as a dangerous, quiet phase
which can lead to detachment, depression and

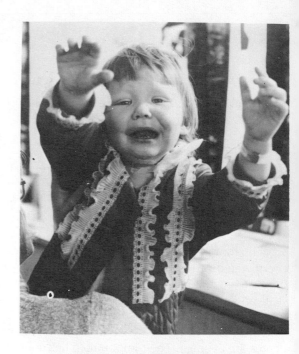

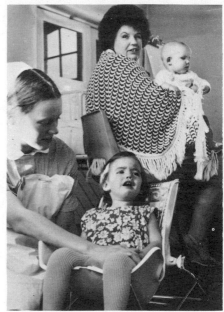

Fig. 11.15   Stress caused by separation from parents.

inability to play (Younger, 1978). There is much
overlap, but symptoms and signs are predictable
and preventable. New policies of ward management, including unrestricted hospital visiting by
parents during the pre-operative and post-operative

periods have been natural developments of child care in hospital during the past 30 years (Figs 11.16, 11.17, 11.18). Parent participation can assist the nursing staff, especially at meal, toilet and bed times, when problems of a functional nature are often added to emotional upsets. These can be compounded by stresses of anaesthetic or surgical treatments, also by blood loss, drugs and infection. When it is certain that there is no physical explanation of the emotional symptoms, sedatives and tranquilliser medication can be used in addition to constant encouragement and reassurance.

Immobilisation

A specific factor influencing the child's psychological reactions when he is in the orthopaedic ward situation, relates to immobilisation. Babies and young children who are nursed on splints with weighted skin traction, or in plaster of Paris jackets, suffer a great deal of discomfort and misery during the first few days. After prolonged anchorage, such infants are at risk of vomiting and can even suffer nutritional problems. Warm relationships with the ward staff must be formed at this time and these include personal contact with various friendly adults in addition to the visiting relatives and family (Figs 11.19 and 11.20).

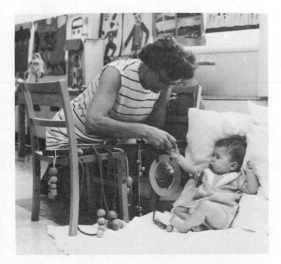

Fig. 11.16   Parental participation.

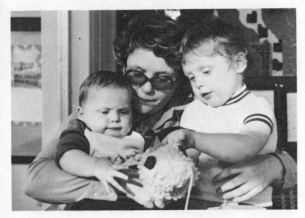

Fig. 11.17   Visits from parents and siblings are very important.

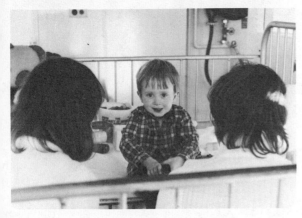

Fig. 11.18   Visits from parents should be frequent.

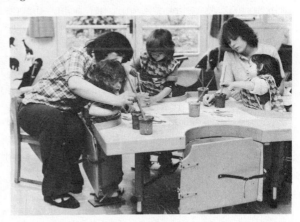

Fig. 11.19   Voluntary helpers can fill the gap of absent parents.

All professional staff need to be vigilant about the possibility of accompanying organic diseases, e.g. vomiting associated with hiatus hernia, haematuria with renal calculi, hypothyroidism with delayed epiphyseal calcification, rickets or hyper-

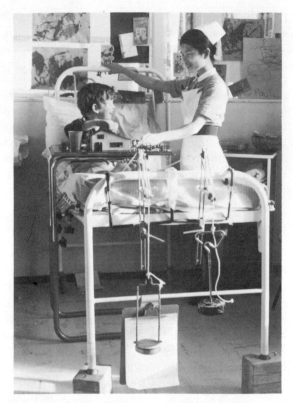

Fig. 11.20 Good relations with ward staff are an aid to recovery.

calcaemia associated with metabolic defects. Remember too that in the case of small babies, anaemia can be associated with repeated venepunctures undertaken for diagnostic purposes. Also that congenital defects can be multiple, e.g. renal pathology with scoliosis, or dislocated hip with aplastic anaemia (Fanconi's, 1960 *Acta Paediatrica*, 49: 518). Hence, appropriate pre- and postoperative investigation is advisable when prolonged immobilisation is an essential part of treatment.

Pre-operative and post-operative emotional states

Preparing children for anaesthetic, or coping with their recovery need nursing staff who have skills in short-term intensive care such as knowledge of intravenous fluids, pulmonary ventilation, bronchial aspiration and use of monitors outside the scope of usual ward services. The emotional preparation for a child's operation warrants the mother's

presence at this critical time, but if this is impossible, suitable mother substitutes (e.g. play ladies) should be available to give children confidence by rehearsing the anticipated procedures (Figs 11.21A, B). In this way, much of the fear of machines and other environmental hazards is removed (Robertson & Robertson, 1973). Children admitted to a predominantly English speaking hospital and whose mother tongue is not English—for example, immigrant and Welsh children—are

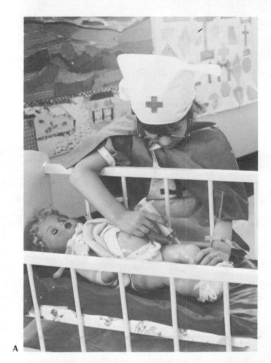

A

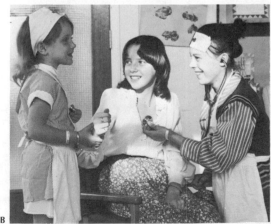

B

Fig. 11.21   A, B. Becoming accustomed to nursing procedures through play helps to reduce anxiety.

likely to suffer a particularly sharp break from their background. In the latter case, Welsh speaking staff (nursing and others) should be available to interpret and explain matters to those bewildered children, faced with frightening circumstances. In the case of the immigrant child where no member of the staff speaks his language, the continuous presence of a bilingual relative is essential.

As an advocate for children, the paediatrician sometimes has to plead with his orthopaedic surgical colleague to give priority to a policy of short-stay care when treating children in high-risk age groups. A sensitive understanding of the child's family dynamics at this time can be provided by a paediatric social worker who could influence the 'timing' of hospitalisation and the wisdom of early discharge home.

Studies of adolescents and young adults in hospital indicate that there are many with poor adaptation to their chronic disorders. Some are inactive, tearful children who show marked dependence on their families from the start. They often lack friends and outside interests and are not willing to take on new responsibilities in hospital. Others are seen to be active, daring young people who deny fears and realistic dangers. These rebel against maternal or other interference and become over-active, defiant adolescents.

NOTES ON GENERAL CARE OF THE CHILD IN HOSPITAL AND IN THE COMMUNITY

Safety in hospital

Responsibility for the care of other people's children require an awareness of dangers. The law demands extremely high standards of care which become a moral and social duty for hospital staff to ensure a safe environment. Nursing staff must feel confident that everything possible is done to avoid accidents or anything which might cause additional anxieties to parents. This is especially the case when babies and young children require in-patient surgical treatment. Meticulous nursing standards must therefore be enforced yet remembering that it is undesirable to impose unnecessary restriction on children.

It is important for the ward Sister to insist on the following safety measures:

1. General ward cleanliness should be maintained.
2. All precautionary measures should be taken to eliminate risk of accidents, when using equipment such as incubators, suction apparatus, resuscitators, etc.
3. All visitors should behave in a safe manner, never leaving the ward unattended or the cot sides insecure.
4. Food trays and large toys which enable children to climb over the side of cots should be eliminated and pillows are not used for children under one-year of age.
5. Gifts and toys should be checked for safety.
6. High chairs should be fixed in the low position and restrainers should only be used in bed if advised by the Paediatrician (pattern recommended HM (66) 11).
7. Cables from television, fans, head phones etc. need to be placed out of the child's reach.
8. Hot water bottles should not be used.
9. Mechanical toys and nylon clothing should not be placed inside oxygen tents.
10. Thermometers must be kept out of children's reach.
11. Babies in incubators should be kept out of direct sunlight to avoid over-heating.
12. Cots should not be placed against radiators without adequate guarding.
13. Steam kettles should not be used unless prescribed. They are safer on the floor, but must be visible and out of the child's reach.
14. Clothing should fit properly so that the child does not trip over it. Marking-ink identifications must be fixed by boiling before garments are used.
15. Plastic bags are not left lying around.
16. Food should not be left in lockers and nuts should not be given.
17. Dummies must be stored in Milton, and food protected from flies.
18. Allergies should be clearly identified on documents.
19. Labelled information for parent co-operation e.g. 'nil by mouth pre-operative', can be placed around the child's neck and also on

the bed. These can stop a kindly visitor from unintentionally giving a child something which is not allowed.

Infection

The important clinical infections of childhood are of viral, bacterial and fungal origin. The respiratory and alimentary tracts are most frequently involved with catarrh, cough, vomiting and diarrhoea as the main symptoms. Classical pictures of the highly infectious virus illnesses such as chicken-pox, measles, rubella and mumps are diagnostic. Pertussis and dysentery of bacterial origin also deserve mention in this group. All these illnesses can interfere with planned, surgical programmes for infants and toddlers in hospital and may even lead to temporary ward closure. Every effort should be made to control cross-infection. Practical hints to effect this include:

1. Selection and screening of all admissions by careful history-taking and clinical observation, using short-stay rooms adjacent to the ward.
2. Microbiological identification attempting to trace the source of infection by taking nose, throat and faecal swab cultures from all patients and contacts on the ward, should preclude specific treatment programmes wherever possible.
3. Meticulous nursing techniques reduce contact and droplet spread of infection. Routines of cubicle nursing include careful hand-washing, gowning, masking, napkin disposal and dressing of open wounds in operating theatres or clean treatment rooms.
4. The avoidance of using drugs empirically, especially broad-spectrum antibiotics which can lead to dangerous, iatrogenic disease. Responsibility for planning medication programmes should rest with a physician, who, adjusts dosage according to body weight and height (expressed as surface areas—see Table 11.3). Life-threatening infections such as septicaemia, meningitis and osteomyelitis normally require intravenous or intramuscular therapy with antibiotics. Dosage is often monitored by frequent blood level estimations.
5. The recognition that small children with infection can present with symptoms, such as diffi-

Table 11.3 Drug doses for children

Age	Mean weight for age		Percentage of adult dose
	lb	kg	
Newborn	7.7	3.5	12.5
2 months	10	4.5	15
4 months	14	6.5	20
1 year	22	10	25
3 years	33	15	33.3
7 years	50	23	50
10 years	66	30	60
12 years	86	39	75
14 years	110	50	80
16 years	128	58	90
Adult	150	68	100

culties with feeding, sleeping and toileting routine. General discomfort can also dominate the picture making their overall progress difficult to assess. A wise nurse is aware that the child's improved appetite, desire to play, smiling response and eagerness to return home can be more important signs of recovery than many laboratory tests. It is in this field that the observations of good nursing staff are invaluable. Attendants who use their eyes, ears and natural senses to elicit responses from their patients are able to make valuable judgements leading to earlier discharge home.

COMMUNICATION WITHIN A MULTIDISCIPLINARY SERVICE

The complexities of sharing professional skills and communicating important data for the benefit of the child and his family are best illustrated diagramatically. Interaction between the services available for orthopaedic children, both inside and outside the hospital, is shown. A remarkable number of agencies, and disciplines concerned with the handicapped family (Fig. 11.2).

All those who make contact with children in hospital should remember *Romans, 12–8*: 'Let those who showeth mercy, do it with cheerfulness'. The nurse with a natural smile, gentle manner and sincerity of purpose is quickly appreciated by children, since they have a gift for recognising the simple things in life.

History-taking from parents prior to the child's admission to hospital demands a trained and tolerant understanding of their anxieties. Care and correct 'timing' are required from medical and nursing staff who are designated to transmit good or bad news. Preparation for such an interview is rewarding. It should take place in a quiet room, away from the distraction of ward noise or telephone interruption. Parents also need adequate time to appreciate the significance of such information. 'One-to-one' discussion is probably best, but the presence of a skilled social worker or health visitor at the interview can be invaluable. Dialogue, which then becomes a means of teaching as well as learning, can thus be encouraged within the children's department.

Writing the formal discharge medical report is an important task. Accurate diagnosis, treatment, prognosis and the reason for any follow-up appointment should be clearly stated in every case. Information already given to the parents should also be included, in order that continuity of care and a consistent policy of management can be assured.

Parents of sick children are willing to talk with any person who can honestly answer their searching questions. It is unhelpful for relatives to be given different view-points by various medical, domestic or nursing staff. The ward Sister is usually the best co-ordinator of this important function. However, the time and depth of transmitting such data can vary, e.g. informing the mother in the delivery room that her baby has spina bifida is done by the midwife, but the information given at the time would need modification soon afterwards. A consultant paediatrician uses experience, and compassion with awareness of the shock that such news has on a particular family. These early discussions can determine a mother's immediate acceptance or rejection of her baby and there is no room for clumsiness in this special area of communication.

Communication within the multidisciplinary team seems to be a more frequently used approach in dealing with abused children and their families. Case conferences need wise, co-ordinated chairmanship for satisfactory rehabilitation programmes to emerge. It is also essential that the various staff involved with discharge procedures know that voluntary agencies such as Parent Associations, as well as Social Services are available to assist families with financial burdens which have been incurred as a result of the child being in hospital.

It should be stressed that to reduce the social and emotional burdens of severe handicap on the child, the family, and society as a whole, there must be proper integration of all services (Fig. 11.22). Moral and ethical obligations in our civilised world could then justify the philosophy—'he's no burden, he's my brother'.

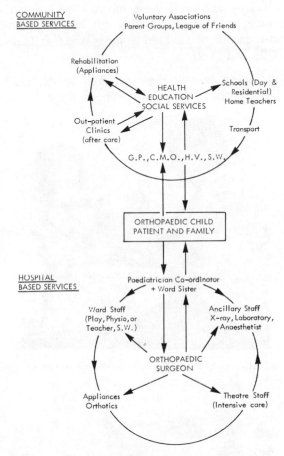

Fig. 11.22 Who communicates?

MOBILITY FOR PHYSICALLY HANDICAPPED CHILDREN

When we accept the developmental concept of there being a 'right time for everything' we will appreciate that it is beneficial for our children to achieve an upright position (sitting) at about 4–5 months of age. They can then free their hands and learn perpendicular hand-eye co-ordination. Similarly, the 12–16 month old is ready to walk; hence, it should be important for spina bifida children to learn standing balance at about this age, despite the fact they are totally paralysed. This is achieved by tailored splintage (Fig. 11.23). With this understanding, the importance of learning bowel and urine control at the age appropriate for the family, is essential for the proper formation of social acceptability.

Having achieved these milestones, it is convenient to consider mobility provisions for three main groups of disabled children (see Figs 11.24, 11.25 and 11.26):

1. *Spina bifida*. These children are generally able to propel standard wheelchairs in their homes

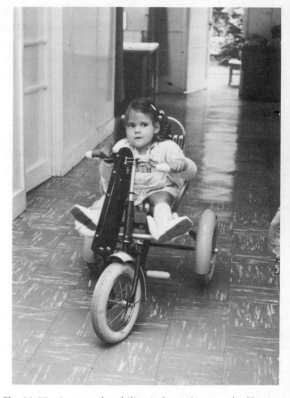

Fig. 11.25 Increased mobility, independence and self-confidence.

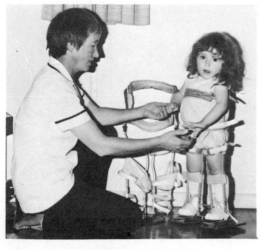

Fig. 11.23 Tailored splintage allows children to learn standing balance.

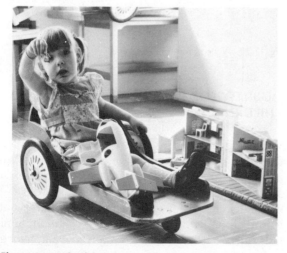

Fig. 11.24 Wheelchair.

and schools. Because of the available arm strength it is desirable to provide a powered unit which has manual steering. Special considerations are given to the seating and leg supports to enable independent access by the children.

2. *Muscular dystrophy and related diseases*. With progressive weakening of the muscles it is likely that a powered mobility aid will be required by the time children reach 12 years of age. For such children joystick steering and control can be conveniently combined by the use of twin motors, one on each driving wheel.

3. *Cerebral palsy*. There is a wide spectrum of handicap in this group and it is particularly difficult to control the many problems which can arise when considering mobility aids for them.

It is important that the design and construction provide good mobility, independence and enjoyment. The primary requirement is independent movement in the house and in the school.

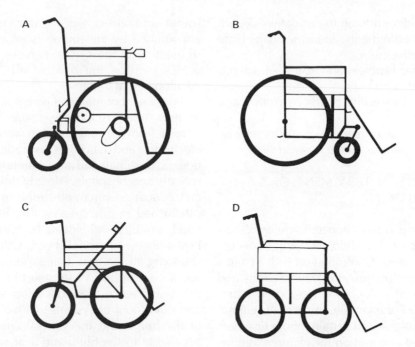

Fig. 11.26 **A.** Power-driven chair for outdoor mobility. **B.** Self-propelled chair, increased mobility, independence and self-confidence. **C.** Hand-lever chair for outdoor mobility and independence. **D.** Transit wheelchair, comfortable and manoeuvrable. (Also available but not shown: commode wheelchair and stair driven models by Meyra-Rehab (UK) Warminster.)

NOTES ON ADDITIONAL SERVICES FOR PHYSICALLY HANDICAPPED CHILDREN

Voluntary helpers

It must be accepted that all services on a children's ward which need continuity of personal relationships should be met by skilled staff and not by volunteers, e.g. organised play and teaching require specialised staff. Escorts in the transport of children to Day Centres should be on a payment for service basis. Mothers of the children could certainly be encouraged to work on a rota basis within the policy of parent-participation programmes.

Voluntary societies (e.g. Spina Bifida, Dystrophy, Cystic Fibrosis, Spastics etc.) always have a dual role; most important perhaps is the self-help function, where parents of handicapped children learn about problems of management from others who have had similar experiences. The other important function is fund-raising, when a Public Relations Officer with business management skills can muster great enthusiasm in money matters.

Before introducing forms of voluntary work with children there must be the closest consultation and co-operation with doctors, nurses and others professionally concerned in the care of the patient, as well as with hospital management, Trades Unions and other voluntary organisations, already providing services.

Suggestions for voluntary services in a children's department include the following:

1. Accompanying mothers and children to and from different Units.
2. Accompanying mothers and children to the hospital; helping them cope with a complicated journey.
3. Bringing parents who are disabled or in poor health themselves to visit their children on the wards, usually by car.
4. Checking toys for breakages.
5. Escorting children to clinics, often by ambulance.
6. In special circumstances, escorting children to their own homes on discharge.

7. Escorting older children to out-patient departments for appointments, when their parents are unable to bring them.
8. Looking after brothers and sisters of patients while parents visit.
9. Marking and mending childrens clothes and bibs.
10. Playing with and reading to children who accompany parents during hospital visits.

NEW CONCEPTS IN TREATMENT OF DISABLED CHILDREN

The nurse working in an orthopaedic children's service should practise the 'child and family' concept of total medical need. Confrontation with a child's variable state developmentally, behaviourally and intellectually often colours the associated orthopaedic problem. For example, in cases of cerebral palsy, myelodysplasia and certain inborn disorders of metabolism, it is common for children to have both mental and skeleto-muscular handicaps with fits, as well as other system disorders; it is, therefore, essential for nurses to be updated with multidisciplinary assessment and treatment programmes involving play specialists, speech and language therapists, clinical psychologists, physiotherapists and pre-school educationists. An appreciation of home environment and the child's progress at school also give guidance about the child's own motivation and 'drive'. These are essential before predicting an accurate prognosis.

Careful history-taking must include pre- and perinatal events as well as information about the usual early milestones, viz: head control, sitting balance, eye-to-eye gaze, hand to mouth transfer, babbling and meaningful word linkage. The developmental stages of normal locomotion are of particular importance. A comprehensive diagnosis leads to early, well-planned intervention and better home management by the family. Day centres, whether hospital or community based, where pre-school children with special needs can be happy with socialising play, toilet training and splint training are also mandatory.

In addition, the early introduction of electronic teaching aids such as the Possum audio-visual units have proved highly successful in the past decade. Achievements of the children are documented by sound and video tapes. They are praised and encouraged by the discovery of new skills. Such stimulation of the central nervous system through achievement is the basis of all good paediatric developmental therapy.

Assessment of maximal potential must now look to new inter-disciplinary research opportunities ranging from play aids, speech synthesisers, micro-electronics and data bases, to modifications for outdoor power-chair and access units for use at special schools and hospitals. Already there are four special education micro-electronic resource centres established in this country. The liberation of isolated, disabled individuals by bringing the Bank, Post Office, Library, School, Office, University, shopping etc. to their living rooms using low cost adaptations to a T.V. set, must be a challenge for the new science. Rapid developments in robotics and other control systems will make various parts of the home and the general environment more accessible to the blind and deaf, with individualised needs being met.

For further reading on this topic, reference may be had from HPRU Directory of non-medical research relating to handicapped people November 1982 and September 1983—Newcastle upon Tyne Polytechnic No. 1, Coach Lane, Newcastle NE7 7TW.

BIBLIOGRAPHY

Beighton P 1978 Inherited Disorders of the Skeleton. Edinburgh: Churchill Livingstone
Bickel H, Stern J 1976 Inborn Errors of Calcium and Bone Metabolism. Baltimore: University Park Press
Bowlby J 1951 Maternal Care and Mental Health. WHO Monograph Series No. 2, Geneva
Brand L, Wisbeach A 1973 Wheelchairs for Children and Adapting Wheelchairs for Children. Tape and Slides—Medical Recording Service Foundation, Kitts Croft, Whittle, Chelmsford, CM1 3EH
Bunnel W P 1983 Angle of trunk rotation: an objective criterion for spinal screening programs. Exhibit at the Scoliosis Research Society, 18th Annual Meeting, New Orleans, Louisiana, USA, 28 September to 1 October
Burwell R G 1978 Biostereometrics, Shape Replication and Orthopaedics. In Conference to mark the opening of the Oxford Orthopaedic Engineering Centre. London: Biological Engineering Society
Burwell R G, Vernon C L 1979 Skeletal Measurement. Ch. 37. In Scientific Foundations of Orthopaedics and the Surgery of Trauma. Owen R, Goodfellow J W, Bullough P G (eds). London: Heinemann
Burwell R G, Dangerfield P H, Vernon C L 1977

Anthropometry and Scoliosis. In Scoliosis. Proceedings of a Fifth Symposium. Zorab P A (ed.). London: Academic Press

Burwell R G, Dangerfield P H, Hall D J, Vernon C L, Harrison M H M 1978 Perthes' disease. An anthropometric study revealing impaired and disproportionate growth. Journal of Bone and Joint Surgery 60B: 461–477

Burwell R G, James N J, Johnson F, Webb J K, Wilson Y G 1983 Standardised trunk asymmetry scores. A study of back contour in healthy schoolchildren. Journal of Bone and Joint Surgery 65B: 452–63

Court S D M (Chairman) 1976 Fit for the Future. Report of the Committee on Child Health Services. London: HMSO

Dangerfield P H, Burwell R G, Vernon C L 1980 Anthropometry and scoliosis, In Spinal Deformities, 2nd edn, ed. Roaf R, Ch. 14. London: Pitman Medical

Francis D, Dixon D 1970 Diets for Sick Children—2nd edn. Oxford: Blackwell Scientific

Hall D J, Harrison M H M, Burwell R G 1979 Congenital abnormalities and Perthes' disease. Clinical evidence that children with Perthes' disease may have a major congenital defect. Journal of Bone and Joint Surgery 61B: 18

Hall A J, Barker D J P, Dangerfield P H, Taylor J F 1983. Perthes' disease of the hip in Liverpool. British Medical Journal 287: 1757–9

Harrison M H M, Burwell R G 1981 Perthes' disease: a concept of pathogenesis. Clinical Orthopaedics and Related Research 156: 115–25

Jolly H 1978 The importance of 'bonding' of new born baby, mother—and father—. Nursing Mirror, 31 August, 19

Marshall N A 1977 Human Growth and its Disorders. London: Academic Press

MOH 1964 Hospital Building Note No. 23

Nicolopoulos C S, Burwell R G, Webb J K 1984 A tall pelvis in girls with adolescent idiopathic scoliosis. Journal of Bone and Joint Surgery. In press. (Proceedings of the British Orthopaedic Research Society, September 1983.)

Noble E 1967 Play and the Sick Child. London: Faber

Report by the British Orthopaedic Association and the British Scoliosis Society 1983 School screening for scoliosis. British Medical Journal 287: 963–4

Robertson J, Robertson J 1973 Substitute mothering. Nursing Times, 29 November

Silk D B A 1978 Parental Nutrition, Hospital Update 4543

Stacey M 1972 Safety of Children in Hospital. Appx 14. Children in Hospital in Wales

Stacey M 1972 Voluntary Work with Children. Appx 34. Children in Hospital in Wales

Vernon D A, Foley et al 1965 The Psychological Responses of Children to Hospitalisation and Illness. Springfield: Charles C Thomas

Watkins A G 1947 Paediatrics for Nurses

WHB 1972 Children in Hospital in Wales. Final report of the Working party on Children in Hospital in Wales. (Margaret Stacey, Chairman)

Younger N R 1978 Children in Hospital. Nursing Times, 16 March, Paediatric News 5

12

Paediatric orthopaedics 2: special considerations

PHYSIOTHERAPY IN PAEDIATRIC ORTHOPAEDICS

INTRODUCTION

The majority of children in an orthopaedic hospital are relatively long-stay and their conditions include congenital abnormalities, Perthes' disease, spinal deformities and various conditions affecting the nervous system and musculo-skeletal system. They share many of the problems common to all children in hospital, but a long stay brings its own special ones, for example, losing a 'link' with the family and home, loss of education, delayed language development, etc. so that the therapeutic team must be constantly aware of these problems and try to compensate as best they can.

PHYSIOTHERAPY TREATMENT

General considerations

This may be given for a child as a group activity or as an individual treatment.

Individual treatments should be short, repeated often, and whenever possible, must be pain-free; the physiotherapist should explain exactly what she is going to do and the object of the treatment. A child is much more likely to be nervous and wary of individual treatment rather than that given in a group; it is often useful to introduce the child to one with a similar condition at a later stage in his treatment so that they can talk together and compare their treatments and progress. A child should be involved in his own treatment as much as possible, for example, if the aim of treatment is to gain mobility in a joint we measure the joint range daily, and let the child—where possible—keep his own record of progress and chart it daily. The nurse can help and encourage the child by asking about his chart, commenting on any increase, and asking the child to show the improved range of movement. Another example of the way in which the nurse can help is where there is a child with scoliosis and respiratory impairment; such a patient should be encouraged to take part in ward activities rather than lie in bed so as to increase exercise tolerance and vital capacity.

Group treatments may include patients with a variety of conditions, for example, those with a physical disability, those with minimal brain dysfunction, or those with both. For example, a child who is fully mobile but has a balance problem and other specific difficulties such as poor hand/eye co-ordination, will benefit from being treated with the child who has had surgery for a nerve injury repair; both can be treated by means of supervised use of play dough or building blocks. The child is then aware only of his own goal—the tower to build, or the picture to paint—so tends to forget his handicap; in this way treatment becomes play and an enjoyable activity.

Physiotherapy for special conditions

These include spina bifida, congenital dislocation of the hip, scoliosis and other conditions such as cerebral palsy.

Spina bifida

Treatment for this condition takes many varied forms, ranging from passive movements from birth onwards to prevent deformities and muscle contractures and deformity, to educating the older child in 'walking' in some form of orthosis. Obviously the parents of the new-born will be taught the basic passive movements so avoiding the need to keep the baby in hospital any longer than necessary; but the baby is often readmitted

at a later date for further treatments, when it is imperative that the child receives treatment as a whole and not just for an affected limb. The nurse can help in the prevention of deformity by correct positioning, perhaps with the use of pillows, and, needless to say, she has great responsibilities in the prevention of other complications such as pressure sores and urinary infection (Ch. 14). A sheepskin splint is often used as being both preventive and corrective with many of the children (Figs 12.1, 12.2 and 12.3).

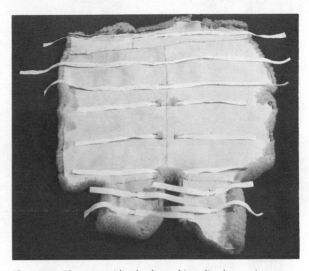

Fig. 12.1 The outer side of a sheepskin splint for use in cases of spina bifida showing laces for tying.

The splint is made from a standard National Health Service natural sheepskin; synthetic 'nursing fleeces' were tried out but found to be unsuitable. The sheepskin splint is made to measure and the appropriate measurements are set out below:

1. Nipple line to great toe with the limbs in a neutral position—(or as near a neutral position as possible). If the child is too young to sit or is unable to do so because of the neurological deficit, a measurement from the waist-line to the great toe is sufficient in length.
2. Inside leg measurement;
3. Girth around nipple line plus approximately 1" overlap;
4. Girth around pelvis at level of greater trochanter plus approximately 1" overlap.

Two or three velcro straps are stitched on so as

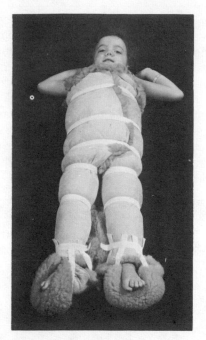

Fig. 12.2 The sheepskin splint *in situ*.

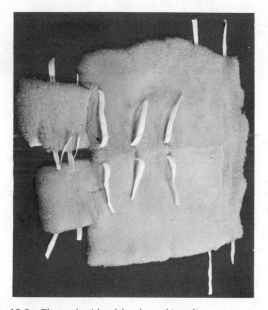

Fig. 12.3 The underside of the sheepskin splint.

to encircle each leg and depending upon the size of the child, are placed at these levels:

a. Upper third of femur.
b. Knee.
c. Lower third of tibia.

A fourth velcro strap is placed beneath the sole of the foot as a stirrup, to maintain the neutral position at the ankle joint.

The sheepskin should cover the skin area completely and the velcro straps must not come into direct contact with the skin at any point. The straps are stitched in such a way as to hold the limb in a neutral position, discouraging external rotation.

Incontinence is not a serious problem so long as waterproof pants are worn. Should the wool side of the sheepskin become wet, it is very easily rubbed dry. Canvas-backed nursing fleeces are definitely *NOT* suitable as they both tear readily and become soiled very easily. The child is nursed in either the prone or supine position and an older child may be able to turn himself while wearing the splint.

The splint is used for many purposes, including following an operation when a child is 'tailored' to a swivel walker orthosis by radical division of active imbalanced muscle groups and excision of contracted tissue (Ch. 14). Pathological fracture, especially of the femur, is a common complication in this condition and this too can often be held in the splint until union occurs. Displacements of a fracture and leg length discrepancy requires treatment with Ventfoam skin extensions and gentle traction, incorporated in the splint. While the splint is worn passive movements are given to the unaffected leg. The splints may often be quite complicated, but by working together, the physiotherapist and nurse will soon become proficient in their use; this is essential because an orthosis often becomes as much a part of the child's daily dressing routine as putting on trousers, socks or shoes etc.

Training in walking and transfer activities using various orthoses is an important aspect of treatment (Ch. 14) and maximum independence is dependent upon the increased field of vision which standing allows. Walking is encouraged by increasing the child's abilities, using toys placed at varying heights, or mobile toys.

Spinal surgery is performed in a child with spina bifida who develops a kyphoscoliosis due to muscle imbalance and loss of stability of the trunk; physiotherapy consists mainly of encouraging deep breathing and increasing a low vital capacity to avoid respiratory complications. Following operation the child may be recumbent for as long as three months and it is important during this time to maintain good posture and prevent muscle contractures so as to enable the patient to return to his orthosis as soon as possible.

Congenital dislocation of the hip (Ch. 14)

The physiotherapist has only a small part to play in the early stages of the total treatment; encouragement of active foot movements and passive movements of the patellae are given when the child is on traction (Ch. 14). Once the affected hip is reduced by means of traction, it may be necessary to give gentle passive movements encouraging flexion and internal rotation of the affected hip and so help the final stage of reduction. If napkins are worn the nurse can be of great assistance by rolling the child on to the unaffected side to remove the soiled napkin and to place a clean one beneath the buttocks; this avoids hyperextension of the hips with anterior dislocation of the head of the femur. In the later stages treatment, especially following immobilisation, exercises to regain mobility of hips and knees may be necessary; graduated muscle-strengthening exercises are begun as soon as the surgeon permits, especially for the gluteal muscles. Hydrotherapy is started as soon as possible as this obviously provides a great deal of pleasure for the child and at the same time enables the physiotherapist to employ many varied methods of treatment, simply as play. Weight-bearing, progressively increased, is allowed once the hips and knees are mobile and muscle power is sufficient to protect the joint. A close watch must be kept for an asymmetrical gait once weight-bearing begins as this may become habitual. Again the nurse can be of great assistance by observing the child as she walks around the ward unaware of being watched, and by reporting any abnormality.

Scoliosis

The child with scoliosis has usually been observed for several years and during this time assessments are made at regular intervals. The physiotherapy assessment consists of charting a series of measurements which include vital capacity, chest expansion, exercise tolerance, weight, total height and arm span. The arm span is measured from one mid-

dle finger-tip to the other with the arms outstretched; in the normal child the measurement is equivalent within one centimetre to the total height of the body so that discrepancy between these measurements indicates the approximate amount of height lost in the spinal curve. The arm span also enables us to assess the vital capacity, comparing it to the normal and informing the surgeon prior to the operation. Another piece of information taken into account is the height of a rib hump, or conversely, the depth of a valley at the site of a low thoracic or lumbar curve. This is measured by means of a gauge placed over the child's back in a forward bending position (Figs 12.4, 12.5 and

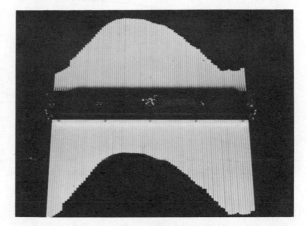

Fig. 12.4 Gauge for measurement of degree of Scoliosis.

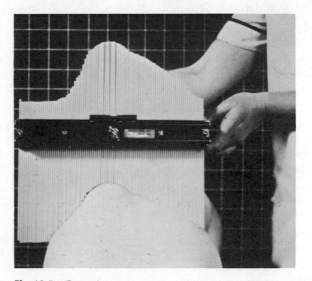

Fig. 12.5 Gauge in use.

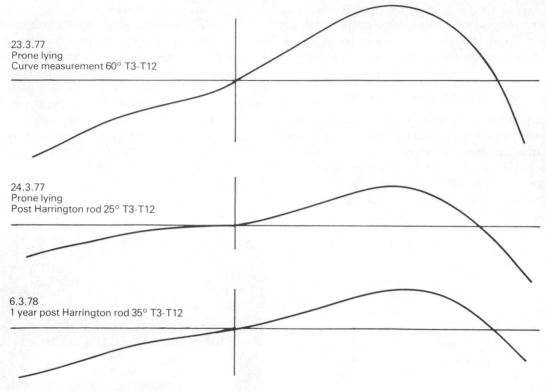

23.3.77
Prone lying
Curve measurement 60° T3-T12

24.3.77
Prone lying
Post Harrington rod 25° T3-T12

6.3.78
1 year post Harrington rod 35° T3-T12

Fig. 12.6   Record on graph paper of the degree of Scoliosis.

12.6) and also in the prone lying position. The outline of the hump is then traced on to graph paper
as a record. All of these measurements are repeated
at regular intervals and any marked change is
reported to the surgeon.

The choice between conservative or surgical
treatment is made by the surgeon depending upon
various factors such as age, degree of curvature
and the general condition of the child. If conservative treatment is instituted this is usually in the form
of a Milwaukee brace (Fig. 15.6) combined with
specific exercises. The exercises are designed to
combine with the brace to prevent further deformity
occurring and maintain good muscle power. They
include exercises aimed at reducing the lumbar lordosis so often seen in children with scoliosis, and
strengthening the abdominal and gluteal muscles.
They are performed initially out of the brace and
once the child is confident, repeated in the brace.
The brace is worn for twenty-three hours a day,
and deep breathing exercises are also included in
the programme. These serve to improve the vital

capacity and also provide active corrective exercises for the rib cage, which is very important in
the child with a thoracic scoliosis. Every effort
should be made by the members of the team to
make the adolescent feel completely normal in her
brace; fashionable, present-day clothing combined
with the services of a proficient orthotist ensures
that the brace is almost unnoticeable.

Surgical treatment. Pre-operative preparation of
the child is of the utmost importance particularly
relating to prevention of respiratory and neurological complications which may arise immediately
following operation. The most commonly used surgical procedure is insertion of Harrington Rods. The
most common neurological hazard is that of cord
damage, the cause almost certainly being due to
ischaemia from excessive stretch on the blood vessels to the cord, the thoracic region being most
vulnerable. Therefore it is vital that the nurse and
the physiotherapist observe very closely for any
changes in active movement and sensation in the
lower limbs. The child should be taught foot and

ankle movements, static contractions of the quadriceps before surgery, and these are gently encouraged after the operation. It is often the nurse who first notices any change in the neurological picture while making the bed or bathing the child, and this must be reported immediately, no matter how insignificant it may seem. Post-operative respiratory problems arise largely due to respiration being inhibited by pain; deep breathing exercises must be taught before operation and again, encouraged frequently afterwards. Where necessary, manual manipulations may have to be given, with assisted coughing (Fig. 23.17). Respiratory function tests are carried out daily from the day of operation until discharge. There is always a dramatic drop in the vital capacity on the day following operation but if the child is progressing normally this will steadily increase, though the normal vital capacity of the child does not appear to return until approximately one year after the operation. A plaster of Paris cast is usually applied about seven to ten days after operation and immediately before applying the cast a rib hump measurement is taken; this usually shows a dramatic improvement in the height (Fig. 12.6). Once the cast is dry, the child becomes ambulant; she is taught to get in and out of bed by rolling into the prone position and 'coming up' backwards, thus using her back extensor muscles. The nurse should be aware of the method and can help the child to become proficient by encouraging her to get in and out of bed while it is made, and at meal times. As the child being treated is often an adolescent it is important that she is given as much encouragement and support as possible during this difficult time. The nurse and physiotherapist work together and must be prepared to offer reassurance and to sit and listen to the girl should she want to discuss her problems.

Perthes' disease (Ch. 15)

Perthes' disease is thought to be a local disturbance of blood supply to the femoral capital epiphysis, thus rendering it necrotic. Revascularisation of the head takes place over a period of two or three years and it is during this time that many varied forms of treatment are being used. The treatments may be divided basically into non-weight-bearing and weight-bearing.

Frame fixation on Jones' double abduction frame is one of the methods used when non-weight-bearing is required (Ch. 10). The child is completely immobilised on the frame, but physiotherapy treatment is given to mobilise alternate legs, twice daily, throughout the period needed for restoration of the shape of the femoral head. Active exercises for hip, knee and ankle joints are given to maintain their range of movement. It is often the case that several young boys are being treated at the same time by this method and this can be an ideal opportunity for group treatments which provide competition and incentive. The disease has no direct adverse affect upon the child's general health and so the prolonged hospital stay must be made as pleasant and normal as possible. In the later stages of femoral head restoration, the boys are allowed daily hydrotherapy, strictly non-weight-bearing, but this allows maximum mobility and freedom and a great deal of pleasure as Figs 12.7 and 12.8 show.

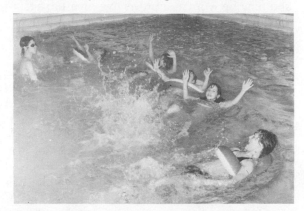

Fig. 12.7 Hydrotherapy: non-weight bearing activity for Perthes' disease.

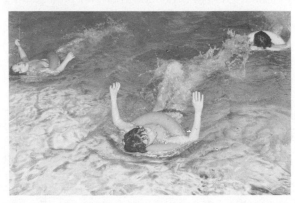

Fig. 12.8 Hydrotherapy is enjoyable as well as therapeutic.

When it is decided to use a Birmingham splint (Figs 7.11, 15.11, 12.12) to treat the condition this is also using the principle of relieving weight-bearing on the femoral head but allows the child to lead a relatively normal life at home, avoiding a long hospital stay. It is necessary to admit the child to hospital when the splint is fitted to educate him in balance and gait and to teach him and his parents the exercises necessary to prevent shortening and muscle-wasting of the affected limb. This usually takes about three weeks in which time the child must become completely independent with crutches, able to negotiate steps and stairs and walk long distances. Before discharge the parents must be taught how to give the strong exercises to the quadriceps and must be told how important it is that these are performed at least three times a day, every day. The splint is worn twenty-four hours a day, unless a night-splint is worn. This may be in the form of bivalved 'broomstick' (Fig. 15.10) and may be worn as a preventive measure against weightbearing during sleep-walking.

Weight-bearing with the hips held in abduction is another method used in the treatment of Perthes' disease, and the position is maintained by the application of broomstick plasters, i.e. long leg plaster cylinders joined by a broomstick at mid-calf level holding the hips abducted and internally rotated. It takes approximately three weeks to teach the children to walk in these and once confident they may be discharged; the physiotherapy mainly involved is teaching the child balance before beginning gait training. The parents are taught exercises to maintain the strength of the gluteal muscles, and since the child walks with flexed hips and knees it is essential to encourage periods of lying prone during the day to avoid hip flexion contractures.

Conclusion

When planning treatment for a physically handicapped child the effect of the handicap is judged not only in relation to the present time but to the probable future of the child; for example, one who is heavily handicapped by spina bifida needs realistic goals in physiotherapy as well as in social, educational and vocational services.

THE EDUCATION OF ORTHOPAEDICALLY HANDICAPPED CHILDREN

HISTORICAL ASPECTS

The education of physically handicapped children began in the early part of this century. It was pioneered by the voluntary effort of men and women of vision who were responsible for the first open-air schools, convalescent homes and schools in hospital. Those people realised that children with orthopaedic conditions, requiring long hospitalisation, needed educational therapy as well as medical or surgical treatment. The emphasis was on handicrafts which, as children became older, had a vocational bias.

The 1944 Education Act, generally regarded as a radical and visionary response to post-war needs, contained a section specifically regarding the education of children unable to attend school. Section 56 made it possible for a group of children or individuals to be taught 'otherwise than at school'. Teaching children in a hospital ward therefore became possible. The existing hospital schools became the responsibility of local education authorities. A Ministry of Education Report in 1954 emphasised the importance of mental stimulus so that the hospitalised child would not fall behind his peers in school work. Later, health authority reports were to highlight the value of play and education, for continuity of harmonious development and the emotional stability of the child in hospital. A committee, set up by the Minister of Health in 1956, made a special study of the welfare of children in hospital, and the subsequent report—The Platt Report—drew attention to the need for considering not only the physical disorder from which the child was suffering but also the social, emotional and environment problems of a child separated from his family.

In 1976, the Court Committee set up to review the needs of children in hospital laid great stress on the importance of play and educational facilities for the hospitalised child. Section 2 (6) of the Court Report states: 'a child immobilised in bed is likely to suffer frustration and boredom and may be unable to cope with his inner feelings and fears unless special help is given to enable him to gain satisfaction and compensation through play'.

The Warnock Committee report was published

in May, 1978. Enquiring into the education of handicapped children a section was devoted to hospital schools. It appreciated the value of education for the short-stay as well as the long-stay child, and also for the very young baby. It stated: 'We consider that education has an indispensable contribution to make in helping them through its very normality to come to terms with a brief but perhaps traumatic period of hospital care. Many of these children would be very young and in keeping with our view that the need for special education may begin at birth, we believe that there should be no lower limit to the age at which education can be provided in hospital.'

Some of the ideas arising from the Warnock Research were crystallised in an Education Act, namely the 1981 Act which deals specifically with special educational needs. Although there are no direct implications for nurses it is important that they should be aware of the obligations that this Act places upon professional medical personnel involved with children who may have special educational requirements.

The main focus of attention is upon the whole child and how he functions, rather than merely upon his disability. The Act states that a child's special educational needs are related to his abilities as well as his disabilities, and to the nature of his interaction with his environment. Assessment is a continuous process and should involve a child's parents. It should be a partnership between groups of professionals and parents in a joint endeavour to discover and understand the nature of the child's difficulties, and to establish which special provision will help to meet the needs which those difficulties present.

For a child under the age of five years, and in some cases at any age, a medical officer may be the first professional to refer the child as having special educational needs. A medical and/or nursing officer designated by the District Health Authority (para. 13 D.H.S.S. Circular HN (82)9) will co-ordinate information from all the doctors who have a contribution to make to the assessment of the child's needs. In the case of an orthopaedically handicapped child advice would be given to the Local Education Authority about specific areas of physical and motor development, about special equipment, specialist facilities or educational

resource requirements. There may be a need to advise on other specialist resource requirements, for example, speech therapy, occupational therapy, physiotherapy or special nursing care as well as specific advice on the physical environment, e.g. access and facilities for non-ambulant children and perhaps special transport needs.

Professional assessment may be organised in a variety of ways according to local circumstances and requirements of individual cases. The most important point is that by bringing together the skills, perceptions and insights of different disciplines there should emerge a clearer picture and a more complete understanding of a child's special educational needs.

This short chapter about the education of children within a hospital setting highlights the need for multi-disciplinary collaboration. The 1981 Education Act adds further weight to this. It is not easy to achieve because it requires a depth of understanding and tolerance, mutual support and continuous dialogue. Each professional must be aware of the roles of colleagues and should seek to reach agreement and understanding of their roles and functions.

IMPLICATIONS OF HOSPITALISATION

When a child enters hospital, he is inevitably placed in a strange and unfamiliar world. He will certainly be confronted by bewildering sights, sounds and smells and by hospital staff who come and go with little continuity. But, even more important, he will be separated from his family, his home and his normal environment perhaps for a protracted period. Research has shown that such separation can have far-reaching psychological effects which may persist months after the child has been discharged from hospital. It is now generally agreed that the continuity of family ties and close contact between mother and child is reciprocally beneficial for their emotional well-being. Education, therefore, is seen in the context of total family care with the teacher, nursery assistant, parent and nurse working in close co-operation especially during the all important settling in period. This team work calls for a high degree of understanding and maturity from the professionals involved since not all parents are adequately equipped to cope or to give positive support to their children when they themselves are under stress.

Successful involvement of parent and child in practical activities in which they are able to become absorbed can often lessen that high intensity of feeling which exists between a mother and her child in hospital. Also, if parents are encouraged to participate rather than just left to sit at the bedside as an observer they will feel welcome, gain confidence and this confidence will ultimately be transmitted to the child (Figs 12.9 and 12.10).

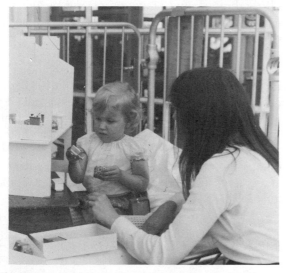

Fig. 12.9 A child confined to bed enjoys a reminder of home by playing with the dolls' house with mother.

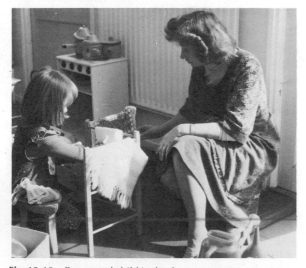

Fig. 12.10 Parent and child in the 'home corner'.

THE SCHOOL AND ITS OBJECTIVES

The type of educational provision in hospital depends on historical factors, geographical position as well as existing attitudes of all disciplines involved in the care of the children. It is desirable that all school-aged children should be placed in a paediatric unit so that they may be grouped for school according to age, ability or length of stay. However, this is not always possible as older adolescents are still sometimes nursed on adult wards. The quality of the educational programme depends upon the ratio of teachers to pupils and this in turn is governed by the policy of the Local Education Authority. An officially designated 'hospital school' comes into the category of special education and as such requires a generous staffing ratio, similar to that provided in a day special school in the community, so that teachers can be flexibly deployed to meet changing needs. A hospital school has a governing body which meets three times each year

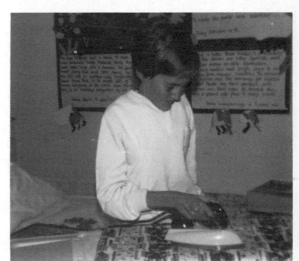

Fig. 12.11 Domestic activity. 'Normalising the ward setting.'

to discuss the problems which arise in the day-to-day running of the school, and to offer support and advice of a general nature so that the head teacher and members of her staff can offer the best possible service in their particular setting. A hospital school often holds the entire school population in microcosm having the full age and ability range amongst its pupils. It is therefore very important that there are enough appropriately trained staff to meet these very different needs.

The teachers themselves must be adaptable and resourceful and they should view their work as educators in the widest sense. A child may regress academically at first, but a sensitive teacher will appreciate that this is inevitable and will help the child in other directions until he has assimilated his hospital experience and become emotionally secure enough to cope with the more academic work. It is desirable for the hospital school to have premises set apart from the ward where children are able to work uninterrupted in a quiet peaceful environment for at least part of each school day. Many local education authorities provide such facilities within the hospital grounds so that children

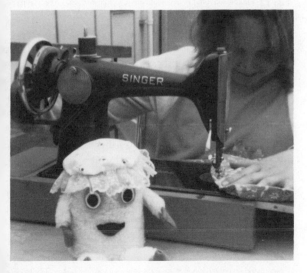

Fig. 12.12 Absorbed in sewing a doll's garment.

can undertake activities such as cooking, pottery, music and drama, all of which are much less easy to pursue in a busy ward (Fig. 12.12).

The teacher and the nurse

Nurses and teachers work alongside each other daily. They are each responsible for the well-being and care of the child in different, yet vitally important ways. The teacher needs to appreciate that a nurse's duties will inevitably interrupt her educational routine whilst the nurse must understand that the educational programme will only be effective

if these interruptions are minimal, especially when children are engaged in more formal lessons. However, creative activities can be enjoyed in a relaxed atmosphere with nurse participation whenever working duties allow (Fig. 12.13). The teacher may

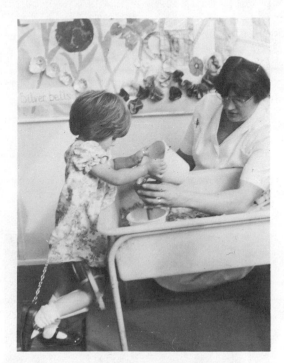

Fig. 12.13 Sand play enjoyed with nurse's help.

take on a caring role, comforting a child after some painful procedure. This interchange of roles helps to promote a deeper understanding of the child's overall personality. Nurses and teachers should always be ready to discuss the children in their care, alerting each other to any underlying emotional stresses which may be hindering the child's progress.

Equipment and apparatus

In order to work effectively children need apparatus which will help to facilitate writing. Special easels may be purchased which fit onto beds, but these are expensive. It should be possible for individual hospital teachers to involve either a local secondary school design team or the hospital carpenters in making easels and cot trays which cater for the precise requirements of particular children (Fig.

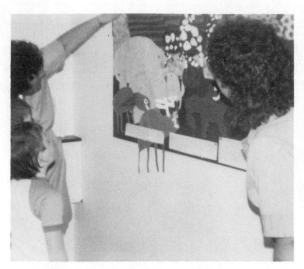

Fig. 12.14 Showing the ward helpers a composite picture the children have produced.

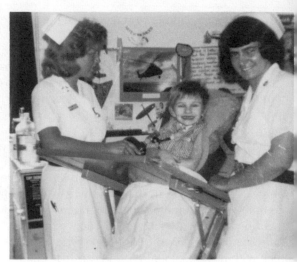

Fig. 12.16 Ready to commence his school work. At ease in the standing frame.

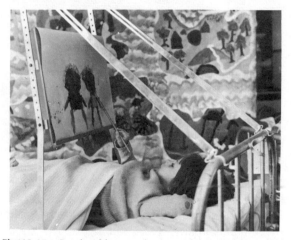

Fig. 12.15 Comfortably at work: an easel designed for a child in supine position.

12.15). Magnetic boards which are more readily available from educational suppliers help if children are immobilised. Flannel-graph material can also be used for teaching purposes as can overhead projectors.

School holidays

The Warnock Report, Section 8.85 contains the recommendation that some educational provision should be made in hospitals during school holidays, particularly for children who are there for a long time. This need has always been appreciated by teachers in hospital schools and several schemes have been tried. Some hospital schools stagger teachers' holidays so that the school year is continuous. However, there are children who resent having formal lessons when their friends are enjoying summer holidays. Also, a long-stay patient who has been working hard at academic subjects needs a rest from formal school work during the holidays.

It must be agreed, however, that some form of educational provision should be provided during the long summer vacation. The emphasis should be on creative activities, hobbies, outings and games so that children are able to enjoy fresh air, companionship and recreational pursuits. This can be provided by employing student teachers, but it is desirable that the usual teaching staff work on a rota basis so that their expert knowledge of the children and of the hospital routine can be drawn upon.

THE LONG-STAY CHILD

The educational programme for long-stay children should include a variety of outings in order to preserve precious links with the environment (Fig. 12.17). It is important that the developing child is able to keep contact with every-day sights, sounds and smells. The orthopaedic child may be

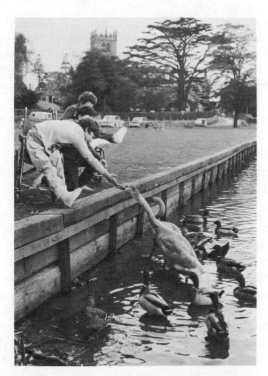

Fig. 12.17 An excursion to the lake to feed the ducks.

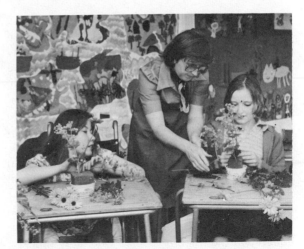

Fig. 12.18 A flower arranging class. A link with the outside environment.

brownie packs or even membership of clubs all come within the scope of the hospital teaching team.

Special problems

In any orthopaedic ward there will be special difficulties when children are not only physically but also mentally handicapped. There will be a range of individual and specific difficulties associated with the nature and type of handicap, its effect on learning ability and on the social and emotional development of the child. In order to plan an appropriate programme, the teacher may sometimes call upon the special expertise of an educational psychologist, who will make a detailed educational assessment.

A teacher must make her own assessment of a child's ability from her observations of his behaviour and general functioning. She must then select an appropriate teaching target applicable to the need. This must be carried out in small steps, each of which the child must fully grasp before she can proceed to the next step. When the child has succeeded he should be praised for effort.

Finally, the teacher will have to make an evaluation of the learning that has taken place to ensure that her objectives have been achieved.

Non-English speaking children

From time to time children may be admitted to an

physically restricted and unable to explore for himself but a trip to a local place of interest in a car or a hospital bus will do much to stimulate interest and provide a topic for discussion in school. A visit to the shops to buy a small item, to the Post Office to post a letter, or to the local library, can bring that element of normality so lacking in a ward setting. Teachers in long-stay hospitals should endeavour to organise visits from interesting people in order to preserve links with the outside community. Films can be shown, puppet theatre groups brought in, for the children's education and enjoyment. Flower arranging can also be a very worthwhile creative pursuit (Fig. 12.18). It may be possible to organise visits from school-children who could bring along a musical programme which might include songs in which the hospital child could participate. It is important that the orthopaedic long-stay child should have opportunities of mixing with healthy children. Such activities help to prevent a child from becoming isolated and institutionalised and help to keep alive his natural inquisitiveness and interest in the outside world. Extra-curricula activities such as organising cubs, orthopaedic hospital from a non-English speaking community. This obviously poses problems of communication which add to the stresses already imposed upon the child by hospitalisation. The teacher must devote individual attention initially so that she may establish contact with the pupil and gain his confidence. She must then help to build up a vocabulary by naming objects which the child perceives around him. If a child is hospitalised for any length of time these communication problems are gradually resolved; since the pupil is constantly exposed to the new language it has been found that a working knowledge of it is gradually acquired. A child who knows his own language will often learn the new one fairly quickly, probably more readily than a non-English speaking child in an ordinary school in the community, because many of these children revert to speaking their first language once they return home to the family in the evening. The child in hospital learns to communicate satisfactorily because there is no alternative language for him to use if he is to be understood.

A very young child who is just beginning to learn his own language is at greater risk than an older one when he comes into hospital where he hears new and incomprehensible sounds. He may become confused and disturbed, and will cease to communicate at all. In such cases it would seem sensible for the parent to be with the child as much as possible speaking the language which he understands.

PRE-SCHOOL AND INFANT EDUCATION

The importance of play

'Play is the very stuff of which a child's life is made. It uses every ounce of energy, it encourages his imagination, it develops skills of both body and mind—it offers healing for hurts and sadness, it breaks down tension and releases pent-up urges towards self expression. Play is the working partner for growth, for activity, and is as vital to growth as food and sleep.'

This quotation illustrates how urgent and indispensable is the child's need to play. The desire for play which dominates the behaviour of all young children and which is essential for normal

development and maturity is inhibited if a child is immobilised in bed. Efforts must be made to provide mental stimulation and to give appropriate play opportunities so that the child has scope for experimentation. A trained play specialist or teacher must have time to talk to the child and to encourage the continuation of play activities most appropriate to the child's developmental level.

Organisation of play in an orthopaedic ward

In an orthopaedic ward there will be children who are purely physically handicapped but others who have multiple handicaps. Both groups will be impeded in movement and in the ability to learn from the environment. These restrictions will hinder both mental and physical development unless steps are taken to compensate. A small child should be carried around, taken out of doors and given an opportunity to make physical contact with objects near him. Tactile experience can be gained from dabbling the hands in sand, soapy water, seeds or salt (Fig. 12.19). The child needs to handle

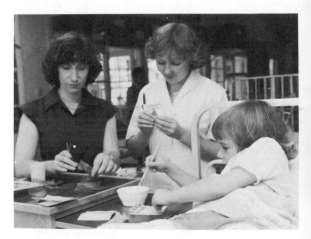

Fig. 12.19 Tactile experience. Nurse, mother and child helping to prepare a collage.

objects of varying shape, size and texture and to have opportunities to discriminate between smells. A child could play on a mattress where he will get opportunities to search and explore for himself. If it is necessary for him to remain in bed on traction, however, stimulation can be given by hanging mobiles within sight, those with music can be especially valuable. Blowing bubbles and following them can also help and a large adjustable mirror so that the child can catch every movement in the room will enrich his experience and keep alive his interest in the environment.

A teacher's skilful provision of play materials can help a child to cope with the tensions and anxieties that he will inevitably feel in the hospital situation. He is not able to find relief in words and instead he uses play materials to give vent to his innermost feelings. Given the opportunity the child works out his problems through his play. Sand and water can have a therapeutic effect and promote long periods of concentration. Clay, wet sand and dough can be banged and pummelled and offer a legitimate means of releasing feelings of anger and resentment. Finger paint can produce bright colours to delight as well as offer satisfying tactile experience. Domestic play inspired by the use of dolls, kitchen equipment and other objects which remind a child of home also help to preserve the attachment he has to mother and family, and at the same time keep alive his past memories.

Language development

Language is acquired long before a child can communicate with words. It develops from birth through his interaction with mother. It is most at risk if family links are broken by a child's admission to hospital. The teacher has an important task here because it is through language that future intellectual development depends. A child's ability to read and write and to verbalise effectively depends upon early language acquisition. 'Language is a preliminary function to reading and is necessary to most school activities . . . In the initial stages of reading, the amount of satisfaction he experiences in responding to the written word will largely be dependent upon the pleasurable association developed in the early language programme.' (Williams, 1970.)

The teacher must help the child to interpret his new environment by giving words to strange objects and equipment the child perceives. She must also help to keep alive his existing vocabulary with nursery rhymes, jingles, finger play and conversation about home. There should be opportunities to listen to stories, indulge in dramatic play,

draw, paint and build with constructional toys (Fig. 12.20). In such play activities the child's skill in

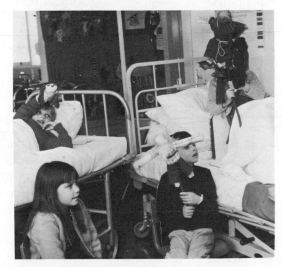

Fig. 12.20 A puppet play. Children act out a story with puppets which they have made.

thinking and communicating will be fostered, because of the meaning such activities have and the satisfaction he gets from them.

It must be emphasised that language is a continuously developing process that must be nurtured for the whole period of childhood. It begins at birth and continues growing in complexity as a young person reaches maturity. Language is essential to the establishment of good human relationships and successful integration into society. Effective use of language provides emotional satisfaction and growth. It is, therefore, immensely important that a hospitalised child has a suitable environment for language development. At the pre-school period, a one-to-one relationship with a teacher or nursery assistant for part of a day is essential so that the child is able to listen, and understand, to talk and be understood and so gain language experience from a conducive environment.

JUNIOR EDUCATION

Social aspects

Junior aged children entering the orthopaedic wards do so from a variety of background. For some families it will be their first experience of hospital, but for others it will be one of a series when school and home life has to be interrupted for orthopaedic treatment. In either case, there is a traumatic break in the continuity of the normal routine and there has to be a period of adaption. Each child will react in a different way and must be given time to settle down and absorb all the unfamiliar and sometimes frightening aspects of his new environment. At this stage in his development, a child is able to anticipate and often has an exaggerated fear of what might happen to him. He relates to people around him and may be unduly worried about the plight of others. He may even feel and say that his parents have rejected him. A teacher needs to exercise skills in coping with these problems. She must identify individual needs and at the same time provide a controlled setting and a familiar work routine into which the child will ultimately fit. A teacher who successfully involves the parent in school activities helps not only to promote parental interest in the child's school work but also provides a welcoming atmosphere into which the parent is able to feel part of the team involved in the child's recovery. The parents presence can also help to reassure a child that he is still wanted.

The teacher and the parent

The Plowden Report, 1966 recommended a closer association between parents and teachers and between home and school. The aim is for information to pass between the two environments which will help to ensure consistency of approach towards a child's progress. In the hospital situation there is an opportunity for teachers to establish and develop a working relationship with parents thereby helping them to understand the educational objectives and the methods being used to achieve them.

The education programme

The junior child has already made friends at his ordinary school, with whom he should be able to keep contact during his stay in hospital either by visits from them or, if that is not possible, by the exchange of letters and cards. It is important that he is able to continue with a similar work programme so that on his return to school he will be

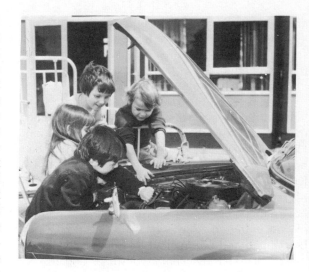

Fig. 12.21   A practical activity out of doors.

able to take his place in class again without too much difficulty. This, however, is not always easy as concentration is affected by anxiety and a child may regress to a stage of development he has already passed through. Although it is desirable to maintain concentration in basic subjects, the emphasis in the hospital school needs to be on a practical approach to learning. The value of cooking, playing with dough, making music, painting and going out into the environment has already been mentioned (Fig. 12.21).

Reading

Books of all kinds should be readily available to the children. These ought to include a child's usual reading scheme but many children get pleasure from a variety of supplementary colourful readers which have only a few pages. Group activities are important for primary school children, since at this age they enjoy competition and the stimulation of working together. Group story sessions are valuable especially as they help to initiate dramatic play and group conversation. Table games can help their social development as also can group participation in artistic projects. The children's art work should always be mounted attractively and if possible displayed in the ward. This helps to inspire conversation and it also adds colour and interest in an otherwise clinical setting.

Mathematical development

In the past, people equated mathematics with the ability to manipulate numbers, learn rules and produce correct answers. During the last thirty years there has been a change in emphasis from the child being taught to the child learning through a practical approach to mathematical experiences. One function of mathematics is to alert a child's mind to the world about him and help him to understand the mathematical aspect of it.

A child is able to understand mathematical concepts only when he has reached a certain level of intellectual maturity. In the early years mathematical ideas grow naturally in an environment of action. The child must be given the opportunity to sort and classify concrete articles according to shape, size or colour. He should be able to make comparisons of size and shape and the teacher should help him to build-up a number vocabulary from such experiences. Many play activities may be used to promote mathematical understanding. A child pouring water from one container to another learns about capacity. Matching cups to saucers in tea party play gives a child experience in matching his counting to objects being counted.

Certain table games offer scope for increasing awareness of number. Games with dice or with packs of playing cards can encourage counting and be of value in developing number sense.

The hospital teacher should try to make maths interesting in a structured, purposeful and practical way, leading children to understand mathematical concepts expressed in concrete terms.

Computers

One important recent advance in teaching aids has been the computer. Computers have been introduced in both secondary and primary schools and also in the hospital schools' setting. Older pupils learn computer programming, opening up career prospects in that field. All pupils benefit from educational programmes designed to suit their requirements, not least those who need to improve basic skills of numeracy and literacy. Children almost always become absorbed in the activities, usually developing increased powers of concentration, of perception, of memory and accelerated responses. Most important, for some orthopaedically handicapped pupils there is an improvement in hand–eye co-ordination and in manual dexterity.

For those severely handicapped, such as children

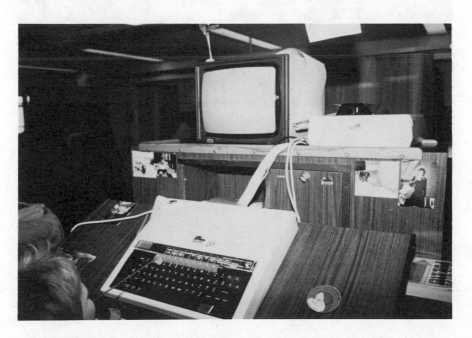

Fig. 12.22 Using a mouthpiece as an aid to press the computer key-board.

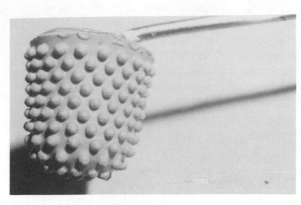

Fig. 12.23 Close-up of rubber end of mouth-piece.

suffering high-level tetraplegia, a computer may provide the only means whereby he can work unaided, in complete and independent charge of his learning. In some cases, where there is no residual arm function, a mouthpiece can be used so that the pupil may press the computer keyboard. A print-out facility may produce a pupil's work (Fig. 12.22).

There are many professional agencies working in conjunction with computer experts to develop and adapt computers for use with handicapped pupils. Computers may help with activities of daily living, but there is great scope for their use as educational aids (Figs. 12.23–26).

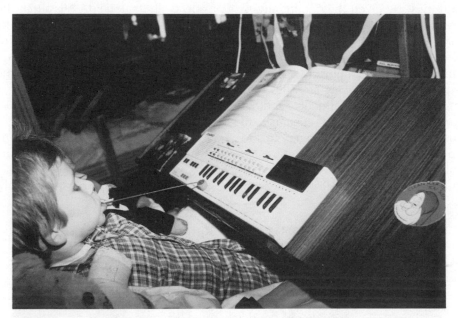

Fig. 12.24 Enjoyment from playing a musical instrument.

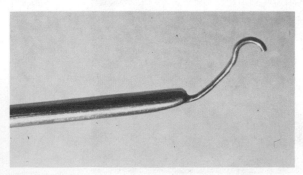

Fig. 12.25 A mouth-piece fitted with a hook to enable pupils to play games.

SECONDARY EDUCATION

Organisation

There are several problems facing a hospital teacher in her endeavour to provide a comprehensive programme for this age group. The requirements of students studying for a variety of specialist subjects in public examinations needs to be met whilst at the same time there must be careful planning for an appropriate programme of work for the less able adolescent or the severely handicapped. The problem is often compounded when adoles-

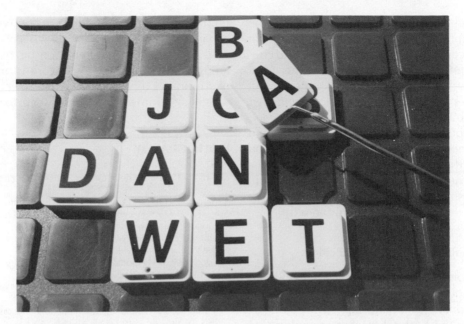

Fig. 12.26 A game of scrabble being played with the use of the hook to lift letter pieces.

cents are placed on adult wards. It is highly desirable that these young people are known to the teaching staff and that there are opportunities for them to be drawn out of the ward to a schoolroom for a period each day when they can meet their peers and participate in an educational programme. Even if they are working at different levels individually there can be social benefits as well as opportunities to voice anxieties and problems.

Problems of adolescence

Adolescence is ordinarily a turbulent period when young people are self-critical, often having doubts about their academic success or their ability to match up to a personal ideal. Their behaviour is unpredictable and their moods change without apparent reason. A period in hospital can only add to the stresses inherent in adolescence and, therefore, the hospital teacher must use skill and understanding in helping the young person through this difficult period. For some there will be very real fears about school-work and examination success. Contacts must be made with a pupil's usual head-teacher and where appropriate a scheme of work obtained from specialist teachers. Close liaison must be maintained with that school, and work passed back for appraisal. Ideally, a report from the hospital school head-teacher should be sent to the pupil's school when he has been discharged. If a return to a normal school routine is not possible immediately, then home-tuition should be arranged and a similar liaison with the school established by the home tutor.

Public examinations

Arrangements can be made for pupils to sit external examinations at the hospital school. However, if admission for treatment is planned and not urgent then it would seem more appropriate to delay such an admission until after public examinations. When this is not possible, examination boards will allow a concession in time if treatment hinders writing. An amanuensis can also be used by those unable to write.

Reluctant scholars

There are some adolescent pupils who appear to have little motivation for formal school-work and who appear content to lie in bed without any active participation in school-work. These pupils have often failed to achieve any academic success and are really lacking self-confidence as a result. The teacher's approach must be skilful. Aware that these adolescent pupils will probably refuse to concentrate on formal written work the teacher must try and draw them into discussions on topics of interest to them, aiming all the time to extend their reasoning powers, widen their vocabulary and learn the art of controversial discussion rather than argument. These pupils are often very insecure and need to feel that the teacher accepts them and listens to their views. They are also probably far more afraid of hospital treatment and separation from parents than they would ever openly admit.

Pupils entering hospital after an accident

When an adolescent enters hospital following sudden illness or an accident and as a result has become permanently handicapped, it will be necessary for the hospital teacher in conjunction with other members of a team to help the young person adapt to a new mode of living, possibly one with many physical restraints. The pupil may need advice about future employment prospects. Here the Disablement Resettlement Officer and Careers Officer can and should be introduced to the pupil to help make a realistic assessment of future prospects.

The adolescent and the community

A handicapped child must eventually take his place in the community. The special educational programme offered in hospital should be seen, therefore, as part of a process of preparation for adulthood, especially for young people whose disability will cause them to experience difficulty in finding their place in society. The emphasis should be on developing self-sufficiency and an independence of spirit whenever possible. An extremely important factor in the education of the physically handicapped is in helping them to develop skills necessary for them to be able to take employment. Many are not ready at the normal school-leaving age of sixteen, so there needs to be an extension of further educational facilities.

The aim should be to help these children to take up useful productive employment within their capabilities so that they are able to feel useful citizens and to enjoy the companionship of a working group. Brown 1954 states: 'Work is an essential part of man's life, since it is that aspect of his life which gives him status and binds him to society.'

BIBLIOGRAPHY

Adams J C 1971 Outline of Orthopaedics. Edinburgh: Churchill Livingstone
Anderson E 1973 The Disabled Schoolchild. London: Methuen
Apley G A 1975 A System of Orthopaedics and Fractures. London: Butterworths
Blount W P, Moe J H 1973 The Milwaukee Brace. Baltimore: The Williams and Wilkins Co
Brown J A 1976 The Social Psychology of Industry. Harmondsworth: Penguin
Cass J 1971 The Significance of Children's Play. London: Batsford
Catterall A 1975 The management of congenital dislocation of the hip. Nursing Mirror 6 March, 44
Downey, Low 1974 The Child with Disabling Illness, Principles of Rehabilitation. London: W B Saunders Co
Harvey S, Hales-Tooke A 1975 Play in Hospital. London: Faber
James J I P 1975 The management of infants with scoliosis. Journal of Bone and Joint Surgery 57B: 422–429
James J I P 1976 Scoliosis. Edinburgh: Churchill Livingstone
Laufer M 1975 Adolescent disturbance and breakdown. Mind
Lindh H, Bjure J 1975 Lung volumes in Scoliosis before and after correction by the Harrington Instrumentation Method. Acta Orthop Scand 46: 934–948, 59
Lloyd-Roberts G C 1971 Orthopaedics in Infancy and Childhood. London: Butterworths
Lorber J 1972 Your Child with Spina Bifida. London: Association for Spina Bifida and Hydrocephalus
Menelaus M B 1971 The Orthopaedic Management of Spina Bifida. Edinburgh: E & S Livingstone
Noble E 1976 Play and the Sick Child. London: Faber
Nordwall A, Willner S 1975 A study of Skeletal Age and Height in Girls with Idiopathic Scoliosis. Clinical Orthopaedics and Related Research 6
Pringle M K 1975 The Needs of Children. London: Hutchinson
Pritchard D G 1963 Education and the Handicapped, 1760–1960. London: Routledge and Kegan Paul
Rowe J, Dyer L (eds) 1977 Care of the Orthopaedic Patient. Oxford: Blackwell Scientific
Thurlbourne T, Gillespie R 1976 Journal of Bone and Joint Surgery 58B: 64
Waldron S 1983 Integration of handicapped pupils. Nursing Times 13 April
Wilkinson A 1971 The Foundation of Language. Oxford: Oxford University Press
Winnicott D W 1968 The Family and Individual Development. London: Tavistock
Woods G E 1975 The Handicapped Child Assessment and Management. Oxford: Blackwell Scientific
Zorab P A 1969 Scoliosis. London: Heinemann

13

The principles of genetics

Genetics is the study of the mechanisms by means of which physical characteristics are transmitted from the parents to the offspring, i.e. the new individual formed by the union of ovum and sperm. Modern genetics stems from the studies, mainly with the breeding of garden peas, which were made by the monk Gregor Mendel in the second half of the last century. As it was Mendel who first clearly enunciated the laws of inheritance, we often refer to genetic principles as 'Mendelian genetics'.

It is now realised that not only are gross physical characteristics inherited, but the whole biochemistry of the individual is controlled by the minute units of inheritance called the *genes*. As disease is very commonly the result of a disturbance of the biochemistry of the body, a genetic basis for many diseases has now been discovered and the number of diseases with a pattern of inheritance is steadily growing. It is thus important for those whose job it is to treat and tend patients with such diseases to understand some of the basic elements of Mendelian genetics.

THE GENE

The basic unit of inheritance is the *gene*. This is an extremely small particle of a very complex biochemical nature. Each gene, of which there are many thousands in the human cell, controls some biochemical process in the cells of the body; a gene may, for example, control the production of a particular type of protein, which in turn is essential for some function such as acting as an enzyme, or by contributing to the connective tissue of the body.

Enzymes are extremely important in the working of the body because they control most of the processes in the cells. In the case of respiration for example, the simple fact that oxygen is converted to CO_2 and energy released, involves a great number of enzymes, each of which control a step of this complicated process.

An example of the importance of genes may be drawn from the tropical anaemia called sickle cell anaemia, which is being met with more and more frequently in this country with the influx of immigrants from Africa and the West Indies. In sickle cell anaemia the red blood corpuscles, which are normally round in shape, become crescentic or sickle-shaped. This is due to the fact that the haemoglobin contained in these cells is not the usual 'A' type but is the abnormal haemoglobin S (Hb-S). This differs from Haemoglobin-A by the replacement of one amino acid in the make-up of the protein globin by another. This occurs because of the existence of an abnormal gene, and because it is due to the action of a gene it is found to 'run in families' or be *inherited*.

Genes are arranged, rather like a necklace of glass beads, upon structures called *chromosomes* which are found in the nucleus of the cell. It is only comparatively recently that it has been possible to actually see the chromosomes by using the microscope (see later), but genes are too small to be seen by present-day methods. It is, however, now possible for organic chemists to 'make' genes by welding together the nucleotide building blocks which make the gene up. There are only four nucleotides in the DNA (deoxyribose nucleic acid) which make up the genes—these are derived from the bases adenine, guanine, thymine and cytosine by addition of sugar (deoxyribose) and phosphate. It is the order of these bases in the DNA sequence of the gene which control the synthesis of the particular protein, the 'gene product', which is produced by the cell. They are the basis of the genetic code which is formed by triplets of bases. At present the base 'sequence' of a gene must be known before the chemist can synthesise it; however, the artificial gene can be put into a simple organism, such as a bacterium, which will then make the protein. This is the basis of so-called genetic engineering.

The chromosomes are important structures because they play a leading part in the process of cell division which results in an increase in cell numbers.

CELL DIVISION

To understand the principles of genetics it is essential to know a little of the way in which the chromosomes behave during the process of cell division. Each cell of the body contains a fixed number of chromosomes, which is the same in all cells from all animals of the same species (with one or two exceptions). Human cells contain 23 pairs of

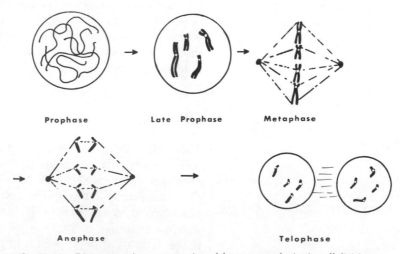

Prophase   Late Prophase   Metaphase

Anaphase   Telophase

Fig. 13.1A   Diagrammatic representation of the process of mitotic cell division.

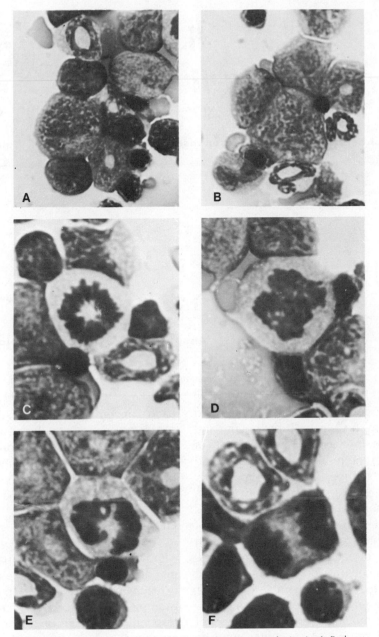

Fig. 13.1B Photomicrographs of cells in various stages of mitosis. **A.** Early prophase. **B.** Prophase. **C.** Metaphase. **D, E.** Anaphase. **F.** Late anaphase.

chromosomes, and in the female each member of the pair is identical, making 46 chromosomes in all. During the process of cell division (or *mitosis*) the chromosomes each replicate themselves and become double structures. The two halves of each chromosome then split and move away from each other to opposite ends of the cell which then divides in half. Each of the daughter cells so formed now contains an identical set of chromosomes, carrying identical genes and each is identical to the original parent cell. This type of division is shown in Fig. 13.1A and B.

A second type of division called *meiosis* also exists which must be explained. During the process

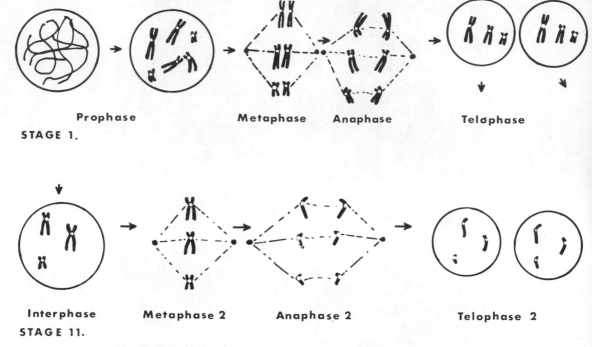

STAGE 1.

Prophase Metaphase Anaphase Telophase

STAGE 11.

Interphase Metaphase 2 Anaphase 2 Telophase 2

Fig. 13.2 Diagrammatic representation of the process of meiotic cell division.

of fertilisation the germ cells from the male and female fuse to form the *zygote*. If both ovum and sperm each contain the full complement of chromosomes then the resulting individual would possess double the number of chromosomes—e.g. 92 in the human. This does not actually happen because during their development the germ cells undergo a special type of division by means of which each daughter germ cell comes to contain only one member of each pair of chromosomes. During this type of cell division each chromosome comes to lie next to the other member of the pair (Fig. 13.2); then, instead of each chromosome splitting and each half moving apart, the members of the pairs repel each other, and move off to opposite ends of the cell which then divides into two. Thus, each daughter cell now contains only 23 chromosomes. This is then followed by a normal division so that eventually from each one germ cell precursor four germ cells are produced and each contains only one representative of each chromosome pair.

When male and female germ cells unite at fertilisation the new individual receives a full complement of 46 chromosomes, one member from each pair coming from each parent. As the chromosomes are paired, so the genes carried on them are paired; it follows therefore that the full complement of genes in the new individual will consist of a representative from each parent.

GENES AND CHARACTERS

Although the members of a pair of chromosomes may look very similar, this is not necessarily true of each member of a gene pair (or *alleles*). For example, a pair of genes which are situated at corresponding positions on a pair of chromosomes in an animal may each control eye colour, but one may produce blue eyes, whereas the other may produce brown eyes. The final eye colour of the individual would depend on the strength of the two genes. Often one type of gene is 'stronger' than the other, in which case it would be called the *dominant* gene and its partner called the *recessive* gene. If the brown-eye gene is dominant the blue-eye gene would not be expressed and the eye colour would be brown. The eyes would only be blue if both genes of the pair were of the blue type. Such an individual who has identical genes at the same point (or *locus*) on a pair of chromosomes is said to be *homozygous* for that gene. If one gene was a blue-eye gene and the other was a brown-eye gene then the individual would be said to be *heterozygous* for the eye colour gene. Sometimes neither type of gene is stronger than the other and they are said to be *co-dominant*. For example, if a plant colour is determined by a pair of genes, one producing a white flower and the other producing a red flower, then those plants with one of each type of gene would be pink if the genes were co-dominant.

The genetic ratios

Having dealt with the basic mechanisms of inheritance we can now see how they may be applied

to studies of families. We may take as an example the inheritance of the ability to taste the chemical phenyl-thio-urea when it is at low concentrations. There are two types of gene at the locus of the chromosome which may determine this ability and we may represent them as 'T' which is the dominant and 't', the recessive. If 'T' is present in the individual he will be able to taste the compound. Let us assume a 'taster' homozygous for 'T' (i.e. TT) marries a non-taster, who must be homozygous for 't' (i.e. tt). Only one 'taster' gene can go into each germ cell of each parent when the chromosome pairs part company during meiosis. This is known as *segregation*. On fertilisation the germ cells will fuse and the baby will have a 'taster' gene from each parent. The possible combinations of germ cells from these two individuals are shown in Fig. 13.3. All children produced by these parents will possess the dominant gene 'T' and will be tasters.

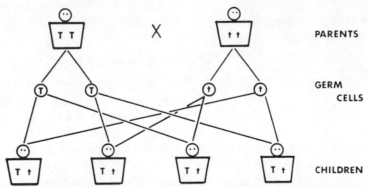

Fig. 13.3 Diagrammatic representation of the possible types of children resulting from the marriage of individuals who are homozygous for the taster gene T and for the non-taster gene t. All children resulting will be herozygous Tt and will therefore be tasters.

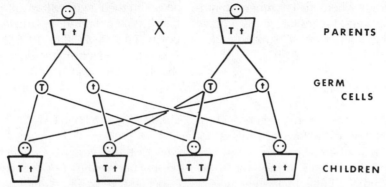

Fig. 13.4 Diagrammatic representation of the possible types of children resulting from the marriage of individuals who are heterozygous for the taster gene. It will be seen that three out of the four children will be tasters but only one of the three tasters will be homozygous. TT for the taster gene.

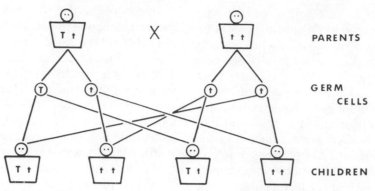

Fig. 13.5 Diagrammatic representation of the possible types of children resulting from the marriage of individuals who are heterozygous for the nontaster gene Tt and homozygous for the nontaster gene tt. It will be seen that two out of the four children will be tasters and these will be heterozygous for the taster gene.

As they will all get the recessive gene 't' from the other parent they will all be heterozygotes as far as this gene is concerned.

If the parents were both heterozygous for this gene then the result will be different, as shown in Fig. 13.4. It will be seen that one child in four could be a non-taster, homozygous for 't'. Only one of the three tasters on the other hand will be homozygous for 'T'.

If one parent is a heterozygote Tt, and the other one homozygous tt, then yet another pattern will emerge (Fig. 13.5). The possible ratio of tasters to non-tasters would 1:1. If instead of being tt the second parent was TT, then all children would be tasters.

These ratios are important because they form the basis of genetics. However, one cannot in practice take them too literally when small numbers of individuals are studied, and before the ratios emerge a large number of individuals must be examined.

THE SEX CHROMOSOMES

It was stated earlier that there were 23 pairs of chromosomes in the human cell. However, this is not strictly true. One pair of chromosomes known as the *sex chromosomes*, are only a true pair in the female cell of mammals. In the male they are not alike. The 22 true pairs of chromosomes are known as *autosomes*. The sex chromosomes come in two types: the X chromosome and the Y chromosome

which is very much smaller than the X and, in man, is also a completely different shape. The female possesses two X chromosomes (XX), whereas the male possesses one of each (XY).

Sex determination

These chromosomes are very important in sex determination. When the germ cells are formed, the sex chromosomes are separated as a pair during meiosis just as are all the autosomes. As the female has two X chromosomes it follows that all ova will have an X chromosome. This is not true of the sperm, however, which can exist as two types: one type contains an X chromosome, the other a Y chromosome. Thus, the sex of a child is determined by the father. If an X-containing sperm fertilises an ovum then a girl will result (XX); if on the other hand a Y-containing sperm fertilises the ovum a boy will result (XY) (Fig. 13.6).

It will be seen from the diagram that the sex ratio should, in theory at any rate, be 50:50.

SEX-LINKED INHERITANCE

Due to this difference between the sexes, genes present upon either X or Y chromosomes may show a special type of inheritance pattern which we call *sex-linked inheritance*.

Genes carried on the X chromosome may, if they are recessive, show a typical pattern of inheritance

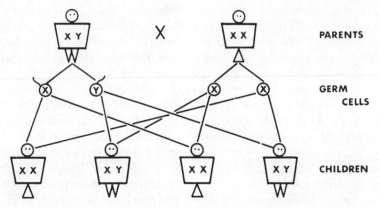

Fig. 13.6 Diagrammatic representation of the sex determining mechanism in man. It will be seen that the theoretical sex ratio of the offspring will be one male to one female.

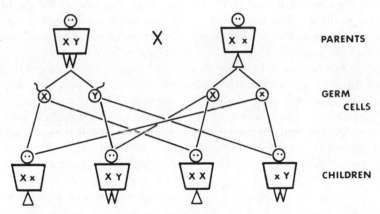

Fig. 13.7 The inheritance of the haemophilic gene. The chromosome carrying the haemophilic gene (represented by x) which is present in the mother may be passed on to daughters and sons. The daughters containing this abnormal gene, however, will be non-bleeders, but carriers, whereas one out of two sons are likely to possess the abnormal gene.

which we call *X-linked inheritance*. A number of genes are now known which are situated on the X chromosome. The colour blindness gene, the muscular dystrophy gene, and the haemophiliac gene are but three. The genes which determine all of these three conditions are all weak or recessive genes, and they therefore are most commonly manifest in the male where there is no second X chromosome. We may take as an example the mode of inheritance of haemophilia. A 'carrier' woman is an individual who carries the haemophiliac gene on one of her X chromosomes but because she has a normal dominant gene at the same locus on the other X chromosome her blood

clotting system will be normal. If such a woman marries a normal man (Fig. 13.7), it will be seen that all her daughters will be normal in that they will not be 'bleeders' but there is a chance that one in two may be carriers of the gene. Of her sons, it is possible that one in two may be normal or, on the other hand, if the X chromosome that the son has received carries the affected gene then he will be a 'bleeder'.

The only circumstances where a woman could be a 'bleeder' would be if both her X chromosomes carried the affected gene, i.e. if she was homozygous for it. This state of affairs could arise if a carrier female married a 'bleeder' male. Such a match would be highly undesirable from the haemophilic point of view, as all daughters would either be carriers or else be 'bleeders', and the chances are that half the sons would be 'bleeders'

Unfortunately the presence of a gene in a carrier female is at present very difficult to detect with certainty. If a 'bleeder' man marries a normal woman, all of their daughters would carry the gene, but all sons would be normal. Sex-linked recessive genes are therefore usually expressed in the male with only very rarely affected females, but they can be transmitted through the female.

The discussion so far has been concerned with the haemophilic gene which is recessive. If an abnormal gene, which is on the X chromosome is dominant it would be very difficult to say with certainty whether or not it was X-linked simply by an examination of a pedigree. The pattern of inheritance would be the same as that of a dominant gene carried on one of the autosomes.

A very rare type of inheritance is that due to a *Y-linked* gene: such diseases are extremely uncommon and, as would be expected, are confined to the male sex. Characteristics determined by Y-borne genes are extremely rare and are passed from father to son and cannot be transmitted through the mother, as can the X-linked gene.

MUTATIONS

Occasionally one finds an individual who possesses a genetically controlled disease or deformity, and yet there has been no previous history of this disease or deformity in the family. One likely explanation for this occurrence is that a *mutation* has taken place. A mutation is a change in the chemical make-up of a gene which alters its whole nature—for example, let us assume a change occurs in the gene on the X chromosome which controls the production of anti-haemophilic globulin. This is the protein present in the blood clotting mechanism. As a result of the mutation this gene may be unable to bring about the production of this vital protein and, should this abnormal gene be on an X chromosome which is present in an ovum that has been fertilised by a normal Y sperm, then the resulting male child will have a defective blood clotting mechanism and will be a haemophiliac or 'bleeder'. Often a mutation is the result of a change in a single base at one place in the DNA of the gene. This will have the effect of altering one of the triplets of the genetic code and thus causing a completely different protein to be produced.

Mutations are occurring at a very low rate in many cells of the body throughout life; however, unless they occur in the germ cell precursors they will not be transmitted to the offspring. It is thought that the cancer cell may have been a normal cell in which mutations have occurred in certain genes, resulting in that cell escaping from the normal control processes of the body, and so it becomes malignant. If a mutation occurs in the germ precursors then the abnormal mutant gene may be passed on to children and so a disease, or characteristic appearance, occurs for the first time in a family. Once the mutation has occurred it can be passed on to succeeding generations. Mutations in germ cells are, however, rare.

A number of external factors can cause mutations, probably the best known of which is radiation. Exposure to high doses of X-rays and other forms of radiation may produce mutations in genes. For this reason it is desirable to keep the dose of radiation to which an individual may be exposed for therapeutic or diagnostic reasons as low as possible. Viruses and some chemicals may also alter genes and give rise to mutations.

GENETICS AND TRANSPLANTATION

In the last ten years there has been a considerable increase in our knowledge of the mechanisms underlying the failure of foreign organ grafts. As a result, organ transplantation has become a clinical reality, with some types of graft, such as kidney liver and heart, giving good results. Whole joint grafts, and even large bone grafts, are now being actively studied in a number of centres. Central to the success of clinical use of foreign grafts was the realisation that rejection of a foreign tissue is due to the recognition by the host's immune system of structures on the graft which are known as *antigens*. These are complex chemical substances which are on the surface of every cell of the body. Their production is under the control of a number of genes and thus they are inherited in the same way as are other features.

The simplest system of such antigens are those responsible for the ABO blood groups. These are not important as *transplantation antigens* however. In the human a group of antigens, which are readily detectable in the laboratory by tissue typing, have been discovered which are very important transplantation antigens and form what is called the *major histocompatibility antigen system* or the *HLA* complex. Similar systems have also been discovered in other species studied which include mouse, rat, dog, pig and sheep. In the human it is clear now that there are in fact at least 4 groups of antigens in the HLA system. The first group form the *HLA-A system*, the second is the *HLA-B system*, the third is the *HLA-C system*, and the fourth is the *HLA-D system*. The antigens of all four systems can be recognised on the white blood cells in the laboratory by means of tissue typing using antibodies recognising the antigens. A fifth group of antigens are those which make up the HLA-DR system. The DR and D antigens cannot be detected easily by conventional tissue typing. Although white cells are used in the laboratory to detect these antigens, they are also present on most cells in the body. In each of these systems there are a series of antigens, each of which is determined by a single gene (alleles). These genes are co-dominant. Thus each human being can have up to ten HLA antigens (two from each of the five systems). The gene loci for HLA systems are situated on the same chromosome and are in fact very close together and so they are inherited *en bloc*.

The inheritance of the HLA genes is governed by the same laws as any other genes. Thus, to take an example, using the -A and -B systems, let us suppose a father has the HLA genes HLA-A1 and HLA-B3 on one of his chromosomes and HLA-A2 and HLA-B4 on the other (this is known as his *genotype*). His cells will show the HLA-A1 and 2 and the HLA-B3 and 4 antigens. Let us next suppose that his wife has the genes for HLA-A3 and HLA-B1 on one chromosome and HLA-A4 and HLA-B2 on the other. Her cells will show the HLA-A3 and 4 and HLA-B1 and 2 antigens. Their children will each inherit one chromosome from each parent, thus they will have one of the following four genotypes:

HLA-A1,B3/HLA-A3,B1
HLA-A2,B4/HLA-A4,B2
HLA-A1,B3/HLA-A4,B2
or HLA-A2,B4/HLA-A3,B1

One of the principles of organ transplantation is that the graft and its recipient should have as many transplantation antigens in common as possible. In addition to the HLA antigens there are also other 'weak transplantation antigen' systems. In practice, however, only the major, HLA, antigens are taken into account and rejection due to differences in the minor antigen systems is checked by drugs which suppress the immune response. There is evidence that if a kidney graft and its recipient have two or less HLA-A and -B antigen differences the graft will survive better than one with more than two differences. A graft between mother and father in the above family would have four antigen differences; the maximum possible difference. It is also clear that a parent's graft can only have two antigen differences if put into one of the children. Grafts between the children may have two *or* four antigens different, *but* there is also a good chance that two children may be identical as far as their HLA genotypes are concerned. This is why the order of preference, from the genetic point of view, of graft donors for an individual would be: his sibling (if HLA-identical); parent; unrelated person. The importance of the HLA-C, -D and -DR systems for graft rejection is not yet clear.

DISEASES AND HLA ANTIGENS

An interesting development which has arisen out of studies of the HLA genes in human populations is the discovery that some diseases are associated with particular HLA antigens. The association of greatest relevance to Orthopaedics is that between ankylosing spondylitis and the HLA-B27 antigen.

In Britain the HLA-B27 is found on the tissue cells of only 5–10 per cent of the general population. However, when individuals with ankylosing spondylitis were tissue typed about 90 per cent of them were found to have the HLA-B27 antigen. About 50 per cent of their first-degree relatives, without the disease themselves, also had this antigen. This association is not seen in other populations such as Japanese, American negroes or Pima Indians. Therefore, care must be taken not to regard the presence of the HLA-B27 antigen as diagnostic of this disease.

Although ankylosing spondylitis is the best example of a disease associated with a transplantation antigen gene, it is not the only one. Reiter's disease, some forms of uveitis, and juvenile rheumatoid arthritis are also associated with the HLA-B27 antigen. Coeliac disease, myasthenia gravis, Graves disease and chronic hepatitis have been found to be associated with HLA-B8; acute lymphoblastic leukaemia with HLA-A2; and breast carcinoma with HLA-A10. The reason for these disease associations is the phenomenon known as *genetic linkage*.

Genetic linkage

As mentioned above the genes are arranged on the chromosome like beads on a necklace. Therefore, a gene for eye colour may be situated on the same chromosome as genes controlling another feature, say, hair colour. If matters were as simple as this then a particular eye colour should always be associated with a particular hair colour in a given population because the genes would always be inherited together. However, this is not always the case. During the chromosomal manoeuvres which take place at cell division, and particularly meiosis in the germ cells, breaks often occur at points along the chromosome and the ends then rejoin but not always with the same chromosome. *Crossing-over* may occur between the members of each chromosome pair and breaks may join again with the wrong chromosome. The effect of this is the separation of the two genes if the break happens to have occurred between them. Thus, if we take two genes 'A' and 'b' which are one chromosome, and their alleles 'a' and 'B' on the other, a break and rejoin may result in one chromosome with 'A' and 'B' together and with 'a' and 'b' together if crossing-over occurred. It will be obvious that the farther apart two genes are on the chromosome then the more chance there will be of them becoming separated. If the genes are very close, however, then crossing-over affecting the part of the chromosome between them will be very rare. A very good example of such genetic linkage is the HLA system

where the two loci, HLA-A and HLA-B are so close together that crossing-over does not happen often, and they appear to behave almost as a single unit when family studies are made. In the case of the diseases associated with HLA genes, it is likely that the gene, or genes, controlling the disease process are situated very close to the HLA locus and so tend to not get separated, in the population, from a particular HLA gene.

THE CHROMOSOMES

Between the years 1958 to 1960 great advances were made in the field of human genetics and these were made possible by the development, at about that time, of various techniques for making the chromosomes of human cells available for study in the laboratory. Up until this time it was generally believed that there were 48 chromosomes in the human cells; it is now well established that there are in fact only 46 chromosomes (23 pairs). Various methods are at present available for the study of human chromosomes, all of which rely upon the availability of cells that are in the process of cell division; this is the only time in the life of a cell when its chromosomes are visible. Small fragments of skin may be grown in tissue culture and the skin cells which divide in the culture can be examined; alternatively, bone marrow may be sampled and its cells also subjected to a short period of tissue culture in order to obtain numbers of dividing blood-forming cells for examination. Both of these procedures, however, are not very convenient and bone marrow aspiration can in fact be quite painful, and healthy individuals rarely wish to be subjected to such a procedure. In about 1960 a new technique was evolved whereby lymphocytes from the peripheral blood, drawn by venepuncture, could be made to transform into large cells which can divide. The transformation is brought about by exposure of the lymphocyte to the bean extract, Phytohaemagglutinin. This technique has been widely used, and in some hospitals is becoming a routine procedure in the investigation of certain congenital disorders.

The tissue cultures containing the dividing cells are treated with a drug, colchicine, which prevents the cells completing their division and they are therefore stopped midway. At this stage the chromosomes are readily visible as double structures and by various forms of treatment the cells are swollen up and spread on microscopic slides. The chromosomes contained within them are spread out and can be easily examined. A preparation such as this is seen in Fig. 13.8.

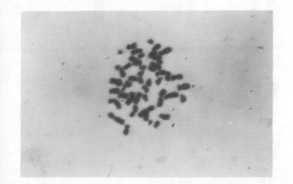

Fig. 13.8 Photomicrograph of human chromosomes obtained from a dividing blood cell and spread out for microscopy.

The chromosomes in the human cell, it will be seen, come in various shapes and sizes, and a conference held in 1960 at Denver laid down a system of classification whereby the chromosomes in a cell are arranged in order of size and then each pair is given a number. A diagrammatic summary of this classification is shown in Fig. 13.9. The procedure used for the analysis of the chromosome complement of a cell is to photograph the chromosomes of a spread-out cell and then cut out each chromosome on the photographic print and arrange them in their pairs. They are then glued on to a sheet of card in the order recommended by the Denver conference. Figure 13.10 shows the appearance of a male and a female cell set out in this way. In very good preparations it is possible to identify a number of individual pairs of chromosomes—for example, the five biggest pairs (1–5) are all readily distinguishable; however, the large group numbered from 6–12, and including the X sex chromosomes, are very difficult to identify separately. Numbers 13–15 are a group of medium-sized 'V'-shaped chromosomes; numbers 16–20 are small and cross-shaped, and 21–22, and the male Y chromosome, are small and 'V'-shaped structures. In more recent years, however, special staining techniques have been developed which have revealed the presence on chromosomes of bands. Each member of a pair of chromosomes will have the same banding pattern, and can therefore be recognised. Using such techniques it is becoming possible to obtain more accurate identification of the autosomes. An even more recent development in this field is the use of computers to scan the chromosomes and then identify them.

DISEASES WITH CHROMOSOME ABNORMALITIES

As a result of being able to examine human chromosomes the genetic basis for a number of diseases has now become apparent.

Sex chromosome abnormalities

One large group are the sex chromosome abnormalities; these are individuals who possess more or

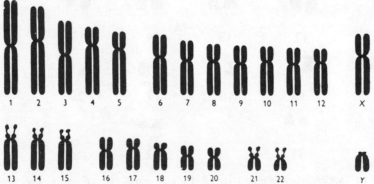

Fig. 13.9 Diagrammatic representation of the arrangement of the human chromosome pairs according to the Denver classification.

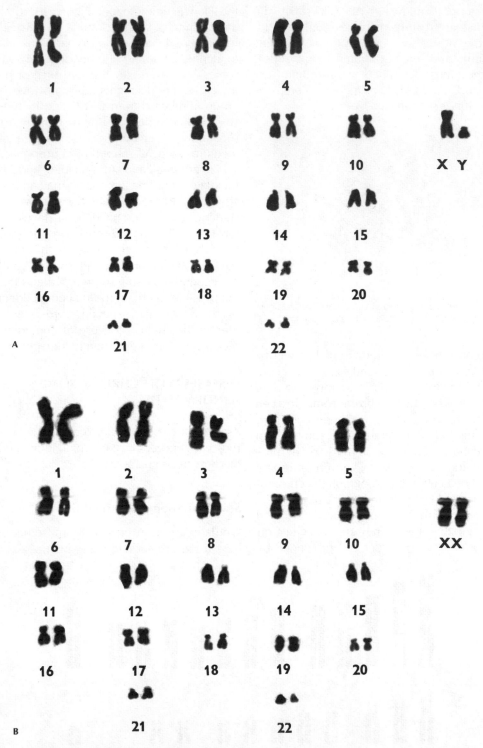

Fig. 13.10 A. Chromosomes from a normal male cell, and **B,** from a normal female cell, cut out of the photomicrograph as in Fig. 13.8. The chromosomes have been paired up and arranged according to the Denver classification in Fig. 13.8.

fewer than the normal complement of sex chromosomes. It is possible, for example, to find an XXY sex chromosome pattern which leads to a characteristic abnormality which is called Klinefelter syndrome. The XXY individual looks like a male but is in fact sexually retarded, sterile and usually mentally subnormal. Individuals are also known to exist who only have one X chromosome (XO); they are apparently female but lack the secondary sex characteristics, are infertile, and again more often than not, they are mentally subnormal. Since the beginning of the chromosome era, many such abnormalities of sex chromosome numbers have been discovered; individuals are now known who are XXX, XXXX, and XXXXX, XXXY, YY and so on. Most of these patients showed sexual abnormalities and a varying degree of mental retardation.

The mechanism by means of which individuals are produced with these sex chromosome abnormalities is not difficult to understand. During the 'reduction division' (meiosis), in germ cell formation (Fig. 13.2) in one of the parents the X chromosomes pair up but the members of the pair fail to separate as normally. If this happens in the mother such an event will lead to two ova being formed, one of which contains two X chromosomes instead of one, and the second ovum lacks an X chromosome altogether. If these ova are fertilised by normal X- or Y-containing sperm, then the various types of abnormal sex chromosome constitutions can arise. This will be seen from Fig. 13.11. When a pair of chromosomes fails to separate during germ formation, the process is known as *non-disjunction*. Such errors in cell division during germ cell formation tend to occur more often in later life and it is commonly found that the mothers of patients

with sex chromosome abnormalities were of late child-bearing age at the time of the child's birth.

Diseases with autosomal abnormalities

Very few diseases are known to have abnormalities of the autosomes; the most common disease due to an autosomal abnormality is Down's syndrome (mongolism). The mongol has three No. 21 chromosomes instead of the normal two and is said to be *trisomic* for No. 21. Each cell would therefore have 47 chromosomes. This state of affairs, like that of the abnormal sex chromosome constitution, is due to the process of non-disjunction which usually occurs in the mother during the formation of the ova. It must be pointed out, however, that the father might be the affected partner, although this is far more rare. In this case, however, instead of the X chromosomes being involved, the No. 21 chromosome pair fail to split up and go their separate ways. This results in one ovum having no No. 21 chromosome and the other ovum has two instead of the usual one. If this ovum is then fertilised by a normal sperm with one 21 chromosome, the resulting individual will have three 21 chromosomes and will be a mongol. Again, it is well known that the mongol children are most commonly born to mothers in their late child-bearing years. The chances of having a mongol child increases with maternal age.

Occasionally one meets the situation where a mongol child is born to a mother in her early or late twenties. When the chromosomes of this child are examined it is found that the chromosome number is normal, i.e. 46 instead of 47 which is usual for the mongol child. However, there is an abnormal chromosome present and one normal autosome is missing. What has happened in this type of situation is that the additional 21 chromosome, associated with mongolism, is present in the cell but has been fused onto one of the other 'V'-shaped chromosomes in either group 13–15 or 21–23. The chromosome with the addition is abnormal in shape and size and is no longer recognisable as its former self but the result is that the cell contains, in addition to the normal amount of chromosome material, the abnormal extra material from chromosome 21 (Fig. 13.12). This phenomenon is known as *translocation* and again

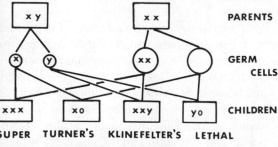

PARENTS

GERM CELLS

CHILDREN

SUPER FEMALE · TURNER'S SYNDROME · KLINEFELTER'S SYNDROME · LETHAL

Fig. 13.11 Diagrammatic illustration showing the origin of the various sex chromosome abnormalities which are most commonly seen as a result of non-disjunction in the mother.

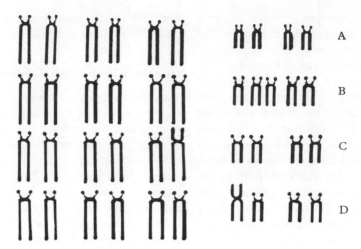

Fig. 13.12 Abnormal chromosomes in mongolism. **A.** Normal chromosomes of group 13–15 and 21–22. **B.** The mongol chromosomes. (NB three No. 21 chromosomes.) **C.** The translocation mongol. Two No. 21 chromosomes are present but one No. 13–15 group chromosome is abnormal and has the missing No. 21 attached to it. **D.** Second type of translocation mongol where two No. 21 chromosomes are joined together.

usually occurs in the mother. If one examines the chromosome constitution of the mother of this child it will be found that she has only 45 chromosomes; the abnormal 'double' chromosome is present but there is only one 21 chromosome. As far as the genetic material in her cells is concerned, the mother is therefore balanced and quite normal. This woman may pass the abnormal chromosome on to her children, however, and it is possible for the geneticist to give such a young mother a fairly good idea of what her chances of having further mongol children are likely to be. Chromosome studies are therefore of great value in this context in the genetic counselling of parents.

Some infants with extremely severe abnormalities affecting the skeletal system, the heart, the connective tissues and other systems have been found to be trisomic for others of the small chromosomes in groups between Nos 16–20. These unfortunate children, however, do not survive longer than a few days or weeks. Trisomy of one of the smaller autosomes therefore leads to very gross defects which are barely compatible with life. No individual has yet been found in which any of the larger chromosomes are trisomic. Also as yet no individual has been found with a completely missing

autosome. Such states of affairs are presumably not compatible with life beyond the earliest embryonic stages and, in fact, chromosome studies of a number of abortuses have shown them to have had very gross chromosomal abnormalities. Chromosome studies may therefore shed some light on the cause of spontaneous abortion.

Another disease which has been found has widespread abnormalities including growth and mental retardation, skeletal and facial abnormalities, and is associated with loss, or *deletion*, of a small part of the No. 5 chromosome. This disease is characterised by a quite distinctive cry of the affected infant and is known as the *cri du chat* (cat-cry) syndrome. Some of these children survive for some time.

With increasingly precise methods of examining human chromosomes, smaller abnormalities are being recognised, e.g. breaks in chromosomes or small deletions (i.e. loss of a part of the chromosome). Sometimes a clinical condition is associated with particular minor chromosomal changes; examples include Fanconis anaemia, ataxia telangiestasia, and xeroderma pigmentosa. All of these diseases are inherited in an autosomal recessive manner.

Chromosomes in leukaemias

Chromosome studies have also thrown light on a number of diseases of the blood. In a type of leukaemia known as chronic myeloid (granulocytic) leukaemia it has been found that some of the blood-forming cells of the marrow have an abnormally small No. 21 chromosome which, instead of being 'V'-shaped, is cross-shaped. Part of the normal 21 chromosome has been lost or deleted. The abnormality is confined to the leukaemia bone marrow cells. This chromosome is known as the Philadelphia (or Ph^1) chromosome, and is present in the bone marrow cells from the earliest stages of the disease. Its presence is of considerable value to the haematologist in diagnosing this type of leukaemia and in distinguishing it from 'leukaemoid' reactions to various stimuli—e.g. infection, which often mimic this kind of leukaemia.

Some patients with chronic lymphocytic leukaemia have an abnormality in the chromosomes of the leukaemic cells—often trisomy for chromosome 12. The presence of this abnormality alone, or with other abnormalities, indicates a poorer prognosis compared with that of patients without any abnormal chromosomes.

Many of the blood-forming cells in acute leukaemias also show damaged chromosomes, loss of chromosomes or additional chromosomes but there is no specific or consistent pattern. Different patients with this disease differ in the chromosomal abnormalities they possess. It is, however, not yet clear whether the chromosomal abnormalities in the acute leukaemias are the cause of the disease or the result of it. Similarly, widespread chromosomal damage is also found in the cells of a number of solid tumours. There is now mounting evidence that chromosomal changes, i.e. translocations or deletions, may be important in causing malignant changes in cells. By these changes genes can be separated from each other, or brought together on the same chromosome. If one of the genes is a so-called 'oncogene', then it may be activated by the new neighbour gene or avoid a 'switching-off' control exerted by a now separated gene. The effect may be to turn the gene on, so that the cell produces the abnormal proteins and becomes malignant.

GENETIC COUNSELLING AND PRENATAL DIAGNOSIS

In this country a number of centres have been established in order to provide expert genetic counselling and advice to couples who have either a family history of a genetically determined disease or who have had a child with such a disease. It is possible, after carefully establishing the diagnosis, to study the pattern of a disease in the patient's family. This often requires a considerable amount of investigation and research. It is then possible for the counsellor to advise the patient about the probability of having affected children. The degree of risk is estimated from a knowledge of the manner of inheritance of the gene; its frequency of occurrence in the population, and some of its other properties such as degree of dominance. In some diseases such as mongolism (Down's syndrome), chromosome analysis is sometimes of considerable help in genetic counselling. The patient is therefore put in a position to judge for himself the risks that are involved in having further children and can act accordingly.

A recent development in medical genetics has been the development of prenatal diagnostic techniques. By a process known as amniocentesis a sample of amniotic fluid and cells can be withdrawn from the womb. Appropriate biochemical tests may then be carried out using this material in order to establish whether or not the fetus has inherited the diseases and is affected. So far this approach is only possible in those genetically determined diseases in which the gene in question gives rise to an error in metabolism such as the mucopolysaccharidoses, Tay Sach disease, phenylketonuria. Using cells obtained from amniotic fluid and tissue culture techniques it is possible to examine the chromosome constitution of the fetus. This is particularly useful in the context of the older mother who is at risk of producing a mongol child.

From information derived from amniocentesis the prospective parents may be counselled and appropriate advice given. With forewarning, corrective action may be planned in some cases. For example, some of the metabolic diseases may be due to lack of a particular enzyme by cells of the body. It is now possible to correct the defect by giving the patient a bone marrow transplant containing normal cells with the enzyme. These cells can, under some circumstances, pass on the enzyme to the deficient cells and so alleviate the condition.

SOME HEREDITARY DEFECTS OF THE LOCOMOTOR SYSTEM

The following is a list of some of the diseases which affect the locomotor system in some way and which are known to have a genetic basis.

Cranio-cleidal dysostosis.
Congenital dislocation of the head of the radius.
Dupuytren contracture.
Polydactyly and syndactyly.
Congenital dislocation of the hip.
Perthes' disease.
Nail-patellar syndrome.
Club-foot.
Achondroplasia.
Diaphyseal aclasis.
Osteogenesis imperfecta.
Multiple epiphyseal dysplasia.

Mongolism.
Arachnodactyly (Marfan syndrome).
Ehlers-Danlos syndrome.
Myositis ossificans progressiva.
Muscular dystrophies.
Peroneal muscular atrophy (Charcot-Marie-Tooth).
Lipoidoses, e.g. Gaucher's disease.
Neurofibromatosis.

BIBLIOGRAPHY

Carter C O 1979 Human heredity. 2nd edn. Harmondsworth: Penguin
Cowell H R 1970 Genetic aspects of orthopaedic diseases. American Journal of Nursing 70, 4 November.
Duthie R B, Townes P L 1967 Genetics of Orthopaedic conditions. Journal of Bone and Joint Surgery 49: 229, 248, May
Jones I H 1978 Genetics and inherited diseases. Nursing Times, 24 March, 392
Matthews D R 1978 Genetics: your fate in your genes. Nursing Mirror, 12 October, 30
Roberts J A F, Pembrey M E 1978 An introduction to medical genetics. 7th edn. Oxford University Press
Systems of Life No. 105 1983 Setting up the Systems 5. Nursing Times, 7 September
Systems of Life No. 106 1983 Setting up the Systems 6. Nursing Times, 5 October

14

Congenital anomalies

In this chapter, we shall discuss congenital anomalies commonly seen in orthopaedic practice. The influence of genetic factors and of those in the maternal environment are included because the nurse will often be called upon to obtain the *history* of patients admitted to hospital with these conditions; moreover it is she who observes and talks to members of the *family* visiting the patient.

The causes of congenital anomaly are varied, complex and as yet, largely unproven and speculative.

A. Genetic factors

These have already been discussed; abnormal genes transmitted from the parents are thought to disturb the function of the embryonic cells. Then there are certain conditions known to be due to recessive sex-linked genes, such as haemophilia and colour-blindness; moreover it is important to remember that the *tendency* to certain diseases appears to be transmitted, and to 'run in the family' especially with regard to various allergies, diabetes, epilepsy and rheumatoid arthritis.

B. Factors in the maternal environment

These are believed to cause congenital anomaly either by their influence on the development of a genetic error in the germ cells as previously described, or by their direct effect on the developing embryo; these factors are listed below:

1. *Nutritional*, including generalised under-

nourishment, lack of Vitamin A or of substances such as iron, calcium and phosphorus.

2. *Infective*, particularly with regard to German measles and influenza.

3. *Temperature changes*, related to the above or to some other febrile condition in the mother.

4. *Circulatory disturbance* to the developing fetus, due to cardio-vascular disease in the mother.

5. *Oxygen deficiency*, due to cardio-vascular disease as described above, or to disease of the placenta.

6. *Hormonal disturbances* due to endocrine disorder in the mother or in the developing fetus itself.

7. *Chemical poisons* taken by the mother, e.g. quinine; thalidomide.

8. *Mechanical causes*; abnormal posture of the fetus *in utero*, breech presentation.

9. *X-ray irradiation* of the mother; recent research also suggests that this may later cause malignant disease, e.g. leukaemia.

10. *Incompatibility between the blood of mother and child* resulting in haemolytic disease of the newborn.

11. *Other factors* thought to be connected with congenital anomaly in the infant are elderly parents and multiple births.

Any part of the body may be the site of congenital anomaly, but the parts most commonly seen to be affected are the cardio-vascular and nervous systems. It is important to remember that multiple congenital anomalies may be present in the same individual, for example, congenital dislocation of the hip may be accompanied by club-foot; it is also important to remember that in some cases there may be an associated mental defect which will influence both the development of the child and the course of the treatment.

GENERAL MANAGEMENT OF CHILDREN WITH CONGENITAL ANOMALIES

During the last decade, and particularly as a result of the social changes referred to in the Introduction to this book, there has been a marked improvement in the whole gamut of treatment of congenital anomalies, not only in the development of surgical techniques but in supervision of the mother during her pregnancy and in early recognition of congenital anomaly in the infant during the neonatal period. Most important of all is the development of techniques to discover the possibility of congenital anomaly and thereby reduce the number of children born with congenital defects (Chs 11 and 13).

There has also been a change of attitude with regard to the child who has a physical handicap

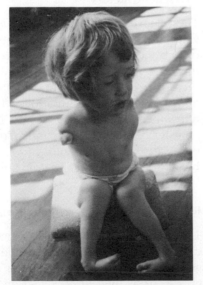
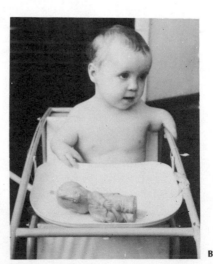

Fig. 14.1 A. Multiple congenital anomalies. Bilateral absence of arms, with rudimentary digits; congenital dislocation of hips and talipes equinovarus of feet. Small trolley with castors gives mobility. **B.** Congenital deformity of upper limbs. (With kind permission from Princess Margaret Rose Hospital, Edinburgh.)

because of a congenital anomaly; many who were previously denied educational opportunities are now received into normal schools.

Team-work is the key to successful treatment, which only *begins* in hospital and must be carried on in the world outside, so that the team not only includes hospital personnel but representatives of the community health and education authorities, the patient's family, and ultimately, the patient himself.

The patient's family requires special consideration; it is not difficult to imagine the agony of mind suffered by the parents of a child with a severe congenital anomaly. Often one or both parents may have feelings of guilt, especially if the child was initially unwanted; then one parent may blame the other for the child's anomaly, and attribute its presence to being 'in' his (or her) 'side' of the family. Sometimes one parent, usually the mother, dotes on a handicapped child to the exclusion of her husband or of her other children; or there may be a frank rejection of the unfortunate one, but this is uncommon and in time most families, especially where there are several children, accept a handicapped member so that he receives the love and security that is essential for his normal emotional development.

Education of the parents is a vital part of the treatment. The surgeon will explain to them, in simple terms, the nature of the child's disability and will outline the programme of treatment. He will explain that, where possible, the aim of treatment is the child's return to normal home life, normal schooling and, eventually, to open employment. The nurse, the physiotherapist, the school-teacher and the medico-social worker will also play their part in the education, reassurance and support required by the parents. The nurse will teach the mother (or better still, both parents) all the ins and outs of the daily care of the child, with special reference to possible complications. If an aunt or an elder sister or brother can also be instructed in the care of the child, so much the better, but in this connection it is important to remember that other children in the family are occasionally overburdened with the care of a handicapped brother or sister, even to the detriment of their own education, activities and friendships. Parents must also know to whom to turn if things go wrong, since apprehension, anxiety and insecurity on the part of the parents is soon conveyed to the child.

Special centres

Children who for some reason cannot be cared for at home are often accommodated in special centres where they receive not only nursing care, but education suited to their condition. It must be borne in mind, however, that the decision to remove a child from the care of his parents, and especially from his mother, who is his natural protector, guide and teacher is a serious matter and one not lightly

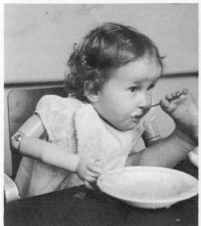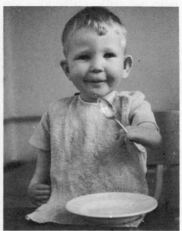

A   B

Fig. 14.2 A, B. shows independence in feeding in spite of congenital deformity. 'Foot feeding' is shown in Fig. 14.2A.

recommended. The natural home environment and the parents' management of a handicapped child may for some reason seem inadequate to us, but the fact remains that no institutional care can equal that of a normal happy home and no affection that of a loving mother; the only children who benefit from institutional care and attention are those for whom, unfortunately, for one reason or another there is no practical alternative.

Sometimes handicapped children can live at home but attend special schools where the educational programmes are adapted to their needs, where each child receives individual attention from his teacher, and where day-to-day treatment of his physical handicap can be supervised.

Because of the special arrangements outlined above, we may see a handicapped child suffering from a congenital anomaly admitted to an orthopaedic ward only when some specific treatment is required, such as an operation; in this discussion we shall confine ourselves to those commonly seen in orthopaedic practice.

MANAGEMENT OF THE CHILD IN HOSPITAL

Chapter 11 deals with the general management of children in hospital. Since a child suffering from a congenital anomaly often needs repeated admission to hospital, sometimes over a period of years, it is advisable to admit him to the same ward on each occasion; it is also desirable that key members of the nursing staff remain unchanged as far as possible; the sight of a familiar face on re-admission is reassuring both to the child and to his parents. When a child is admitted to hospital from the care of his parents, we must be prepared to accept their advice on some aspects of his management, for example, with regard to the stage reached in toilet training or in feeding; parents suffer great anxiety if their account of their child's 'little ways' is ignored. We must always remember that the child *belongs* to his father and mother and not to us, so that our responsibilities must embrace not only the patient but the family unit to which he rightly belongs.

It is quite simple to lay down a pattern of treatment for a specific condition, but in the case of children, we have to remember that we are dealing with a growing, developing individual so that constant re-assessment of progress is required, and changes must be made to suit the changing demands of the individual child. A decision to alter a course of treatment or even to suspend it is made in the light of the surgeon's knowledge not only of the progress of the individual child but of his temperament, his mental status, and his home environment. For example, a régime which might be suitable for a very young child may be quite unsuitable once he reaches school age; in some cases, a fixed unalterable régime may actually prevent the patient from learning to do things for himself, or from using his own initiative. Long periods of treatment, particularly in hospital, sometimes destroys the child's natural urge to experiment for himself so that he becomes over-docile and, in the process, over-dependent on those around him.

CONGENITAL DISLOCATION OF THE HIP

This is a partial or complete displacement of the femoral head from the acetabulum in the newborn. It may be unilateral or bilateral; it is more common amongst girls and in certain parts of the world, notably in Northern Italy and in Japan, and where babies are swaddled with extended hips as by Indians in North America. Conversely it appears to be less common where babies are carried in the frog position on the back or on the hip (Fig. 14.3A and B). Experience indicates that it is hereditary in that the daughter of a mother who has had a congenital dislocation of the hip is herself very likely to demonstrate the condition. It is believed that there may be a combination of genetic factors and of those in the maternal environment which cause undue laxity of ligaments and predispose the hip to dislocation, or the factor may be inherent in the formation of component parts of the hip itself, notably a poorly developed acetabular lip and anteversion of the femoral neck. There is often a history of breech delivery with extended legs; since early diagnosis is the key to successful treatment, the midwife, the obstetrician, the general practitioner, or the paediatrician will call on the orthopaedic surgeon to examine a new-born baby if there is any suggestion of hip dysplasia; in many

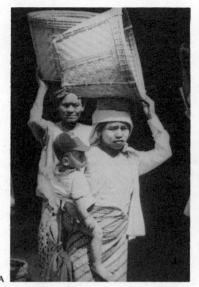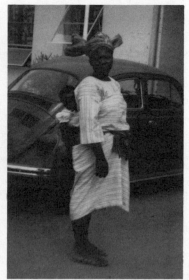

A   B

Fig. 14.3 **A.** Burmese child carried on mother's hip. (Courtesy Aga Photo Agency (Pte) Limited.) **B.** Baby carried on mother's back (From the National Orthopaedic Hospital, Lagos, Nigeria.)

areas, this team-work is deliberately organised as part of the maternity service.

Pathological changes

1. *In the bones.* The femoral head is displaced upwards and backwards to a greater or lesser degree and since it is not in its normal relationship to the acetabulum this too fails to develop normally and becomes shallow and shelving. A 'false acetabulum' develops with weight-bearing if the femoral head is so displaced as to rest on the dorsum of the ilium. The femoral head may be large in comparison with the acetabulum and is often flattened; the neck is shortened and anteverted (i.e. bent forwards) and coxa valga is present.

2. *Changes in soft structures.* The capsule is stretched and elongated and there may be a constriction which may prove an obstacle to reduction. The adductor muscles, tensor fasciae femoris and sartorius shorten, while the obturators and quadratus femoris are stretched. Gluteus medius and minimus become shortened and are at a mechanical disadvantage.

Symptoms and signs

1. *In early life, before weight-bearing.* As already stated, *early diagnosis* is the key to successful treatment; the *history* is important and the baby whose family reveals, even remotely, any suggestion of 'hip disease', is examined with this fact in mind. In the new-born baby gentle manipulation of the flexed abducted hips may reveal a palpable or even audible 'click' (*Ortolani sign*), and the presence of any other congenital deformity (e.g. club-foot) is also significant. *Barlow's sign* may be elicited by carrying the flexed hips into abduction while the fingers press on the great trochanter and thumbs are pressed into the groin. A click or 'slip' may be seen or felt as the femoral head is levered over the acetabular rim. Otherwise, the observant nurse or mother may notice that the legs cannot be fully abducted. The perineum is abnormally broad, and the buttocks flattened. Sometimes a swelling in the gluteal region denotes the displaced position of the femoral head.

Radiography in special positions will show the degree of displacement of the head, and a small, ill-developed acetabulum.

Arthrography is usually advised, when radio-opaque material is injected into the joint and obstacles to reduction such as an inverted limbus or hypertrophied ligamentum teres are more clearly revealed than by ordinary X-ray films.

2. *In later life, after weight-bearing has commenced*, there is a limp which may be slight at first and becomes more marked as the child grows. In unilateral cases, the limp takes the form of a dip to the affected side, and there will be shortening of the limb. If the condition is bilateral, there will be a dip to both sides, resulting in a waddling gait, and the legs will appear short in comparison with the trunk. The perineum is wide, the buttocks broad and flattened, and there is a lumbar lordosis due to the forward tilt of the pelvis. In both unilateral and bilateral cases there is prominence of the great trochanter, limitation of abduction and external rotation, and flexion deformity. There may be a hollow in the groin which is normally filled by the femoral head, and the femoral vessels may be difficult to palpate.

Telescoping may be elicited, i.e. the limb can be moved upwards and downwards in its long axis.

Trendelenburg sign. This can be elicited by asking the patient to stand on first one leg and then the other. When standing on the affected side, the pelvis drops on the sound side, due to the failure of the gluteus medius and minimus to keep the pelvis level. This is due to their shortening and inability to contract when weight is borne on the affected side. In bilateral cases, this sign is present on both sides.

Treatment

Treatment is aimed at reduction of the dislocation, maintenance of reduction and preservation of the normal contours and function of the joint. *The earlier it is instituted the better*, since once the femoral head is reduced in the acetabulum normal growth and development will proceed. Different surgeons adopt different techniques, and each case is treated on its own merits, bearing in mind the age of the child and the degree of dislocation; treatment may also be influenced by social factors, e.g. the extent of co-operation expected of the parents.

CONSERVATIVE TREATMENT

1. Von Rosen splint

This consists of malleable metal which is so bent by hand as to fit the child's trunk and limbs as shown in Figs 14.4A and B. Nursing care is simplified by the design of the splint and the child is easily cared for at home, with regular supervision as an out-patient, on a weekly basis.

The splint is usually removed only under supervision, and the mother and baby are together when adjustment of the splint, washing of the parts and care of the skin is carried out. The splint must not become outgrown; in an uncomplicated case, it is usually worn for 8–12 weeks.

2. Pavlik harness (Fig. 14.5A and B)

This device allows the baby to move the hips within a constrained range of flexion and abduction, and is the least rigid of the splints. The child's activity promotes spontaneous reduction of the dislocated hip and remodelling of the acetabular dysplasia. Unlike the former splint, which is applied to the newborn baby after passive reduction of the dislocation, the Pavlik harness can be used with success up to the age of 6 months. It is worn continuously until the femoral head is reduced and stable. Hygiene and nursing care is the same as for other abduction splints.

3. Reduction by traction and cross-pull on double abduction frame

A double abduction frame with C-shaped cross-bar and two saddles is required. One saddle is the ordinary type, while the other has leg-portions abducted to 180 degrees (Fig. 14.6).

Method. Skin extensions are applied and the child is immobilised on the frame as described in Ch. 10. At first, the hips are held in about 20 degrees abduction, and steady traction is exerted. It is usually necessary to tie the frame to the foot of the bed, which is elevated so that counter-traction is provided and the pressure of the groin-strap is relieved. It is important to remember that over-powerful traction and rough handling may result in interference with the blood-supply to the femoral head. When check X-rays show that the femoral head is opposite the acetabulum, gradual abduction is commenced, increasing it a few degrees every second day. When the 80 degrees or 90 degrees position has been reached and further X-rays show that the head still remains opposite the

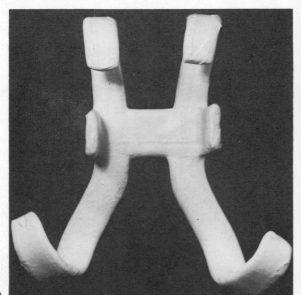

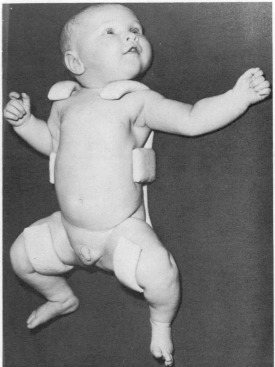

A B

Fig. 14.4   A, B. Van Rosen splint is easily moulded to fit the infant and is covered in rubber so that it can be worn at bath-time. (With kind permission from the *Institute of Orthopaedics*, Royal National Orthopaedic Hospital.)

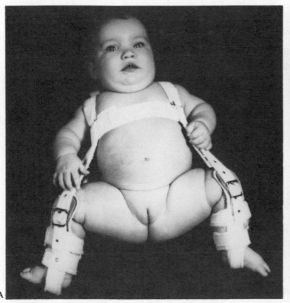

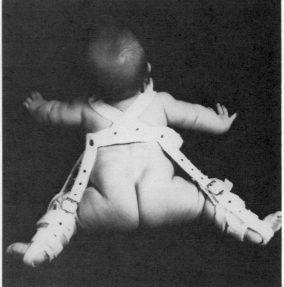

A B

Fig. 14.5   A, B. The Pavlik harness.

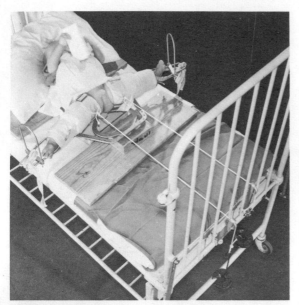

Fig. 14.6 Cross-pull applied by means of weight and pulley. (With kind permission of the Nuffield Orthopaedic Centre, Oxford.)

acetabulum, abduction is further increased and cross-pull commenced.

Cross-pull requirements: A small metal gutter-splint moulded to the shape of the patient's thigh; a piece of felt and a strong bandage or piece of ticking.

Method of application: Cover the gutter-splint with felt, and place it on the outer side of the patient's thigh. Slip the bandage under the limb,

bring it round the gutter-splint and tie it to the frame on the opposite side. Alternatively, cross-pull may be exerted by passing a canvas sling around the thigh and attaching it to a weighted cord which travels over a pulley fixed to the opposite side of the bed.

In bilateral cases, the same procedure is adopted on the other side. The degree of abduction is further increased, traction and cross-pull always being maintained, until the 180 degrees position has been reached. At this stage, there should be clinical and radiological evidence that reduction is complete (Fig. 14.7).

Nursing care

This is similar to that described in Ch. 10 for a patient on an abduction frame. The following special points should be noted.

General care. In older children, sedatives may be necessary for the relief of pain. This method of treatment is not as a rule ordered for patients over the age of 6 years.

Daily care of splintage. (1) Extension tapes and cross-pull must *always* be kept taut. (2) Be sure that the cross-pull is exerted as *high up on the femur as possible*, and does not merely exert strain on the knee-joint. (3) See that pressure-sores do not occur under the gutter-splint. (4) Bandaging must not interfere with the blood or nerve supply to the limb.

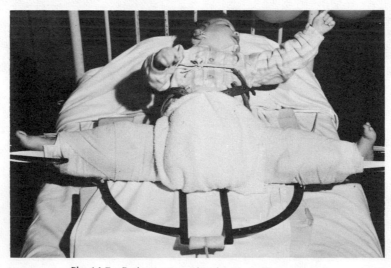

Fig. 14.7 Reduction completed; cross-pull removed.

4. Reduction by Alvik traction

This method of treatment was described by Professor Ivan Alvik and was first used at Overlege Sophies Minde Ortopedisk Hospital, Oslo. The object is to use the infant's body weight as counter-traction, to overcome friction and at the same time allow the child more movement than that permitted by the abduction frame previously described. The patient can be turned prone without disturbing the traction force.

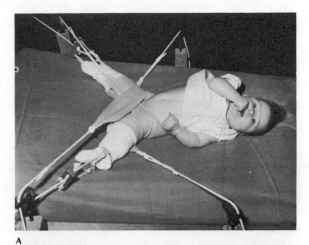

A

Method of application

Above-knee skin extensions are applied in the usual manner (Ch. 10) and attached to a spreader which will carry a cord and weight running over pulleys fixed to the bed. The legs are abducted and the weight attached according to the surgeon's orders. The two-way cross-pull is now applied by using two bandages to which weighted cords are afterwards attached, as shown in Figs 14.8A and B. The bandage at the top of the thigh is applied from without inwards so that the rotation force is applied from the front of the thigh, and the lower one from without inwards from the back of the thigh. The arrows in Fig. 14.8B show the direction of the force applied; in simple words, 'the top bandage *goes inwards from the front*, and the bottom bandage *inwards from the back*'. In the case shown in the illustrations a single 'Vent-foam' backed by calico bandage was used for each leg. Lampwick extension loops are sewn to the ends of the bandages and cords and weights are attached as shown. The amount of weight used is decided by the surgeon and will vary with the patient's body weight; not more than 1–1.5 kg is generally used, and the foot of the bed is elevated to provide counter-traction. The case shown is one of bilateral congenital dislocation of the hip; if the condition is unilateral, longitudinal traction is applied to both legs, and Alvik traction to the affected leg only.

Nursing care. The extensions and rotation bandages require daily inspection and care as described in connection with an abduction frame (Ch. 10). In babies still at the 'nappy' stage, frequent and regular 'changing' and protection by plastic pants ensures cleanliness of the bandages and extensions. Older children can be taught to use

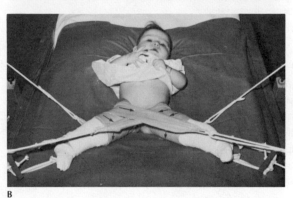

B

Fig. 14.8   A, B. A case of bilateral congenital dislocation of the hip under treatment by Alvik traction (see text).

a receiver as a urinal, and a bedpan is easily placed beneath the patient in the usual way.

It is imperative that the child is maintained in such a position that the degree of abduction is not lost, and turning on the side or sitting up is not permitted. In older children, it may be necessary to apply a restrainer (Fig. 14.9).

5. Reduction by means of hoop traction

This is shown in Fig. 14.10 when the hips are flexed, and the extensions tied to an overhead hoop fixed to the bed—the hip joints are gradually abducted. Gillow (1980) describes this form of treatment together with nursing care.

Note that any form of 'gallows' traction carries the risk of neurovascular damage, and constant vigilance is required to prevent this complication.

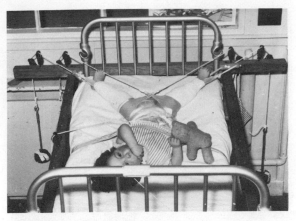

Fig. 14.9 One method of reduction by traction and cross-pull. Movement of the child's trunk resulted in loss of traction force; hence the restrainer.

Later treatment

Splintage is maintained until the femoral head and acetabulum are reconstituted and reduction is stable. Any of the methods of splintage about to be described may then be used to maintain reduction, either a plaster cast, Denis Browne splint, or Forrester-Brown splint. Eventually the child is allowed to mobilise the legs in bed and weight-bearing is resumed.

Other forms of splintage

Various other methods of splintage will now be discussed; the nurse will seek specific instruction from the surgeon as to whether the particular splint ordered is to be worn continuously, or whether it may be removed daily for bathing, exercise, etc. Any of the splints mentioned may be used with or without manipulative reduction.

1. Putti's mattress

This consists of a solid triangular wedge which is inserted between the child's legs. It is secured by a series of straps, and the degree of abduction is gradually increased. It is removed daily for cleansing and the limb is meanwhile gently manipulated into abduction and internal rotation. This method of treatment is useful during the first year of life.

2. Denis Browne splint (Fig. 14.11)

This consists of leather cuffs which lace around the thighs and joined by a metal bar which is prevented from slipping downwards by canvas braces over the shoulders. A pad of sponge-rubber over the sacrum acts as a fulcrum against which the hips are

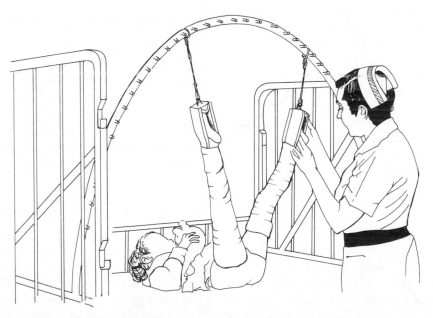

Fig. 14.10 Note that the nurse is inspecting the patient's feet (see text). This illustration is based on one that originally appeared in *Nursing Times* on April 7, 1982.

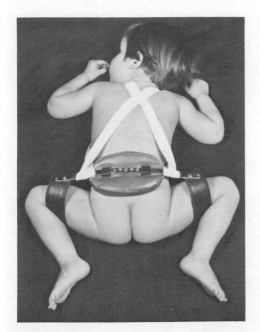

Fig. 14.11 Posterior view of Denis Browne splint.

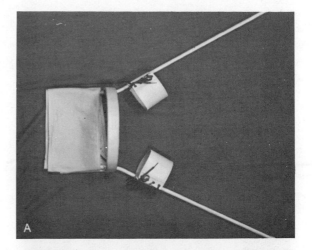

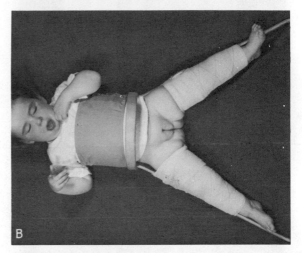

Fig. 14.12   A, B. Forrester-Brown splint. (With kind permission from the Princess Margaret Rose Hospital, Edinburgh.)

abducted in the leather cuffs. So long as reduction is maintained, the child is encouraged to kick and even to stand and walk in the splint, since muscle-action encourages normal development of the hip-joint. The horizontal metal bar holding the cuffs must be kept at full length as the child grows. Other-wise nursing care proceeds on the same lines as described for a patient wearing a frog plaster.

3. Forrester-Brown splint

This consists of a metal frame supporting a canvas corset which encloses the child's trunk, and leather cuffs which enclose the thighs (Fig. 14.12). The child is laid in the corset, the cuffs are laced, the legs bandaged to the metal struts as shown in Fig. 14.12. Nursing care proceeds as already outlined.

4. 'Bloodless' reduction and plaster fixation

Preliminary traction is applied for two or three weeks, usually with the hips in flexion (Fig. 14.35), and abducting slowly to a position 10 degrees short of the maximum range of the dislocated hip. The dislocation is then reduced by manipulation under general anaesthesia. The reduction is confirmed by X-ray, and plaster fixation may be by:

(a) Frog plaster—extreme abduction may cause avascular necrosis of the femoral head, and is avoided.

(b) Batchelor plaster.

a. Frog plaster

This extends from the nipple-line to the ankles and is applied on a hip-prop with the hips in full abduction and external rotation, and the knees flexed to the right angle.

Immediate nursing care. When the plaster is wet, it is supported on three firm pillows, covered first with waterproof material and then with towelling. A suitable receptable such as a kidney-dish is kept in position to prevent soiling of the plaster until regular habits are established, or a folded napkin can be tucked between the legs and changed frequently. Other nursing details will be found in Chs 6 and 10.

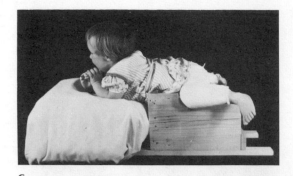

C

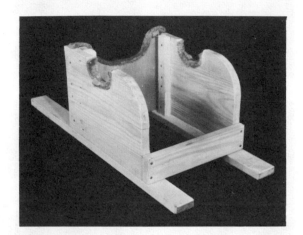

A

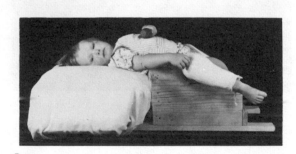

B

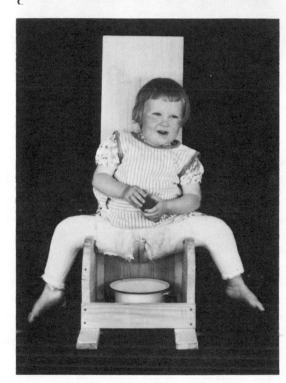

Fig. 14.13 A–D. A useful home-made wooden perch for use with frog plaster.

Daily nursing care. These patients are usually healthy children and should be allowed to develop as such. Once the plaster is dry, and so long as it remains in good repair, activity within the limits of splintage is encouraged; for example, the child is allowed to crawl about the floor. If of a suitable age, he should sit at a table for meals, and should be encouraged to play with other children. Contamination of the plaster is avoided by the following means:

1. Training the child in regular habits, e.g. 'holding out', or 'potting', in children who are accustomed to it. Figs 14.13A, B, C and D show a useful wooden 'perch' (the Plowden perch) for use with a frog-plaster, which can be made by a hospital carpenter or by any handyman. The patient enjoys being raised from the bed for lessons, meals or play and a back-rest is easily fitted for 'potting' purposes, as seen in Fig. 14.13D.

2. In very young children, a suitable receptacle

is kept in position until such time as regular habits are established.

3. It is sometimes advisable to cover the plaster with jaconet or plastic material in the region of the genitals, or to arrange a piece so that it falls from the buttocks into a receiver and forms a watershed. Otherwise, a frequently-changed 'nappie' folded under the child or worn with plastic pants is satisfactory. Further advice is given in Ch. 6, and the booklet *Your child in an immobilising plaster* (Greenwood, 1980) gives useful advice to parents.

Later treatment. The frog plaster is retained for about nine to eighteen months, or until it is thought that reduction is secure. The child may then be allowed to kick free in bed over pillows, or, successive plasters are applied at four monthly intervals, reducing the angle of flexion and abduction each time.

b. The Batchelor plaster

After reduction, the legs are encased in plaster from the groins to the ankles, in abduction and internal rotation. The plasters are then attached to a broomstick. Fixation is thus achieved whilst allowing flexion and extension at the hip-joint.

N.B. A double spica in the same position is sometimes preferred.

Nursing care is similar to that required for broomstick plasters (Ch. 15).

Treatment on removal of plaster consists of free mobilisation and exercises in bed, followed by re-education in walking. Supervision is continued until growth has ceased.

OPERATIVE TREATMENT

1. *Open reduction*, with removal of an inverted limbus or of some other obstacle to reduction.

2. *Derotation osteotomy* at the sub-trochanteric level, with fixation of the fragments by means of a plate and screws.

3. *Varus osteomy*, sometimes combined with a derotation osteotomy, may be required to correct a valgus deformity.

4. *Shelf operation*, when a portion of the ilium above the acetabulum is turned down to contain the femoral head; it is supported by a bone-graft.

5. *Acetabuloplasty* (Pemberton) which consists of an osteotomy of the roof of the acetabulum, which is turned down and supported by bone-grafts, to contain the femoral head.

6. *Pelvic osteotomy* (Salter) is a procedure when the whole of the lower pelvis is hinged downward over the femoral head, and the osteotomy is supported by a bone-graft.

7. In later cases, where instability persists, *deepening of the acetabulum* may be performed; the femoral head is covered by a portion of the

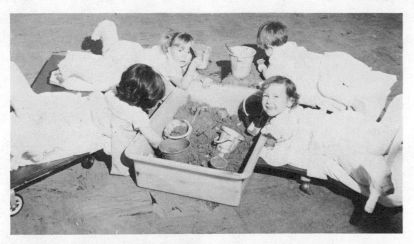

Fig. 14.14 Children in plasters lie prone on wheeled trolleys for mobility and play. (With kind permission from the *Nursing Mirror*.)

capsule before being replaced in the prepared ace-tabulum (Colonna).

8. *Lorenz bifurcation osteotomy* consists of an oblique osteotomy which displaces the lesser trochanter into the acetabulum.

9. *Schanz ostotomy* divides the femur to form a pelvic support.

10. In later life, where other methods have failed and osteoarthritis of the joint has supervened, some form of *cup-arthroplasty* may be required; in unila-teral cases in the younger age-group *arthrodesis* may be preferred.

Post-operative fixation consists of a single or dou-ble plaster spica; nursing care proceeds on the lines already discussed. When the plaster is discarded, the child is allowed to kick about in bed, until weight-bearing is resumed and the patient is dis-charged home. Supervision as an out-patient is usually continued at intervals until growth has ceased.

Conclusion

Early diagnosis, advances in anaesthesia and in operative techniques have greatly improved the outlook for patients suffering from congenital dislo-cation of the hip, and straight-forward cases are soon restored to normal life. More complicated cases, such as those seen in arthrogryposis con-genita multiplexa, myelomeningocele and cerebral palsy, may need longer periods of treatment in hos-pital, and there are a few where other defects are present and where some degree of permanent dis-ability has to be accepted.

CONGENITAL TALIPES EQUINO-VARUS (Club-foot)

This deformity consists of plantar-flexion at the angle-joint, inversion at the sub-talar joint, and adduction at the mid-tarsal joint. In extreme cases, the foot is so turned inward as to bring the sole into contact with the inner border of the tibia (Fig. 14.15).

Most cases of club-foot are termed idiopathic, as no satisfactory cause is known; increased intra-uterine pressure and development error is blamed. Other causes may be *osseous*, as when there is a major bony defect such as congenital absence of the tibia; *nervous*, as in spina bifida; or *muscular*, as in arthrogryposis congenita multiplexa. In this

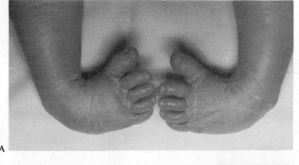
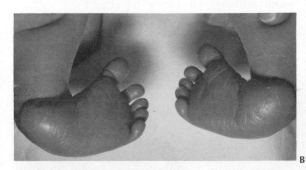
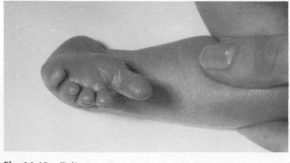
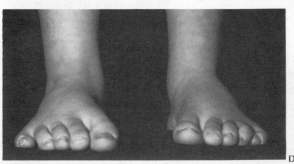

Fig. 14.15   Talipes equino-varus. **A, B** and **C,** the newborn child; **D,** same child aged 7. (By courtesy of Donald Neale (1985) *Common Foot Disorders*, Churchill Livingstone.)

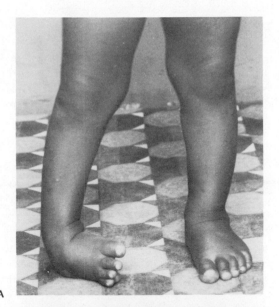

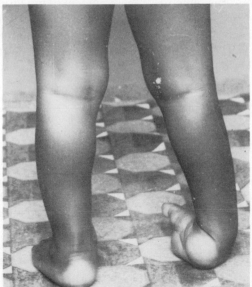

Fig. 14.16 **A** and **B.** Right congenital club-foot (from the National Orthopaedic Hospital, Lagos, Nigeria).

smaller and less well-developed than its fellow. The deformity is at first one of soft tissues only, but bony changes eventually occur. The muscles and tendons are poorly developed; they are tensely contracted on the inner side of the foot and stretched on the outer side; the tendo Achilles is shortened. The talus can be seen and felt on the dorsum of the foot, and that part which escapes from between the malleoli becomes broadened. The calcaneum is tilted medially, so that the heel is small, poorly developed and tucked-up, and navicular and cuboid become displaced inwards. The skin on the dorsum of the foot is stretched and thin and there are abnormal creases on the inner border and on the sole.

In many cases, there is genu-valgum. If weight-bearing is attempted, bursae and callosities develop along the outer side of the foot, and the gait is stumbling and difficult.

Treatment depends upon the stage at which the deformity is first seen. *Ideally, it should commence as soon as possible after birth.* In a young baby, treatment consists of correction of the deformity by frequently repeated manipulation.

Method of manipulation

The baby lies on the lap of an assistant or on a convenient table. In the case of a new-born baby, the mother may not at first be in a fit state to see the manipulations, but once the baby is completely in the care of his mother her co-operation is essential. Manipulation is often difficult because of the smallness of the baby's foot, and it is most essential that the assistant protects the knee from strain by grasping the calf in both hands. Failure to support the leg may result in genu valgum, damage to the upper tibial epiphysis, or even fracture of the tibia. *The inversion and adduction of the foot is corrected first, and the plantar-flexion last.* We will now assume that the right foot is to be corrected. Whilst an assistant protects the knee, place both thumbs on the head of the talus, pressing it back into the mortice of the tibia and fibula; the fingers of the left hand pass round the outer side of the foot and grasp the heel, and the fingers of the right hand pass round the inner side of the foot. Whilst exerting pressure with the thumbs, draw the foot *downwards*, then *outwards* and *upwards*, so that the toes

condition, the muscles of the body fail to split up into the normal groups, and by their malfunction many deformities arise. This type of club-foot is exceedingly difficult to treat.

Clinical features

In bilateral cases, one foot is usually worse than the other. In unilateral cases, the affected leg is describe a complete semi-circle. Unless this manoeuvre is carried out, the talus will not be replaced, correction will occur at the mid-tarsal joint only, and a boat-shaped foot will result. As the foot is drawn outwards, the adduction and inversion is corrected; when it is certain that this is accomplished, the fingers which grasp the heel, pull it slowly downwards, and the foot is dorsiflexed. During the procedure, do not release your grasp or allow the foot to fall back into the deformed position, even for a moment. The manoeuvre must be performed, as it were, in one fell swoop, not in a series of disjointed movements. Allowing the foot to fall back only increases reactionary swelling.

Methods of maintaining correction

After manipulation the foot is held in the over-corrected position by one of the following:

1. Adhesive strapping—the Robert Jones method (Fig. 14.17).
2. Denis Browne splints (Figs 14.18–14.20).
3. Bell-Grice splints (Fig. 14.19A).
4. Plaster fixation.

In very young babies, adhesive strapping is generally advised. After the age of 3 months, when the child is able to kick, Denis Browne splints may be used. Later still, plaster fixation may be employed.

Application of strapping

Prepare beforehand a strip of adhesive tape about 5 cm wide, according to the size of the foot, and long enough to extend up to the knee. Place a piece of lint on the strapping to protect the skin, leaving about 3 cm free at each end. Lay the sticky piece on the dorsum of the foot; carry the strapping round the inner side of the foot, under the sole, then encircle the foot and whilst maintaining full correction, attach it to the outer side of the leg just below the knee (Fig. 14.17). In older children, the strapping may be carried above the knee. A further strip encircles the leg just above the ankle. The strapping must pass directly beneath the calcaneo-cuboid joint. Failure to support this joint will result in a boat-shaped foot. Strapping is renewed at two or

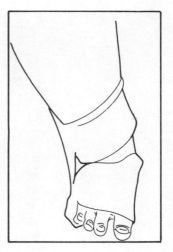

Fig. 14.17 Method of applying corrective strapping in congenital club-foot.

three day intervals, and the manipulation is repeated each time; further strapping can sometimes be applied over the original application. J-shaped aluminium 'banana' splints may be used in conjunction with the strapping.

Application of Denis Browne splints

Remove the foot-pieces from the cross-bar. Pad the outer side of the sole-piece with adhesive felt in such a way as to elevate the outer side of the sole of the foot and produce eversion. In severe cases, it is better to apply the felt directly to the foot rather than to the splint (Fig. 14.18), taking particular

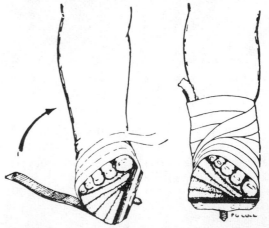

Fig. 14.18 shows the method of applying Denis Browne splint. (By kind permission of Sir Denis Browne and J.B. Lippincott and Co.)

pains to support the calcaneo-cuboid joint; failure to support this joint will inevitably result in a boat-shaped foot. After manipulation, apply the sole-pieces, strapping them on firmly. The leg piece projects outwards from the leg. This in turn is strapped on, and pulls the foot into valgus. Both sole-pieces are then fastened to the cross-bar pointing outwards in as much external rotation as can be gained. If there is a normal foot, it is arranged in a normal position, but pointing outwards about 20 degrees. The child is encouraged to kick and stand in the splint. It provides correction whilst allowing development of the musculature. Re-manipulation and re-application is generally required about once weekly. Later, Denis Browne boots may be worn. They unlace completely so that the toes stick out of the open ends as the child grows (Fig. 14.19B).

Application of Bell-Grice splint

This splint, shown in Fig. 14.19A, is similar in construction to a Denis Browne splint but it has certain advantages in that the metal foot plate is so moulded that packing with felt is not required and

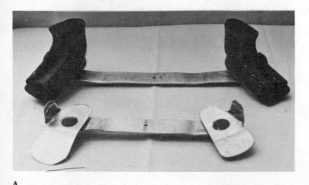

A

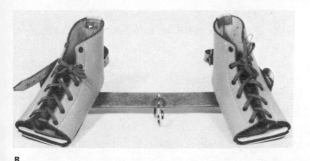

B

Fig. 14.19 A. Bell-Grice splint. B. Denis Browne boots (Taylor).

'boating' of the foot does not occur; another advantage is that there is no lateral metal prolongation to press on the outer side of the leg, on the very muscles where wasting should be avoided as far as possible, i.e. the evertors.

The footplate of the splint is detached from the cross-bar and covered with a thin layer of adhesive felt; two pieces of 2 cm wide strapping are then applied to the sole-piece above the screw, one passing from within outwards from beneath and the other within outwards from above, as shown in Figs 14.20A and B. An assistant steadies the limb as before and the baby's foot is placed on the sole-piece; the strapping is now applied, passing over the dorsum of the foot, upwards and inwards over the ankle as shown in Fig. 14.20B; the second piece is applied in the same manner. A third piece of strapping is then used to hold the heel on to the foot-piece as shown in Fig. 14.20C, and secured by a piece of strapping encircling the limb as shown in Fig. 14.20D. If there is a normal foot it is held in the neutral position, but the affected foot is everted as much as possible and both feet are bolted to the foot-plate.

Nursing care is discussed later.

Application of plaster

The plaster may be skin-tight, but it is usual to cover the limb with wool roll. While correction of the deformity is maintained, apply the plaster in the usual way, carrying the bandage from within outwards. Firm pressure is applied beneath the calcaneo-cuboid joint. In young children, the knee is usually flexed to a right-angle and included in the plaster; this tends to prevent the child kicking the plaster off. A strip of Elastoplast applied round the leg beneath the top of a below-knee plaster will prevent the child kicking it off. Plasters are changed when necessary.

Nursing care

Whatever method of fixation is chosen, the nursing points to be observed are summarised under one heading.

1. These children are generally treated as out-patients. *Never allow the child to leave the hospital*

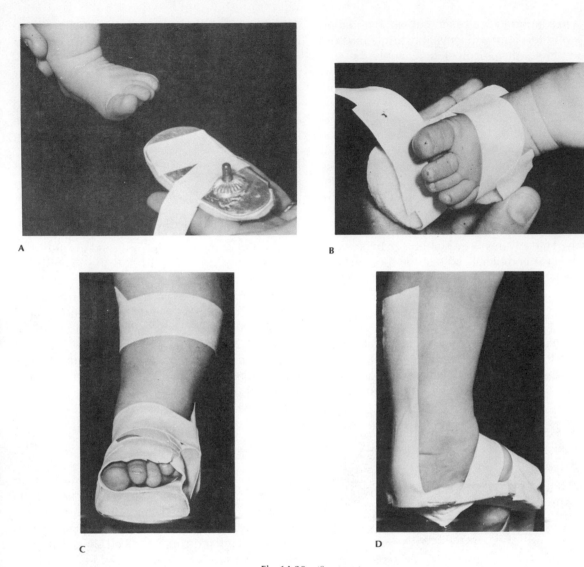

Fig. 14.20 (See text.)

or clinic until you are satisfied that the circulation in the toes is adequate. Instruct the child's mother to observe the toes and to get in touch with you *at once* should anything untoward occur. Some swelling of the toes is to be anticipated, but they should be pink and flush rapidly with blood on release of digital pressure. Gross swelling combined with discolouration is a matter for concern. *The fixation may have to be renewed, but it is never removed altogether, and there is no excuse for losing the correction gained.* A posterior plaster shell in the corrected position can be applied as a temporary measure.

2. The skin must be kept clean and dry. During renewal of splintage, wash the leg and foot carefully, always maintaining the correct position. Pay special attention to areas which have received pressure. Make every effort to keep the splintage dry. A small piece of felt or cardboard may be used to protect the base of the great or little toe from pressure. Always put strapping on a slightly different area of skin each time it is renewed. *Never*

cease the splinting because of pressure-sores or skin irritation. A partly corrected foot that is set free will become more resistant to treatment than one which has never been touched. As already stated, a posterior plaster shell can be used to maintain the corrected position.

Later treatment

Treatment commenced soon after birth results in complete correction at the age of 3 months in approximately two-thirds of cases. Denis Browne boots or plaster shells may be worn at night. As soon as he is old enough to co-operate, *muscle re-education* is commenced, with special reference to the evertors and dorsiflexors of the foot. Re-education in walking is essential. An inside-iron, outside T-strap, with outside raising to the heel of the shoe is occasionally ordered, especially in those cases in which there is weakness of the evertor muscles. When examining the child at an after-care clinic, note whether the tendo Achilles retains its length. Contracture of this tendon is the first sign of relapse. Supervision is continued until growth has ceased, as relapsed cases are difficult to treat.

Operative treatment

If repeated manipulation and splinting has not produced significant correction of the deformity by 6 to 12 weeks of age, operative correction is usually undertaken. This consists of a posterior and medial release of contracted soft tissues and elongation of the tendo Achilles. Later, as the foot grows, operations on bone such as wedge resection of the calcaneum and cuboid (Dillwyn Evans), or calcaneal wedge (Dwyer); tendon transfers are occasionally needed. Several operations over a period of years may be necessary to control the deformity, and supervision is continued until growth has ceased. Old untreated cases may require stabilisation of the foot.

CONGENITAL TALIPES CALCANEO-VALGUS

In this deformity, the foot is dorsiflexed and everted, and the tendo achillis is lengthened. The deformity is the exact opposite of that seen in club-foot, but it is more amenable to treatment. There may be a club-foot on the opposite side.

Treatment consists of a complete plaster or an anterior plaster shell holding the foot in equinovarus. Inside raising to the heel of the shoe and foot exercises may be ordered when the child begins to walk.

CONGENITAL VERTICAL TALUS
(Congenital 'Rocker-Bottom; Flat-Foot)

This is a condition in which the talus is displaced downwards and inwards, forcing the foot into a valgus position and flattening the foot so that it appears boat-shaped; the talus can be seen and felt as a prominence on the inner and lower border of the foot.

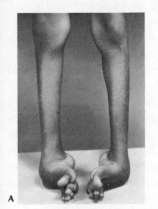
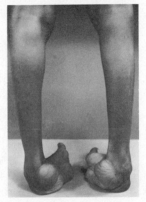
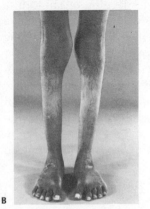
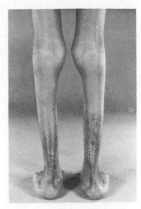

Fig. 14.21   A–B Club-foot. Before and after surgery. (From the Jawaharal Institute for Post-graduate Medical Education and Research, Pondicherry, South India.)

Treatment consists of a soft tissue release operation, with manipulative correction of deformity to restore the normal relationship of the navicular, calcaneum and talus, followed by Kirschner wire fixation and immobilisation in plaster of Paris for 3 to 4 months. Supervision is continued until growth has ceased. A tendon transplant may be required.

CONGENITAL DEFORMITIES OF DIGITS

Dorsal displacement of 5th toe. This condition can be treated by strapping the displaced 5th toe to the 4th toe; by plastic operation; or, in the adult, by amputation of the digit.

Syndactyly ('web-digits') is a congenital anomaly in which the fingers or toes are fused together. *Treatment* consists of an operation to separate the fingers, and skin grafting to cover the resulting defect may be necessary.

Polydactyly is a condition in which there is an extra finger or thumb. *Treatment* usually consists of amputation of the supernumerary digit.

SPINAL DYSRAPHISM

SPINA BIFIDA, MENINGOCOELE, MYELOMENINGOCOELE, DIASTEMATOMYELIA

Spina bifida

This is a developmental defect of the spinal column, where the posterior elements of the spine are deficient and either fail to develop or fail to fuse together. Failure of fusion is called *spina bifida occulta* (Fig. 14.22A). Often the only presenting sign is a dimple, a fatty swelling, or a tuft of hair over the part; the spinal cord is intact and neurological changes in the limbs are not always present.

Treatment is rarely necessary; surgical removal of a swelling or of a disfiguring tuft of hair is sometimes considered if it is subject to pressure from clothing, a waist-belt or a girdle or for cosmetic reasons.

Meningocoele

This is the name given to a more serious condition

when failure of fusion of the vertebral arches posteriorly results in protrusion of the membranes of the spinal cord as a sac over the spinal bony defect and which is often covered only by thin, bluish membrane (Fig. 14.22B). Neurological signs vary according to the degree of the spinal defect.

Treatment may consist of early surgical removal or cover of the sac, closure of the defect and treatment of other presenting symptoms, as outlined below.

Myelomeningocoele

This is an even more serious defect, where the spinal cord forms part of the sac over the spinal bony defect (Fig. 14.22C). The spinal cord elements are adherent to the skin surface. Since patients suffering from this condition are sometimes seen in orthopaedic wards, treatment and nursing management is outlined below. It is important to remember that patients suffering from such a serious handicap require a team approach with treatment from time to time not only by the orthopaedic surgeon but by the paediatrician, the paediatric surgeon, the neurologist, and the urologist; moreover some of them cannot be cared for at home, so that a sheltered environment in a special centre may be recommended. Many patients will proceed to a special school for the physically handicapped where they receive appropriate care from nurses, teachers and physiotherapists.

The most common site for a myelomeningocoele is in the lumbo-sacral region; there may be a large bulging swelling over the spinal defect which contains the protrusion of the spinal cord and its membranes, and which is very liable to break down and ulcerate, so that infection may spread to deeper tissues and result in *meningitis*. The baby's head may become abnormally large, indicating *hydrocephalus*; this may arrest spontaneously, or if untreated, the head may become progressively larger, so that there is pressure on the brain by excess cerebro-spinal fluid and the intellect is impaired; sometimes there is also malformation of the brain itself. As the child grows in utero, traction on the spinal nerves results in *flaccid paralysis* of the lower limbs. *Sensory loss* can cause trophic changes in the skin: *paralysis of the bladder and*

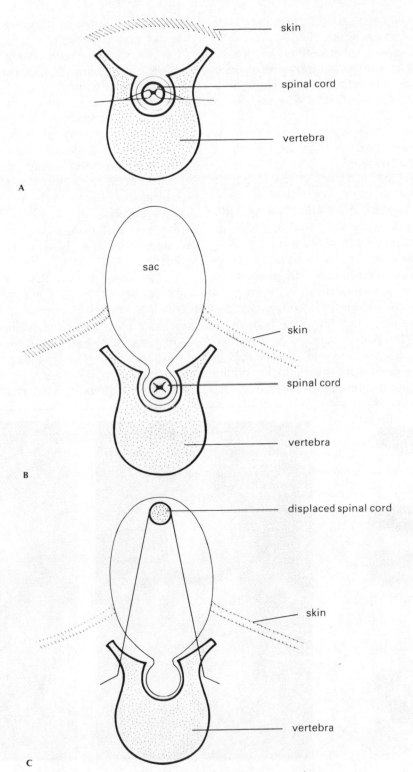

Fig. 14.22 **A.** Spina bifida. **B.** Meningocoele.
C. Myelomeningocoele.

bowel becomes apparent, adding to the tragic clinical picture so evident at birth.

As the child grows, other deformities may be manifest, such as flexion of hips and knees, or dislocation of the hips; the feet may either dangle helplessly or assume the position of equino-varus or calcaneo-valgus.

Spastic paralysis is sometimes seen in the lower limbs secondary to the spinal damage. The upper limbs may also be involved.

Treatment begins in infancy; each patient requires expert evaluation at birth (Lorber, 1974) and thereafter, individual consideration, periodic reassessment as development proceeds, and constant vigilance to prevent complications.

In the infant. Initial treatment may consist of protection of the mass on the back by a large soft dressing carefully applied and arranged in the shape of a circle, square or oblong to accommodate the defect to prevent pressure by clothing, bedclothes or the mattress. The baby is handled carefully and turned regularly from side to side; at each napkin change, the skin of the back, the buttocks and the perineum is cleansed gently and powdered lightly;

any sign of breakdown of tissue over the protruding mass is reported promptly.

Operative treatment consists of skin closure over the defect, preserving the spinal cord and the spinal nerves emerging from it.

Treatment of the hydrocephalus consists of a 'shunt' operation when a polythene tube is inserted, above into the distended lateral ventricle of the brain, and below, into the peritoneum, where excess cerebro-spinal fluid is reabsorbed into the circulation; reflux of fluid into the ventricle is prevented by a Hakim valve connecting the tubes and placed under the skin behind the child's ear at the level of the mastoid process. Blockage of the system needs early recognition and surgical revision.

As the child grows. Paralysis of the limbs, impaired sensation and incontinence become increasingly evident; there is a grave danger of burns from fires, hot objects such as hot-water bottles or domestic dishes, and scalds from hot liquids, or sores from splints or plaster casts, if used. Other deformities such as kyphosis or scoliosis become increasingly evident. It is noticeable that the child

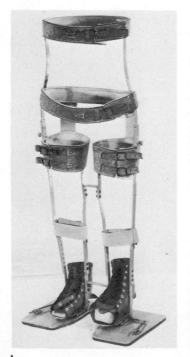
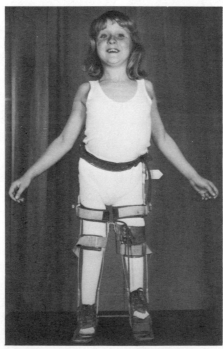
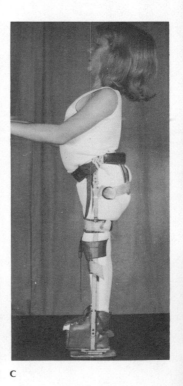

A   B   C

Fig. 14.23   A–C. The Shrewsbury or 'clicking' splint.

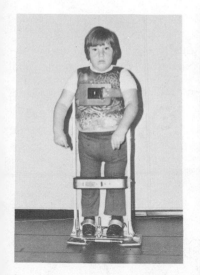

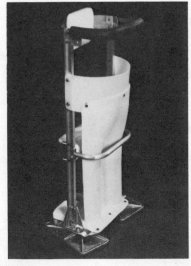

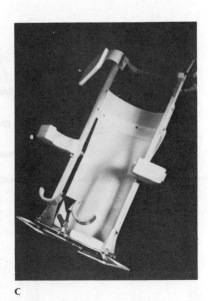

A B C

Fig. 14.24   A–C. The Orlau swivel walker. Orthosis for locomotion.

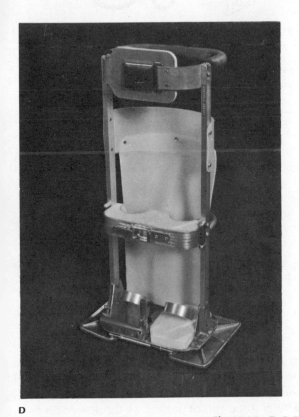

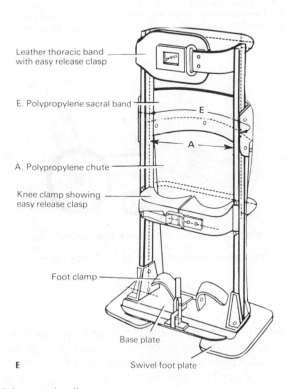

Leather thoracic band
with easy release clasp

E. Polypropylene sacral band

E

A

A. Polypropylene chute

Knee clamp showing
easy release clasp

Foot clamp

Base plate

Swivel foot plate

D

E

Fig. 14.24   D, E. The Orlau swivel walker.

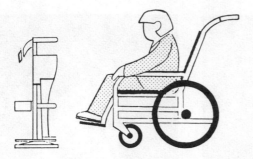

1. Preparation for transfer. Splint with foot clamp, knee clamp and thoracic band opened.

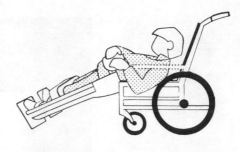

4. Child lying back in chair fastening the thoracic belt.

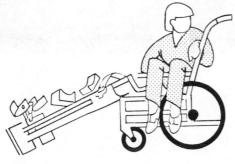

2. Leg over side of chair. Splint lowered into place with back thoracic bar resting on cushion or seat canvas. Child is now ready to place legs into the splint and slide down the shute.

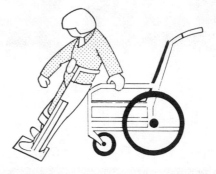

5. Having applied the splint the child levers up with both hands on the arms of the wheelchair drawing the foot plates nearer to the chair with small wriggling movements. Finally the push off with one arm into the standing position.

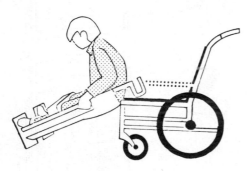

3. Child in sitting position on the polypropylene shute having locked the foot clamp and knee clamp. Child supports trunk with one arm while fastening the clamps with the free hand.

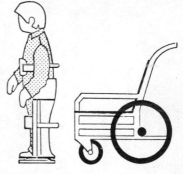

6. Showing child standing clear of the chair in splint ready to move away. Reverse the sequence of illustrations for return transfer to the chair.

Fig. 14.24F

makes no attempt to stand or walk and normal toilet training is impossible because of paralysis of the sphincter muscles of bladder and bowel.

Splintage at the age of 12–18 months may consist of plaster gutter splints to help less-affected children to stand. More heavily handicapped children can be fitted with a swivel walker which mimics normal walking progress (Figs 14.24A, B and C). In patients where some motor power in the lower limbs is spared, band-topped above-knee calipers, or single or double below-knee irons or plastic below-knee splints may be sufficient to support the limbs. Such splints control deformity from muscle imbalance and allow ambulation with or without the use of crutches or walking sticks.

Severe cases, however, usually require splintage such as the 'clicking' splint as shown in Figs 14.23A, B and C. Kennedy describes the gait pattern in this splint (see Bibliography). As the child grows, efforts to preserve muscle length, to prevent contractures and deformity and to strengthen normal muscles are redoubled provided the child is thriving and wishing to walk.

Figures 14.24A–E show the latest type of orthosis first developed by Mr G. K. Rose at Oswestry—the Orlau swivel walker. This enables the patient not only to walk but to transfer to/from a wheelchair. The method of application and transfer into Orlau swivel walker from a wheelchair is shown in Fig. 14.24F.

Activity and play is encouraged from infancy, not only to improve the physical condition but in the interests of the mental development; a crash helmet is worn for play sessions to protect the head. Since some patients may eventually rely on the use of crutches for ambulation, every effort is made to develop the power of the upper limbs. Figure 14.25 shows the hip guidance orthosis and a recent model is shown in Fig. 14.25D.

Sheepskin splints have already been discussed in Ch. 12.

The Orlau swivel walker

The Orlau swivel walker (Figs 14.24A–E) is a further development from the clicking splint and has been designed to improve function and encourage independence (Stallard et al, 1978).

The mechanics incorporating three point fixation at thoracic, pelvic and knee level combined with rigidity of frame, give the child security in the upright position. The design of foot clamps, knee clamps and thoracic band has been carefully planned to enable quick transfer with relative ease. The polypropylene back chute enables the child to slide into the splint from a chair, bed or bench.

The foot plate mechanisms have been strengthened so that progression can be made on to crutches and a swing-through gait achieved. The device will enable many children to transfer in and out at will, to ambulate, stand and work with arms free.

METHOD OF APPLICATION AND TRANSFER INTO ORLAU SWIVEL WALKER FROM A CHAIR

A stage-by-stage guide to this procedure is shown in Fig. 14.24F.

Hip guidance orthosis (HGO)

The hip guidance orthosis (Fig. 14.25) comprises a thoracic/pelvic body brace and leg calipers. The leg calipers are attached to the body brace through a hinge joint positioned adjacent to the patient's anatomical hip joint. The hip hinge joint has a flexion stop set at 5–15 degrees which allows forward progression of the leading leg during ambulation. The orthosis has a rigid structure which ensures lateral stability so that one foot at a time can be raised easily from the ground, using crutches combined with a downward and backward pushing motion. These features of the hip guidance device enable the paraplegic child to walk with a relatively normal gait and a considerable saving of energy expenditure.

The hip guidance orthosis is also being developed for adolescents and adults. This orthosis is called the 'Parawalker' and offers possibilities for low-energy walking to the older patient.

Management of the paralysed bladder

Constant wetting leads to excoriation and maceration of the skin of the buttocks and perineum, and bulky napkins can interfere with the application of splintage and with ambulation. *Credé expression* of the bladder is taught as soon as possible. The child sits on potty or toilet and the parent or helper assists the procedure. In a young child, emptying the bladder is carried out once or twice daily, but as the child grows expression is performed at hourly intervals, increasing to two- or three-hourly if possible.

Urological assessment is required to determine the amount of residual urine left in the bladder after

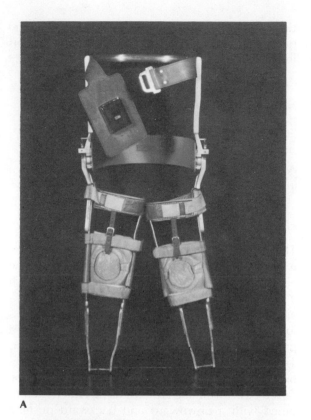

A

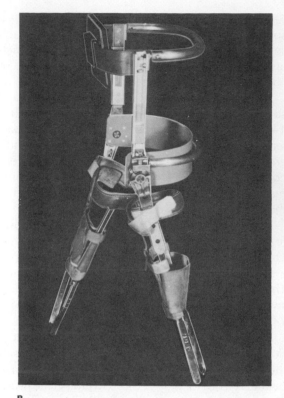

B

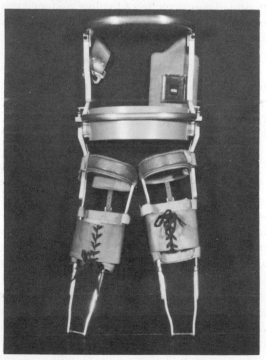

C

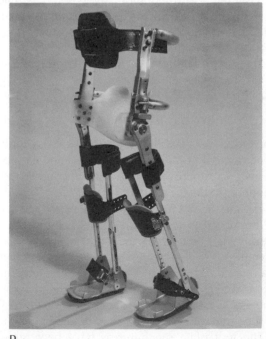

D

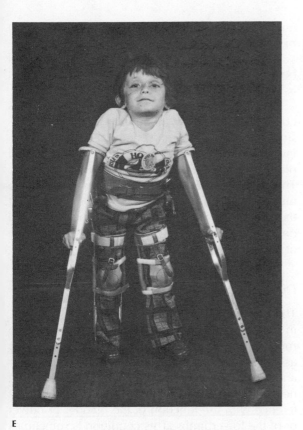

E

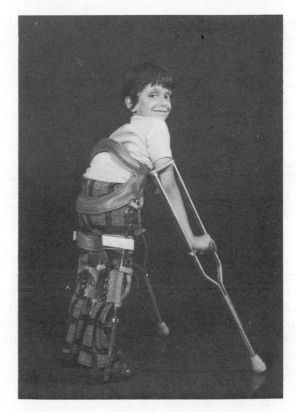

F

voiding. A high level of residual urine requires intermittent catheterisation to prevent a stagnant 'pool' of urine in the bladder which might become infected. This leads to retrograde reflux of urine up the ureters, carrying infection to the kidneys. This in turn leads to pyelonephritis and ultimately to kidney failure. Intermittent catheterisation is now very successful (Preston, 1983) and can be performed by parents or even by the patient herself.

In male patients, condom drainage of the bladder is the mainstay of treatment. Alternatively male patients may wear a urinal similar to those seen in Fig. 23.16A—D.

Urinary infection is treated by the administration of the appropriate antibiotic drugs, and by ensuring a bladder which empties completely and by preventing ureteric reflux.

G

Fig. 14.25 A–G. An early hip guidance orthosis. **A–C** show detailed views of the orthosis. **D** shows a recent model of hip guidance orthosis. **E–G** show the orthosis in use together with a more recent model.

Management of the paralysed bowel

There is complete lack of control because of paralysis of the anal sphincter. Constipation is often marked but if it is not marked, passage of a stool on alternate days is usually satisfactory. Strict attention must be paid to *diet*, and the use of suppositories and rectal washouts may be advised. Intractable dribbling incontinence may mean that there is faecal impaction, which is revealed on rectal examination. The régime best suited to the individual patient can only be found by trial and error.

Treatment of deformities. Dislocation of a single hip is treated on the lines discussed elsewhere in this chapter. If the condition is bilateral, the dislocation (which is painless because of loss of sensation in the part) is accepted, and surprisingly, causes few problems to the spina bifida child.

Hip surgery is approached with caution but flexion-adduction deformity of the hip from muscle imbalance may require release or transplant (Sharrad operation) especially where there are powerful unopposed hip-flexors which also cause an increase in the lumbar lordosis. Club-foot requires soft tissue release operations or operations on bone such as osteotomy or arthrodesis, as described elsewhere. A fixed calcaneo-valgus deformity or progressive scoliosis requires surgical intervention.

Nursing care

These patients require unremitting nursing attention and vigilance, as outlined below:

1. *Vigilance.* The nurse, when attending to the child, notes the general condition, the appearance, and the behaviour; report anything unusual at once. Refusal of food, nasal discharge, vomiting, reluctance to play, rise of temperature, fretfulness, restlessness, lethargy or drowsiness may indicate a full bladder, a loaded colon, the onset of a childish ailment, or more serious complications such as a chest or urinary infection, meningitis or blocking of a Hakim valve.

2. *Care of the skin* over the spinal defect, the buttocks, the perineum and the lower limbs involves scrupulous cleanliness, relief from pressure and avoidance of trauma. Any sign of infection is reported at once; always bear in mind that anaesthetic skin can be damaged by rough treatment, by pressure from clothing, splintage, foreign bodies or toys, and by heat or cold.

3. *Care of the bladder and bowel* is an important nursing duty; neglect may lead to urinary infection or to faecal impaction.

4. *Care of splintage.* Splints must fit perfectly and be kept in good repair; cleanliness of the splint as well as the skin beneath it is essential.

5. Finally, a patient suffering from this serious condition requires, in addition to unremitting physical care, a happy atmosphere, acceptance as an individual, love and security, companionship and play; education, and later, vocational training. Throughout the early years of treatment the nurse must counsel and support not only the patient, but the parents as well. Family stress and strain and divorce proceedings are very common in the home of the spina bifida child.

Diastematomyelia

This is a condition in which the spinal cord (or, in the lumbar region, the dura mater and nerve roots), is divided by a fibrous band or a bony bar; as the child grows, the cord is tethered by the bar and subjected to traction resulting in changing neurological signs in the limbs. There may be interference with the function of the bladder or bowel or of the lower limbs. This condition is sometimes associated with spina bifida and congenital scoliosis.

Treatment consists of investigations (e.g. myelogram) and surgery to relieve the constriction of the spinal cord.

Congenital scoliosis

This is due to architectural defects of the spine such as hemivertebrae, absence of some vertebrae and fusion of ribs.

Treatment proceeds on the lines discussed in Ch. 15.

CONGENITAL TORTICOLLIS (WRY NECK)

This is a deformity of the neck in which there is rotation of the head to one side and lateral flexion to the other. It may be congenital or acquired; the congenital type is by far the more common and will be discussed here.

The cause may be (1) in the cervical spine itself, or (2) in the muscles controlling it.

1. *Causes in the cervical spine* may be due to hemivertebrae or spina bifida. *Acquired* torticollis may be due to an inflammatory lesion such as tuberculosis or osteomyelitis. This is discussed elsewhere (Chs 16 and 17).

2. *Causes in the muscles controlling the cervical spine* may be due to injury to the sterno-cleido-mastoid muscle at birth causing a haematoma called a 'sterno-mastoid tumour'. This may later result in an ischaemic contracture in the muscle.

Clinical features

The child is brought to the surgeon because the parents notice that he 'holds his head on one side'.

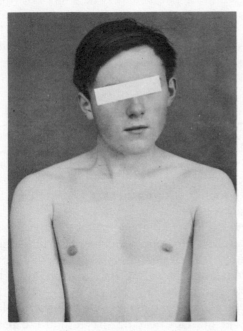

Fig. 14.26 Right torticollis.

On examination, it will be seen that the head is rotated to one side and flexed to the other, and on this side the shoulder may be raised. This is due to contracture of the sterno-cleido-mastoid muscle on one side, which turns the head so that the chin points towards the normal side, and the neck flexes laterally towards the affected side. On attempting to correct the deformity the sterno-cleido-mastoid stands out as a tight band, the maxi-

mum contracture being in the clavicular head of the muscle. In patients in whom the deformity is of long standing, there will be facial asymmetry due to an attempt on the part of nature to maintain the eye-level. This results in the features of the affected side being smaller than those of the other.

Treatment

No treatment is advised until disease of the cervical spine itself has been excluded by clinical and by radiological examination. It may be conservative or operative. Operative treatment is undertaken in late cases or when conservative measures have failed after a reasonable period. In older patients, if the deformity is not severe, interference is not as a rule advised, as the facial asymmetry will persist and become more noticeable, and there may also be complications such as headache and giddiness following alteration of the eye-level.

Conservative treatment

In early life, passive stretchings to the affected muscle are given as soon as possible after birth. The mother is usually taught to do this by a physiotherapist, but the nurse may be called upon to assist. The baby lies on a firm couch, and while its shoulders are held by an assistant the head is gently but firmly flexed away from the affected side and rotated towards it. Great care must be taken in handling the baby's head. The baby may also wear a collar made of newspaper rolled in a handkerchief or other soft material. Re-education is commenced when the child is old enough to follow moving objects with his eyes.

Operative treatment

In an older child, the most usual treatment is open or percutaneous tenotomy of the sterno-mastoid muscle, followed by fixation in the over-corrected position, either between sand-bags with a towel over the forehead, or by plaster fixation. A plaster jacket may be applied immediately after operation or after twenty-four hours. If sand-bags are used post-operatively, it is the nurse's duty to see that the head is held continuously in the over-corrected position, i.e. flexed away from the affected side and rotated towards it—'chin towards the dressing'. The arm on the affected side may be tied down to the bed. Passive stretchings and active exercises are introduced immediately. The patient must be fed and washed and is not allowed to sit up. The position is maintained for about ten days, when a collar may be applied and the patient is allowed up. In addition to the special stretchings and exercises, the child is given general postural exercises and taught self-correction in front of a mirror. The collar is worn until the patient can voluntarily hold the over-corrected position.

Plaster fixation. The plaster is dried as described in Ch. 6 and the same care is needed. The cast is worn for about six weeks.

CEREBRAL PALSY (Spastic paralysis, Little's disease)

Cerebral palsy is a lesion of the upper motor neuron, resulting in stiffness and inco-ordination of movement of the limbs. It is believed to be due to brain damage, from causes already discussed earlier; there may be a history of prematurity, difficult labour, haemolytic disease of the new-born, or anoxia.

There are two main types, characterised by:

1. *Spasticity* of the limbs, and
2. *Athetosis*, meaning inco-ordinate involuntary movement of the limbs, often of a writhing nature.

Other forms of the condition result in ataxia, generalised rigidity, or tremor. The type of lesion commonly seen by the orthopaedic nurse is of the *spastic* variety and even then, only when admitted to hospital for specific treatment, such as an operation. The vast majority of these patients, if they cannot be cared for at home and attend normal or special day-school, are treated in special centres which combine programmes of both physical care and of education, particularly if in addition to the physical handicap, there is associated deafness, blindness, difficulty in swallowing, impairment of speech, drooling at the mouth, facial tics, convulsions and mental deficiency. Since the *spastic type of cerebral palsy* is the one most commonly seen in orthopaedic practice we will confine ourselves to discussion of this condition.

Clinical features

In early life, the first thing to be noticed may be that the infant is a so-called 'floppy baby'; fits are sometimes seen. The baby may be unduly fretful or unduly placid, or there may be feeding difficulties. As the baby grows, slight stiffness of the limbs may be noticed, for example, when putting on nappies. The normal milestones of progress are not reached at the usual time, for example, the mother (or grandmother) may notice that the baby does not smile and begin to gurgle and coo at the time when this is normally expected; i.e. after about the sixth week of life. He may be slow to grasp objects, such as a feeding bottle, cup or toy. Sitting up and other normal milestones may be delayed; crawling and walking may be delayed or not accomplished at all; there may be a limp, or wasting of a calf-muscle with limb shortening. Other defects may become obvious, including the most disastrous one of all, i.e. impairment of the intellect, indicated by an expressionless face and lack of an intelligent gleam in the eye.

Distribution of disability

One limb only—monoplegia.
    One upper and one lower limb—hemiplegia.
    Both lower limbs only—paraplegia.
    All four limbs—tetraplegia (sometimes called quadriplegia).

Though this condition is often spoken of as 'spastic paralysis' it is not in fact paralysis but a failure of control of certain muscle-groups so that they do not relax and allow the smooth working of their opponents.

When special movements are attempted, all the affected muscles become spastic and the patient cannot use one set of muscles without another being stimulated, so that movements are stiff and inco-ordinate.

It may be helpful to compare this condition with poliomyelitis, in which the patient is unable to perform a movement because a group of muscles is paralysed. The spastic patient is unable to perform a movement, not because a group of muscles is paralysed, *but because there is insufficient relaxation of opposing muscles.* For example, the 'polio' may not be able to extend the knee because of paralysis of the quadriceps; the 'spastic' cannot extend it because there is insufficient relaxation of the hamstrings. In both conditions, a muscle which is not balanced by an opponent of equal strength will not only pull a limb into a deformed position, but will contract until the deformity becomes fixed.

Deformities

As the child grows, flexion contractures increase, the normal muscles atrophy, and deformities become fixed. The limbs assume a characteristic position, as described below.

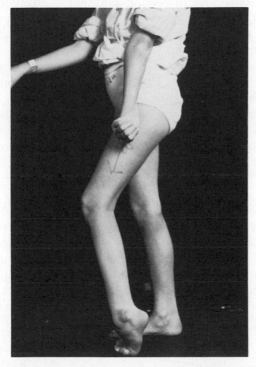

Fig. 14.27 Cerebral palsy with left hemiplegia.

Upper limbs. The elbow is flexed, the forearm pronated, the wrist is flexed, and the thumb may be adducted and pressed into the palm by the flexed fingers, so that when asked to perform a movement the patient uncurls his hand finger by finger.

Lower limbs. The hips are flexed, adducted and internally rotated. The knees are flexed and the feet held in equino-varus. Any attempt to straighten a limb is resisted by muscle spasm and if one succeeds in straightening it, the spasm returns imme-

diately it is released. The reflexes are exaggerated and there are circulatory changes in the limbs so that they become cold and blue.

The gait. Sometimes the first thing to be noticed is that the child 'walks on his toes'; spasm of the adductors may result in 'scissors gait', one leg crossing over the other as the patient attempts to walk.

Dislocation of the hip is not uncommon.

Treatment in severe cases requires the co-operation of a number of people, as outlined earlier in connection with the general care of physically handicapped children. Treatment of co-existing conditions such as deafness or blindness, periodic reassessment, alteration of régimes to meet new demands, arrangements for special education, and above all, support and help for the patient's family are as vital in patients suffering from cerebral palsy as in any other disabling condition. In connection with these patients, however, three members of the team spring to mind as having key positions, outlined as follows:

The child's mother. Not only is she the natural guardian of his early years but his natural teacher. Stimulation from earliest infancy to school age is essential; as soon as is practicable every effort should be made to encourage the child's mobility.

The physiotherapist. During the last two decades the treatment of the cerebral palsied child has become the concern of certain 'schools of thought' in physiotherapeutic treatment, exact details of which need not concern us here but all of which use different techniques aimed at the improvement of function; for example, the work of the Bobath school is based on teaching relaxation and on the use of conditioned reflexes; the Temple Fay school teaches forms of primitive movement; knowledge of these techniques concerns us only when working with a physiotherapist using them, in order to ensure that the effect of treatment begun in the Physiotherapy Department is not neutralised in the ward.

The teacher. With the older cerebral palsied child the teacher has a special rôle, since successful treatment of the child's physical condition is of no avail if he is unable to read and write; on the other hand, teaching, in common with other forms of therapy has to be regulated by the demands of the individual patient, particularly if there are other handicaps, such as deafness.

Other workers who may have a prominent part to play in the treatment programme are the speech therapist and the educational psychologist, and, as in related problems, the Health and Education Authorities in whose area the afflicted child and his family live.

General management of the patient

This will obviously depend upon the severity of the condition, having regard not only to the physical condition but to the mental state; on the other hand, these are not always proportionate; a severely physically affected child might have high intelligence which is masked by the physical defect; conversely a mildly physically handicapped child may be of low intelligence, and many patients exhibit some evidence of emotional instability for which due allowance must be made in our dealings with the child. The degree of intelligence must not be under-rated; improvement of the physical state is usually matched by corresponding improvement in the intellect. It is important to remember that appearances are often deceptive and that the patient may not be so feeble-minded as he may appear.

Patients who can be cared for at home have the irreplaceable advantage of a normal family life and normal companionship at school; more severe cases may need special education at a day school or as boarders at a residential establishment.

The aim of treatment

This is the improvement of function, by correction of deformity, if required, and by physical and mental re-education of the patient.

A happy family life in the company of other children is the ideal background to treatment and, as already explained, these patients are only admitted to orthopaedic hospitals when some specific deformity requires operative correction. On the other hand they may be admitted pending transfer to a special centre, or they may be mild cases which can be cared for at home and attend a normal school but for whom a period of training is indicated. On admission to a children's ward, it is important that the patient is included in the conversation, lessons, games and other activities of his fellows. Patience, perseverance and unfailing good humour on the part of the nurse is essential; she has an important rôle in re-educating the patient in the ordinary acts of living, so that he may become independent of others. On admission, the patient, if neglected, may be dirty, difficult and refactory. The nurse, with other members of the team, will set herself out to win his confidence and to teach him obedience and self-control. It is important to remember that in most cases progress will be very slow; as already stated fits may be present and defective sight or hearing must be treated; speech therapy is often necessary. The patient must never be frightened; spastic limbs must be handled gently, firmly and smoothly, never in an abrupt or jerky manner. A nursing care study in the *Nursing Mirror* (Turner, 1980) gives a good description of the care of a spastic child.

Pressure sores are very liable to occur because of the impaired nourishment and mobility of the limbs. These patients are very sensitive to cold, and bear pain badly.

Outline of re-education

Enterprise and ingenuity is often required to devise suitable aids to function for each individual patient, and endless tact and patience to teach him to use them. Often it is less disturbing to ward routine if the patient is treated as a helpless individual and everything done for him. Unless he is otherwise ill, such as when recovering from an operation,

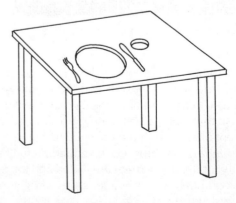

Fig. 14.28 Holes cut for plate and cup prevent them from sliding about the table when eating is attempted.

this should be discouraged. For example, eating a meal may be a lengthy and messy procedure and the nurse is sorely tempted to feed the child. Except in very severe cases, training in the use of special equipment, if indicated, such as a spoon with a large handle, will enable the patient to feed himself. In this connection, it is important to see that food is not 'bolted' and that the patient does in fact receive an adequate diet.

Toilet training is important; if the patient is confined to bed for some reason bedpans are given in the usual way, otherwise regular visits to the lavatory are instituted. Control of the bladder and bowel is often learned very slowly; it is best to ignore a wet bed, and praise a dry one—these patients respond well to encouragement and praise. Sometimes special equipment such as a toothbrush with a padded handle or a long-handled brush or comb is required, and the patient is encouraged to take an interest in his appearance.

Aids to walking. Sometimes splintage is required such as a caliper or a double-iron. The indication for these will be discussed later. The patient may commence re-education in walking between parallel bars, or in some form of walking machine; since mobility is so essential, a powered aid might be ordered (Ch. 11).

Physiotherapy

This plays a very important part in the treatment, as previously outlined. In the absence of the special techniques already mentioned, simple rhythmic exercises are given and the patient is taught to relax as far as possible. Warm baths and hydrotherapy are very valuable. As improvement begins, simple games and exercises which require purposeful coordinated movements are introduced. As in all children, *play* is a vital element in treatment. Fatigue must be avoided, and several short sessions daily are usually better than a single one which is prolonged.

Passive movements, as such, are never given as they cause severe pain and increase the spasm, though special manipulations may be employed to coax a joint into a corrected position during treatment by the physiotherapist. A limb may be passively stretched for splintage to be applied, and

retained in the desired position but, in general, intermittent stretch is never put on a spastic muscle.

Education

This has already been mentioned and is of vital importance; the school-teacher has an important part to play. Again, special equipment is often required, for example to enable the patient to sit at a table for lessons and games. Figure 14.29

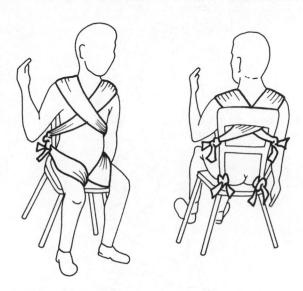

Fig. 14.29 A good sitting posture can be achieved by means of stockinette slings passed round the shoulders and thighs, as shown.

shows how a patient can be seated on an ordinary low chair and the limbs held in a good posture by means of old stockings, scarves, or strips of stockinette such as is used to cover the skin beneath plaster casts. Or the thighs are held to the seat of the chair by straps as shown in Fig. 14.30, or separated by a wooden bar as in Fig. 14.31. In this illustration the patient is shown wearing below-knee irons and a wooden strut is placed on either side of each foot to maintain good alignment. If he is able to stand (and this should be encouraged for at least a short time each day) a 'standing-table' with a cut-out portion as shown in Fig. 14.32 is useful. Alternatively he may stand in a circle cut in the centre of a wooden table. This is very useful for play-time. As in the normal child, play is necessary to development and toys are specially chosen

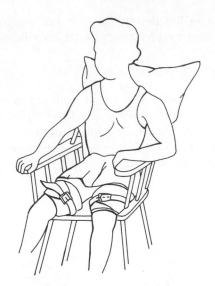

Fig. 14.30 Adductor spasm can be overcome by means of straps fixed to the seat of the chair.

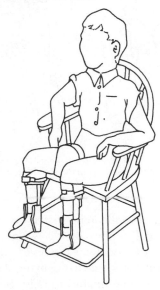

Fig. 14.31 In this illustration the thighs are separated and the leg held in good anatomical alignment by means of wooden struts fixed to the chair. The patient also wears double below knee irons.

for the individual patient. For example, he may handle large building blocks to begin with and progress to smaller ones; he learns to use a large thick pencil and then one of normal size.

Correction of deformity

This is approached with caution. As a rule, interfer-

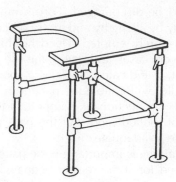

Fig. 14.32 A standing-table. The child is placed in the curved portion, facing the table, and his back is supported against a wall.

ence is indicated only if a deformity seriously interferes with function. For example, adduction contracture at the hip or contracture of the tendo Achilles may prevent the patient from walking.

Retentive splintage may consist of one or two calipers combined with T-straps and posterior stops. Sometimes, elbow-crutches are ordered which later may be exchanged for walking-sticks as co-ordination improves. Correct balance must always be taught before walking is attempted. Above-knee night shells may be worn, and in cases where equino-varus of the feet is the main problem, double or inside below-knee irons may be ordered, with outside T-straps and posterior stops, and plaster shells for night-wear. In any case, splintage is never so rigidly applied as to produce permanent stiffness of the joints, thereby defeating the whole object of the treatment, i.e. improvement of function.

PHYSIOTHERAPY IN CEREBRAL PALSY

Physical treatment for cerebral palsy is very specialised, requiring post-graduate training and experience. What can the physiotherapist do to help the nurse in the management of the patient? Probably it is best to try to help the nurses and parents understand the nature of the child's difficulties. These are so varied in type, distribution and severity that no case is 'typical'. The physiotherapist makes a clinical assessment of functional abilities and the contributory factors causing disabilities. This includes observation and testing and should clarify aims of treatment.

Function

This may be subdivided into (1) communication, (2) self-care, (3) gross motor function (mobility), and should reveal the degree of dependence.

1. *Communication.* The child requires to express his needs and comprehend instructions. Speech may be impossible or unintelligible but parents, attendants, nurses, teachers and therapists should try to learn to interpret the sounds or signs which the child makes. If intellect is impaired this may further handicap the child's ability to communicate; sign language may be used, if so there is an obvious need to understand the method.

On admission to hospital, those who know and understand the child should be consulted about his condition, e.g. the parents, school-teacher. Assessment of function is carried out on the lines set out below;

2. *Self-care.* This includes feeding, dressing, washing, toilet in lavatory and when resting, change of position to relieve pressure. A preliminary survey is also made at this stage as to how function can be improved and with what aids.

3. *Gross motor activity* (mobility). This means the ability to take and hold positions, change to others, transfer from place to place, e.g. bed to wheelchair, chair to lavatory. Also in some cases, the method of walking should be assessed, in others the methods and skill in wheelchair use; the difficulty and speed of achievement should be noted.

Contributory factors causing dysfunction must be analysed as treatment differs in relation to these. Spasticity is the term used when mature selective controlled movements are not possible; the patient can produce only mass primitive movements involving the whole limb or body. The position of the head in space and in relation to the trunk may also influence the position and movement of trunk and limbs. These 'tonic reflexes' are present in the normal infant and are soon modified but may persist in cases of brain damage. The patient with spasticity cannot control isolated movements at individual joints or combine joint positions in a normal way to sit, kneel, roll, crawl, stand or walk. Affected hands may make manual skills impossible. Effort, i.e. simply trying harder to achieve a movement actually increases spasticity. The distribution and severity of spasticity should be recorded.

Failure to develop stability to counteract the effect of the force of gravity and other external forces occurs either because of the focal brain damage, or because lack of normal stimulation and sensory input prevents maturation of undamaged parts of the brain. The child may show lack of controlled co-ordinated movements and balance reactions because of brain damage. Lack of normal postural reactions and presence of excessive unwanted movements results from various lesions in the extra-pyramidal system whose centres are in the basal ganglia and brain stem. Combinations of types of motor disorders exist in some cases. Sensation, including sight, hearing, kinaesthetic sensation (awareness of body position and movement) and cutaneous sensation may be defective. The brain lesion may cause perceptual defects such as inability to recognise spatial relationship, body image etc. Language centres may be affected or the control of breathing and/or lips and tongue may be defective so that swallowing and speech are abnormal. Secondary contractures and bone deformities may develop as a result of spasticity.

Having analysed factors contributing to dysfunction, treatment can be planned to try to overcome these, provide a more normal sensory input and elicit more normal motor responses; this may improve function, aid the development of undamaged parts of the brain and help to prevent secondary complications such as contractures.

Physiotherapy is traditionally concerned with gross motor function but if posture and ability to take and hold more normal positions is improved, self-care, swallowing and voice production will also be facilitated. *The physiotherapist, speech-therapist and occupational therapist work in co-ordination as does the teacher with the school-aged patient.*

Many methods of treatment are too specialised to describe here; However, the most helpful positions, stimuli and instructions for each patient can be demonstrated by physiotherapists to help nurses and others in the management of the child (Fig. 14.33A and B).

Human beings at birth can move but cannot hold even their heads steady. Basic control of posture and movement is gradually acquired automatically by maturation of the nervous system. Thus normal babies reach physical 'landmarks' at approximately

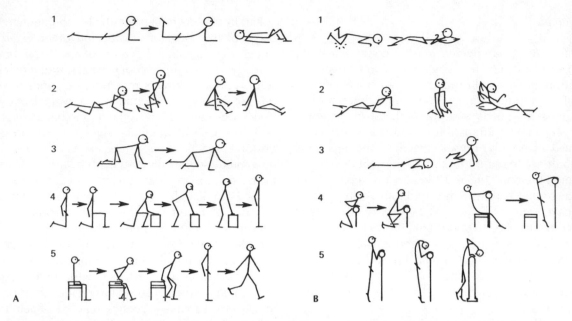

Fig. 14.33 **A.** Useful patterns to be encouraged. These are useful because they are functionally sound, give a balanced combination of flexor and extensor synergies and relate to the normal developmental milestones. **B.** Useless patterns which should be discouraged. These are useless because they can never lead to independent function, involve total flexor or total extensor synergies instead of balanced elements of each, and do not relate to normal developmental milestones. (Reprinted by permission of Faber and Faber, from *Neurology for Physiotherapists*, 2nd Edn.)

the same ages throughout the first years of life (Illingworth et al, 1975). We take this automatic control for granted and do not realise how dependent we are on the background of control of our skeleto-muscular system for all automatic postural reactions and so called 'voluntary' skilled movements.

The nurse must realise that in severe cerebral palsy such basic activities as rolling and sitting up in bed are not possible; the child either cannot keep still, maintain balance, or combine the necessary joint positions to achieve even simple supported sitting or half-lying positions. He must not be blamed if he cannot move normally or obey requests; effort increases unwanted activity especially pathological reflex activity such as spasticity; stress also increases the disability and the harder the child tries to move the less likely he is to achieve normal function. Having found the best positions and methods of handling each patient, the physiotherapist can show these to all other personnel, and to the mother or guardian.

In an orthopaedic unit, cases of cerebral palsy are usually admitted only for consideration of sur-

gery or to try out orthotic devices. The need for physiotherapist and nurse to understand the patient's problems is emphasised by the hazards of attempting to immobilise spastic or athetoid parts by splintage. In contrast to cases with flaccid paralysis, those with hyperactive primitive reflexes and defects of control are more likely to develop sores from pressure or friction and increase in malalignment rather than correction.

On removal of a plaster cast or other splintage, great care is needed in handling to prevent uncontrolled movements which are very painful and may negate benefits of surgery; again, physiotherapists and nurses should co-operate in selecting stimuli and methods of handling to avoid eliciting reflex action. Bivalved plaster shells or other splints should be retained, except during treatment sessions, until some control is achieved by the patient. The position of the patient in bed and later in a wheelchair should be carefully considered. If it is possible and permitted by the surgeon, prone lying is usually preferable to supine, side-lying or half-lying. If a wedge is used so that the child's head and shoulders are raised and his hips are in extension he will have better head and arm control, speech, breathing, swallowing, and hand activities will be facilitated. The patient's head should face the centre of the ward, rather than a blank wall so that he can enjoy seeing what is going on.

All cerebral palsy cases need thoughtful, careful, slow handling; hurried abrupt movements by child or nurse produce unwanted reflex activity.

Further reading is suggested in the Bibliography.

Operative treatment

This is undertaken with caution; operations on bones, joints, muscles and nerves are aimed at correction of deformity with improvement of the function and of the appearance of the affected limbs, as outlined below:

1. *In the upper limb, arthrodesis of the wrist* is performed for correction of flexion deformity and subsequent improvement in the appearance and function of the hand. *Muscle releases* can correct a flexion contracture at the elbow and the pronated posture of the forearm.

2. *In the lower limb*, where adduction deformity is the prime disability, *adductor tenotomy* or *obturator neurectomy* may be advised; flexion contracture may require a *release operation*; where dislocation of the hip is the main problem, *transplantation of the iliopsoas tendon* to the postero-lateral aspect of the greater trochanter (Sharrard) may be advised; *de-rotation osteotomy* of the femur is sometimes required. Flexion deformity of the knee may be treated by means of *Egger's operation*, when the hamstrings are transplanted to the posterior part of the femoral shaft above the condyles.

3. *Foot deformities* may require open elongation of the tendo achillis, osteotomy of the calcaneum (Dwyer) for persistent clawfoot, or triple arthrodesis.

Occasionally, several operative procedures are performed in combination; post-operatively, the limbs are held in the corrected position by means of plaster casts. Special vigilance is required in the prevention of sores and in reporting any sign of circulatory disturbance, as described in a previous chapter. On removal of plaster, retentive splintage such as a caliper or below-knee iron may be required; *re-education* commences as soon as pos-

sible, since correction of deformity is only a prelude to the *real* treatment, which is the continuous process of physical and mental re-education in an effort to prepare the patient as far as possible for normal living. Those unable to walk with or without appliances require *aids to mobility* (Fig. 14.34),

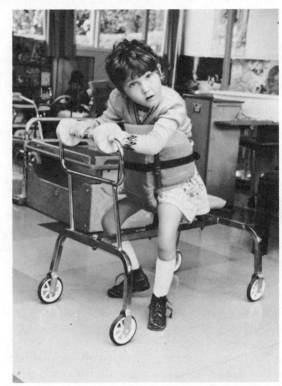

Fig. 14.34   Aids to mobility are devised to suit the individual child.

for example, a conventional wheelchair, electrically-propelled wheelchair (Hancox, 1978) or suitably converted motor car.

Help for the child suffering from cerebral palsy can be obtained from The Secretary, The Spastics Society, 12 Park Crescent, London W1 and very often, from local associations as well.

BIRTH TRAUMA

In the preceding section we have discussed congenital anomalies which are probably due to genetic factors, or to factors in the maternal environment; but we have also seen that during the second stage of labour the infant is exposed to the risk of hypoxia, hypoglycaemia and often hazards which might result in other conditions, notably cerebral palsy. Other birth injuries to the locomotor system are also seen, such as bony damage, brachial plexus palsy, and lesions to peripheral nerves, such as sciatic palsy which might occur as result of injections given into the umbilical vein, or to the radial or lateral popliteal nerves due to trauma.

Brachial plexus lesions

Erb's palsy

This is due to a traction injury to the fifth and sixth cervical nerve roots during birth. There is paralysis of deltoid, biceps, supra-spinatus, infra-spinatus, and the supinators of the forearm. The arm hangs by the side in a position of internal rotation at the shoulder, and extension and pronation of the forearm—the characteristic 'porter's hand'. If the condition is untreated, contractures occur and the deformity becomes fixed.

Treatment. In very young babies the arm may be tied to the top of the cot as a temporary measure. *Splintage* is applied to hold the limb in full external rotation and abduction at the shoulder, right-angled flexion of the elbow and full supination of the forearm. Alternatively, a comfortable and convenient splint is easily made of padded Cramer wire. *Physiotherapy* is commenced at once, and is directed towards preventing contractures at the elbow and shoulder. As the child grows, re-education of muscles is commenced. The mother is taught to encourage abduction and external rotation of the shoulder and supination of the forearm when playing with the child. Later, active use is encouraged by bandaging the sound arm to the side or by keeping it beneath the clothes. The prognosis is good.

Klumpke's palsy

This is a lesion of the eighth cervical and first thoracic nerve roots. There is paralysis of the intrinsic muscles of the hand, the flexors of the thumb and wrist, and of the muscles of the thenar and hypothenar eminences. The fingers cannot be spread out or approximated and become clawed.

Treatment. Splintage as for an ulnar palsy may be applied in an effort to prevent claw-hand deformity. *Physiotherapy* is always ordered. Later, active use of the hand is encouraged, but the prospect of recovery is not good.

Birth fractures

The shafts of the humerus, the clavicle, the femur and the tibia are the commonest sites of fracture in the newly-born baby. They are usually sustained during delivery of the infant. Multiple fractures may be present if there is congenital fragility of bone.

Fracture of the humerus

A pad of wool of sufficient size to maintain a moderate degree of abduction is placed in the axilla, and the arm is bandaged to the side.

Fracture of the femur

This may be treated by the application of skin extensions to both legs, which are then flexed to the right angle and tied to a bar fixed over the cot. The extension ties must be fastened at sufficient tension to lift the buttocks only just clear of the bed (Fig. 14.35). If domestic circumstances permit, the child can be nursed at home on a portable gallows frame (Fig. 14.36).

Nursing care. This proceeds on the lines described in Chs 5, 10, and 11; in addition, it is *imperative* that the feet and legs are inspected regularly with special regard to the circulation, which may be impeded by the position in which they are held or by a tight bandage. Swelling of the feet or any other adverse sign is reported to the surgeon without delay. Toileting is no problem since a napkin can be placed under the buttocks; feeds are given with caution while the baby becomes accustomed to the position.

Fracture of the tibia—congenital pseudarthrosis of tibia

This may be present at birth, or manifest itself in early life as a result of apparently trivial violence. The affected bone may show cystic changes, or one or both of the bone ends are sclerotic; the con-

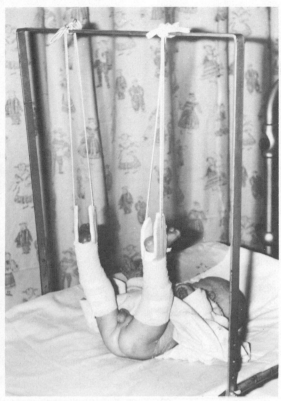

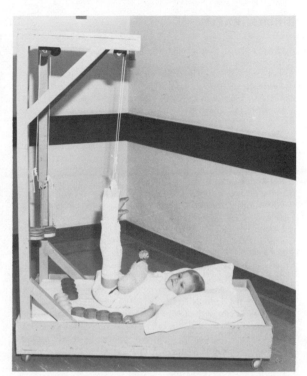

Fig. 14.36 The High Wycombe portable gallows traction frame.

Fig. 14.35 Birth-fracture of femur is treated by extensions fastened to an overhead beam. (Bryant's traction.) *NB* Note once more that this form of traction can interfere with blood/nerve supply to the feet.

dition is thought to be connected with neurofibromatosis or fibrous dysplasia.

Treatment. Early operation is usually advised in an attempt to prevent progressive deformity and shortening of the limb.

Internal fixation is usually employed, either in the form of a bone-graft using the child's own contralateral tibia or his ilium, or, bone taken from a parent or from the bone-bank. A 'by-pass' operation is sometimes performed when the fibula is used to bridge the angle formed by the pseudarthrosis; alternatively, fixation is achieved by means of an intramedullary nail inserted either from above, or from below across the ankle joint.

Re-fracture is common, so that repeated attempts at fixation and bone grafts may be necessary; plaster casts are used post-operatively and protection by means of a caliper may be required for a long period.

In cases where union is not achieved and where there is progressive deformity and shortening of the limb, amputation may finally be advised.

OTHER CONGENITAL ABNORMALITIES

In this chapter, we have discussed only those congenital anomalies commonly seen in orthopaedic practice. There are, of course, other congenital conditions which from time to time may come under the care of the orthopaedic surgeon, including achondroplasia, arthrogryposis multiplexa congenita, osteogenesis imperfecta, amytonia congenita, muscular dystrophy, cranio-cleidal dyostosis, Klipper-Feil syndrome, Sprengel shoulder, club-hand and congenital dislocation of the knee. A detailed description of these conditions is outside the scope of this book and treatment of specific deformities and disabilities which might arise as a result of these conditions proceeds on similar lines to those discussed in preceding pages.

BIBLIOGRAPHY

Adams J C 1971 Outline of Orthopaedics. Edinburgh: Churchill Livingstone

Anderson E M 1977 The Child with Spina Bifida. London: Methuen, p 26

Apley A G 1977 A System of Orthopaedics and Fractures. London: Butterworths

Barsky A J 1958 Congenital Anomalies of the Hand and their Surgical Treatment. Charles C Thomas

Bleackley R (ed) 1974 Despite Disability. Reading: Educational Explorers

Bleck E E 1977 Congenital clubfoot. Clinical Orthopaedics and Related Research 125: 119–130

Bowley A H, Gardner L 1972 The Handicapped Child. Edinburgh: Churchill Livingstone

Carter M J 1975 Congenital clubfoot. Nursing Mirror, 141, November 1975, 58–62

Cotton E 1974 The Basic Motor Pattern. London: The Spastics Society

Curtis C 1968 A child with a signoid colonic urinary conduit. Nursing Times, 11 October, 1370

Day H 1977 The early referral of children with congenital limb deficiencies. Health Trends 9(1): 12–13

DHSS 1973 Care of the Child with Spina Bifida. Prepared by the Standing Medical Advisory Committee. London: DHSS

Eckstein H B 1968 Complications of ventricule-atrial drainage for hydrocephalus. Nursing Mirror, 31 May, 29

Fairbrother C 1982 Reporting work of M Delaney. One nurse's bright idea. Nursing Times, 7 April

Fanshawe E et al 1978 Disability without handicap. Nursing Times Supplement, 17 August, 3–20

Farrow R, Forest D 1974 The Surgery of Childhood for Nurses. Edinburgh: Churchill Livingstone

Finnie N 1974 Handling the Young Cerebral Palsied Child at Home. London: Heinemann

Gilchrist M I 1969 Posterior ilio-psoas transplant. Nursing Times, 11 December, 1575

Gillow J 1980 Congenital dislocation of the hip—Conservative treatment of a child, using hoop traction. Nursing Care Study. Nursing Times, 28 August

Goel K 1981 An old enemy returns. Nursing Mirror, Jan 8, 16–18

Greenwood A 1980 Your child in an immobilising plaster. London: National Association for the Welfare of Children in Hospital

Hancox V F 1978 Bomber put the world at my feet. Nursing Times, 24 August, 1428

Hilt N, Schmitt E W 1975 Paediatric Orthopaedic Nursing. Mosby, pp 28–32

Hosking G 1982 Treating the untreatable. London: Nursing Mirror, 16 June

Hunt P (ed) 1966 Stigma—the Experience of Disability. London: Geoffrey Chapman

Illingworth R S 1975 Basic Developmental Screening 0–2 yrs. London: Blackwell Scientific

Kennedy J M 1974 Orthopaedic Splints and Appliances. London: Ballière Tindal

Ling C 1972 Sternomastoid tumour and muscular torticollis. Clinical Orthopaedics and Related Research 86: 144–150

Lorber J 1973 Management of Spina Bifida Cystica, Parts 1, 2 & 3. Nursing Mirror, 12, 19, 26 October, 21, 33, 35

Lorber J 1974 Myelomeningocele—new approaches to its management. London: Nursing Times, 21 February, 272

Lorber J 1976 Ethical problems in the management of myelomeningocele and hydrocephalus. Nursing Times, Key Clinical, 26 February, 5; 25 March, 9

McCarthy J 1976 Congenital malformations. Nursing Mirror, 24 June, 26

McHugh A 1978 Nursing Care Study. Congenital Dislocation of the Hip. Nursing Mirror, 6 April, 19–21

Neale D 1985 Common Foot Disorders, 2nd edn. Edinburgh: Churchill Livingstone

Nichol C 1977 Congenital dislocated hip. Canadian Nurse 73(7): 14–19

McKibbin B 1970 Sources of Error in Early Recognition of Congenital Dislocation of the Hip

McRae R 1976 Clinical Orthopaedic Examination. Edinburgh: Churchill Livingstone

Preston E T 1977 Congenital idiopathic clubfoot. Clinical Orthopaedics and Related Research 122: 102–109

Preston S 1983 Catheterising Mary. Nursing Times Community Outlook, 15 September

Roaf R, Hodkinson L J 1976 Textbook of Orthopaedic Nursing. London: Blackwell Scientific

Rose G K 1971 Splintage for Spina Bifida cystica. Nursing Mirror, 20 August, 20

Rose G K 1979 The principles and practice of hip guidance articulations. Prosthetics and Orthotics International 3: 37–43

Rose G K et al 1979 Orthotics. Physiotherapy 63: 78

Rowe J, Dyer L (eds) 1977 Care of the Orthopaedic Patient. Oxford: Blackwell Scientific

Savage J H 1975 The red arrow. Nursing Times, 20 November, 1869

Shaw N E 1977 Treatment and prognosis in clubfoot. British Medical Journal 6055: 219–222

Sheridan M D 1975 Children's Developmental Progress from Birth to Five Years; The Stycar Sequences, 3rd edn. London: NFER Publishing Co

Spraggon C M 1975 Urinary Diversion Stomas. Edinburgh: Churchill Livingstone

Stark G D 1975 Spina Bifida: Problems and Management. Oxford: Blackwell Scientific

Stallard J, Rose G K, and Farmer I R 1978 The Orlau swivel walker. Prosthetics and Orthotics International 2: 35–42

Stone E, Pinney R 1978 Orthopaedics for Nurses. London: Ballière Tindall

Turner J 1980 A case for careful handling. Nursing Mirror, 10 June

Waechter E H 1975 Developmental consequences of congenital abnormalities. Nursing Forum 14(2): 108–129

Weiner D S 1976 Congenital dislocation of the hip associated with congenital muscular torticollis. Clinical Orthopaedics and Related Research 121: 163–165

Williams E, Innes et al 1965 Urinary diversion in children. London: Nursing Mirror Symposium, 17 December, 1–5

Wilson J S P 1969 Some observations on the treatment of congenital abnormalities of the hand. The Hand 1: 63–66

Young D G, Weller B F 1971 Baby Surgery. London: Harvey Miller and Medcalf, 155–157

Younger N R 1978 Children in hospital. Nursing Times, 16 March, Paediatric News, 5

15

Growth disorders

DEFORMITIES OF THE SPINE, THE HIP, THE KNEE AND THE FOOT

Disorders which occur during the growth period are frequently seen in orthopaedic practice. Some of these conditions are initiated by a congenital lesion, e.g. scoliosis associated with a wedged vertebra, while others follow disease, e.g. the kyphos of Pott's disease of the spine (Ch. 16), or injury, e.g. growth arrest of epiphyses of limb bones. Other disorders are due to muscle imbalance, e.g. the short leg of poliomyelitis, while some are idiopathic, i.e. the cause is unknown; these include Perthes' disease and many cases of scoliosis, genu valgum, hallux valgus, and muscular dystrophy. Finally, certain diseases during growth are due to dietary deficiencies, e.g. rickets; or to endocrine disorders, e.g. cretinism and gigantism; or to metabolic disease, e.g. renal rickets.

THE SPINE

The spine is an organ of great flexibility, subservient to the motor functions of the whole body. Its mechanical function can be summarised as follows:

1. It is a sustaining rod, maintaining the upright position, and carrying the weight of the body.
2. It is an anchorage for powerful muscles, not only for those of the trunk, but for those of the shoulder and pelvic girdles.
3. It is a buffer spring receiving in endless and rapid

sequence innumerable jars and jolts associated with the function of the body.

4. It is a casing of safety for the spinal cord and nerves.

Disorders of the spine during growth include the following: spondylolisthesis; kyphosis; lordosis; and scoliosis.

A. SCOLIOSIS

Scoliosis comes from the Greek meaning 'a curvature of the spine'. It is now used specifically for lateral spinal curvatures of the spine in excess of 10 degrees. The pathological description is clear; scoliosis is seen as deformed vertebrae where the vertebral body shifts towards the convexity of the curve and the spinous processes deviate towards the concave side (Fig. 15.1). If the deformity involves the thoracic spine the result is a diminution of the entire volume of the thoracic cage leading

ultimately to respiratory impairment. The spinal deformity will be reflected in a distortion of the spinal canal itself which may be responsible for cord compression, particularly in congenital curvatures.

Scoliotic deformities are classified according to their magnitude, direction, location and aetiology. 90 per cent of scoliosis is so-called idiopathic; treatment thus remains empirical and speculative. There are two basic points to remember; (i) the younger the patient the worse the prognosis, and (ii) curves which rapidly deteriorate and/or are painful will need surgery.

School screening

Prevention is better than cure and the recently popular schoolscreening programmes which were started in North America over 20 years ago and introduced first to the United Kingdom in 1976 involve the routine survey of all children in the age group 10–14 by use of the Forward Bending Test (Fig. 15.2). A positive incidence of 3 per cent is observed which compares exactly with the overall results from North America. The screening is

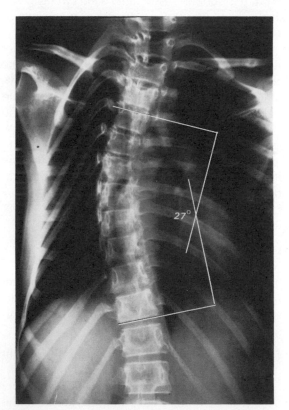

Fig. 15.1 Radiograph showing a typical scoliosis curve; the extent of the curve is measured by the Cobb method.

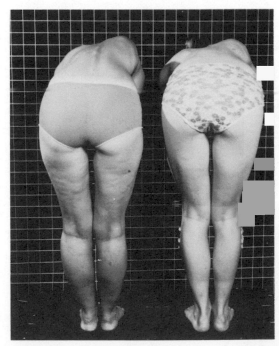

Fig. 15.2 The forward-bending test. Two sisters both with a 'positive' result. Note the uneven rib hump.

carried out in schools by visiting community nurses or physical education teachers who have been trained to assess asymmetry of the spine and trunk with the child bending forward. Children with so-called 'positive forward bending tests' are asked to attend a hospital clinic where they will be seen by a doctor and if necessary a radiograph will be taken. This is the most vulnerable age group for scoliosis precipitated by the growth spurt. The introduction of school screening has meant that children with adolescent idiopathic scoliosis are detected earlier.

Team-work

This is essential to maintain close links with the families involved from their first appearance at the clinic, which may be traumatic and frightening, through the general conservative care and, if all else fails, into surgical treatment and post-operative care. Most of the general public are uninformed about scoliosis and need positive education and reassurance if the treatment programme is going to work. Many spinal centres now produce a book-let informing the child and the family about scolio-sis and what may happen at every stage.

The curve

There are three main types of scoliotic curve which account for most cases of scoliosis:

    idiopathic
    paralytic
    congenital

However, there are numerous less well known causes of scoliosis: neurofibromatosis, metabolic bone disease, osteogenesis imperfecta and others.

Idiopathic scoliosis

Idiopathic means 'of unknown pathology' and there is no obvious reason for the onset of this sco-liosis which is the largest group in scoliosis. The sub groups are classified according to the age of onset of the curvature.

Infantile (onset birth to 3 years)

This is rare in North America but common in the United Kingdom. In 85 per cent of cases there is spontaneous resolution without treatment. Mostly male children are affected, and the curve is to the left side. A major area of concern is the progressive form of infantile scoliosis where the curve con-tinues to deteriorate relentlessly in spite of bracing. In some cases surgery will be necessary to prevent inevitable serious deterioration.

Juvenile (onset between 3 and 10 years)

The prognosis is poor in this group as they have had a longer period of growth and development in which to deform and deteriorate (spinal defor-mity tends to deteriorate maximally during the growth spurt).

The management of these patients, if the curve is severe enough, is by bracing. This should delay the need for fusion; however it is sometimes essen-tial to fuse the spine in order to prevent a severe deformity. Fusion at an early age will result in a shortened stature at maturity as it eliminates growth over the fused segments.

There is currently an encouraging surgical deve-lopment in the form of subcutaneous rodding of these immature curves without simultaneous fusion. This requires occasional lengthening of the rods so that the spine is kept straight and vertebral growth can continue with the child held in a well fitting brace. Although it is a recent advance the results are promising for such a difficult problem.

Adolescent (onset between 10 to 20 years)

More effective school screening programmes result in earlier detection of scoliosis in this group. Most are treated by bracing and few need surgery.

Adult (onset over 20 years)

Scoliosis may occur in the older age group as a result of disc degeneration. Mild scoliosis, if present, is said to deteriorate at the rate of one degree a year. An acute deterioration, that is up to 20 degrees in a year, is occasionally seen associ-ated with pregnancy.

Adults often have several other problems not seen in the younger age groups. Severe pain in the lumbar scoliosis may be the reason why the patient seeks medical attention. Scoliosis in the adult is associated with an increased incidence of respiratory impairment and a higher rate of complications if surgery is required.

Paralytic scoliosis

The three commonest causes of paralytic scoliosis are:

poliomyelitis
cerebral palsy
spina bifida

Post-poliomyelitis scoliosis. The vaccines of Salk and Sabin have dramatically reduced this disease, although it still remains very common in the Third World. 25 per cent of children affected with paralytic poliomyelitis will develop a scoliosis. This is a serious problem as it is inevitably progressive (muscle imbalance) and it has the associated problems of pelvic obliquity, limb paralysis, severe deformity and respiratory impairment.

Cerebral palsy has a commonly associated scoliosis due to muscle imbalance, and surgery should be considered if it will improve the child's level of function.

Spina bifida scoliosis is common. The curvature is complicated by the associated anaesthetic skin below the neurological deficit and in some cases with a paralytic bowel and bladder.

Congenital scoliosis

Most congenital curvatures are apparent and visible at birth. Some milder congenital anomalies, however, may not appear until much later, usually at the time of the adolescent growth spurt. There is a high incidence of associated genito-urinary abnormality and lesions within the spinal canal such as fibrous bands, diastematomyelia, etc. The use of a brace in these curves is ineffective and if the curve has been demonstrated to progress, surgery will be required.

The curve

1. The extent of the curve is recorded in degrees and measured by the Cobb method (Fig. 15.1). It is commonly regarded as significant if it measures 10 degrees or more. All surgeons would regard curves measuring over 60 degrees as an absolute indication for surgery. Complications with respiratory impairment are usually apparent with thoracic curves over 60 degrees.

2. Curvature can be convex to the left or right side or in the case of a double curve it will be left and right-sided. For reasons not fully apparent 90 per cent of adolescent curves are convex to the right side and most commonly seen in females.

3. Scoliotic curves are named from the apex of the curvature, namely:

Cervical scoliosis, apex between C1 and C6
Cervico-thoracic scoliosis, apex at the cervico-thoracic junction
Thoracic scoliosis, apex between T2 and T11
Thoraco-lumbar scoliosis, apex at the thoraco-lumbar junction
Lumbar scoliosis, apex between L2 and L4
Lumbo-sacral scoliosis, apex at the lumbo-sacral joint

A curve may thus be described as 'idiopathic, right-sided thoraco-lumbar scoliosis measuring 60 degrees'.

Curve progression and the iliac apophysis

Scoliosis deteriorates most rapidly during the period of spinal growth. The cessation of spinal growth coincides with completion of growth of the iliac apophysis (Fig. 15.3). It usually takes about one year from the time the iliac apophysis appears at the front of the iliac crest on the radiograph until the time it completes its growth in the posterior part of the iliac crest. This is known as the Risser sign. Risser '5' indicates complete fusion of the iliac apophysis and this coincides with the completion

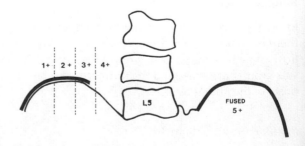

Fig. 15.3　Risser method of assessing maturity of the spine.

of spinal growth which usually indicates the end of significant rapid deterioration of the deformity.

Clinical management—conservative

The assessment of the patient with scoliosis will include a detailed case history with physical examination, appropriate radiological examination of the spine and myelography when indicated (all cases of congenital scoliosis).

1. Observation

If the curve is mild (say less than 20 degrees) then a half-yearly clinical appointment for radiograph and clinical photograph will be adequate in the first instance.

2. Brace management

Brace management will be decided when the curve is of the appropriate aetiology and not severe enough to warrant surgery. Bracing may in some cases be used to hold the child's spine until he

is a more suitable age for surgery (Fig. 15.4A,B, and C). When the curve is not suitable for bracing or when the brace is not tolerated by the patient, or, occasionally, when he refuses to wear the brace, then surgical correction and fusion will be required.

Again a team approach is vital for the assessment of the child; depending upon the decision of the surgeon regarding the nature and level of the curve either a Milwaukee or Boston brace is used. If a Milwaukee brace is prescribed following casting and preliminary fitting as an out-patient, the child is admitted to hospital for final fitting of the brace and to learn from the physiotherapists how to do the brace exercises proficiently. Over the next 5 days, there is gradual increase of usage aiming at a total of 23 hours a day, the brace only being removed for bathing.

The Boston braces are modular and can be selected off the shelf in the out-patients. In many centres these are often fitted in out-patients and the child and parents instructed in skin care and appropriate exercises at that time (Fig. 15.5).

For both the braces all normal activities are to

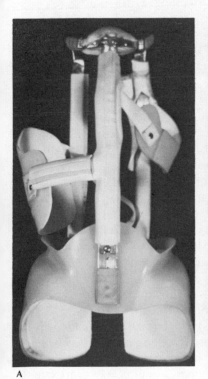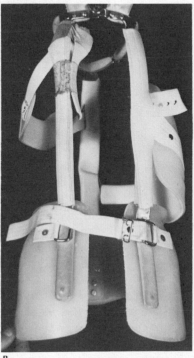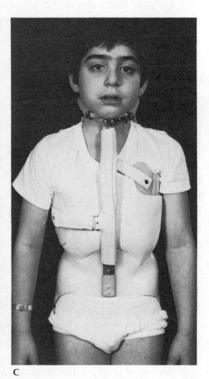

A   B   C

Fig. 15.4 The Milwaukee brace. **A.** Anterior view. **B.** Posterior view. **C.** Fittted.

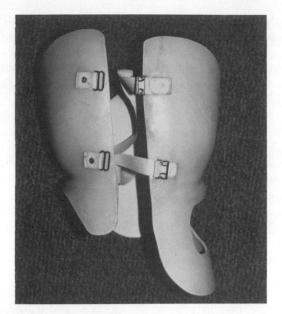

Fig. 15.5 The Boston brace. This is a most recent development in scoliosis bracing and is very well tolerated by the patient because she does not require the brace extending underneath the jaw and the back of the head.

be strongly encouraged so that the patient does not feel a freak; with a well-fitting brace and fashionable clothes the brace should almost be unnoticeable.

Clinical management–surgery

Surgical procedures for scoliosis

Indications for surgery

Cord compression
Progression of the curve
Pain
Respiratory impairment
Cosmetic

The use of preliminary traction

There are two forms of spinal traction; skeletal and non-skeletal, depending on whether pins are used in the skull and lower limbs or pelvis to achieve strong traction. It is important to remember that traction not only stretches and corrects the deformed spine but it also stretches the spinal cord

and therefore when traction is used it must be monitored with regular neurological assessment.

The various forms of spinal skeletal traction include halo-femoral traction, halo-pelvic traction (see Sister Redempta's account) and halo-wheelchair traction (Fig. 15.6), the latter because it is

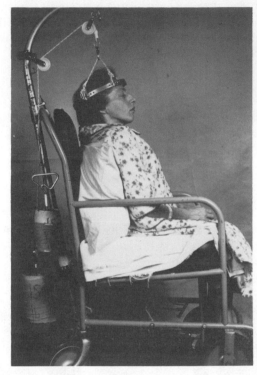

Fig. 15.6 The halo-wheelchair traction.

well tolerated by the patient and is becoming increasingly popular. The non-skeletal traction system most common is that developed by Dr Yves Cotrel.

With halo-femoral traction, it is essential that the lower limb joints be put through a full range of motion every day, especially the hip joints, in order to avoid avascular necrosis. Strong forces being applied to the hip joints distract the hip joint, probably interfering with its blood supply, and over a period of several weeks this is likely to produce avascular changes in the femoral head with resulting hip stiffness and significant disability.

Pre-operative skeletal traction should only be used when indicated because of the risks involved. In lesser degrees of deformity there is little to be gained with preliminary traction. A typical example of a case which would benefit from preliminary traction would be a paralytic scolosis measuring 100 degrees, associated with pelvic obliquity.

Methods of surgical fusion of the spine include:

1. *Posterior fusion only* (without correction). This may be considered when correction of the curve is regarded as dangerous, for example, some mild curves with diastematomyelia (a bony spur within the spinal canal). Most surgeons would prefer to fuse the spine and use internal fixation, for example, a Harrington Rod, without gaining correction but using the rod as an internal splint to encourage healing of the bone grafts.

Fusion without fixation may be considered in the young child under 7 or 8 years where the implants themselves are too large for the soft neural arches. In these cases, the surgeon may consider fusing the spine and then obtaining correction one or two weeks later after surgery by a plaster technique using the traction table.

2. *Posterior instrumentation and fusion of the spine*. This is the most commonly accepted form of treatment for idiopathic scoliosis and the implant most commonly preferred is that designed by Harrington.

The principles of posterior fusion are as follows:

(a) A subperiosteal dissection to expose the entire length of the deformed spine.
(b) Insertion of hooks one or two levels above and below the spinal deformity.
(c) Removal of autogenous bone graft from the posterior aspect of one iliac crest.
(d) Removal of the facet joints over the length of spine to be fused and the addition of the supplementary bone graft.
(e) The addition of the Harrington rod using safe, corrective forces.
(f) The function of the spinal cord can be checked using the 'wake-up' test or by the increasingly popular spinal cord monitoring equipment.
(g) Application of a plaster of Paris jacket (using a traction table), to be worn until the spinal fusion is confirmed to be solid both by clinical and radiographic means. This usually means 6 to 9 months in a plaster jacket, changing the jacket at about 3 months.

3. *Luque instrumentation*. This is a new method which involves the use of two malleable rods and multiple wires affixing each lamina to the rods. The multi-level fixation does away with the necessity for post-operative plaster of Paris immobilisation; this has a very real benefit in patients with respiratory insufficiency such as those with muscular dystrophy (Fig. 15.8).

4. *Nylon straps*. This is a development from the Luque technique. The idea developed because of the danger of complications with the use of wires to hold the laminae. In Oswestry the wires have been replaced with strong plastic straps, which are easily laced beneath the posterior elements and avoid any complications with the spinal cord (Fig. 15.9).

5. *Posterior and anterior fusion*. For the more complex cases, such as paralytic scoliosis with pelvic obliquity, a combined posterior and anterior instrumentation is used; and sometimes if the curvature is severe, preliminary halo-pelvic or halo-femoral traction will be used. The anterior correction and fusion is done employing the screw and cable technique of Dwyer, and this is supple-

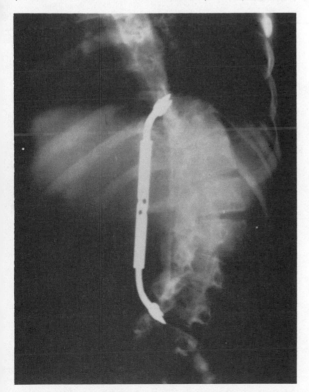

Fig. 15.7 Radiograph showing posterior instrumentation and fusion of the spine using 'Allen Jack' instrumentation.

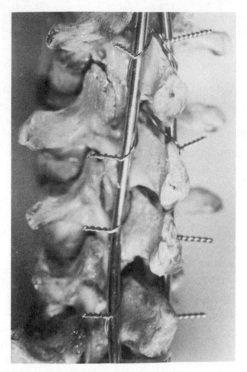

Fig. 15.8 Model of spine with Luque instrumentation.

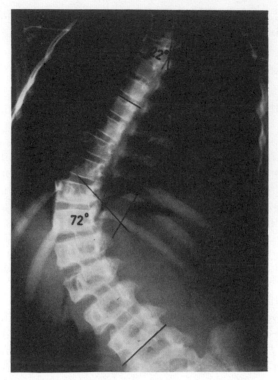

Fig. 15.10 Radiograph showing pre-operative paralytic scoliosis.

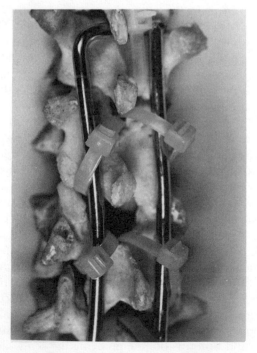

Fig. 15.9 Model of spine nylon straps in position.

mented two weeks later by an extensive posterior fusion with a Harrington rod. The Dwyer operation involves the radical removal of the intervertebral discs, and this mobilises the curve significantly so that greater correction of the deformity is obtainable than by the use of a posterior instrumentation alone. The combined Dwyer and Harrington rod technique is particularly successful when deformity is associated with pelvic obliquity and this is commonly seen in paralytic scoliosis (Figs 15.10 and 15.11).

B. KYPHOSIS

A kyphosis is less common than a scoliosis but in some types it is more dangerous because it is very likely to progress and, in some instances, to compress the spinal cord with resulting paraplegia.

The general shape of a kyphosis may be:

(a) a gradual roundback deformity as with ankylosing spondylitis, or

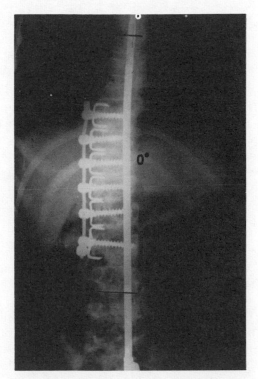

Fig. 15.11 Radiograph of same patient as Fig. 10 showing correction of the paralytic scoliosis by combined anterior and posterior instrumentation and fusion using a Harrington Rod and the Dwyer screw and cable instrumentation.

(b) acute or hunchback deformity as with tuberculosis of the spine (Fig. 15.12).

A simple classification of kyphosis is as follows:

Gradual curvature

1. These include adolescent kyphosis which is a result of wedging of the vertebral bodies during the phase of growth and is usually confined to the thoracic spine.

2. Scheuermann's disease is also commonly seen in the thoracic spine and is obvious in the adolescent with a round back deformity. The radiograph will demonstrate abnormal changes in the vertebral growth plate.

3. Ankylosing spondylitis. A syndrome commonly seen by rheumatologists in its early stages, but as the spinal curvature progresses and the patient is no longer able to look forwards and there may also be spinal pain, the matter will be referred to a surgeon for surgery. Correction of these defor-

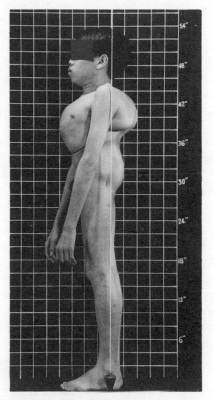

Fig. 15.12 Patient with severe tuberculous kyphosis.

mities usually transforms the patient who can now look people in the eye, will have regained some height and the sense of balance will have been restored.

4. Acute angulation of the spine is seen in tuberculosis of the spine and in congenital kyphosis (hunchback deformity). Any pathological process causing destruction or absence of part or all of the vertebral bodies will produce a kyphosis (a kyphosis is, by definition, a shortening of the anterior column of the spine-vertebral bodies and intervertebral discs).

5. There are a range of syndromes which may produce kyphosis: the most common is senile osteoporosis where there is a gradual collapse of the vertebral bodies with an increasing curvature. These patients may have significant pain from collapse of the cancellous bone of the bodies.

Treatment of kyphosis

1. *Bracing*—is most effective in the treatment of Scheuermann's disease, the appropriate brace

holds the spine in an extended position, thus unloading the growth plates and allowing them to recover from the abnormal growth pressures. In other types of scoliosis bracing is not effective.

2. *Surgical treatment of kyphosis.* A progressive kyphosis is likely to compress the spinal cord (Fig. 15.13); thus myelography is an essential investigation.

In the whole field of kyphotic deformity it is the congenital and tubercular lesions which are most likely to lead to severe problems because of spinal cord involvement. The principles of treatment for these acutely angled kyphotic deformities are:

(a) Detailed preliminary investigations including respiratory function tests and myelography.
(b) Spinal cord decompression through an anterior surgical approach when compression has been indicated with preliminary investigations.
(c) Correction of the deformity if this is safe and feasible. This may mean gradual controlled

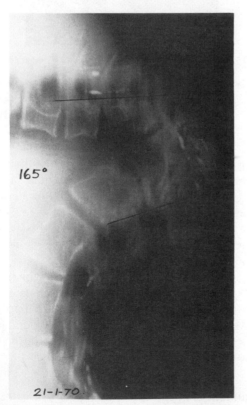

165°

21-1-70

Fig. 15.13 Radiograph of patient in Fig. 15.12. *Note* vertebral body destruction and cord compression at the apex of the deformity.

traction over several weeks using some system already referred to in the section on scoliosis.
(d) Final stabilisation of the spine using bone grafts in order to preserve the correction of the kyphosis obtained with traction.

These deformities are most commonly seen in the thoracic spine where there will be inevitable impairment of respiratory function and where the spinal cord is most vulnerable. This group presents one of the most difficult problems in spinal deformity work.

C. SPONDYLOLISTHESIS

An unusual deformity in adolescents is spondylolisthesis or dislocation of the lumbo-sacral joint. All degrees of forward shift of the body of L5 on the first sacral body may occur, but spondylolisthesis refers mainly to congenital maldevelopment of the neural arch of L5. The end result is a grotesque posture, kyphosis at the lumbo-sacral joint and significant anterior trunk shift. There are often serious neurological problems because of the compression of the nerve roots at the lumbo-sacral level. Some of these patients may have minimal deformity and little pain; others are severely disabled with pain and severe deformity.

The surgical treatment generally recommended for severe spondylolisthesis of lumbar 5 in the adolescent is fusion in situ, in other words, accepting the deformity and obtaining stability through arthrodesis. Recent efforts in Oswestry have been aimed at the safe correction of the deformity, reduction of the dislocation and fusion of the lumbo-sacral joint. This new surgical technique includes the following stages:

1. Laminectomy of L5 with simultaneous lateral fusion of L5 to the sacrum (McPhee & O'Brien, 1979).
2. A period of skull femoral traction lasting 10 to 14 days with regular detailed neurological observation because of the possible risk of injury to the lumbo-sacral nerve roots. The reduction is achieved by hyperextension combined with longitudinal pull. The degree of elevation of the trunk platform is determined by radiographs. Gravitational oedema may be a problem, and

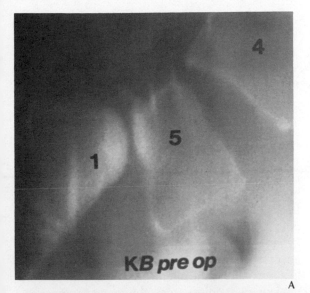

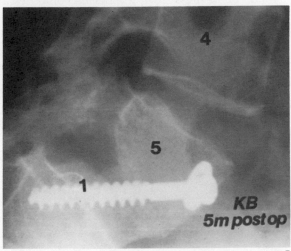

Fig. 15.14 A, B. A. Pre-operative lateral radiograph showing severe spondylolisthesis Grade 4. **B.** Post-operative lateral radiograph showing reduction and fusion of the spondylolisthesis.

support stockings should be worn as well as intensive ankle and knee movements being encouraged. The traction is removed twice daily for vigorous exercises to be given to the lower limbs; hip flexion beyond 60 degrees must be avoided.

3. When reduction has been achieved, removal of the lumbo-sacral disc through an anterior approach and its replacement with bone graft from the iliac crest (Fig. 15.14A and B). The

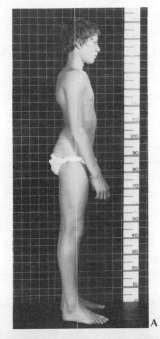

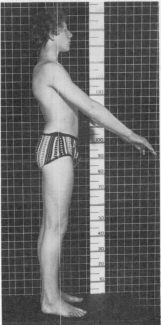

Fig. 15.15 A, B. A. Pre-operative photograph of patient with spondylolisthesis. **B.** Post-operative photograph of same patient.

available evidence suggests that the spine then grows straight (Fig. 15.15A and B).

Clinical features may be minimal with the patient complaining of slight low back pain; on examination it is often possible to palpate the 'step' due to forward displacement. Surgical measures are advised.

4. Post-operatively the patient is log rolled for about 10 days after which a plaster of Paris jacket is applied; to be worn for a minimum of 6 months until fusion is radiographically solid.

D. TORTICOLLIS

Torticollis occurs with congenital spinal abnormalities, fibrous shortening of the sterno-mastoid muscle or severe infections of the throat which is just anterior to the upper part of the cervical spine.

The treatment will depend on the cause of the deformity in which the head is twisted and rotated to one side (Fig. 15.16). The diagnosis is made after

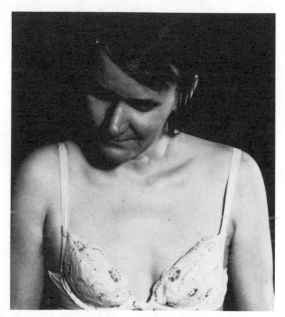

Fig. 15.16 Patient with torticollis.

detailed history and a good clinical examination. Radiographs of the cervical spine will demonstrate the presence of a congenital deformity which may be corrected with spine surgery but this is extremely risky. Shortening of the sterno-mastoid is the commonest cause of torticollis and the tight bands can be easily felt and divided at surgery.

Infections in the throat may soften the ligaments uniting the atlas to the axis and lead to displacement of this joint, a condition which was common in Hong Kong and led to the development of surgery of the upper cervical spine through the mouth approach.

Patients are maintained in a neck collar until the fusion is radiographically solid.

Treatment by means of halo-pelvic traction

(This account was written by Sister Redempta, Ward Sister, Duchess of Kent Hospital, Sandy Bay, Hong Kong.) The halo-pelvic device is a form of external skeletal fixation by means of which traction can be put on the spine between two fixed points. It is used in the correction of scoliotic and kyphotic deformities of the spine. As well as achieving correction by traction, it also serves to maintain fixation of the spine after fusion.

Made of stainless steel, the device comprises a halo, which is attached to the skull by means of four threaded pins; a pelvic hoop, to which are attached the two pelvic pins which transfix both iliac crests; four extension bars, attached to the halo above and to the pelvic hoop below (Fig. 15.17A and B).

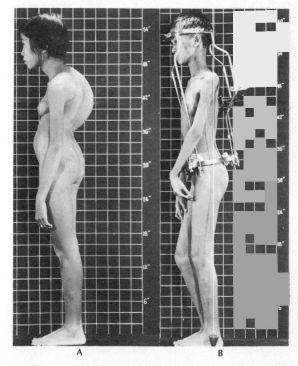

Fig. 15.17 A, B. (See text.) (with kind permission of the *Nursing Times* and Dr J. O'Brien.)

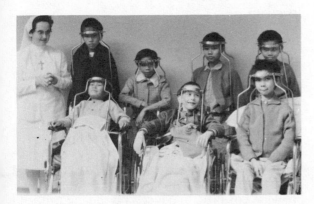

Fig. 15.17 C shows the writer of this section with some of her patients. (With kind permission of the *Nursing Times* and Dr J. O'Brien.)

Investigations. Before application of the device, several routine investigations and procedures are carried out. They include, measurement of the patient for the device, clinical photography, X-rays, myelography, tomography, respiratory function assessment, dental examination, shaving the head. These investigations necessitate the admission of the patient a week or so in advance of the application. This has the advantage of giving him time to grow accustomed to the apparatus, seeing it on other patients. It is also a valuable time for the nursing staff, who should try to put the patient at his ease by explaining the nature, purpose and advantages of the halo-pelvic apparatus to him.

Application. The apparatus is fitted under general anaesthesia, endotracheal intubation being necessary. First the halo is attached by means of four pins which pierce the outer cortex of the skull. Using the torque screw-driver a force of 2.5 kg is exerted on each pin thus firmly fixing it in the skull. The pelvic pins are inserted with a hand brace. They are attached to the pelvic hoop by means of special fittings. Finally the extension bars are added. They attach to the halo by means of Allen screws, and to the pelvic hoop by means of special screws there for that purpose. The whole fitting takes about half an hour.

Nursing care. Patients whose rib hump or kyphus projects beyond the posterior extension bars are better nursed on a bed of foam-rubber sections, the adjustment of which allow him to lie supine without any pressure on the deformity. A pillow is used to support the legs and two to support the arms when in this position. A very small pillow is placed behind the neck, in front of the posterior extension bars. The patient may also lie on either side.

For the first day or two the patient may feel rather frightened in his rigid frame. No matter how well prepared he is, it is nearly always frightening to the patient to discover that he cannot move his neck or bend his back. In some patients, especially children, vomiting is not an uncommon feature during the first 24 hours after the application. By the third day the patient is accustomed to his appliance, and even feels secure in it.

After 24 hours, the patient may sit out of bed, and by the following day he is able to walk. The fact that the patient can walk while in the device is a great advantage over other forms of spinal traction, e.g. distraction casts, halo-femoral traction and such. It dispels at once any feeding or toilet problems, and the possibility of pressure sores does not arise. It is of special advantage in the case of children, to whom long weeks in bed are tedious. The halo-pelvic device does not prevent them from attending school, and they are able to enter into nearly all the fun and games of their companions.

The pin-holes are dressed daily, using Cetremide 1 per cent and an antibiotic spray. The hair around the occipital pins is kept cut close to the skull. Small keyhole dressings are put on the pelvic pin-holes. All the nuts and screws on the apparatus are checked daily, as any movement predisposes to infection. Any looseness of the pins is reported and dealt with immediately. If infection of the pins does occur, a swab is taken for culturing, and the patient is put on a course of antibiotics. In some cases it may be necessary to change a pin. For this reason a supply of sterile halo pins should always be at hand. The halo pin may be changed in the ward under local anaesthetic. The changing of the pelvic pin will of course require a general anaesthetic.

Distraction. Several days after the application, distraction of the spine is begun. Sometimes a posterior release or vertebral osteotomy is required first, and in this case distraction is postponed until the wound is healed. Distraction is carried out by screwing nuts on the extension bars with a wrench, at the level of the pelvic hoop. The usual rate of distraction is a twelfth of an inch daily. The time and amount of distraction are noted and a record kept. Close surveillance of the patient is of major importance throughout the period of distraction, and it calls for good team work among the staff.

Daily neurological investigations are carried out. Any signs of spasticity, hand weakness or jerky gait (signs which are indicative of cord traction) are at once reported and traction stopped. The patient is also examined for a squint, which could occur due to lateral rectus muscle palsy, X-rays of the spine are taken every third day to see the correction being realised.

In order to reduce the rotation aspect of a scoliotic deformity, a pressure pad which attaches to the posterior extension bars may be applied. Force on the rib hump is increased daily through this attachment. It may also be used on those patients with a kyphotic deformity. In order to avoid skin necrosis pressure is released one hour in every three. Distraction is continued until the maximum correction is reached or until the patient starts complaining of continuing neck pain. When this happens the sternomastoids are seen to be very taut on either side, and may be in spasm. In this case tension is reduced by shortening the bars.

Full correction having been achieved the patient is ready for spinal fusion.

Fusion of the spine. The posterior extension bars are removed to allow access to the spine for posterior fusion. In some cases further correction may be realised post-operatively by continuing distraction. The patient is left in the apparatus until the fusion is solid. Daily pin-hole dressings and checks are carried out as usual. Within a week or so of having his spine fused, the patient is ambulant and able to continue a normal daily routine. The halo-pelvic device maintains rigid immobility of the spine, allowing the fusion to knit. It is of great advantage to those patients with poor respiratory reserve.

When the fusion is intact, the halo-pelvic apparatus is removed with the patient anaesthetised. The most usual complaint, and usually the only one, after removal of traction, is neck pain. A felt collar may be worn until the patient becomes accustomed to spinal mobility again. He is nursed flat in bed for a few days, and dressings are applied to the pin-holes, which dry in a matter of days. He is then ready for home.

THE HIP

COXA VARA

The normal adult femur presents an angle between the femoral neck and shaft of between 120 degrees and 140 degrees. In coxa vara, this angle is decreased. There is depression of the femoral neck, normal opposition of joint surfaces is lost, and the femoral head becomes ill-fitting. The great trochanter is displaced upwards and there is limitation of abduction and internal rotation at the hip joint. Bilateral coxa vara produces a waddling gait, and a dip to the affected side is present in unilateral cases. There may be real shortening of the limb, with external rotation deformity.

Coxa vara may be *congenital* or *acquired*.

Congenital or *infantile coxa vara* is due to constitutional or development diseases, such as achondroplasia.

Acquired coxa vara may be due to the following conditions:

1. Rickets, or other bone dystrophies.
2. Separation of the upper femoral epiphysis (adolescent coxa vara).
3. Other causes include fracture of the femoral neck, or osteotomy for osteoarthritis of the hip.

Treatment of the congenital type may be by osteotomy. The acquired type requires treatment according to the cause.

Coxa valga is present if the femoral neck-shaft angle is increased. It occurs in congenital dislocation of the hip, and in conditions where there is muscular imbalance.

PERTHES' DISEASE
(Legge-Calve-Perthes' Disease, Pseudo-Coxalgia, Quiet Hip Disease)

This is an affection of the upper femoral epiphysis occurring mostly in boys between the ages of 5 and 10 years. It may be unilateral or bilateral, and is characterised by certain changes in the femoral head and neck. It is thought that these changes are due to impairment of the blood-supply to the femoral head. The cause is unknown. Other conditions which predispose to such damage to the femoral epiphysis include femoral neck fracture, septic arthritis of the hip, and forcible manipulation of a congenital dislocation of the hip joint.

Symptoms and signs

The general health and vigour is unimpaired. A limp is usually the first thing to be noticed, and is of a carefree 'stomping' nature, as opposed to the painful hesitant limp which occurs in true inflammation of the hip joint. Pain is not a marked symptom, though it is usually present in some degree and may be referred to the knee. On examination, there will be limitation of *abduction* and *internal rotation*, as opposed to infective lesions of the hip joint in which there is limitation of *all* movements. In addition, pain and muscle spasm is never so marked. In cases of very long standing, there may be flexion contracture of the hip joint.

X-ray changes

Serial X-rays of a typical case of Perthes' disease will show three stages:

1. Sclerosis.
2. Fragmentation and mushrooming.
3. Recalcification and healing.

The three stages merge gradually into each other, and the whole disease process, from the time of onset to complete recalcification, is thought to occupy from two to three years. Most cases are treated in hospital for at least two years.

Stage 1: Sclerosis. In early Perthes' disease, the femoral head will be of *increased density* in the X-ray film. This is due to the impairment of the blood supply with local death of the head. Increased density on an X-ray is described as 'sclerosis'. There may be flattening and broadening of the femoral head, and, sometimes, changes in the neck and acetabulum.

Stage 2: Fragmentation and mushrooming. As the blood supply begins to be re-established, islands of rarefaction appear in the dense bone, giving it a moth-eaten appearance. If weight is borne on the femoral head, gross flattening and distortion will occur, which is aptly named 'mushrooming' (Fig. 11.11).

Stage 3: Recalcification and healing. The blood supply is re-established and the areas of rarefaction and sclerosis are gradually replaced by normal bone.

Treatment

This is aimed at the prevention or correction of deformity, and the preservation of the normal contours and function of the hip joint. The initial treatment consists of bed rest and skin traction until the presenting pain and muscle spasm have disappeared. This takes two or three weeks in the majority of patients. Subsequent treatment varies according to the X-ray signs and surgeon's wishes.

There are two treatment principles, which are sometimes used in combination. The first is the prevention of weightbearing and relief of pressure on the affected femoral head. The second principle is called 'containment', and consists of placing the damaged portion of the femoral head fully into the acetabulum. This acts as a mould which retains the spherical shape of the head.

1. *Recumbency without traction.* Some surgeons maintain that to keep the child off his feet is sufficient, but as the period of recumbency must necessarily be uninterrupted and prolonged in any case, some form of splintage is usually ordered (Fig. 15.20).

2. *Recumbency with traction.* In early cases, prolonged fixation and traction followed by re-education usually produces a very satisfactory end-result. Even in cases where treatment has been instituted very late, a good functional result is to be expected. If, however, there is gross flattening and distortion of the femoral head with disorganisation of joint surfaces, arthritic changes most certainly will supervene in later life, giving rise to such pain and stiffness as to necessitate arthrodesis or arthroplasty of the hip. (a) *Jones double abduction frame* with skin extensions is occasionally ordered. The application and nursing care is exactly the same as that described in Ch. 10. The degree of abduction is decided by the surgeon. Frame fixation is usually continued until pain and spasm have disappeared (perhaps 3 to 6 months) and sometimes, until revascularisation of the femoral head is established (generally 18 months to 2 years) when the patient is either allowed free in bed, with the legs

supported on pillows; or some less stringent form of fixation is substituted for the frame. (b) *Pugh's traction*. This is applied and nursed as described in Ch. 9.

3. *Thomas patten-ended caliper* (Fig. 15.18). A pattern (usually 7.5 cm at the heel sloping to 5 cm

They are applied in full abduction and internal rotation in order to contain the head fully in the acetabulum. It is thought that the recalcifying femoral head is moulded by the movement of the pelvis on the femora as the patient sits up (Fig. 15.19A, B).

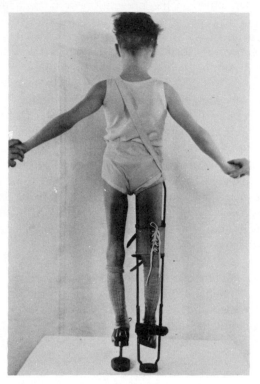

Fig. 15.18 Thomas patten-ended caliper.

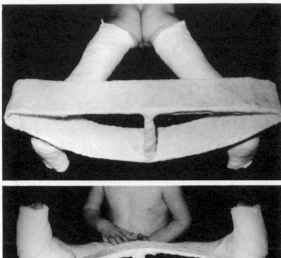

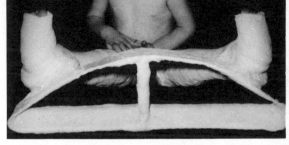

Fig. 15.19 A, B. Broomstick plaster.

at the sole) is applied to the boot of the unaffected side. It should compensate exactly for the length of the caliper. Apply as for a walking caliper. See that the knee is properly supported and that the affected limb hangs free in the splint. Fasten the webbing band on the opposite shoulder.

Daily care. Care of the skin under the ring as for an ordinary caliper. Watch the patient closely for signs of scoliosis, as this quickly develops due to the pull of the webbing band on the shoulder.

At first, standing and walking are taught by a physiotherapist, correct balance is first taught, followed by re-education in walking. Exercises and games are continued throughout.

4. *Broomstick plasters*. These are occasionally ordered in those cases in which the femoral head has commenced to 'flow' out of the acetabulum.

Application. Well-moulded plasters are applied to both legs from the toes to the groin, and fixed to a broomstick by means of a plaster bandage. Sitting-up is gradually introduced, and flexion of the hip joint regained.

Nursing care. The plasters are inspected daily for cracks and for signs of pressure-sores. Broomstick plasters can give rise to certain complications unless the patient is nursed with unceasing vigilance.

1. *Scoliosis*. If the child sits up unsupervised or too soon, he will rotate the pelvis forwards on the unaffected side, due to limitation of flexion in the affected hip. A curve of the lumbar spine will then follow, with a compensatory thoracic curve above, and scoliosis results.

2. *Kyphosis*. The general musculature is always weak after frame-fixation. If sitting-up is unsu-

pervised and the back muscles are not strong enough to maintain the upright position, the child crouches in bed and a kyphosis results.

3. *Lordosis* may be compensatory to kyphosis or flexion contracture of the hip, or to stretching and weakness of the abdominal muscles.

4. *Flexion contracture of the hip*. In the sitting position, the hip flexors are shortened and prolonged sitting in any splint will lead to contracture of these muscles.

5. *Genu recurvatum*. Some laxity of the knee joints is almost certain to occur, as the hamstrings are constantly on the stretch in the sitting position, but genu recurvatum can be largely prevented by the application of very carefully moulded plasters holding the knees in slight flexion.

6. *Genu valgum* or *genu varum* can be prevented by correctly moulded plasters.

7. *Foot deformities* can be prevented by correct moulding of the plasters and by free movement of the toes.

Exercises for the spinal, abdominal and gluteal muscles are practised intensively, and the patient should spent part of each day lying on his face (Fig. 15.19A). When flexion of the hip has been regained, the patient is allowed to kick free in bed with pillows under the knees, and is eventually allowed up with or without splintage.

For further information on physiotherapy for this condition, please see Ch. 12.

Convalescence. When recalcification of the femoral head is complete, all splintage is removed and the child allowed to kick free in bed, with a pillow under the knees to prevent hyperextension. Non-weight-bearing exercises for all muscle groups are practised, but kneeling or standing is strictly forbidden. When the musculature is good and the bone-texture of the femoral head is normal, weight-bearing is gradually introduced. A caliper is occasionally ordered, or, a Thomas patten-ended caliper as already described.

5. *Operative treatment* may consist of osteotomy of the femur (varus-derotation) or pelvis (Salter osteotomy) in order to contain the damaged portion of the femoral head fully in the acetabulum. Following boney union of the osteotomy, the child is usually allowed to weightbear normally and there are no constraints on hip movement.

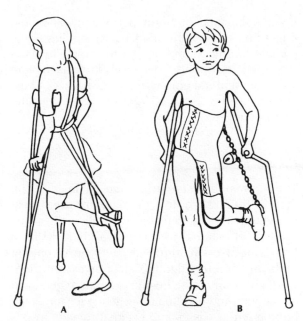

Fig. 15.20 **A.** The Snyder sling. When worn it provides total relief from compression of the hip joint but is only suitable for unilateral disease. **B.** The Birmingham splint. It is suitable for unilateral disease where containment of the hip is also required.

SLIPPED UPPER FEMORAL EPIPHYSIS
(Epiphyseal Coxa Vara)

This is a separation of the upper femoral epiphysis occurring mostly in boys and less commonly in girls, at or around the time of puberty, i.e. between the ages of 11 and 17. It is due to a disturbance of the complicated mechanism whereby the sex hormones are secreted by the gonads in response to the gonadotrophic hormone in the anterior lobe of the pituitary, which at the same time also secretes the growth hormone. At puberty, these hormones are both active since growth is rapid and at the same time the sexual characteristics are beginning to appear. In some patients who present with slipped epiphysis, there is a lesion of the pituitary gland itself, resulting in obesity and delay in development of the sexual characteristics—Fröhlich syndrome. Some patients are overweight and sexually infantile—the 'Fröhlich type'—or there may be overgrowth of the skeleton indicating over-activity of the growth hormone. On the other hand, many patients appear quite normal and the level of development is normal for their age.

An imbalance of hormonal activity, therefore might be due either to inadequate supplies of the gonado-trophic hormone, or to over-activity of the growth hormone. This results in weakening of the upper femoral epiphysis so that it slips and the femoral head is displaced from the shaft to a greater or lesser degree.

Clinical features

The slip may be *acute* or *gradual*. In an acute slip there is usually a history of injury and the patient presents with a painful hip which is held in the position of external rotation. In a gradual slip, a limp is the first symptom, with pain which is present in the hip or referred to the knee; on examination, the hip is found to be held in external rotation and abduction, and on attempting gentle flexion of the hip the femur passes into external rotation as it is flexed. All movements are limited by muscle spasm and there may be real or apparent shortening.

X-rays are taken in both the antero-posterior and lateral planes. The articular surface of the femoral head is displaced downwards and backwards, and in advanced cases, it may lie loose in the acetabulum.

Treatment

The aims of treatment are to replace the displaced epiphysis, to maintain reduction until fusion takes place, and to retain the function of the joint.

Treatment is determined by the following factors:

1. The *degree* of separation.
2. The *duration* of the separation.

It may be conservative or operative.

Conservative treatment

1. Manipulative reduction followed by plaster fixation in the desired position.
2. Traction with internal rotation may be used alone as the patient lies in bed.

N.B. The sound hip is examined from time to time, as the epiphysis on that side is very likely to slip, even during immobilisation.

Operative treatment

This may consist of the following:

1. *Reduction and internal fixation.* Manipulation and insertion of Moore's pins, which are inserted in three different places across the epiphysis. Weight-bearing is not allowed for six weeks, and it is usual to remove the pins after fusion of the epiphysis to the metaphysis.
2. *Subtrochanteric osteotomy* may be advised in those cases in which fusion has occurred in deformed position.
3. *Arthrodesis* of the hip joint may be performed in those cases in which arthritis has supervened, as when interference with the blood supply has produced aseptic necrosis of the femoral head.

Later treatment. Recumbency is continued until reduction and fusion of the epiphysis has taken place. Exercises for the general musculature are commenced and weight-bearing is gradually introduced.

THE KNEE

GENU VALGUM

This deformity (knock-knee) is present when the medial malleoli cannot be brought together except by the knees overlapping each other (Fig. 15.21). The medial collateral ligament becomes stretched and the knees unstable. The degree of deformity is generally assessed by the amount of intermalleolar separation when the knees are in contact with each other.

Causes

These include the following:

1. Bad posture and gait.
2. Weak musculature.
3. Flat-foot, which alters the line of weight-bearing; knock-knee often accompanies weak valgoid feet in children.
4. Obesity.
5. Traumatic lesions, such as a sprain or fracture.
6. Poliomyelitis.
7. Rickets and other bone dystrophies.
8. Inflammatory lesions of the knee.

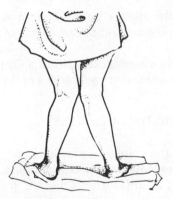

Fig. 15.21   Bilateral genu valgum.

9. Knock-knee may be secondary to flexion-adduction deformity of the hip, especially in patients wearing a short single spica.
10. A large number of cases are idiopathic.

Treatment

This is determined by the cause and by the degree of deformity. Attention to the general health and nutrition may be required, with avoidance of fatigue and over-exertion. Mild cases require inside raising to the heels of the shoes, and exercises. *The altered shoes are worn constantly. No other shoes are worn; weight-bearing without shoes is not permitted.* The object of the inside raising is to relieve the strain on the medial collateral ligament, and prevent overgrowth of the internal femoral condyle. Exercises are aimed at strengthening the musculature of the leg, particularly the quadriceps. Re-education in walking is essential.

A Girdlestone mermaid splint may be ordered (Kennedy, 1974).

Application. This splint is worn only at night. It is placed between the child's legs, a firm pad of wool is placed between the inner side of the knee joint and the splint, and the straps are fastened. The application is described by Kennedy (see Bibliography), who also describes an adaptation for bow-legs (genu varum). The limbs are covered with a piece of splint-wool and a firm bandage is applied around both legs and the splint between them. The bandage must extend to the groin and include the foot to the toes; it is essential that the legs and feet lie exactly parallel to each other and that the feet and patellae point straight forwards. External rotation of the limb results in loss of the corrective force. During the day, the patient wears altered shoes as already described.

Manipulation and plaster fixation. Successive plasters are applied, without anaesthesia, gaining more correction each time. Alternatively, wedged plasters may be used. This is followed by altered shoes, exercises, and re-education in walking.

Operative treatment usually consists of an osteotomy, followed by fixation in a bed-splint or a plaster spica. Sometimes staples are inserted into the epiphysis on the side of the deformity; they are removed when correction is obtained. Gross deformity due to paralysis or an inflammatory lesion, may require arthrodesis of the knee.

GENU VARUM

Genu varum (bow-leg) is present when both knees and both medial malleoli cannot be brought together. It may be confined to the tibia, or it may affect the whole leg (Fig. 15.22).

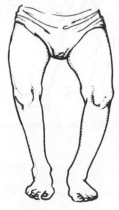

Fig. 15.22   Bilateral genu varum.

Causes

These include the following:

1. Bad posture and gait.
2. Rickets.
3. Diseases of bone such as osteomyelitis.
4. Injuries.

Treatment

Conservative treatment consists of manipulation without anaesthesia, and successive plasters;

wedged plasters may be ordered. Physiotherapy and re-education in walking is introduced when the plaster is discarded.

Operative treatment consists of an osteotomy at the site of election, and plaster fixation until union is sound. A stapling operation is sometimes advised.

GENU RECURVATUM

Genu recurvatum (back-knee) is present when the knee is hyper-extended (Fig. 15.23).

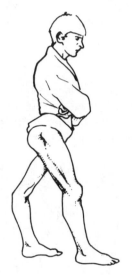

Fig. 15.23   Genu recurvatum of severe degree.

Causes

These include the following:

1. Generalised ligamentous laxity which allows joint hypermobility.
2. Weak musculature, especially following long periods in recumbency when the knee is inadequately supported.
3. Paralysis of the hamstrings, as in poliomyelitis.
4. Inflammatory lesions, such as tuberculosis.
5. Injuries to the knee joint.

Treatment

Exercises may be sufficient in mild cases. Splintage, such as caliper or knee-cage may be ordered. In nursing inflammatory lesions and injuries, special attention must be paid to *prevention* of this deformity.

Operative treatment consists of an osteotomy of the femur or tibia or an arthrodesis of the knee.

OTHER EPIPHYSEAL LESIONS

Lesions of the epiphyses may affect a single bone and be of unknown origin, or, multiple lesions may be present, as in Gaucher's disease, multiple epiphyseal dysplasia and haemoglobinopathies. The *cause* is often obscure, though there may be associated infection or metabolic disturbance, and there is sometimes a history of trauma; avascular necrosis as a complication of the treatment of congenital dislocation of the hip has already been mentioned.

Osteochondritis dissecans

This is a condition in which a small flake of bone becomes detached from the femoral condyle, or from some other part of the articular surface. More rarely, another joint is affected, e.g. the elbow joint.

Conservative treatment. So long as the fragment is not detached from its bed, immobilisation in a plaster cylinder for six to eight weeks may be advised.

Operative treatment may be required to remove a detached fragment or, to re-attach it in its bed by means of a needle (Smillie).

Osgood-Schlatter's disease

This is an osteochondritis of the epiphysis of the tibial tubercle, occurring mostly in boys in the 10 to 15 age group. It is nearly always associated with trauma or over-exertion. There is pain and difficulty in walking with oedema and local tenderness referred to the tibial tubercle. X-rays show fragmentation, and sometimes, separation of the epiphysis.

Treatment. In most cases the acute symptoms settle by avoiding strenuous physical activities for a few weeks. Minor residual symptoms usually remit at skeletal maturity. Very occasionally symptoms are troublesome and require rest in a plaster cylinder for several weeks.

Operative treatment may take the form of drilling of the epiphysis.

Köhlers disease

This is an osteochondritis of the tarsal navicular, and occurs mostly in boys of the 5 to 10 age group. There is pain in the foot, exaggerated by weight-bearing, with swelling and tenderness over the navicular. A limp is present and weight is borne on the outer border of the foot. X-rays show a scler-osed navicular which looks like a coin placed on edge.

Treatment. A walking plaster until recalcification occurs, followed by foot exercises and re-educa-tion in walking. The heel of the shoe may be raised on the inner side. Possible septic foci are investi-gated and treated.

Sever's disease

This is an osteochondritis of the epiphysis of the calcaneum. It is of gradual onset, and occurs in the 5 to 10 age group. There is pain in the heel on weight-bearing, which is exaggerated by exer-cise and by wearing low-heeled shoes. A limp is present and the patient walks with short steps, avoiding putting the heel to the ground. X-rays show irregularity of the epiphysis of the calcaneum.

Treatment. A walking plaster until recalcification takes place, usually four to six weeks, followed by exercises and re-education in walking. A piece of sorbo-rubber may then be worn in the heel of the shoe.

Freiberg's disease

This is an osteochondritis of the head of the second metatarsal, and occurs in adolescents. There is pain, swelling, difficulty in walking, and local ten-derness over the second metatarsal head. X-rays show irregularity of his epiphysis.

Treatment. A plaster slipper or walking plaster until recalcification occurs, followed by foot exer-cises. A metatarsal bar to the shoe or an insole with bar or button may be ordered.

Operative treatment consists of removal of the metatarsal head.

Kienboch's disease

This is an osteochondritis of the carpal lunate; it occurs in adolescents and is often associated with trauma. There is aching pain, swelling, loss of func-tion of the hand, and local tenderness on pressure. X-rays show increased density and irregularity of the epiphysis.

Treatment. Plaster fixation in the optimum posi-tion for two to six months or until recalcification has occurred. This is combined with finger exer-cises and free use of the hand. Resulting osteoarthri-tis may later necessitate arthrodesis of the wrist.

INEQUALITY IN THE LENGTH OF THE LEGS

This is related to many orthopaedic conditions; it is discussed here because it may be due to interfer-ence with normal growth of the limb, especially in conditions where there is disturbance of blood supply. Inequality in leg length may be due to the following:

1. Congenital anomaly, such as congenital hypo-plasia of the femur or congenital absence of fibula.
2. Diseases of the nervous system, such as polio-myelitis or spastic hemiplegia; in these condi-tions, the blood supply is disturbed because of deficiencies in the neuro-muscular mechanism.
3. Destructive disease of bone, such as suppura-tive or tuberculous arthritis of the hip.
4. Injuries, particularly those resulting in damage to the epiphyseal cartilage and subsequent inter-ference with growth.
5. Operative interference; arthrodesis of the hip or knee before growth is complete.
6. Overgrowth of one leg due to a congenital arter-iovenous aneurysm may produce a relative shortening of the opposite leg.
7. Many otherwise normal people are found to have shortening of one leg, sometimes as much as 2.5 cm. As a rule this gives rise to no disability though strains of the back may be encountered in later life.

Conservative treatment by means of raised foot-wear is described in Ch. 17. This is satisfactory during childhood, but in adult life, particularly in the female, a raised shoe may be considered clumsy and unsightly.

Operative treatment

Leg shortening may be carried out on the sound limb by means of bone resection of the femur or tibia or, in the growing limb, by stapling the lower femoral and/or upper tibial epiphyseal growth plates. An early permanent fusion of these epiphyses may be achieved by an operation called 'epiphyseodesis'.

Leg lengthening is carried out by means of distraction apparatus such as that shown in Figs 15.24 and 15.25. Though this appears to be a formidable procedure, nursing care is surprisingly simple but *vigilance* is required; the limb is suspended so that

the limb moves as one unit and movement of the pins in their tracks is prevented. Dry dressings are applied at the point of exit of the pins and the temperature chart and the circulation in the limb is closely watched.

Complications. These include infection, over-distraction and non-union and interference with blood or nerve supply to the limb.

GENERAL GROWTH DISORDERS

Rickets

Rickets is a deficiency disease of childhood. It is due to lack of Vitamin D, either because of inadequate diet or insufficient sunlight. It is characterised by skeletal deformities, which are, however, only

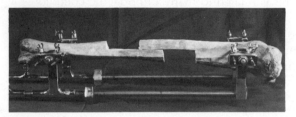

Fig. 15.24 A. Shows the action of a leg-lengthening distraction apparatus on the skeleton. Note that the tibia and fibula have been divided in two places and fixed at each end by skeletal pins, which in turn are attached to a longitudinal bar. The divided bone-ends are gradually separated by a turn-buckle device. (*From the Princess Margaret Rose Hospital, Edinburgh.*)

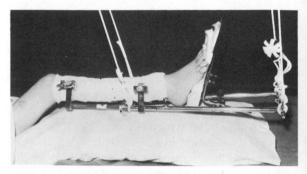

Fig 15.24 B, C, D. Show the limb comfortably suspended after operation for leg-lengthening.

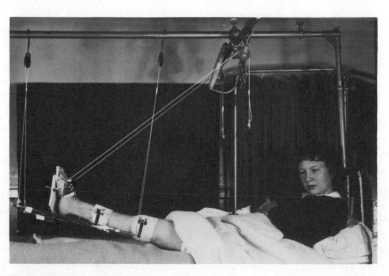

Fig. 15.24C

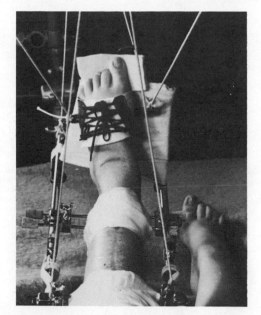

Fig. 15.24D

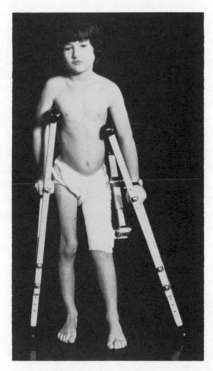

Fig. 15.25 Lengthening by application of a Wagner external fixator. With this technique the child is mobile.

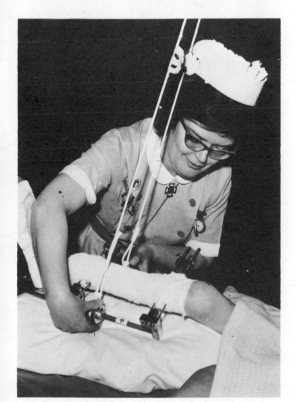

Fig. 15.24 **E.** The distraction device is opened a few centimetres each day according to the surgeon's order.

one aspect of a general constitutional disorder. At one time it was common in industrial areas, but since the introduction of cod-liver oil for children in 1917, rickets in its active state is rarely seen, though some children may pass through a mild attack. It has been noted, however, that immigrants to Britain are in danger of this condition (Ford, 1979; Goel, 1981).

Vitamin D is found in cod-liver oil and in certain fatty foodstuffs; it is also manufactured in the skin by the action of ultra-violet rays, as found in sunlight. Its role is to promote the absorption of fats from the alimentary tract, and thereby facilitate the absorption of calcium salts. When this process is disturbed, bone formation is impaired; the orderly replacement of cartilage by bone in the metaphysis is upset, with the result that this region becomes expanded and the bone formed is soft and pliable. Under the stress of weight-bearing and muscular activity, the bones become bent and curved, and the whole skeleton may become stunted.

Symptoms and signs

The child is usually between the ages of 6 months and 2 years; thereafter activity of the disease ceases, but the effects of the skeleton may be permanent. The child may appear well-nourished, and in fact is often heavy, flabby and pale. He is disinclined to move or be moved, and standing and walking is attempted late; dentition is delayed. Recurrent bronchitis and diarrhoea are common, and there may be nervous symptoms, such as convulsions. There is excessive sweating of the head and upper part of the body, with disturbed sleep and fretfulness. In severe cases, muscle wasting and muscle weakness are marked. The glands and spleen may be enlarged and anaemia may be present.

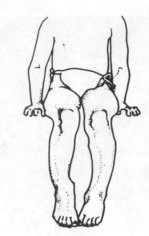

Fig. 15.26 Rachitic tibial bow-leg.

Skeletal deformities

The skull is broadened, the forehead is square, broad and bossy, and the fontanelles are late in closing.

The thorax. There is enlargement of the costochondral junctions, producing the so-called 'rickety rosary'. The ribs bend with respiration and a 'pigeon-chest' may be present, especially if there is also kyphotic deformity of the spine.

The lower ribs may be sucked in, forming a groove known as 'Harrison's sulcus'.

The spine. Kyphosis is the most common deformity, though scoliosis is sometimes seen.

The femur. The normal forward and outward bowing becomes exaggerated. The femoral neck yields to weight-bearing, producing coxa vara.

The tibia is bent fowards and outwards. Bowing of both femur and tibia may be present, producing genu varum (bow-leg) (Fig. 15.22) or bowing may be confined to the tibia only, when it is spoken of as 'tibial bow-leg' (Fig. 15.26). On the other hand, genu valgum (knock-knee) may be present (Fig. 15.27), or the deformities may be combined (i.e. knock-knee on one side and bow-leg on the other) in a child who has been carried on his mother's arm (Fig. 15.28). In addition, there is broadening of the metaphyses, especially of the lower ends of the radius of the tibia. Gross deformity is shown in Fig. 15.29.

The pelvis assumes a trefoil shape; it is flattened

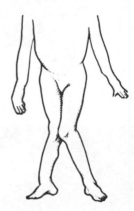

Fig. 15.27 Rachitic knock-knee. Note the pot belly and enlargement of the epiphyses.

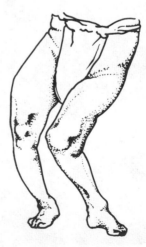

Fig. 15.28 The result of untreated rickets. Right leg: genu varum. Left leg: genu valgum.

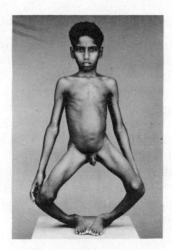

Fig. 15.29   Gross tibial bow-leg due to rickets. This was corrected by surgery. (From the Jawarharlal Institute of Post-graduate Medical Education and Research, Pondicherry, South India.)

and its diameter is lost. This may prove a serious obstacle to child-bearing in later life.

X-rays during the active stage show broadening and blurring of the metaphyses. Later, the bone-ends are broadened and have a scooped-out appearance and deformities such as coxa vara may be evident.

Treatment

Preventive measures include breast-feeding, followed by a full adequate diet, rich in those foods containing Vitamin D, especially milk and butter. The administration of cod-liver oil should be continued at least until the age of 3 years, and the growing child should be exposed to fresh-air and sunlight. Treatment of the established condition is both *medical and orthopaedic*.

Medical treatment

This is aimed at restoring the Vitamin D content and arresting the disease.

1. *Rest* is essential during the active stage; sitting up, crawling or walking is not allowed.
2. *The diet* will be as ordered by the physician, and will be rich in those foods containing Vitamin D.
3. *Sunlight*, either real or artificial, will be given in carefully graduated doses.

4. *Cod-liver oil* or halibut-liver oil will be given on the advice of the physician. Other preparations may be ordered.
5. *Treatment of other manifestations of the disease*, e.g. bronchitis or anaemia, will be carried out according to the instructions of the physician.

Orthopaedic treatment

This is aimed at the prevention or correction of deformity.

Mild cases, with little or no deformity, require just sufficient splintage to prevent the child sitting up or standing. An ordinary 'restrainer' may be used in conjunction with either metal or plaster gutter-splints for the lower limbs. These are removed several times daily for treatment of pressure points and for gentle exercises to preserve the musculature.

Severe cases, in which the bones are still soft, but there is established deformity, are treated according to the part affected.

Deformity of the spine may require immobilisation on a plaster bed. The application and care is already described in Ch. 9.

Deformity of the pelvis may necessitate a Jones abduction frame with skin-traction.

In most cases, deformity of the lower limbs presents the greatest problem.

Knock-knee or *bow-leg* may be treated by gradual correction by manipulation and plaster fixation, or by wedged plasters.

Gentle exercises are commenced as soon as possible. Weight-bearing is resumed when activity of the disease has ceased.

Operative treatment

This may be undertaken when the bones are no longer soft and deformities have become fixed.

Osteotomy may be performed for correction of deformity. The limb is then fixed in plaster until union is sound.

Renal rickets

Renal rickets is also a disease of calcium metabolism due either to chronic renal failure or to a specific tubular insufficiency in the kidneys themselves (Ch. 30).

Treatment consists of medical measures to correct the metabolic disturbance, including the administration of Vitamin D.

Orthopaedic treatment is related to the skeletal manifestations as they arise.

Adult rickets

Adult rickets (osteomalacia) is due to disturbance of the normal deposition of calcium salts, due to poor absorption from the small intestine; it may be nutritional or follow gastrectomy or adult coeliac disease (sprue) (Ch. 30).

Scurvy

Scurvy is rarely seen nowadays. It is due to lack of ascorbic acid (Vitamin C) in the diet, or inability to assimilate it. The normal calcification of bone is disturbed and the patient is presented to the orthopaedic surgeon because the epiphyses become broadened and irregular, and eventually, collapsed and dislocated.

Treatment consists of medical measures, including the administration of Vitamin C. Treatment of the epiphyseal lesions consists of plaster fixation of the part until healing takes place.

Cretinism

Cretinism is due to insufficiency of thyroid hormone during fetal life or during early infancy, so that there is retarded development of the skeleton and other systems of the body.

Gigantism

Gigantism is a condition in which there is overgrowth of the skeleton before the epiphyses have fused and which is due to excess of the growth hormone secreted by the anterior lobe of the pituitary gland.

Treatment of these conditions (apart from medical measures which are outside the scope of this book) is symptomatic; shortening of limb bones may be performed.

Pseudo-hypertrophic muscular dystrophy

This is a familial disease of unknown origin, affecting mainly male children and characterised by progressive loss of muscle function; there is enlargement of some muscles, notably those of the calf of the leg, with wasting of others, notably those of the shoulder girdle. Early diagnosis is aided by enzyme estimations of the blood (aldolase and creatinekinase).

Treatment is palliative and aimed at preserving activity for as long as possible in an effort to combat the increasing helplessness; a wheelchair is eventually required.

THE FOOT

FOOT DEFORMITIES
(Pes Planus, Pes Valgus, Talipes Equinus, Pes Cavus, Talipes Calcaneus, Talipes Varus, Metatarsus Varus, Hallux Valgus, Hallux Rigidus, Hammer Toe, Metatarsalgia)

The foot is an elastic yet powerful structure, consisting of a number of small spongy bones arranged in a series of arches. In standing, the foot receives and transmits the entire weight of the body, and in walking, provides a resilient spring for its forward propulsion.

The arches of the foot

The longitudinal arch consists of an inner and outer portion which rest on a common pillar posteriorly, the tuberosity of calcaneum. The inner portion is the higher, and extends from calcaneum behind to the head of the first metatarsal in front, the remaining constituent bones being talus, navicular and the inner three metatarsals. The talus is spoken of as the keystone of the arch. The outer portion is much lower, and extends from calcaneum to the outer two metatarsal heads, the cuboid intervening.

The transverse arch extends from behind the first to the fifth metatarsal head.

The supports of the arches

The arches are maintained by the following structures.

1. *The shape of the constituent bones:* at one time they were likened to stones used in masonry but this theory no longer holds good.
2. *The interosseus ligaments,* which bind the individual bones together.
3. *The long ligaments of the foot;* the *spring ligament* supports the inner side of the foot, passing from calcaneum to navicular, and thereby supporting the talus. The *long and short plantar ligaments* support the outer portion, passing from calcaneum to cuboid and the fourth and fifth metatarsals. The *plantar fascia* is a powerful support as are the *transverse ligaments* of the metatarsal heads.

Muscular supports

The *tibialis posterior* passes under the spring ligament to its attachment on all the bones of the foot except talus, and acts as a supporting sling. *Tibialis anterior* also helps to maintain the inner side of the foot. These muscles are balanced on the outer side by the *peroneus longus,* which passes across the sole of the foot to its attachment on the plantar surface of the first metatarsal. The long flexors of the toes and the intrinsic foot muscles also help to support the longitudinal curve. The intrinsic foot muscles and the peroneus longus act as support to the forefoot.

Foot deformities are therefore due to the following causes:

1. Alteration in the shape of the bones.
2. Ligamentous changes.
3. Failure of the muscular supports.

In a great many cases, the primary cause of deformity lies in weakness or imbalance of the muscles. Ligaments then become stretched and weakened, and bony changes eventually occur.

Pes planus (Flat-foot)

Flat-foot is a deformity in which the arch of the foot appears flattened to a varying degree. In childhood and adolescence it may be due in the first instance to congenital ligamentous laxity and later, to failure of the muscular support of the foot; the ligaments then become stretched, the shape of the bones altered, and the deformity becomes fixed.

In later life, there may be arthritic changes in the joints of the foot.

Predisposing causes include congenital vertical talus, congenital rocker-bottom foot (Ch. 14), contracture of tendo-Achilles, calcaneo-navicular bar, poliomyelitis, genu valgum, and obesity.

Types of flat-foot

There are four main types. (1) *Acute foot strain.* (2) *Mobile flat-foot.* (3) *Spasmodic flat-foot.* (4) *Rigid or permanent flat-foot.*

1. Acute foot strain

This is generally seen in adolescents or young adults who have undertaken a job or recreation which taxes the foot-musculature too heavily, as for example in the student nurse or week-end hiker.

Clinical features. The patient complains that the feet are hot and uncomfortable, that they burn and sweat, and that they swell towards the end of the day. Aching pain is felt on the front of the leg and under the base of the toes. The gait becomes stiff and clumsy, and the pain may be so severe that the patient is confined to bed. Areas of local tenderness may be found, for example, under the spring ligament. There is no deformity.

Treatment. Rest in a below-knee plaster cast in very severe cases. Alternatively, a Rose-Schwartz meniscus or a polypropylene shoe insert made to a cast of the foot may prove effective. *Change of occupation* is occasionally advised.

Flat-foot exercises are often ordered. These should be non-weight-bearing at first, and should be simple and easily practised at home; two examples are given below:

a. The patient stands with the feet together and turns them over so that weight is borne on the outer borders. The toes are curled under. The position is held for a few moments and *slowly* relaxed.
b. Sitting with the knees bent and the feet together, the patient reforms the arch and draws the heel towards the toes in a 'caterpillar' movement.

Other forms of physiotherapy. Faradic foot-baths may be ordered to stimulate the muscles. *Contrast baths* improve the circulation and help to reduce swelling. The patient sits in front of two bowls or buckets containing hot and cold water respectively. The feet are plunged into first one and then the other.

Altered shoes. The inner side of the heel, and in most cases of the sole as well, of the shoe is raised 0.3 cm, 0.4 cm or 0.6 cm, according to the surgeon's orders. A 'float-out' heel may be advised or a Thomas heel may be ordered (Ch. 7). The shoe must be flat-heeled, well built and well fitting, with a straight inner border.

The patient receives the following instructions:

a. Foot exercises must be carried out several times daily.
b. Altered shoes or the appropriate insoles only must be worn. Wearing carpet slippers and gym shoes is discouraged.

N.B. *Correct heel-and-toe walking and general postural training is essential in all cases.*

2. Mobile flat-foot in children

This is frequently seen in conjunction with knock-knee deformity, torsion of the tibia and a short tendo-Achilles, particularly in children with long, narrow feet and poor musculature. It is often symptomless, though walking may be delayed; the child's mother may complain that the child tires easily and stumbles and falls a great deal. There may be associated laxity of other joints.

Treatment

a. Shoe alterations.
b. Rose-Schwartz heel insole (Fig. 15.30A and B);
c. Helfet heel cup moulded insole (Fig. 15.31A and B);
d. An outside or double iron with inside T strap. (Fig. 7.7.)

In adults with a similar condition, a sponge-rubber insole is sometimes recommended.

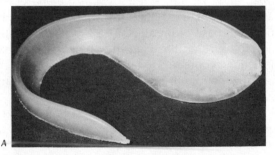 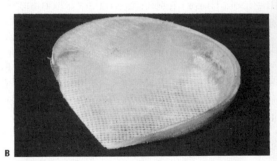

Fig. 15.30 **A.** The fundamental shape of the Rose-Schwartz meniscus insole. **B.** Space has been filled in to give strength and an adhesive area. (Courtesy of Mr G. K. Rose.)

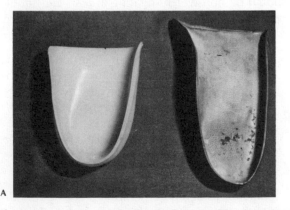 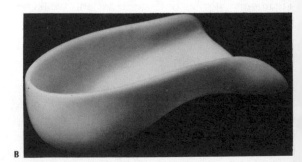

Fig. 15.31 **A.** Corrective insoles are worn inside the shoes; the shorter insole is the Helfet heel cup. The longer plastic insole is effective. **B.** Polypropylene insole to correct a valgus deformity made on a cast of the foot. (Courtesy of Mr G. K. Rose.)

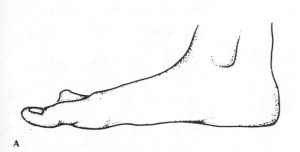
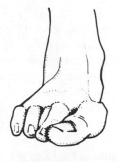
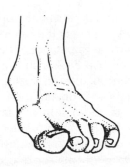

A　　　　　　　　　　　　　　　　　　　　　　　　　　　　　　　　　**B**

Fig. 15.32　A, B. Rigid flat-foot. Note the eversion of the feet, and co-existing hallux valgus and hammer-toes.

3. Peroneal or spasmodic flat-foot

This deformity is not, as the name suggests, associated with spastic paralysis. The foot is everted due to spasm of the peroneal muscles; it is thought that this spasm is protective in nature and associated with congenital anomalies, e.g. talo-calcaneal bar, calcaneo-navicular bar, or with inflammatory conditions, e.g. tuberculosis or rheumatoid arthritis.

Clinical features. This condition is generally unilateral; the foot is very painful and walking is difficult. On examination, the foot is strongly everted, and the peronei can be seen to stand out as a tight band behind the lateral malleolus.

Treatment

1. Manipulation under anaesthesia followed by plaster fixation in the corrected position. The plaster is worn for six to eight weeks and may be followed by the application of an outside iron and inside T-strap, and in any case is followed by foot exercises.

2. *Operative treatment* may be:
a. Tenotomy of the peronei, followed by plaster fixation.
b. Excision of an abnormal bar.
c. Stabilisation of the foot is often the ultimate fate.

4. Rigid or permanent flat-foot

This may be the end result of untreated congenital vertical talus or spasmodic flat-foot. The arch is so flattened that it rests on the ground and cannot be either voluntarily or manually reproduced.

Clinical features. Pain and disability is usually due to adhesions or to osteo-arthritic changes in the joints of the foot. Eventually, the pain may disappear but the foot becomes comletely stiff. The arch may be so flattened that the tubercle of scaphoid or the head of talus is prominent on the inner side of the foot. The feet may be so everted as to assume the 'quarter to three' position, and the gait is plodding, awkward and devoid of spring. There is often co-existing hallux valgus or hammer-toe (Fig. 15.32).

Treatment

a. Any of the measures already described may be advised.
b. Manipulation under anaesthesia, followed by plaster fixation in the corrected position.
c. As a last resort, stabilisation of the foot may be performed.

Talipes equinus (Drop-foot)

This deformity is said to be present when the foot cannot be dorsiflexed (Fig. 15.33). It may be postural deformity, and due to pressure of bedclothes or neglect of foot exercises, especially in very ill

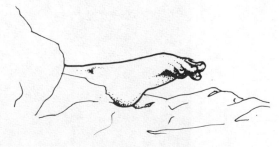

Fig. 15.33 Equinus deformity of the foot following poliomyelitis.

or debilitated patients, or it may be caused by diseases of the central nervous system in which there is muscle imbalance, notably in poliomyelitis and spastic paralysis. In the former, it is due to weakness of the dorsiflexors of the foot, when the plantar-flexors are functioning; in a flail limb it may be due to the action of gravity. In spastic paralysis it is due to spasm of the calf-muscles and contracture of the tendo-Achilles.

Drop-foot may be due to injury to the lateral popliteal nerve, which may be pressed upon by tight bandages, splints or plasters, or the nerve may be damaged during injury to the knee joint. Other causes include injury or disease of the ankle joint.

Treatment. This depends upon the cause. Postural and paralytic drop-foot requires support in a club-foot shoe or plaster shell, with the foot at a right-angle. Physiotherapy is employed to re-educate weak muscles and to stretch contracted ones, and to restore muscle balance.

Contracture of the tendo-Achilles may require fixation in successive plasters to overcome the deformity.

Method of application. The patient lies on a table, an assistant grasps the knee, protecting it from strain and *maintaining it in right-angled flexion.* The limb is covered with wool-roll, the foot grasped in both hands and pushed into as much dorsiflexion as the patient can stand. The plaster is then applied in the usual way.

The following important points should be noted:

1. The foot must be in neutral rotation, neither in varus nor in valgus.
2. Correction must take place at the ankle joint, not at the mid-tarsal joint.
3. The knee remains flexed to the right-angle. The plaster is applied below the knee first; when it has set firmly, slowly straighten the knee and incorporate it in the plaster. A few turns of wool-roll at the junction of the upper and lower portions of the plaster will prevent pressure-sores.

The plasters are changed at weekly intervals until full correction is obtained.

If conservative methods fail, open or percutaneous elongation of tendo-Achilles may be performed.

Permanent drop-foot requires a double iron with posterior stops, or some other form of splintage with plaster shell for night wear.

Operative treatment may consist of tendon transfer or certain forms of stabilisation.

Pes cavus (Claw-foot)

Claw-foot is a deformity in which there is exaggeration of the longitudinal arch of the foot, dropping of the metatarsal heads, and clawing of the toes (Fig. 15.34). Idiopathic claw-foot is the most common, but it may be associated with disease of the

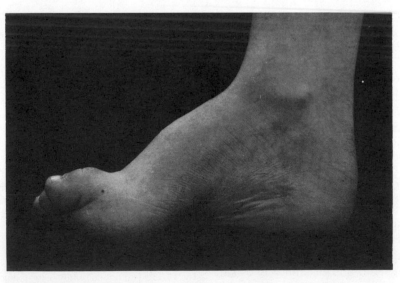

Fig. 15.34 Claw-foot.

nervous system, such as poliomyelitis, spina bifida, Friedreich's ataxia or peroneal muscular atrophy, when the foot muscles are weakened. Claw-foot sometimes follows disease or injury of the bones of the foot.

Clinical features. The patient tires easily and the gait is clumsy. Painful callosites form beneath the dropped metatarsal heads, and corns appear on the interphalangeal joints of the clawed toes. On dorsiflexing the foot, the tight plantar fascia can be seen and felt.

Treatment. Conservative treatment in mild cases consists of a metatarsal bar to the shoe, manual stretching and foot exercises.

Operative treatment. Numerous operations are employed, often in combination.

1. Excision of plantar fascia and stripping of plantar muscles from calcaneum; plaster fixation for four months (Steindler). Weight-bearing in plaster is allowed in a few days. Foot exercises are commenced on removal of plaster and a metatarsal bar is sometimes ordered.

2. Correction of clawing of the toes by tenotomy of the flexor tendons, plaster fixation for six or eight weeks.

3. Multiple tendon transfer (Girdlestone); transfer of extensor hallucis longus through 3rd metatarsal head (Jones). Plaster fixation is required for six or eight weeks.

4. In later life, correction can be obtained only by bone resection, some form of stabilisation may be required. Arthrodesis of the interphalangeal joints of all the toes. In extreme cases, amputation of all the toes ('pobble' operation) is sometimes advised.

Talipes calcaneus (Long-heel)

This is a deformity in which the calf muscles are weakened and the tendo-Achilles is lengthened, so that the heel is at a lower level than the forefoot. It is sometimes combined with a cavus deformity (Fig. 15.35). Causes include poliomyelitis affecting the calf muscles, stretching of the tendo-Achilles from any cause, or injury to the tendo-Achilles in childhood.

Treatment. Conservative treatment consists of a heel-elevator (a piece of cork or sorbo-rubber is inserted inside the heel of the shoe) and exercises.

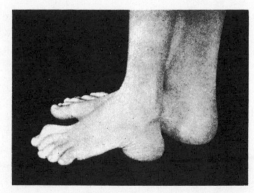

Fig. 15.35 Paralytic calcaneo-cavus deformity of the left foot.

Operative treatment may consist of transfer of active muscles to the tendo-Achilles; this is often combined with stabilisation of the foot.

Heel varus

This is a deformity in which there is inversion of the foot. It is due to muscle imbalance, as in poliomyelitis, when the evertors are paralysed and the invertors functioning normally; in spastic paralysis it is due to spasm of the invertors. It may be combined with an equinus deformity. Other causes include disease or injury of the bones of the ankle or foot.

Treatment. Conservative treatment may be:

1. Plaster fixation in the corrected position.
2. Inside iron, outside T-strap.
3. Physiotherapy, to restore muscle balance.

Operative treatment may consist of transfer of tendons from the inner to the outer side of the foot, wedge resection of the calcaneum (Dwyer), or, some form of stabilisation.

Metatarsus adductus

This deformity, in which there is adduction of the forefoot at the mid-tarsal joints, remits spontaneously in the majority of patients.

Treatment. When present in the newborn, mild cases are treated by repeated manipulations undertaken by the mother, and the more rigid deformities are corrected by moulding in successive plasters. The deformity can also arise during the first year of life as the result of a persistent prone sleeping posture with the feet inturned. This position can be countered by the application of Denis Browne boots and a bar (Fig. 14.19B) as a night splint. Surgical correction is rarely required.

Hallux valgus

This is a deformity of the great toe, in which it is abducted away from the midline of the body (Fig. 15.32). It may pass under or over the second toe, which often develops a 'hammer' deformity. An exostosis develops over the first metatarsal, and friction from the shoe eventually produces a bursa covered with horny skin; this is commonly known as a bunion, and it may eventually break down and suppurate.

In the early stages, hallux valgus may give rise to no trouble, apart from its unsightliness and difficulty in wearing shoes, but in later life, osteo-arthritic changes give rise to increasing pain, stiffness and difficulty in walking.

Treatment. Conservative treatment is advised in early cases, particularly if it is associated with flat-foot. It consists of soft wide shoes with straight inner border, manual stretching and foot exercises.

Operative treatment may consist of the following:

1. Transfer of the adductor hallucis from the proximal phalanx to the metatarsal (McBride).
2. Simple trimming of the metatarsal head (Bonnin) is undertaken if there are no osteo-arthritic changes. A simple dressing and bandage is applied, foot exercises are commenced in a few days and weight-bearing in seven to ten days.
3. Osteotomy of the metatarsal, with correction of deformity.
4. Arthroplasty, either by trimming of the first metatarsal head and excision of the proximal half of the first phalanx of the great toe (Keller's operation) or, more rarely, by excision of the head of the first metatarsal (Mayo). After-care consists of a simple dressing and bandage; gentle exercises are commenced about the fifth day and weight-bearing in about three weeks. Kirschner wire fixation with plaster fixation for three weeks is sometimes used.
5. Arthrodesis of the first metatarso-phalangeal joint.

Hallux rigidus

This is a deformity in which the big toe becomes stiff. In extreme cases, dorsiflexion is completely lost, and the toe assumes a flexed position; this condition is known as 'hallux flexus'. The patient is unable to rise on the toes, and there is pain and difficulty in walking.

Treatment. Conservative treatment in mild cases consists of a metatarsal bar to the outside of the shoe, or, a metal plate worn inside the shoe. Foot exercises are also ordered.

Operative treatment usually consists of a Keller's operation or an arthrodesis.

N.B. *In both hallux valgus and hallux rigidus correct foot-wear, foot exercises, and re-education in walking are an essential part of the after-care.*

Hammer toe

This deformity consists of dorsiflexion of the proximal phalanx, plantar flexion of the second, and either flexion or extension of the distal phalanx (Fig. 15.32). The second toe is most commonly affected. The head of the first phalanx is subjected to pressure from the shoe and painful bursae and corns appear. It is commonly associated with other foot deformities, especially hallux valgus and pes cavus. It may be caused by squeezing the toes into ill-fitting shoes. The corn over the first phalanx gives rise to more symptoms than the deformity itself, and there is difficulty in fitting shoes, with pain and difficulty in walking.

Treatment. Conservative treatment consists of manual correction and foot exercises. Strapping may be used in mild cases to maintain correction, especially in children. In adults, small felt pads arranged to relieve pressure on the toe may alleviate the symptoms.

Operative treatment consists of an excision and arthrodesis, often by the 'spike' or 'wire' method, of the joints of the offending toe, with correction of the deformity, followed by fixation in plaster for about four weeks. Alternatively, a 'filleting' operation may be performed, when the proximal phalanx of the offending toe is completely excised. This procedure requires only a simple dressing and bandage and weight-bearing is allowed as soon as the sutures are removed. Dorsal displacement of the toe may require amputation.

Metatarsalgia

Metatarsalgia is the name given to a pain experienced under the metatarsal heads. In many cases it is due to weakness of the intrinsic foot muscles, and may be combined with foot-strain; painful callosites develop under the metatarsal heads and the toes are sometimes clawed. In 'Morton's metatarsalgia', there is lancinating pain between the third and fourth toes and the condition is then due to a neuroma of the interdigital nerve.

Treatment consists of intensive foot exercises to strengthen the intrinsic muscles, combined with some device to relieve the weight taken by the metatarsal heads. This may consist of a pad of white felt placed behind the metatarsal heads and retained by strapping as shown in Fig. 15.36. Alternatively, an insole with metatarsal bar or button

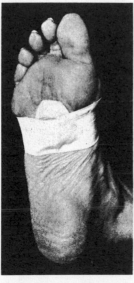

Fig. 15.36 Felt pad and strapping applied for metatarsalgia (Farquharson).

may be advised, or a metatarsal bar attached to the shoe itself (Fig. 7.13). Experiment may be necessary to determine the exact situation of the bar or button and rational foot-wear is essential.

Morton's metatarsalgia requires removal of the neuroma between the third and fourth toes.

General care of the feet

It is important to remember that the general characteristics of the feet and legs follow the same pattern as the rest of the patient's body, so that their appearance is likely to be similar; for example, the person of slender build is likely to have slender legs and feet; similarly the person with powerful general musculature is likely to have equally powerful legs and feet. It is also important to remember that the function of the legs and feet is not only static but dynamic, and a posture which appears abnormal at rest may disappear on movement, as for example in the case of the longitudinal arch of the foot. Furthermore, in the case of children we recall that all babies appear to have bowed legs and chubby 'flat' feet. Parents will often seek advice on account of their child's 'deformity' of the legs or feet which might very well disappear as the child grows, whether treated or not. This does not mean, however, that a thorough examination is not made to exclude serious causes of deformity or serious conditions, for example, congenital dislocation of the hip or spina bifida.

Patients sometimes seek advice not because a deformity interferes with function but because it is unsightly, for example, a bunion may be painless but prevent the patient from wearing fashionable shoes.

Finally, we must remember that the tissues of the legs and feet, in common with other structures, are affected by abnormal metabolic processes and also that they deteriorate with age, so that generalised skeletal change, deterioration in muscle tone, laxity of ligaments or circulatory change in other parts of the body is reflected in turn in the tissues of the lower limbs.

Foot hygiene

It goes without saying that the feet require the same standard of general hygiene as the rest of the body, if only for aesthetic reasons; on the other hand, many people in the habit of taking a daily bath neglect to *wash* the feet, much less dry them thoroughly, particularly between the toes; in fact, most people ignore them until they become troublesome, as is often the case in middle-age when diminution in muscle tone and in circulation is often combined with an increase in body weight; obesity overloads the feet as it overloads other structures (Fig. 15.37).

Toe-nails should be cut straight across, and 'ath-

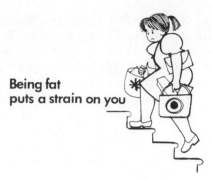

**Being fat
puts a strain on you**

Fig. 15.37
(Courtesy of Dr Thomson and Lancashire Health Board.)

lete's foot', corns, callosites and other disorders which are not serious enough to warrant surgical treatment but which cause discomfort and disability are dealt with by a chiropodist. In this connection, elderly patients and those so handicapped as to be unable to care for their own feet require special consideration.

Patients suffering from conditions which impair their circulation and therefore the nourishment of the tissues of the feet must care for their feet as they would their hands, particularly where there is loss of skin sensation. Conditions where special care is required include poliomyelitis, cerebral palsy, traumatic paraplegia, metabolic and peripheral vascular disease. Care must include protection from cold, avoidance of chafing or constriction by foot-wear or by splintage, and avoidance of injury, including burns and scalds.

Foot-wear

It has been shown that many foot deformities e.g. hallux valgus have a very high familial incidence unrelated to the type of shoe worn or even where shoes are not worn at all. A shoe which forces the foot into an unnatural shape however is blamed for foot deformities, particularly one with a high heel and a pointed toe, especially if it is too short for the foot and is worn continuously; on the other hand, if the general health, musculature and ligamentous support is good, faulty foot-wear is unlikely to be the sole cause, though unsuitable shoes undoubtedly contribute not only to foot troubles but to others which may be associated with abnormal postures, e.g. back-ache. The ideal shoe,

therefore, should be a perfect fit and have a flat heel, a straight inner border, a firm shank, and an upper which embraces the foot firmly. It is important that shoes are kept in good repair and that socks or stockings are of such length as not to constrict the toes. Children's shoes and socks must not become outgrown, and running about barefoot in suitable surroundings is encouraged.

ACKNOWLEDGEMENT

Figures 15.3, 15.11, 15.12, 15.13 and 15.14 have appeared in *Cash's Textbook of Orthopaedics and Rheumatology for Physiotherapists* and are reproduced by permission of the publishers, Faber and Faber Ltd.

BIBLIOGRAPHY

Adams J C 1971 Outline of Orthopaedics. Edinburgh: Churchill Livingstone
Apley E G 1977 A System of Orthopaedics and Fractures. London: Butterworths
Beck M E 1978 Nutrition and Dietetics for Nurses. Edinburgh: Livingstone Nursing Texts
Briggs D, Evans 1982 An 11-year-old girl with spondylolisthesis. Nursing Times, 24 March
Disabled Living Foundation 1971 How to adapt existing clothing for the disabled. Clothing Project Staff. London: Disabled Living Foundation
Farrell J 1977 Illustrated Guide to Orthopaedic Nursing. Oxford: Blackwell Scientific
Farrow R, Forrest D 1974 The Surgery of Childhood for Nurses. Edinburgh: Churchill Livingstone
Fawns H T 1978 Vitamin D and rickets. Nursing Times, 5 October, 1648
Fixsen J A 1972 Common postural deformities in children. Nursing Times, 31 August, 1086
Flanders A 1983 Tracey's curve. Nursing Mirror, 2 November
Forbes G 1971 Clothing for the Handicapped Child. London: Disabled Living Foundation
Gilchrist M I, Blockley N J 1971 Paediatric Orthopaedics. London: Heinemann
Jackson C 1982 Scoliosis. Nursing Times, 7 April
Kennedy J M 1974 Orthopaedic Splints and Appliances. London: Ballière Tindal
Kessel I 1976 Essentials of Paediatrics for Nurses. Edinburgh: Churchill Livingstone
Lobo, E de H 1978 Children of Immigrants to Britain. London: Hodder and Stoughton
McPhee I B, O'Brien J P 1979 Reduction of severe spondylolisthesis—a preliminary report. Spine 4, 5 430–434
MacRae R 1976 Clinical Orthopaedic Examination. Edinburgh: Churchill Livingstone
Neale D 1985 Common Foot Disorders, 2nd edn. Edinburgh: Churchill Livingstone
Nott M 1973 Painful feet. Nursing Times, 13 September, 1190
Pearson J R, Austin R T (1973) Accident Surgery and Orthopaedics. London: Lloyd-Luke

Roaf R, Hodkinson L J 1975 A Textbook of Orthopaedic Nursing. Oxford: Blackwell Scientific
Rose G K et al 1977 Orthotics. Physiotherapy 63: 78
Rowe J, Dyer L (eds) 1977 Care of the Orthopaedic Patient. Oxford: Blackwell Scientific
Scoliosis self-help group, 20 Prince Edward Mansions, Moscow Road, London W2 4EN

Sodha U 1980 Congenital scoliosis. Nursing Times, 28 August
Stone E, Pinney E 1978 Orthopaedics for Nurses. London: Ballière Tindall
Thomson W 1978 Health Education. 1–6. Nursing Times, 14 September, 1561; 21 September 1561; 28 September, 1614; 5 October, 1652; 12 October 1692; 19 October, 1728

16

Pyogenic infections of bones and joints

ACUTE HAEMATOGENOUS OSTEOMYELITIS

This is an acute inflammation of bone, occurring mostly in boys under the age of sixteen years.

Before the advent of antibiotics this condition was the cause of much chronic illness and many deaths. In developed countries, it is still a serious challenge simply *because* it is less common than it used to be, and early manifestations of the disease are easily overlooked so that effective treatment is instituted too late. Indeed, in one instance damages amounting to a very large sum of money were awarded to a child whose parents claimed that osteomyelitis was not diagnosed (*The Guardian*, 6 November, 1980). In less developed countries, it is still a dreadful scourge, and people do not always know when to seek medical advice for their children, even if it is readily available; poor transport arrangements, long distances from centres of medical help and shortage of trained doctors results in ineffective treatment and many cases of chronic bone disease with consequent suffering and disability. The invading organism is in most cases the *Staphylococcus aureus* though the streptococcus is sometimes responsible, especially in very young children, and there is frequently a history of a lesion in the skin, such as a boil or infected abrasion, or, an infected tooth or upper respiratory tract infection. The organism becomes blood-borne, and septicaemia is present even in mild cases. The most common site of local infection is the metaphysis of a long bone. There may be mild trauma, such as a blow or an epiphyseal strain, producing a local haematoma in that part of the bone where the blood supply is already abundant and relatively sluggish, i.e. the metaphysis. In these ideal surroundings the bacilli and their toxins increase and multiply; blood vessels become thrombosed by infection and by pressure, the blood supply to that part of the bone is cut off, and necrosis results. If the disease is unchecked, pus forms in large quantities, and spreads through the Haversian systems. It then tracks upwards and downwards under the periosteum, thus separating it from the bone and further depriving it of blood supply. Spread is limited by the epiphyses, but occasionally a neighbouring joint becomes involved (septic arthritis). Sometimes the nutrient vessel becomes thrombosed, resulting in necrosis and death of the entire diaphysis of the bone, and if the progress of the disease is unchecked, pus eventually tracks through the tissue planes to the skin (Fig. 16.1). Meanwhile,

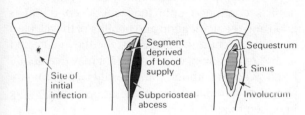

Fig. 16.1 The sequence of events in acute osteomyelitis. (From Stone and Pinney *Orthopaedics for Nurses*, by courtesy of authors and publishers.

bacilli and their toxins are rapidly multiplying in the local abscess and in the bloodstream and a severe general illness results.

Symptoms and signs

There may be a history of a skin lesion as already mentioned, and of a minor injury, followed by a few days general malaise.

General symptoms and signs

There is pyrexia, often 40°C (103–104°F) and the disease may be ushered in by a rigor. The pulse is rapid, the face flushed and the tongue furred. There is fretfulness, headache, disturbed sleep, and sometimes delirium; anorexia and constipation are usually present; the urine contains albumin, and examination of the blood reveals raised blood-sedi-

mentation rate and an increased white-cell count. Anaemia quickly occurs in severe cases. Many cases are acutely ill in the early stages, and chronic cases are seen occasionally, especially in those patients who develop resistance to antibiotics.

Local symptoms and signs

The patient resents examination and the limb is held in the position he finds most comfortable. Neighbouring joints may be held in flexion to accommodate effusion. There is excruciating pain, with local heat and swelling; **an area of exquisite local tenderness is an important diagnostic sign**; if pus is present fluctuation may be elicited.

X-rays of an early case may reveal no abnormality.

Note. Osteomyelitis can occur in sickle cell disease.

TREATMENT

Conservative treatment consists of chemotherapy, relief of pain by means of rest of the whole body and of the affected part, and the maintenance of fluid and electrolyte balance.

Operative treatment may be carried out in conjunction with the above measures.

Nursing care

General care. The patient is received into a warm bed in a quiet corner of the ward. A fracture-board supports the mattress and a cradle is used to support the weight of the bedclothes. The temperature, pulse and respiration are recorded four hourly. A light nourishing diet is given, the bowels are regulated and the mouth cleansed. Pressure points are treated by change of position, and the affected limb must be handled with the utmost gentleness. If the patient is in great pain, apply a simple splint, e.g. a well-padded gutter-splint or piece of Kramer wire; this will rest the part and relieve pain whilst awaiting definitive treatment.

Fluid balance

The maintenance of fluid balance is of vital importance. If large quantities of fluid cannot be taken by mouth, it must be given intravenously, and if anaemia is present, transfusions of whole blood may be necessary.

Chemotherapy

Penicillin is the drug of choice and the modern approach to chemotherapy is described in Ch. 2.

Rest of the affected part

Splintage is applied according to the part affected and should allow of free inspection and palpation. Plaster shells are frequently ordered, for example, in the case of the tibia. Osteomyelitis of the femur usually requires immobilisation in a plaster spica with a window. As soon as the acute symptoms have subsided and the convalescent stage entered, fixation in a closed plaster may be advised.

Operative treatment

This may be undertaken early in the treatment, if an obvious sub-periosteal abscess is present, or after a few days, when local tenderness persists. It is directed towards the removal of pus and the relief of tension in bone, and consists of drainage of a sub-periosteal abscess with or without drilling of the bone. In severe cases, the wound may be left open to allow free drainage; in others, it may be closed. Continuous suction drainage of the wound may be advised.

No operation is performed unless or until the general condition allows, and chemotherapy, maintenance of fluid balance, and splintage is continued throughout. As a rule, chemotherapy is continued until the temperature has been normal for about 12 days, and in some cases for as long as 6 weeks.

Treatment by closed plaster

After incision and drainage of an abscess a complete padded plaster cast may be applied. This may quickly become stained with pus, but so long as the patient remains apyrexial and well, it is not changed more often than is absolutely necessary. Meddlesome dressing of the wound will prevent healing, not accelerate it. Simple dry gauze dressings are advised; saline or Cetavlon is used for cleansing the skin, and strong antiseptics should not be used. Before the advent of prompt treatment by chemotherapy and surgery, many of these plasters had a disagreeable smell, but this problem is rarely met nowadays.

Later X-rays may reveal patchy decalcification, and the formation of sub-periosteal new bone. This is called the involucrum. Later still, sequestra may be present.

Discharging sinuses may appear spontaneously, or at the site of an operation wound. These should be dressed as infrequently as possible. Occasionally, a sequestrum is extruded from a sinus.

Convalescence

Rest in bed and immobilisation (usually plaster fixation) is continued until the general condition is good and recalcification and healing of the affected bone has occurred. Exercises for the unaffected limbs are commenced. The patient may eventually be allowed up without splintage (after a preliminary period of graduated exercises) or, weight-bearing in plaster may be advised.

CHRONIC OSTEOMYELITIS

This is said to be present when full healing and recalcification does not take place. Relapses may occur when the general health becomes poor and the patient's powers of resistance lowered. Discharging sinuses may be present, and deformity may occur from interference with bone growth or instability of joints. Pathological fractures may occur. Occasionally, a cavity filled with pus and surrounded by sclerosed bone appears. This is known as a Brodie's abscess.

Chronic osteomyelitis is sometimes seen following an injury, e.g. an open fracture, or following orthopaedic surgery.

It should be noted that the patient with a draining sinus is a source of infection to others.

Treatment

This consists of the maintenance of a high level

of general health, and splintage to prevent deformity or to relieve weight. Chemotherapy is discussed in Ch. 2.

Operative treatment. The following operations may be performed: sequestrectomy; evacuation of a Brodie's abscess; osteotomy to correct deformity; bone grafting; very rarely, amputation of the limb. In resistant cases operative débridement may be followed by continuous closed irrigation-suction of the wound using a solution containing a detergent, and the administration of the appropriate antibiotics.

Other complications include the following:

persistent discharging sinuses leading to chronic ill-health and amyloid disease;
pathological fracture and deformity;
interference with bone growth;
malignancy in an ulcer or a sinus track.

PYOGENIC ARTHRITIS

This is due to the infection of a joint cavity by pyogenic organisms. The staphylococcus is most frequently found, especially in children; other organisms are the streptococcus, the pneumococcus, the gonococcus, or more rarely the bacillus typhosus. The organism may be blood-borne, and gain entrance as in acute osteomyelitis, or, it may enter the joint from a wound or open fracture or, following an injection into the joint. Pyogenic arthritis may occur as a complication of acute infections such as pneumonia.

The reaction of the joint depends on the virulence of the infection and the resistance of the individual. In all cases, there is distension of the joint by an exudation of fluid; in early cases this may be serous and due to a simple synovitus. Later, the joint becomes filled with sero-fibrinous exudate, and in severe cases, frank pus may be found. If the disease is unchecked, destruction of joint-surfaces will occur, and sometimes, pathological subluxation. In early cases, good function is often preserved, but gross destruction generally leads to ankylosis of the joint.

In the neonate, osteomyelitis of the upper end of the femur may break through into the joint causing permanent damage (Eyre-Brook, 1960).

Symptoms and signs

There is pain, swelling, local heat and tenderness. Movements of the joint are impossible because of pain and muscle spasm, and the joint is fixed in flexion. The systemic upset is great, and the clinical picture is similar to that of acute osteomyelitis which may be an accompanying feature. There is pyrexia and the patient is of toxic appearance. Dehydration and anaemia rapidly occur. As in osteomyelitis, the mortality and morbidity in this disease has been greatly reduced since the discovery of penicillin but there is an equal need for prompt recognition of the condition and for effective early treatment to save the joint from destruction.

TREATMENT

Treatment proceeds on the lines already described for acute osteomyelitis—relief of pain by means of rest, both general and local, combined with chemotherapy and the maintenance of fluid and electrolyte balance, and correction of anaemia.

Aspiration of the joint is sometimes performed, and in cases where frank pus is present, this may be followed by drainage, when pus is evacuated and the joint washed out.

Splintage is applied according to the joint involved and ideally should permit of free inspection. *Traction* is usually ordered. An affected hip requires immobilisation by means of Pugh's traction or weight-and-pulley traction (Ch. 2). A great disadvantage, however, is that this form of treatment permits movement at the hip-joint, which might be very painful during nursing attention, e.g. bedmaking or giving bedpans. A plaster hip spica provides better immobilisation but does not permit inspection of the part. A Jones double abduction frame, if available, provides ideal immobilisation in the acute stage when the hip is very painful (Ch. 10). A Thomas bed-splint with skin-extensions, may be used for the knee-joint; or, a plaster cast from the toe to the groin (Ch. 6).

Later treatment consists of free mobilisation in bed, with graduated exercises and eventual weight-bearing. Gross destruction rendering ankylosis certain may necessitate protected weight-bearing in splintage, e.g. a plaster spica for the hip, or a caliper for the knee.

SOME OTHER AFFECTIONS OF JOINTS

1. Transient or toxic synovitis of childhood

It is thought that this may be secondary to infection of the tonsils. The hip or the knee is commonly affected, and the symptoms and signs may simulate a tuberculous or other infective arthritis in its early stages.

Treatment is instituted as if this is in fact the case. If, after two or three months' treatment, the condition has subsided and x-rays show no change, the surgeon may advise gradual mobilisation in bed. This is followed by gradual weight-bearing, and if there is no return of symptoms, the child is allowed home. On discharge, the parents are asked to communicate with the hospital if there is a return of the symptoms, *and supervision is continued until it is certain that the condition has in fact subsided.*

2. Syphilis of joints

Syphilis of joints is usually symmetrical, e.g. affecting both knees; it is accompanied by other signs of the disease, and the Wasserman reaction is positive.

Clutton's joint is the name given to the painless effusion in the knees of the congenital syphilitic.

Charcot's joint is the name given to the swollen, deformed and disorganised joints which may accompany tabes dorsalis or general paralysis of the insane.

Treatment consists of medical measures for the systemic disease. Splintage to prevent deformity or to relieve weight may be ordered, e.g. a caliper or knee-cage.

Physiotherapy to strengthen the musculature may be advised. In rare cases, arthrodesis of the joint may be performed.

3. Gonococcal arthritis

This may be acute, affecting one large joint, or many joints may be affected, when the condition resembles rheumatoid arthritis. There is pain, stiff-ness and swelling of the joint; eventually the articular cartilage is dissolved and ankylosis occurs.

Treatment consists of medical measures for the systemic disease. Splintage and physiotherapy may be ordered.

4. Haemophilia

Haemophilia is a hereditary sex-linked disease in which the clotting of blood is retarded. Extravasation of blood into a joint may follow a trivial injury. The knee is most commonly affected, and becomes swollen, hot and painful. Flexion contracture may occur.

Treatment consists of rest and splintage to the affected joint. Bleeding may be arrested, if necessary, by transfusion of fresh plasma or of anti-haemophilic factor. Physiotherapy is begun when haemorrhage has ceased, and deformities may require correction by means of traction, manipulation under anaesthesia or by operation. Correction of flexion deformity of hip and knee is described in Ch. 10. Sometimes splintage such as a caliper is required to protect the joint.

BIBLIOGRAPHY

Adams J C 1971 Outline of Orthopaedics. Edinburgh: Churchill Livingstone

Apley E G 1977 A System of Orthopaedics and Fractures. London: Butterworths

Bentley G 1975 Haemophilia. 1 and 2. Nursing Times, 4 December, 1926; 11 December, 1984

Catterall R D 1975 A Short Textbook of Venereology. London: English Universities Press

Cauthidge J 1984 Haemophilia. Nursing Mirror Clinical Forum, 15 February

Eyre-Brook A L 1960 Septic arthritis of hip and osteomyelitis upper end of femur in the infant. Journal of Bone and Joint Surgery 42–311

Forrest D, Farrow R 1974 The Surgery of Childhood for Nurses. Edinburgh: Churchill Livingstone

Fountain E J 1981 Orthopaedic management of haemophilic arthropathy. Nursing Times, 25 November

Gilchrist M I, Blockley N J 1971 Paediatric Orthopaedics. London: Heinemann

Handbook on Sickle Cell Disease. A Guide for Families. A Sickle Cell Society Publication c/o Brent Community Health Council, 16 High St., Harlesden, London NW10 42X

Kessel I 1976 Essentials of Paediatrics for Nurses. Edinburgh: Churchill Livingstone

MacRae R 1976 Clinical Orthopaedic Examination. Edinburgh: Churchill Livingstone

Mollan R A B 1977 Acute osteomyelitis in children. Journal of Bone and Joint Surgery 59B: 2–7

Norton T H, Tait J M 1971 Orthopaedic Surgery. London: Heinemann

Raw Anne Y 1982 Home therapy for patients with haemophilia and Christmas disease. Nursing Times, 14 April

Reynolds V J 1978 Eyes on joints in sexually transmitted diseases. London. Hospital Update 16: 11, 1331

Roaf R and Hodkinson L J 1975 Textbook of Orthopaedic Nursing. Oxford: Blackwell Scientific

Rowe J, Dyer L (eds) 1977 Care of the Orthopaedic Patient. Oxford: Blackwell Scientific

Schofield C B C 1975 Sexually Transmitted Disease. Edinburgh: Churchill Livingstone

Sickle-cell. Menace in the Blood 1978 Nursing Mirror, 20 July

Stone E, Pinney E 1978 Orthopaedics for Nurses. London: Ballière Tindall

Susman, Shaw A 1981 Home treatment for children with haemophilia. Nursing Times, 23 September

Upton M 1983 Young Winston. Nursing Mirror, 10 August

Waldrogel F A, Medoff G, Swartz M N 1971 Osteomyelitis. Springfield, Illinois: Thomas

17

Tuberculosis of bones and joints

MODES OF INFECTION

Tuberculosis of bones and joints is caused by the invasion of the body by Koch's bacillus, and occurs most frequently in childhood. It is influenced by economic and hereditary factors, in that bad living conditions and poor nutrition resulting in a low state of general health predispose the subject to tuberculosis, and overcrowded dwellings encourage its spread. In many cases there is a family history of tuberculosis. At one time, our orthopaedic hospitals were filled with patients suffering from skeletal tuberculosis. This is no longer the case. The incidence of the disease has been greatly reduced by improvement in living conditions, in safe milk supplies, in nutrition, in public health services, and by vaccination of persons who show a negative reaction to tuberculin skin tests with BCG (Bacille Calmette Guérin). In addition, treatment has been revolutionised by the discovery of streptomycin and other antibiotics and by advances in surgical techniques. Nevertheless, cases such as are described in the following pages with all their terrible attendant complications are still quite common in some countries, and serious cases (e.g. affecting the spine) are still seen in our own hospitals. Varieties of tuberculosis—tuberculous peritonitis, osteomyelitis, meningitis—that were becoming rare in Britain are now seen again in immigrant children or adults (de Lobo, 1978).

The invading organism may be one of two types:

1. *Human* type, which is acquired by inhalation from persons suffering from tuberculosis of the lung or by ingestion of infected food-stuffs.

2. *Bovine* type, which is ingested in milk from infected cows.

The infection, by either route, spreads via the lymph vessels and bloodstream; lymph glands become infected, and may send showers of organisms into the lymph and bloodstreams from time to time. In joints the local lesion frequently commences in the synovial membrane, especially near its reflection from bone. In many cases, there is a history of injury, producing a haematoma which is the ideal breeding ground for invading organisms. In children, if the resistance is high and treatment efficient and prolonged, the lesion may remain confined to the synovial membrane.

The local reaction of tissue to the presence of tuberculous bacilli is known as a *tubercule* or *tuberculous follicle*. This is seen microscopically to consist of lymphocytes surrounding clumps of bacilli, and a typical feature is the presence of a giant-cell. Toxins are liberated by the bacilli which destroy the protective cells; in this process, which is called caseation, the damaged cells soften and liquefy, and as the disease progresses, various tuberculous follicles fuse together in a cheesy mass, which may become obvious as a 'cold abscess'. Further changes depend on the virulence of the infection and the degree of resistance of the individual. If the progress of the disease is arrested, fibrous tissue is laid down, which eventually walls off the disease and healing takes place, calcification in abscess walls often marking its site permanently.

Changes which occur in affected joints

The synovial membrane becomes thickened and the synovial fluid increased in amount. The cartilage becomes dull, disintegrated and eroded, and may become separated from, the bone. The bone at and around the lesion becomes decalcified, due to the increased blood supply, and appears less dense than normal bone on X-ray examination. As the disease progresses there is erosion and destruction of bone, with the formation of cavities, and sometimes, sequestra (fragments of dead bone). The soft tissues undergo degenerative changes. Ligaments and tendons become swollen, stretched and lax, muscles atrophy, and cold abscesses may appear as fluctuant swellings.

DIAGNOSIS

The diagnosis of a tuberculosis is made from the following points:

1. History.
2. Clinical signs.
3. X-ray signs.
4. Skin tests, e.g. Mantoux or Heaf test.
5. The presence of tuberculous bacilli in pus, if obtainable.
6. The presence of tuberculous glands in the abdomen of a guinea-pig killed six weeks after it has been injected with suspected pus. This is the most sensitive test, but suspected early cases are diagnosed and treated on clinical grounds alone, even in the absence of X-ray and other signs.
7. In some cases, biopsy of synovial membrane or of neighbouring lymph glands may help to establish the diagnosis.

General symptoms and signs of tuberculosis of joints

The patient is pale and listless, and does not enjoy his work or play. He is tired on slight exertion and there may be marked loss of appetite and loss of weight. There may be rise of temperature in the evenings, with night sweats and disturbed sleep. Later, the blood-sedimentation rate may be raised.

Local symptoms and signs

There may be aching pain, sometimes referred to neighbouring parts, swelling, local heat and local tenderness on palpation. There may be protective muscle spasm around the part, and later, muscle wasting from disuse. Movements of an affected joint are limited in all directions and deformity may be present.

Aims of treatment

1. *To save life.*
2. *To induce healing of the diseased part in the best possible functional position.*

These aims are achieved by:

1. *General treatment*, including chemotherapy and attention to the general health, and improvement in nutrition and social conditions where indicated.
2. *Local treatment* consists of rest of the affected part. Severe cases of joint tuberculosis may require prolonged treatment in hospital, sometimes for some months, e.g. in massive infection of the spine.
3. *Surgery* is used increasingly, e.g. synovectomy, eradication of a local focus.

General treatment

Before the discovery of specific antibiotics, general treatment of these patients could only consist of measures aimed at raising the natural resistance of the body, namely rest, combined with good nutrition, exposure to fresh air and sunlight in clean, healthy and happy surroundings. Though no longer of primary importance, these measures are still the essential background to successful treatment and are therefore listed below.

1. *Rest in bed* is often ordered in the early stages; even if the particular lesions allow the patient to remain ambulant, adequate sleep is essential. Rest for the body must also include *rest for the mind*; attention to social and economic problems is part and parcel of treatment and includes both the patient and his family.

2. *Exposure to fresh air*, to sunlight and to changes of weather stimulates metabolism and promotes a sense of well-being, though in the early stages indiscriminate sun-bathing must be prevented.

3. *Liberal diet*. A high protein diet is often ordered, and food must be well cooked, varied and pleasantly served. The nurse must not allow a patient rendered helpless by immobilisation to struggle ineffectually with his food. She must report any patient refusing food and exercise charm and tact in feeding children and old people.

4. *Fluids*. In recumbency, a high fluid intake is essential to minimise the risk of renal stones. The nurse will explain to the adult patient the necessity for taking more fluid than he wants, and gently insists on it in the case of a child.

5. *Treatment of co-existing disease*. Investigations such as radiographs of the chest and examination of the blood are carried out to exclude conditions which may hamper the patient's recovery, and the appropriate treatment is instituted.

CHEMOTHERAPY OF TUBERCULOSIS
(Hopkins, S. J.)

This section appeared as an article in the *Nursing Mirror* (29 July 1981) and is reprinted by kind permission of the editor.

For several years, streptomycin, isoniazid and para-aminosalicylic acid (PAS) were the standard drugs in the treatment of tuberculosis and many different dosage schemes were devised to produce the maximum response with the minimum of side-effects.

Streptomycin is usually given by intramuscular injection in doses of 0.75–1 g daily. Toxic effects, such as giddiness and deafness, may require a reduction in dose. It is no longer regarded as a first-line drug except in unusual circumstances. PAS must be given in large doses and is not always well tolerated.

First-line treatment

For the initial phase or first-line treatment, rifampicin (Rifadin, Rimactane) together with isoniazid and ethambutol are preferred.

Rifampicin is a derivative of an antimicrobial substance isolated from a strain of *Streptomyces mediterranei*, and is one of the most effective antituberculous drugs now available. It is given orally in doses of 450–600 mg daily (10 mg/kg) as a single dose before breakfast, because administration on an empty stomach promotes absorption and gives higher blood levels.

It is reddish brown and patients should be warned it may colour their urine, sputum, tears and other secretions. It is relatively well tolerated, but gastrointestinal upsets, drowsiness and disturbances of liver function may occur. It may also increase the liver breakdown of some drugs, such as corticosteroids, warfarin, digoxin and oral hypoglycaemic agents. In women taking rifampicin together with an oral contraceptive, unexpected pregnancies have occurred because the increased breakdown of the steroid contraceptive resulted in a lower degree of protection.

Ethambutol is a synthetic drug with a bacteriostatic action against *M. tuberculosis*. It is valuable in combined therapy because it prevents the emergence of drug-resistant strains of the organism during treatment. It is given orally in doses of 15–25 mg/kg daily, but the dose should be reduced in cases of impaired renal function.

It may cause a retrobulbar neuritis with reduction in visual acuity and partial colour-blindness. This effect is linked with a gradual loss of copper and zinc, and patients taking this drug should be warned to report any visual disturbances as soon as possible. These ocular disturbances are usually reversible if the drug is withdrawn promptly. An allergic rash and gastrointestinal disturbances may be associated with higher doses.

Isoniazid is usually given concurrently with rifampicin and ethambutol in the initial phase of treatment in doses of 200–300 mg daily. It has a bacteriostatic action, but unlike many other drugs used in infectious diseases, it has virtually no activity against any organism other than *M. tuberculosis*.

It is also of interest because it is normally excreted in the urine largely unchanged, and only a small proportion of the dose is excreted as an acetyl derivative. This derivative is much less active than the parent drug. Certain ethnic groups are capable of acetylating the drug much more rapidly than others. Slow acetylators of isoniazid have a higher serum level of the parent drug than rapid acetylators, but the incidence of hepatitis as a side-effect is more likely with the latter group. Conversely, slow acetylators are more likely to develop peripheral neuropathy, due to a deficiency of pyridoxine, and this may be prevented by administering pyridoxine in doses of 50–100 mg daily.

As a rule, a three-drug regimen along the above lines should be continued for two to three months, after which a two-drug dosage scheme should be continued for at least another six months. The drugs of choice are usually rifampicin and isoniazid, but ideally the choice should be based on drug-sensitivity tests. With controlled long-term therapy, there is a high rate of conversion of sputum to tuberculosis negative, and the relapse rate may be as low as one per cent.

Second-line treatment

The so-called second-line drugs are used mainly in cases of drug resistance or when first-line drugs are poorly tolerated.

Pyrazinamide (Zinamide), like isoniazid, is bacteriostatic and only effective against *M. tuberculosis*. It is useful for short-term treatment in doses of 25–35 mg/kg daily, usually in association with streptomycin, and is useful in the treatment of tuberculous meningitis as it easily penetrates the cerebrospinal fluid. Care is necessary in cases of liver dysfunction and hepatitis has been known to occur with higher doses. It may also initiate latent gout but the gouty attacks can be controlled by drugs which reduce hyperuricaemia such as probenecid or allopurinol.

Capreomycin, an antibiotic obtained from *Streptomyces capreolus*, has some of the properties of streptomycin. It is given in doses up to 1 g daily by deep intramuscular injection in cases where streptomycin is not tolerated or in drug-resistant infections, but always in association with other antituberculous drugs.

Cycloserine is another antibiotic that is sometimes effective in resistant infections, but it may cause convulsions and other toxic effects even with relatively low doses.

Prothionamide (Trevintix) is a synthetic drug with similar actions and uses to ethionamide and is sometimes a useful alternative.

Thiacetazone is an older synthetic antituberculous and antileprotic drug given in doses of 2 mg/kg daily, but it is now seldom used because of the high incidence of side-effects. However, it is very cheap when the cost is compared with that of most first-line drugs. Thiacetazone is still used in those countries where tuberculosis is common and the cost of large-scale therapy is a severely limiting factor.

Even with effective and relatively well-tolerated drugs, the treatment of tuberculosis is a long process, and regular and continuous treatment is essential for recovery. Patient compliance with treatment is of paramount importance, as erratic dosage or occasional omission of treatment results in higher relapse rates and increasing risk of drug resistance. In consequence, even more intensive therapy with a wider range of drugs may become necessary.

The causes of non-compliance are numerous and the psychology behind it is a fascinating and still largely unexplored area. Much can be done by warning the patient beforehand of possible side-effects—although cynics might say such warnings ensure the side-effects occur!—and, above all, making sure the patient understands the course of treatment. Doctors and nurses should not only instruct the patient on the dose and frequency of administration but also take the trouble to ask the patient to repeat the information he has been given.

There is a reluctance at times to prescribe combined products, which could reduce the number of tablets to be taken, often on the grounds that the dose should be adjusted to the patient. How many doctors take a patient's weight into account when assessing a dose and, if they do, how often is a tablet with an adjusted dose available? This need for dose adjustment is often more apparent than real, except in the very young or elderly. In the case of the tuberculous patient, mixed products such as Mynah (ethambutol and isoniazid), Rifinah and Rimactazid (rifampicin and isoniazid) have advantages.

Administration at fixed time intervals is another method of ensuring regular treatment and with the increased interest of some patients in their diet, vague directions such as 'three times a day after meals' should be avoided. Some patients do not take three 'meals' daily and, even if they do, the intervals between meals may vary so widely that the drug serum levels also do.

Another disadvantage of antituberculous therapy is that the results are not dramatic and patients easily lose the incentive to continue treatment on a regular basis. Nurses should remember that every patient, no matter how well-intentioned, is a potential defaulter where drug treatment is concerned. The surprising response to schemes for returning unused and unwanted drugs to a local chemist is ample proof of poor instructions and even poorer patient compliance. Nurses could play their part by ensuring that instructions are understood and patients comply and co-operate with treatment.

COMPLICATIONS OF TUBERCULOSIS OF JOINTS

The following complications may occur in *any* case of tuberculosis. Special complications for each region will be enumerated later.

1. Deformity of the affected part

This may be due to protective muscle spasm, destruction of bone, or ankylosis of joints, and can be seen on examination.

2. Abscess formation

When the tubercle bacillus invades the body it is immediately assailed by the special cells in the bloodstream whose function it is to combat infection (i.e. the lymphocytes). The battle which ensues causes the formation of pus, containing dead and dying bacteria and dead or dying blood and tissue cells. If the invading organism is of such a virulent nature as to set up a severe systemic reaction (as for example in acute osteomyelitis), pus is formed in large quantities and quickly comes to the surface as an abscess. In most cases of tuberculosis, however, the battle is slow and sustained and the formation of pus may give rise to little or no systemic reaction. Such a collection of pus is spoken of as a 'cold abscess'. It may remain adjacent to the affected bone, or, taking always the line of least resistance through the surrounding tissues, track to the skin and appear as a fluctuant swelling. Abscess formation is often quite symptomless, or it may be indicated by pain, rise of temperature, loss of appetite, disturbed sleep, and finally by the appearance of a fluctuant swelling, which may be at a very great distance from the site of the disease. The pus is evacuated by repeated aspiration through healthy skin under strictly aseptic conditions. This is to prevent the abscess breaking down and the formation of sinuses. Incision and drainage of an abscess may be carried out in certain selected cases.

3. Sinus formation

In some cases the skin over an abscess becomes so thin, reddened and devitalised that it yields and breaks down in spite of repeated aspirations, and a passage between the skin and the deeper tissues appears. A sinus must be dressed with meticulous care and aseptic precautions always observed, no matter how small and innocuous a wound it may appear. One carelessly applied dressing will be sufficient to introduce other micro-organisms into the wound, so that the patient has two infections to combat instead of one. This may result in a severe general illness, and the condition may become chronic with the attendant evils of long continued sepsis.

Penicillin or some other antibiotic may be ordered in cases where an abscess has become cross-infected.

4. Amyloid disease

In cases of long-standing, and particularly in those where there are multiple sinuses and long-continued sepsis, waxy deposits are laid down in the vital organs (for example, the liver, kidneys, spleen and intestines.) This results in a gradual replacement of vital cells by lardaceous material, with degeneration of solid organs, consequent slowing-down of metabolic processes and a gradual decline in the patient's general condition. Discharging sinuses result in loss of albumin and plasma protein, resulting in oedema. There may be periodic vomiting, diarrhoea alternating with constipation, and albuminuria. There is progressive loss of weight, the skin becomes yellow and dry, and the features haggard and drawn. The patient may live for months in an emaciated, exhausted state until death supervenes. Mercifully, since the advent of the antibiotic drugs the miserable lingering death which was formerly the fate of the patient suffering from this condition is now a rare occurrence. In addition to the nutritional and other general measures already described, intravenous infusion of concentrated plasma may be given in suspected cases; as a last resort, and in suitable cases (e.g. the ankle) amputation of the affected limb may be advised.

5. Tuberculosis of other parts (other than the primary lymphatic infection)

This is a common complication, as the bacilli are carried all over the body by the blood and lymph stream. The part attacked may be another joint, the lung, the kidney, or the mastoid cells. Such lesions may be manifested by pain in another joint, by rise of temperature, by cough, by urinary symptoms or by digestive upsets, according to the part attacked. Any indication of a tuberculous lesion elsewhere must be promptly reported and dealt with.

6. Deformity of other parts

These are most commonly due to bad nursing and will be enumerated later.

7. Renal complications

When bone is decalcified and destroyed by disease, the liberated calcium salts are eliminated by the kidneys. Prolonged immobilisation in the lying position during the course of treatment prevents adequate drainage of the kidneys, and this, combined with insufficient fluid intake, results in the retention of salts within the renal pelvis. This may lead to the formation of stones, which predispose the urinary tract to infection. The urine must be tested at regular intervals as changes in its composition (e.g. the presence of albumin) may indicate urinary complications. If this is suspected, a fluid intake and output chart must be kept and it will be necessary to obtain a sterile specimen of urine for bacteriological examination. Elevating the head and foot of the bed alternately for short periods assists in drainage of the kidneys, or, frequent change of position in those cases in which it is not injurious.

Renal complications may be (a) renal stones; (b) renal colic; and (c) renal infection.

a. Renal stones

These may be symptomless or there may be haematuria on turning.

Treatment. (i) Frequent change of position (e.g. turning) within the limits of correct orthopaedic treatment. (ii) Copious fluids. (iii) Surgical intervention.

b. Renal colic

The passage of a stone down the ureter may produce renal colic, with vomiting, pain in the loin or abdomen or referred to the groin, the testicles or the labia. Albumin and blood is found in the urine.

Treatment. (i) Morphia and atropine, or pethidine is ordered for the relief of pain, with attention to the general comfort. (ii) Surgical intervention.

c. Renal infection

This may be either (i) pyelitis, an inflammatory condition of the renal pelvis or (ii) pyonephritis, in which the kidney substance is involved. The infection may be blood-borne or it may ascend from the bladder, and is commonly associated with renal stasis. It is indicated by the following *general symptoms*: malaise, pyrexia, headache and vomiting. The *local symptoms are*: pain in the loin, frequency of micturition, and burning pain on micturition which is referred to the urethra. The urine contains pus and organisms.

Treatment. Medical treatment, which includes the administration of drugs, fluids, and dietary measures as ordered by the physician.

8. Pott's paraplegia

This is a complication of tuberculosis of the spine and is described under that heading.

9. Tuberculous meningitis

This may be characterised in the prodomal stage by loss of appetite, apathy and general loss of interest in life. There is then severe headache, restlessness, neck rigidity, and intolerance to light, with pyrexia, vomiting and sometimes, delirium. The patient finally relapses into unconsciousness, and death supervenes. *Streptomycin* is usually ordered and, in cases diagnosed early, holds out hope of recovery.

10. General miliary tuberculosis

The patient's body becomes the seat of multiple virulent tuberculous lesions, manifested by any or all of the signs and symptoms previously enumerated, and death supervenes.

TUBERCULOSIS OF THE SPINE (POTT'S DISEASE)

The spine is more often attacked by tuberculosis than any single joint. The vertebral bodies in the thoracolumbar region are most frequently affected, because it is in this region that most weight is borne and most movement takes place. The vertebral body becomes eroded, and collapse occurs due to muscle-spasm and weight-bearing on diseased bone. This is always marked in the thoracic region as, owing to the normal backward convexity of the spine in this area, most weight is thrown on the front of the bodies, predisposing them to collapse. In cervical and lumbar caries, collapse is never so marked, as the spine is convex forward in these areas and weight is borne chiefly on the articular processes and the back of the bodies respectively.

SYMPTOMS AND SIGNS OF TUBERCULOUS DISEASE IN PARTICULAR REGIONS OF THE SPINE

The general symptoms and signs are set out in the previous chapter.

Cervical region

The patient will walk carefully, with short steps, and if the condition is advanced he may support his head in his hands. There is limitation of neck movement in all directions. Pain will be present, sometimes referred to the top of the head. There will be loss of the normal forward cervical curve, and swelling denoting an abscess may be palpated in the suboccipital region, or a retropharyngeal abscess may be present. If the condition is far advanced, there may be signs of cord pressure, varying from exaggerated reflexes to actual spastic or flaccid paralysis. The arms will be affected first, and the legs follow.

Thoracic region

The spine is held stiffly, the gait is erect and careful, and the patient dislikes sitting. Spasm of the erector spinae muscle may be visible. Collapse of the affected vertebral bodies will cause the spinous processes to protrude, causing a bony projection called a kyphos or gibbus. This is frequently the first thing to be noticed. The kyphos may be tender on palpation and hot to the touch. Pain may be referred around the chest wall (girdle pains) or may be described as aching in character. There may be fullness or swelling in the loins or along the ribs indicating an abscess, though as a rule tuberculous abscesses in this region remain peri-spinal and do not escape to the skin. It is because of this that paraplegia is most common in thoracic lesions. In early cases, cord pressure may be indicated by ataxic gait and exaggerated tendon-reflexes and, later, paralysis of the legs may occur. In the most advanced cases sensory changes may be present below the lesion.

Lumbar region

There is rigidity, a careful gait and the patient will not stoop. Pain radiates down the legs and there may be flexion of the hips due to spasm of the psoas muscle. Kyphos is not often marked, but there is obliteration of the normal lumbar lordosis. There may be abscess formation in the loin, or the abscess may track down the sheath of the psoas muscle and appear in the groin or in front of the thigh. A psoas abscess is the most common complication of tuberculous disease of this area.

X-ray examination is carried out in all cases. It may reveal diminution of the joint-space between two adjacent vertebrae or evidence of bony destruction.

TREATMENT

1. *General treatment* as already described.
2. *Local treatment*, i.e. rest of the affected part.
3. *Surgery*.

Splintage

Splintage is applied according to the part affected and each case is considered individually. All splintage described here is subject to variations according to the surgeon's wishes, the age, build, and general condition of the patient, and his particular lesion. As time goes on, immobilisation as a means of treatment is used less and less, but it is mentioned here because of the nursing problems involved. Children require more stringent immobilisation than adults because of their greater activity. Immobilisation is carried out by means of a *plaster bed*.

Splintage for different regions of the spine

1. *Cervical region* (first to seventh cervical vertebrae). A plaster bed with sunken headpiece; a collar may be ordered.
2. *Upper thoracic region* (above the sixth thoracic vertebra). A plaster bed with sunken headpiece; a collar may be ordered.

N.B. *In all lesions of the cervical or high thoracic region, a tilting mirror must be fixed to the bed.*

Mid-thoracic region (between the sixth and ninth thoracic vertebrae). A plaster bed with a sunken headpiece, no pillow allowed.

Lower thoracic region (between the ninth and twelfth thoracic vertebrae). A plaster bed with one pillow.

3. *Lumbar and sacral region*. A plaster bed with or without a pelvic-band. *An anterior plaster shell in which the patient is turned is usually ordered in all these cases.*

Nursing care in cases where this type of immobilisation is ordered is described in Ch. 9.

Alternative methods of splintage for different regions of the spine

All those named in Ch. 9 may be used from the outset, or in the later stages of treatment when the patient becomes ambulant, or following operative treatment. As healing takes place splintage may be gradually discarded.

1. *Cervical region.*
   a. A doll's collar, either plaster, leather or polythene (Fig. 19.26).
   b. Minerva jacket (Fig. 19.25).
2. *High thoracic region.*
   a. Plaster jacket including the neck, in some cases the head too.
   b. Spinal support with collar attached.
   c. Block-leather jacket with collar attached.
3. *Lower thoracic region.*
   a. Plaster jacket from clavicles to hip joints.
   b. Jones spinal support.
   c. Block leather.
4. *Lumbar and sacral region.*
   a. Plaster spica including one leg (above knee).
   b. Block-leather spica including one leg.
   c. Supporting belt (Fig. 28.12).

Operative treatment

Operative treatment may consist of excision and clearance of a local focus and drainage of an abscess, with or without spinal fusion.

POTT'S PARAPLEGIA

Paraplegia is one of the most serious complications of tuberculous disease of the spine. It is also one of the most distressing to the patient—'in an infant most melancholy to see, in an adult most miserable to endure' (Percival Pott). It is caused by pressure on the spinal cord, which may be due to one of the following factors:

1. abscess formation;
2. sequestra;
3. sudden collapse of a vertebra;
4. vascular catastrophe.

As the spinal cord extends only to the level of the second lumbar vertebra, paraplegia occurs most commonly in caries of the cervical and thoracic regions.

Paraplegia may be roughly divided into two types;

1. that of early onset, i.e. manifest within eighteen months from the commencement of disease;
2. that of late onset, i.e. manifest later than two years from the commencement of disease. This division is made chiefly from the point of view of prognosis, the likelihood of recovery being greater in cases of early onset.

Paraplegia may be either partial or complete, and consists of an interruption of normal transmission of impulses along the spinal cord. The earliest sign is usually spasticity of the lower limbs, and incoordination of voluntary movement. This is due to diminution of the inhibitory effect of the higher centres on the lower reflex arcs. The ankle and knee jerks are increased, the abdominal reflexes are lost, and the Babinski sign may be positive. Passive movements of the limbs are accompanied by some resistance and there may be clonus of the ankle and patella. Voluntary power may be at first weak and, later, absent. One leg may be involved before or to a greater extent than the other. If the condition progresses voluntary power may be completely lost, together with loss of control of the bladder and rectum and, finally, anaesthesia may develop. When this stage is reached, the patient is virtually 'cut in half' so that the lower part of the body, i.e. that part supplied by nerves arising from the spinal cord below the lesion, is governed only by its reflexes and is no longer under the control of the higher centres in the brain. Any stimulus of the skin initiates violent spasm, often in the nature of a mass reflex in which the limbs are flexed and the bladder and rectum emptied.

N.B. *As the onset of paraplegia is usually insidious all cases of tuberculosis of the spine, particularly those with lesions in the cervical and thoracic regions, must be carefully watched and systematically examined for the above signs and treatment instituted at once.*

TREATMENT

Conservative treatment. This consists of general measures as already laid down and may be combined with immobilisation of the patient as a whole.

Operative treatment. Surgery is frequently performed and includes costo-transversectomy; anterolateral decompression or laminectomy. Many operations may be performed by the anterior (trans-thoracic) approach, to relieve pressure on the spinal cord. This is discussed fully by Mr D. Ll. Griffiths in *Recent Advances in Orthopaedics*, No 3, McKibben, 1979.

Notes on post-operative nursing care

General post-operative and post-anaesthetic care is axiomatic (Ch. 9). The following special points should be noted:

1. If the patient is not immobilised by means of a plaster bed, he is received on to an ordinary bed with a firm base, and the spine is supported on pillows in a comfortable supine position.
2. Note any discharge from the wound. Any wound or chest cavity drainage system is watched closely.
3. Keep a close watch on the respiratory state.

4. Look for abdominal distension; this is not only a danger sign in itself but aggravates respiratory distress.
5. Pain may be severe for the first 24 or 48 hours and analgesics may be ordered.
6. In the initial stages, pain in the back will preclude the normal use of bedpans. Male patients can use a urinal but female patients must pass urine either into a special female urinal (Fig. 5.4) or, into a receiver pressed against the vulva. Training in this method of emptying the bladder is part of preparation for operation (Ch. 9). Defaecation may also be performed into a flat receiver rather than into the conventional bedpan, or, the stool may be received into an incontinence pad.
7. After 24 to 48 hours, the surgeon may allow the patient to be turned gently into the side-lying position for attention to the back. Specific instructions are sought in this respect. Gradually, the pain improves and the patient is able to tolerate movement in bed. Recumbency continues until the surgeon allows the patient to get up; some form of spinal support may be ordered.

TUBERCULOSIS OF THE HIP-JOINT

The hip joint is more often attacked than any other single joint, and is second only to the spine. The lesion may be synovial only, especially in childhood, or it may be situated in any of the constitutent bones of the hip joint, with erosion, destruction and formation of cavities.

Symptoms and signs

1. *The general symptoms and signs.* These have already been described.
2. *Local symptoms and signs.* A limp is almost always the first symptom, and becomes more marked when the patient is tired. Pain may be felt in the hip joint itself or it may be referred along the course of the obturator nerve to the knee, especially in children, in whom this is a very common and misleading symptom. In childhood, when the cartilage has been eroded and sub-chondral bone exposed, there will be a history of disturbed sleep

and night-cries. This is due to the relaxation of protective muscle spasm during sleep. Muscle spasm is an effort on the part of nature to immobilise an inflamed joint. During sleep, the muscles relax their guard, the sensitive joint surfaces rub together and the child wakes with a characteristic sharp cry. Immediately, protective spasm reappears and the child drops off to sleep again. *The nurse on night-duty must always be on the alert for such cries, and must report them because their occurrence during treatment may indicate inadequate immobilisation.*

Examination

Examination of a suspected hip is carried out in the following manner:

1. Inspection.
2. Palpation.
3. Test of movement.
4. Measurements.
5. X-rays.

Inspection. The patient lies on a firm couch; *in an early case* the hip will be held in flexion, abduction and external rotation. This is due to protective muscle spasm, and to the fact that it is in this position that there is most room in the inflamed joint; it is the position of rest, gives maximal synovial space, and pressure within the joint is relieved.

Palpation. This may reveal swelling and thickening around the hip, and perhaps local tenderness.

Test of movement. This will reveal limitation of all movements in all directions by pain and muscle spasm.

Measurements. Comparative measurements at this stage often reveal apparent lengthening. Measurements taken round the thighs at the same level may reveal muscle-wasting, and there may be wasting of the buttock.

X-rays. In a very early case, there may be no X-ray changes at all, but as the X-ray appearances always lag behind the inflammatory process, the case is diagnosed and treated on the clinical signs only. *Both hip joints must be X-rayed for purposes of comparison.*

X-rays. Osteoporosis (the bones appear decalcified, i.e. less dense to X-rays than normal bone) is an important early sign. It may be present throughout the joint, or be confined to the site of the original focus.

In a later case, where muscle spasm has continued over a longer period, the pull of the powerful adductors combined with habitual lying on the unaffected side, produces adduction and internal rotation, but the flexion remains. Palpation may reveal swelling and tenderness, or even abscess formation. Measurements at this stage usually show apparent shortening. X-rays may show evidence of osseous foci. Later still, in addition to any or all of the above signs, there may be an extreme lumbar lordosis, indicating flexion contracture of the hip. The surgeon will determine whether or not this is present by the Thomas test, as described in Ch. 10.

Measurements may reveal real shortening, indicating destruction or dislocation of the hip (Ch. 10). Gross destruction of the acetabulum causing it to 'wander' may result in a pathological subluxation of the femoral head.

TREATMENT

1. *General treatment*, including chemotherapy, has already been described.
2. *Local treatment* may consist of immobilisation of the affected joint in the position of choice.

Splintage

1. A Jones abduction frame with skin extensions (Ch. 10). (Rarely used nowadays.)
2. A plaster bed, with extension-bows and a bar to provide fixation for the groin-strap incorporated; skin extensions.
3. A plaster spica, either single or double (Ch. 6). If used in the early stages of treatment, a double spica is usually ordered as a single spica does not prevent adduction deformity. In the later stages weight-bearing in plaster with patten and crutches may be ordered.

Operative treatment

This may consist of one of the following: *biopsy*, in an attempt to confirm the diagnosis; *excision of a local focus*, in an attempt to limit its spread; *osteotomy*, to realign the joint and increase its sta-

bility; *arthrodesis*, to render the joint stiff, but stable and painless; *arthroplasty*, to provide movement in a stiff joint.

TUBERCULOSIS OF THE KNEE JOINT

Like all other tuberculous lesions in bone, this is always part of a generalised infection. As in tuberculosis of the hip joint, the original site of infection is often in the synovial membrane, and may remain synovial only. Later, infection may spread to the constituent bones of the knee joint, with ulceration of the cartilage and destruction of the joint surfaces.

In time the infection may spread to the constituent bones of the knee joint, with ulceration of the cartilage and destruction of the joint surfaces.

Symptoms and signs

1. *General symptoms and signs* are as already enumerated.
2. *Local symptoms and signs*. In an early case, loss of function is usually more noticeable than pain. The patient avoids putting his heel to the ground and the knee is held in slight flexion. Examination may reveal a hot and swollen knee, and the thickened synovial membrane feels peculiarly 'doughy' on palpation. Wasting of the thigh muscles renders the appearance of the swelling more noticeable, and gives the limb a fusiform appearance. Movements of the joint are limited by pain and muscle spasm, and there may be local tenderness over bony points. *X-rays* may reveal generalised decalcification of the knee joint or the presence of an osseous focus. In a later case, pain will be increased and continued muscle spasm may result in flexion contracture of the knee, or pathological subluxation may occur.

TREATMENT

As in the hip joint, the knee, being a weight-bearing joint, is safe only when either freely moveable or soundly ankylosed.

Splintage

1. Thomas bed-splint with skin extensions with or without guarding splints (Ch. 10).

2. A plaster spica from the toes to the waist (Ch. 6).

Splintage in the later stages may consist of a weight-relieving caliper. *Measurements* for a caliper are as described in Ch. 7.

Operative treatment

This usually consists of excision of diseased synovia and bone, with or without arthrodesis. Plaster fixation is usually ordered post-operatively, and sometimes, a caliper with or without guarding plaster (Ch. 10). Splintage is discarded when union is sound.

TUBERCULOSIS OF THE SACRO-ILIAC JOINT

Tuberculosis of the sacro-iliac joint is frequently combined with other tuberculous lesions. Young adults are most commonly affected. The disease may commence in the synovial membrane; the lower part of the sacro-iliac joint is most often attacked when the lesion becomes osseous.

Symptoms and signs

The general symptoms and signs are already described. The onset is insidious, and the presence of an abscess is frequently the first thing to be noticed. This may be seen over the sacro-iliac joint, or it may track forwards under the iliopsoas and point in the groin. There is pain, aggravated by sudden movements, and by strain, such as prolonged stooping. The gait is careful, and there is sometimes a list of the spine towards the unaffected side. There may be local tenderness on pressure over the affected joint.

X-rays may show generalised osteoporosis and blurring of the joint outlines, followed by destructive changes, and, sometimes, the formation of sequestra.

TREATMENT

Conservative treatment

This consists of immobilisation of the affected joint, with general measures as already described.

Splintage. A plaster bed or a double plaster spica.
Nursing care is carried out on the lines already described in Chs 9 and 10.

Alternative splintage which may be ordered consists of: (1) a plaster corset from the costal margins to the hip joints, with or without groin-straps incorporated, or, a plaster spica incorporating the leg to the knee on the affected side, (2) a sacro-iliac belt.

Operative treatment

This consists of arthrodesis of the sacro-iliac joint. Preparation and after-care is as for any other operation on the spine.

TUBERCULOSIS OF THE SHOULDER JOINT

Tuberculosis of the shoulder is comparatively rare, especially in children. There is commonly a pulmonary lesion on the same side. The lesion may be synovial or osseous; it is sometimes of the atrophic type, which is known as 'caries sicca'.

Symptoms and signs

The onset is insidious; in an early case inflammation of the synovial membrane gives rise to pain, swelling, local heat, tenderness, and limitation of movement.

X-rays may show osteoporosis without erosion. Later, the arm is held to the side and there is muscle wasting, particularly of the deltoid. The patient cannot raise his arm from his side and there is extreme limitation of movement. X-rays may then reveal gross osteoporosis with loss of joint outline and perhaps the presence of osseous foci.

TREATMENT

As the shoulder is not a weight-bearing joint, the surgeon may be satisfied with a fibrous ankylosis, which would be dangerous in joints subjected to such stresses and strains as the hip or the knee. In cases where gross destruction of bone has not occurred, a useful degree of movement, aided by the movements of the scapula on the chest-wall, may be recovered.

Conservative treatment

1. *General treatment* with chemotherapy is carried out in all cases.
2. *Local treatment* may consist of immobilisation of the affected shoulder in the position of choice.
3. *Operative treatment* is carried out when neither a strong fibrous union nor the recovery of a useful range of movement is expected.

Splintage. In the early stage a plaster shoulder spica is usually ordered (Fig. 6.6). *In the later stage* splintage may be (a) plaster spica with removable lid or (b) an abduction splint.

Operative treatment

This usually consists of an arthrodesis of the shoulder, followed by application of a shoulder spica (Ch. 6).

TUBERCULOSIS OF THE ELBOW JOINT

The elbow joint is more frequently attacked by tuberculosis than the shoulder or the wrist, and more often in adults than in children. As in other joints, the lesion may be synovial in the first instance. An osseous focus is most commonly found in the ulna.

Symptoms and signs

The onset is insidious; pain, aggravated by movement, may first be confined to the joint itself, and later may be referred to the forearm. There may be swelling, local heat and tenderness, movements are limited by pain and muscle spasm, and the joint eventually becomes stiff at a mid-position. Muscle wasting is pronounced, and as in the knee joint, exaggerates the appearance of the swelling. *X-rays* may show generalised osteoporosis of the joint, and a bony focus in one of its constituent bones.

TREATMENT

Early and efficient treatment usually preserves a useful joint, especially in children. As in the shoulder, a fibrous ankylosis is regarded as satisfactory.

General treatment has already been described. *Local treatment* consists of immobilisation in the position of choice. *Splintage* in the early stage may be a plaster spica including the shoulder, or an above-elbow plaster and sling. In the later stage, splintage may be a posterior plaster slab with collar and cuff, a collar and cuff only, an elbow-cage, or a block-leather or celluloid splint.

1. *Plaster spica.* In very acute cases a plaster spica may be ordered, and is applied as already described for the shoulder joint.
2. *Above-elbow plaster.* A plaster is applied from the axilla to the web of the fingers. The position of the limb is decided by the surgeon. As a rule, the elbow is held in just above right-angled flexion, the forearm is mid-position and the wrist dorsiflexed. The plaster is supported in a sling or collar and cuff, but free movement of the shoulder and fingers *must* be maintained.

Alternative splintage

1. *Plaster slab and collar and cuff:* a well-moulded posterior slab may be applied and graduated exercises commenced.
2. *Collar and cuff.* This may be ordered in the quiescent stage and is applied with the elbow held in the required amount of flexion. *Application.* Thread two short lengths of bandage through two leather shoulder guards. Tie one round the neck and the other round the wrist. Join them with a third piece of bandage (Fig. 20.5). Improved versions of the collar-and-cuff are now available from manufacturers of medical supplies.
3. *Elbow-cage.*
4. *Block-leather or celluloid splint.* Either of these may be ordered in the quiescent stage to protect the joint. A cast must be taken.

Daily care

Whatever form of splintage is adopted, it is the duty of the nurse to inspect it daily, and to see that all other joints are not becoming stiff. The patient is usually allowed up and may even be treated as an out-patient.

Operative treatment

This may consist of excision of the joint with or without subsequent arthrodesis in the position of choice, followed by plaster fixation until union is sound. Chemotherapy is continued.

TUBERCULOSIS OF THE WRIST JOINT

Tuberculosis of the wrist is relatively uncommon, especially in children. The synovial membrane may be first attacked, or an osseous lesion may be found in one of the constituent bones of the wrist joint, usually in the lower end of the radius.

Symptoms and signs

There may be pain, swelling, local heat and tenderness, limitation of movement and deformity. The wrist is usually held in palmar flexion. Abscesses are superficial and quickly break down and form sinuses. X-rays may show generalised osteoporosis or the presence of an osseous focus.

TREATMENT

1. *General treatment* as for other tuberculous lesions.
2. *Local treatment* consists of immobilisation in plaster.

The plaster extends from the knuckles to just below the elbow, or, above-elbow plaster may be ordered for more stringent fixation. Particular attention must be paid to the position of the wrist. About 30 degrees dorsiflexion is usually ordered, and if the thumb is included it must be held in opposition. Unless otherwise ordered, the plaster extends only to the transverse creases in the palm, as shown in Fig. 6.4. The plaster is inspected daily for cracks or softening as described in Ch. 6.

Later treatment

Plaster fixation and chemotherapy are continued until the disease is quiescent.

Retentive splintage may be ordered, consisting of a leather or celluloid moulded splint made on a cast of the wrist. A watch must be kept for pressure sores on such bony prominences as the ulnar styloid.

Operative treatment is undertaken when the lesion is quiescent and usually consists of an arthrodesis. The wrist is immobilised in plaster in the position of choice until union is complete.

TUBERCULOSIS OF THE ANKLE JOINT

The clinical picture of tuberculosis of the ankle joint is similar to that of the wrist, and as in other joints, the lesion may be synovial or osseous. Abscess formation is common.

TREATMENT

1. *General treatment* is standard.
2. *Local treatment* consists of immobilisation in a well-moulded below-knee plaster cast; occasionally, an above-knee cast is necessary. Recumbency may be ordered in the acute stage; weight-bearing in plaster is gradually introduced when the disease is approaching quiescence, or, crutches may be ordered.

Daily care is as for any tuberculous joint immobilised in plaster. Retentive splintage, may be (a) a double iron, either fixed in the boot or held by contrary stops, and a plaster shell for night wear or (b) Thomas patten-ended caliper, and a plaster shell for night wear.

Measurements for these splints will be found in Ch. 7.

Operative treatment

This may consist of an excision and arthrodesis of the joint, followed by plaster fixation until union is sound. In rare cases, amputation of the limb may be necessary.

TUBERCULOSIS OF THE CARPAL OR TARSAL BONES

Treatment consists of general measures combined with immobilisation of the hand or foot in a plaster cast, care being taken to maintain the normal palmar or plantar arches and the function of the fingers or toes. Tuberculosis of the tarsal bones in adults usually indicates a severe infection and amputation of the foot may be necessary.

TUBERCULOSIS DACTYLITIS

This is confined to young children and affects the metacarpals, metatarsals, or phalanges of the fingers or toes. The fingers or toes become stiff, swollen, and painful, and abscesses quickly break down and form sinuses.

TREATMENT

1. *General treatment* as for other tuberculosis lesions.
2. *Local treatment* is conservative or operative.

Conservative treatment. If the foot is affected, plaster fixation in recumbency is usually ordered. In the case of the metacarpals or phalanges of the fingers, fixation is not as a rule ordered because of the resulting stiffness and impairment of use of the hand, though a light plaster splint may be ordered for a short time if the condition is very acute and the patient ill. The prognosis is good with efficient and prolonged general treatment.

Operative treatment. This consists of excision of a local focus, or amputation of an affected finger or toe.

BIBLIOGRAPHY

Adams J C 1971 Outline of Orthopaedics. Edinburgh: Churchill Livingstone
Apley E G 1977 A System of Orthopaedics and Fractures. London: Butterworths
Forrest D, Farrow R 1974 The Surgery of Childhood for Nurses. Edinburgh: Churchill Livingstone
Gilchrist M I, Blockley N J 1971 Paediatric Orthopaedics. London: Heinemann
Harold A J 1977 Bone and joint disease. British Medical Journal, 1071–1073
Helel B 1977 Bone and joint disease. British Medical Journal, 276–280
Kessel I 1976 Essentials of Paediatrics for Nurses. Edinburgh: Churchill Livingstone
Lobo E H de 1978 Children of Immigrants to Britain: their Health and Social Problems. London: Hodder and Stoughton
MacRae R 1976 Clinical Orthopaedic Examination. Edinburgh: Churchill Livingstone
Pott's disease 1982 Nursing Mirror, 14 July
Radha T G 1978 Miliary tuberculosis. Nursing Times, 17 August, 1362
Roaf R, Hodkinson L J 1975 Textbook of Orthopaedic Nursing. Oxford: Blackwell Scientific
Roaf R, Kirkaldy-Willis H 1959 Surgical Treatment of Bone and Joint Tuberculosis. London: E & S Livingstone
Stone E, Pinney E 1978 Orthopaedics for Nurses. London: Ballière Tindall

18

Acute anterior poliomyelitis

(INFANTILE PARALYSIS)
MODE OF INFECTION

Acute anterior poliomyelitis is an acute infectious disease occurring sporadically and in epidemics, usually in the late summer and autumn. It is caused by the invasion of the central nervous system by a minute filtrable virus, of which there are at least three known varieties. The incubation period is thought to be from 5 to 30 days. In the past, children were most frequently attacked, hence the name 'infantile paralysis', but no age group is immune.

Active immunisation by means of a vaccine has virtually eliminated this disease from western countries (Fig. 18.1) and the only cases now seen are those with residual paralysis from an attack many years ago. In less developed parts of the world however, severe deformities are still seen (Fig. 18.2).

The virus is believed to enter the body via:

1. the respiratory tract (by inhalation) or
2. the alimentary tract (by ingestion).

There are two main types:

1. the *bulbar* type, affecting the brain-stem,
2. the *spinal* type, affecting the spinal cord.

It is the last-named which chiefly concerns the orthopaedic nurse, though both types may be present in the same individual.

The virus is believed to enter the spinal cord via the nerves and the bloodstream. There is hyperaemia of the cord with extensive inflammatory exudate and oedema. The anterior horn cells are either pressed upon by the products of this inflammation,

LANARKSHIRE HEALTH BOARD

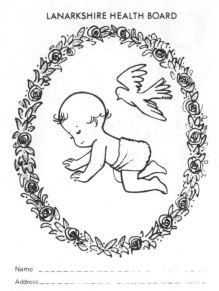

Name _____

Address_____

Be wise – immunise

IMMUNISATION RECORD CARD

Fig. 18.1 Health Education poster to encourage parents to have their children immunised. (By courtesy of Dr William Thomson and the Lanarkshire Health Board.)

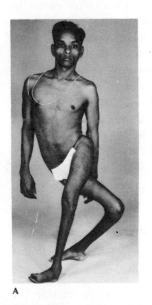 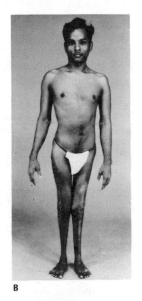

A   B

Fig. 18.2 A, B. Poliomyelitis. Before and after surgery. (From the Jawaharlal Institute for Post-graduate Medical Education and Research, Pondicherry, South India.)

or, they may be partially or completely destroyed by the toxic action of the virus. As a result, the nerve from the affected cell degenerates, the muscle supplied by it is partially or completely deprived of its nerve-supply, and flaccid paralysis ensues. The cranial nerves may be affected; there are no sensory changes. 'Abortive' or 'nonparalytic' cases occur, and persons who have been in contact with the disease but do not contract it may become carriers.

SYMPTOMS AND SIGNS

These may be so slight at first as to be confused with a feverish cold or some other disease of childhood. Sore throat and enlargement of the cervical lymph-glands is usually present. There is pyrexia, and the patient is flushed, irritable and apprehensive. He dislikes being touched, and complains of pain in the back and limbs. *Muscle tenderness* may be present and is an important diagnostic sign; there may be tremors, weakness and unsteadiness of voluntary movements, and sometimes, spasm of muscles not affected by paralysis. Meningeal symptoms include headache, convulsions, drowsiness, or even delirium. Neck rigidity is an important diagnostic sign. Gastrointestinal upsets are common, and there may be anorexia, nausea, vomiting, diarrhoea or constipation. Retention of urine frequently occurs. Lumbar puncture may reveal the presence of increased cells and protein in the cerebrospinal fluid.

Paralysis commonly occurs from one to three days from the time of onset, and varies from weakness of one muscle to complete paralysis of the trunk and limbs; the respiratory muscles or the muscles of deglutition may be involved. Certain muscles are particularly liable to be picked out, notably the quadriceps, the anterior tibial group, the peronei and the deltoid. The last-named rarely recovers. As the inflammation in the spinal cord subsides, those nerve cells which are not actually destroyed are released from pressure, and the muscles supplied by them gradually recover.

PREVENTIVE MEASURES

Poliomyelitis is an infectious disease and *isolation* of suspected cases and of contacts should be instituted immediately. *Investigations* include examination (virus studies) of cerebro-spinal fluid, blood and stools. Persons in contact with known or suspected cases should remain in the environs of their own home. Strict personal hygiene, particularly with regard to washing the hands, is imperative; it should be borne in mind that the virus is excreted in the stools. Food should be protected from flies and during the months when poliomyelitis is prevalent unwashed fruit and vegetables should not be eaten. If an outbreak is suspected, it is advisable to avoid crowded places, particularly swimming pools. Children and young adults who are feverish and unwell should be kept in bed; rest in the early stages of an attack may minimise its severity; violent exercise is known to increase it. It has been noted that an attack of poliomyelitis may follow tonsillectomy, so that this operation is usually avoided during the epidemic season. Inoculation (e.g. against diphtheria) is also discontinued during this time because it has been noted that in the event of an attack of poliomyelitis the most severe paralysis is seen in the limb which was the site of injection.

Active immunisation by means of a vaccine has already been mentioned.

Aims of treatment

1. To limit the spread of infection.
2. To prevent deformity and minimise disability. If there is respiratory involvement, the use of life-support equipment might be required.
3. To rehabilitate the patient as far as possible for normal living.

Treatment of acute stage

As a rule, acute cases are not received in an orthopaedic hospital, but are sent to a specialist hospital for infectious diseases where there are facilities for practising full isolation technique. Occasionally, however, particularly during an epidemic and where complications such as respiratory paralysis do not exist, they are transferred early to an orthopaedic unit. There is still some doubt as to the actual period of infectivity, but *barrier nursing* is usually carried out for at least three weeks from the time of onset, and the stools are regarded as infected for six weeks. Gowns and masks are worn by all personnel attending the patient and by his

visitors; scrupulous attention to the toilet of the hands is essential. Excretions and soiled linen are dealt with as for typhoid fever and all crockery is boiled after use.

The patient is received into a warm bed in a warm, well-ventilated room, or into a ward reserved for these cases, and is nursed on a Dunlopillo or other soft yet firm mattress, which is slightly shorter than the bed itself. A footboard covered with felt or with a pillow is placed at the end of the bed so that the feet are supported at a right-angle to the leg and the heels rest in the space between the mattress and the footboard. The footboard also serves to support the weight of the bedclothes; if one is not available a bed cradle must be used. Other requirements are regulated by the extent of paralysis, but if this is not known it is as well to prepare the following: soft pillows of various sizes, lint for making shoulder pads, knee pads and hand rolls, sand-bags. If respiratory involvement is feared, a respirator is prepared and the anaesthetist is asked to stand by. Respiratory failure might require treatment by means of a tank respirator, or by intubation, or tracheostomy and intermittent-positive-pressure. Bulbar involvement may call for the use of an electric sucker; an oxygen cylinder should be kept in the ward and if the diagnosis is still in doubt a lumbar puncture may be advised.

GENERAL NURSING CARE

Until the extent of the paralysis is known, the patient is not left unattended, particularly if there is any sign of respiratory or bulbar paralysis. If the patient is nursed in a single room, a bell system whereby he can summon his nurse is fixed up immediately. In cases where the upper limbs are paralysed, the hospital engineer will fit a foot-operated bell. In extensive paralysis one which can be operated by a very light touch or even by the pressure of the chin or the temple may be required.

The temperature, pulse and respiration is recorded four-hourly, and the slightest sign of respiratory or bulbar involvement is reported at once.

Complete rest in bed is absolutely essential at this stage. If the patient is restless, sedation may be required, and if the patient is old enough to co-operate the necessity for complete rest is explained to him. Everything must be done for the patient; he is fed, washed and turned by the nursing team; at the same time it should be remembered that the muscles may be acutely tender and all nursing procedures are carried out with the utmost gentleness. A daily blanket bath is given and areas subjected to pressure are inspected regularly. In acute cases, however, handling should be reduced to the minimum and each case varies in the amount of disturbance tolerated. When giving a bedpan, the patient is lifted by one or two nurses and the bedpan slipped beneath him; a pillow is then placed under the lumbar spine and under the thighs, so that good alignment of the trunk is not lost.

Retention of urine is common and catheterisation may become necessary.

Abdominal upsets will be dealt with on the advice of the surgeon. Constipation is common, and may require the administration of glycerine suppositories or enemata. Liquid Paraffin may be ordered. Abdominal distension may require the use of a rectal tube and injections of Pituitrin. Acute dilation of the stomach sometimes occurs. A light nourishing diet is given and fluids administered freely. The mouth should be cleansed after each feed.

The relief of pain. Sedatives are usually ordered, though these are administered with caution if respiratory or bulbar involvement is suspected. Change of position is helpful, both in this connection and in preventing chest complications. Warmth is an important factor; an even temperature is essential, and *the limbs must never become cold.* Well-covered hot-water bottles may be indicated, or the use of an electric blanket. Hot packs are helpful in relieving pain, particularly before physiotherapeutic treatment, and the value of warm baths will be discussed later.

Meningeal symptoms necessitate a quiet, darkened room. Analgesics are given with caution because they mask the symptoms. It should be borne in mind that irritability may herald complications such as respiratory involvement.

Careful handling is important at all stages of the treatment, especially in the acute stage when muscle tenderness and spasm may be marked. The limbs should always be supported in their entirety, e.g. never lift a leg by grasping the foot only. At the same time, the fingers must not dig into tender muscle bellies. It is also borne in mind that joints deprived of their muscular supports are easily subluxated or even dislocated.

Position in bed. The patient is nursed in a position which is comfortable yet posturally correct (Fig. 18.3). A soft pillow is placed beneath the head; many patients are made more comfortable by placing a small roll of soft material under the neck. The head should be held in a central position; paralysis of one sterno-mastoid muscle may result in torticollis. The chin is not allowed to poke forward. If the upper limbs are involved, they are supported on soft pillows with the shoulders in a comfortable degree of forward flexion and the elbows comfortably flexed. The hands are conveniently supported by lint rolls made to fit the grasp. The trunk is held in a central position; sometimes a small flat pillow or folded blanket is needed to support the 'hollow of the back'. Low backache is often severe in these cases. The lower limbs are held in the neutral position, the knees are held in 5°–10° of flexion and a pillow, sand-bag or roll of blanket material may be needed to control rotation at the hip-joints. The feet are supported at a right-angle to the legs by the footboard or by sand-bags as already described. In the later stages, light plaster splints may be ordered to support the hands or feet.

Turning. The patient is turned from side to side and from the supine to the prone position, two, four, six or eight hourly according to the needs of the individual case. Change of position helps to releive pain, and to prevent chest complications and pressure sores. Patients can be nursed in various positions. At first, the prone position may not be well tolerated but it should be introduced as soon as possible, if only for a short period each day.

Prevention of pressure sores

These are prevented by the use of a soft mattress, by changing the position of the limbs and by ensuring that prominent bony parts such as the heels, malleoli, and elbows are protected from pressure by the use of pillows, lint rolls or pads. In the stage of acute muscle tenderness, handling is reduced to a minimum and inspection of pressure areas by massage is carried out with the greatest care. Need-

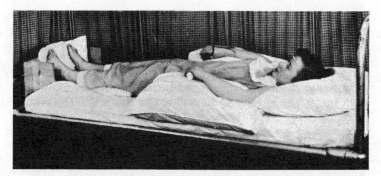

Fig. 18.3 A. The patient is nursed in a position which is comfortable yet posturally correct. Note the position of the footboard, and the lint rolls supporting the hands.

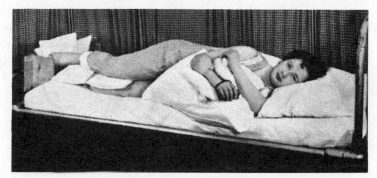

Fig. 18.3 B. Regular turning helps to relieve discomfort and prevents bed-sores and chest complications.

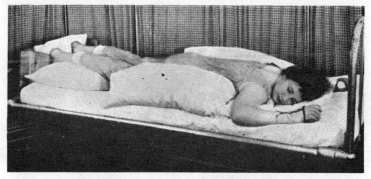

Fig. 18.3 C. The prone position is introduced as soon as possible for at least a short period each day. Note that correct anatomical alignment is still maintained. The patient is wearing a glove splint on the right hand.

less to say, a dry, smooth bed and scrupulous cleanliness of the skin are essential factors in the prevention of pressure sores.

Prevention of deformity

Deformity is due to the following:

1. *Bad posture:* a paralysed limb which is constantly held in a certain position will eventually adopt that position permanently.

2. *The action of gravity:* for instance, an unsupported paralysed foot assumes the drop-foot position, which may eventually become fixed.

3. *Muscle imbalance:* if one muscle or group of muscles is paralysed or weak, and its opponent functioning normally the healthy muscle will pull the limb into a deformed position; for example, if the peronei group is paralysed and the tibialis anticus and posticus functioning normally, the foot is held in the inverted position.

4. *Muscle contracture:* if, as in the example given above, the unopposed invertors were allowed to become contracted, the inversion deformity would become fixed.

Deformity can therefore be prevented by the following measures:

1. Maintaining correct position of the limbs.
2. Eliminating the action of gravity by supports.
3. Preventing overstretching of paralysed muscles and the contracture of healthy ones by:
   a. support;
   b. preserving full mobility of the joints;
   c. re-education of the weakened or paralysed muscles.

Splintage

This is applied according to the surgeon's orders, and should be as light and simple as possible, and unless there is incipient deformity, either from the action of gravity or from muscle imbalance, the use of pillows and sand-bags is sufficient, though light plaster shells or gutter-splints for the hand or foot are sometimes ordered. It must be remem-

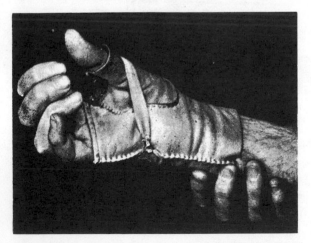

Fig. 18.4 A simple glove splint for paralysis of the muscles of the thenar eminence.

bered, however, that stiffness of joints must be prevented at all costs, and splintage must *never* be so rigidly applied as to produce this.

PHYSIOTHERAPY IN POLIOMYELITIS

INTRODUCTION

In the early stages of the disease, the motor nerve cells infected by the poliomyelitis virus are in varying stages of degeneration; cells showing mild degeneration may completely recover provided they are rested by reducing their activity in generating nerve impulses for muscle contraction; increased activity causes progressive degeneration and death of the cells with corresponding increase in the final paralysis; during the acute inflammatory stage when the patient is febrile, active exercises are contra-indicated, and the patient is encouraged to relax and not to attempt movements.

Early treatment

Passive movements are started as soon as the fever has subsided; muscles which are not repeatedly stretched to their full length will shorten; the shortened muscles then develop fibrous contractures and at a later stage there is joint stiffness with contractures of joint capsules and ligaments; in a child the deformity of the joints increase as the bones grow in length (Fig. 18.5). Ideally the joints are

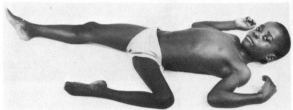

Fig. 18.5 Hip, knee and ankle contractures of left lower limb due to untreated poliomyelitis.

moved from the beginning through a full range but in the early stages the muscles may be painful. Stretching of the painful muscles at the end of the range increases the reflex motor nerve activity to produce the muscle contraction which is nature's protective response to pain. Because of the danger of increasing the damage to the motor nerves, the movement is only performed in the pain free range. The limbs are handled carefully and supported under bony points such as the knee and the heel to prevent pressure on the tender muscles. Hot packs may be given before the passive movements to aid muscle relaxation. The commercial type of hot pack used for treatment of painful joints is too heavy to be suitable for the treatment of painful muscles; pieces of blanket are soaked in boiling water, then passed twice through a wringer and shaken, or spin-dried and wrapped around the tender muscles; a piece of waterproof material and an outer covering of dry blanket retains the heat and moisture.

The physiotherapist co-operates with the nurse in the positioning of the patient paying particular attention to the lower limbs, the joints of which should be maintained in the positions needed for standing. At the shoulder, contractures tend to fix the joint in adduction; even if the patient is finally unable to move the shoulder due to extensive paralysis, lack of the movements of abduction and elevation makes dressing very difficult though in some cases a limited degree of contracture can be a positive advantage in providing a stable joint not liable to subluxation.

Management of the stage of recovery

After two to three weeks, the patient is feeling better. The fever has subsided and the pain and muscle spasm is less or may have disappeared. The paralysis reaches its maximum about one week after onset and recovery of muscle power is now in evidence.

The physiotherapist assesses:

1. Joint range. Limitation at this stage is due to muscle shortening and not joint stiffness.
2. Muscle power. Muscle power is graded on the 0 to 5 Oxford scale.

0 = No palpable muscle contraction.

1 = Flicker of contraction but no movement of the part.

2 = Movement through full range with the part supported to counterbalance the pull of gravity.

Grades 1 and 2 indicate very weak muscles but

at this stage it may be a hopeful sign in that further recovery can take place.

3 = Movement through full available range against gravity. Grade 3 means a muscle of fair power which would be functional for the upper limbs but not sufficiently strong for large weight-bearing muscles of the lower limb.

4 = Movement against gravity and resistance.

Grade 4 is a muscle with good power.

5 = As 4 but the resistance is increased to equal the amount which could be overcome by normal muscle.

Grade 5 = Normal power.

The muscle chart is repeated at monthly intervals and is kept as a record of progressive recovery. The extent of the initial paralysis is no indication of the final result. A very rough assessment of the amount of final recovery of muscle power can be made by adding two grades to the assessment at six weeks or one grade after three months. Muscles of 0 and 1 at three months are unlikely to progress any further. It is of value if the nurse understands these gradings. The physiotherapist can then encourage the patient in a realistic way by drawing his attention to the improvement in muscles but not engendering false optimism about very weak muscles which are unlikely ever to be functionally useful.

Babies and young children

The same gradings are used but they are obtained by utilising stimuli such as stroking or tickling the skin to elicit reflexes which would be present at the particular age level. Reflexes such as the Landau reaction which depend on positioning show up muscle weakness which can also be determined by watching the child at play.

Further treatment

Following the acute stage, there is a period of varying time when the patient tires easily and there may still be some tenderness in the muscles. Although the inflammation has subsided, the motor nerves are still not fully recovered. The patient must not be fatigued; he may be allowed to get up but must go back to bed and resume the lying position at the first sign of tiredness. This is especially important if the trunk muscles are weak because of the danger of scoliosis; for patients with extensive paralysis a tilt table or standing frame may be used; the angle of the tilt table is increased very slowly to the upright position to avoid 'blackouts' and 'dizziness'.

The physiotherapist starts active assisted exercises for the weak muscles and free active exercises for muscles of grade 3 or over. At this stage, the muscles are never worked to the point of fatigue as it is possible by doing so for muscles which were showing signs of recovery to become completely paralysed. Passive movements can now be given in a full range. Exercises in the hydrotherapy pool are started.

Hydrotherapy

The warmth of the water is a useful part of the treatment as the heat is maintained throughout the passive stretching or active exercises. It relaxes muscles for passive stretching and induces a better muscle contraction for the active exercises. The upthrust of the buoyancy of the water may be used to assist a weak muscle, act as a support as the patient moves the part on the surface of the water, or be used as a resistance for a stronger muscle (Figs 18.6A, B and C). By the use of floats and altering the speed of the movement to create turbulence finer gradings of exercises are possible. In deep water, the patient supported by floats can 'cycle' or walk in the water (Fig. 18.6D). In the Bad Ragaz type of exercise the patient is supported on the surface of the water and pushes away from or pulls towards the physiotherapist (Fig. 18.6E). The physiotherapist moves towards or away from the patient and the sequence is repeated, patient and physiotherapist moving together around the pool. The patient is now doing mass movements of the limbs rather than concentrating on individual muscle groups as in Figs. 18.6A, B and C. This

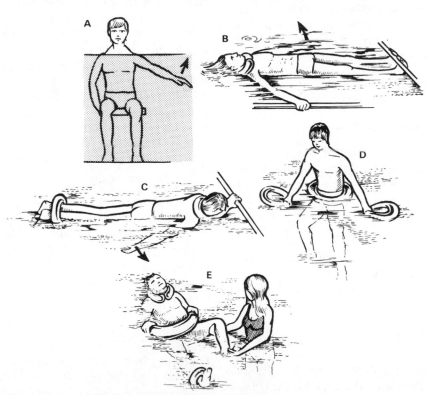

Fig. 18.6 **A.** Shoulder abductors assisted by buoyancy. **B.** Shoulder abduction supported by buoyancy. **C.** Shoulder abductors resisted by buoyancy. **D.** Deep water exercises for legs and trunk. **E.** Bad Ragaz exercise: extension and knee against resistance of physiotherapist.

is very valuable for muscle co-ordination and the patients enjoy travelling movements especially if they are confined to bed or to a wheelchair.

Sitting and standing balance is aided in the pool by the hydrostatic pressure which is exerting an even force on all sides of the body; walking in the water may be difficult for a polio patient; the upward force of buoyancy may swing the leg in an upward direction out of control of the patient when he tries to take a step; a weighted sandal is then used. In the later stages, swimming is a source of great satisfaction to severely handicapped children and adults who otherwise lead a wheel-chair existence. It is their only means of indepen-dent movement.

Progression in exercises

The exercises are gradually progressed in strength until the affected muscles are being worked to the maximum of their capability; the number of repeti-tions of the exercises are progressed for endurance.

Muscles of Grade 0, 1 and 2. Since these muscles are unable to move the part of the body against the force of gravity, the part will be supported by the physiotherapist's hands, sling suspension or by a polished table.

Muscles of Grades 3 and 4. These muscles will be exercised against increasing resistance. The resistance may be manual, weights or springs. Trick movements are encouraged such as laterally rotat-ing the shoulder to achieve abduction when deltoid is paralysed. Facilitation techniques are used to excite motor neurons which are not active but might be with a higher level of stimulation. The techniques are reflex stimulation of muscles super-imposed on the patient's own maximal effort to per-form a strong muscle contraction. Each time the motor neuron 'fires' it is easier for the next impulse to be initiated.

Functional assessment. A full assessment is made of the patient's ability to:

1. Roll over.
2. Sit up from lying.
3. Stand/sit.
4. Transfer from bed to
   a. standing;
   b. standing to bed;
   c. chair to standing;
   d. standing to chair;
   e. floor to chair;
   f. floor to standing;
   g. W.C.
      (i) On;
      (ii) Off;
   h. Bath (i) In; (ii) Out.
5. Walking or wheelchair activities.
   a. Forwards.
   b. Backwards.
   c. Turning.
   d. Slope.
   e. Varying surfaces.
   f. Door.
   g. Stairs.
6. Transport.
   a. Bus.
   b. Car.
7. Hand.
   a. Grip.
8. Personal activities.
   a. Wash.
   b. Dress.
   c. Hair.
   d. Shave.
   e. Eat.
   f. Drink.
   g. Write.

Code—A = Able to perform
   U = Unable to perform
   H = Needs help

Having studied the functional assessment and the 0–5 muscle chart, the physiotherapist decides which muscle groups need special strengthening to enable the patient to perform the activity and if any splints or aids would be helpful. Much of the functional activity is taught on mats on the floor.

Re-education of gait. Whenever possible, walk-ing is started in the parallel bars rather than in a walking machine because it more nearly resembles normal walking. With a walking machine, constant support is given by the arms, whereas with parallel bars there is a moment of time during each step when the support of the arms is lost.

Crutches are of three types—elbow, Canadian, axilliary (Fig. 18.7). From experience, Canadian type crutches are very satisfactory. A strap may be

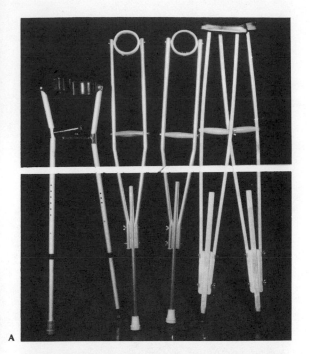

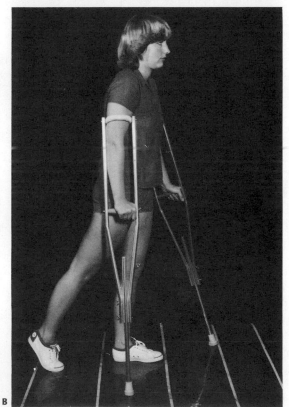

Fig. 18.7 **A.** Elbow, Canadian and Axilliary crutches. **B.** Four point crutch walking.

fastened to the side bars above the elbow if the triceps are paralysed. A four-point gait (Fig. 18.7) is taught and activities as described in 'functional assessment'. In developing countries, crutches can be made from inexpensive local materials, as described by David Weiner (1978) in his book *Where there is no doctor*.

Wheelchair activities. The paraplegic polio patient has the advantage over the spinal injury paraplegic in that he has no loss of skin sensation or of bladder and bowel function; usually some trunk muscles are functioning to give better balance. He is often able to walk with the use of crutches but needs a wheelchair because of the considerable energy expenditure in this type of walking. He is taught to use the wheelchair (as 'functional assessment') and may participate in many sporting activities such as wheelchair basketball, table tennis, archery, etc.

The patient with additional upper limb involvement may require a powered wheelchair; maximum use is made of any remaining functioning muscles; even if the patient can only use his neck muscles he can paint with a brush in his mouth and type on an electric typewriter using a mouthstick; these patients are likely to have respiratory involvement and may need assistance with coughing (Fig. 23.21A, B). If the abdominal muscles are paralysed, deep breathing and coughing is often improved by fastening an abdominal binder around the lower abdomen.

'Frog' breathing. Patients with very weak respiratory muscles may sleep in a tank respirator and use a cuirass respirator in a wheelchair. The physiotherapist can teach these patients glossopharyngeal (frog) breathing which enables them to breathe without any mechanical aid, often for a number of hours.

Physiotherapy for children

Children should be given physiotherapy in a department especially made for them with scaled-down parallel bars and steps and a selection of toys. A useful piece of equipment is a stool with castors fixed to the legs. The physiotherapist can sit on the stool propelling it backwards with the feet leaving the hands free to support a child learning to walk. Much of the activity is given in the form of play and a knowledge of child development is essential for the selection of suitable play activities (Chs 11 and 12). Handling techniques to elicit movement by automatic reflex reactions are also used. It is important that parents are encouraged to join in the sessions so that the treatment can be continued at home, especially passive stretching of tight structures, and walking. For the older child, education is a priority since employment is limited for the physically handicapped; physiotherapy must be co-ordinated to fit in with school activities (Chs 11 and 12).

Untreated polio patients in developing countries

Children and adults are frequently seen who are only able to hop or crawl on all fours (Figs 18.8 and 18.9). The surgeon performs release operations

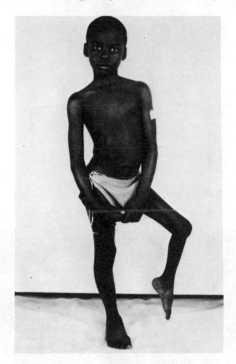

Fig. 18.8   Hopping as a means of locomotion—untreated poliomyelitis. (Same patient as Fig. 18.5.)

and corrective procedures and the physiotherapist will then teach the patient to walk.

In young children it is possible to correct the deformities in the lower limbs by a gradual strong passive stretching. Following this the correction must be maintained by calipers, serial plasters or

removable splints. Since this is a forced movement it should only be carried out or taught to parents by the physiotherapist because careless handling can damage joints or even fracture the brittle bones of a poliomyelitis patient (Fig. 18.10A, B and C).

Calipers should be strong, cheap, and where possible, made locally; (Fig. 18.11); knee joints are not included in children's calipers because they are quickly damaged and workshop facilities may not be adequate to keep them in repair; boots made without toe-caps have a longer life because they allow for growth of the foot. Children find walking sticks easier to manage if they are fixed in a wooden block (Fig. 18.12).

NURSING MANAGEMENT OF THE CONVALESCENT STAGE

This is directed towards improving the function of the limbs, and during this time the patient should be viewed not only as an orthopaedic problem but

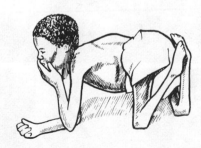

Fig. 18.9   Severely deformed by crawling on the elbows and knees for fourteen years without treatment. (With kind permission of Huckstep (1970) and Makenene Medical Journal, 14:9.)

as a social and economic one. Every effort must be made to prepare the patient for the resumption of normal life.

When the patient is allowed to sit up, a wind-up bed of the Hoskins type is very useful. It is important to make haste slowly, especially where there is paralysis of the spinal and abdominal muscles; sitting up too early or unsupervised may result in spinal deformity such as scoliosis, and correct anatomical alignment must be insisted upon no matter what the position adopted.

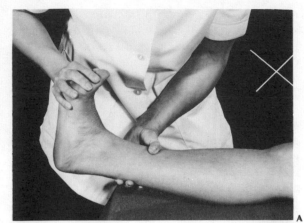

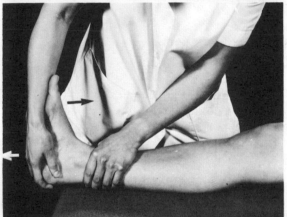

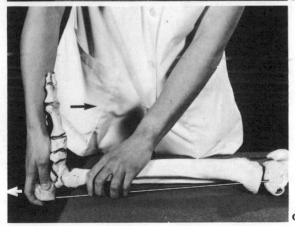

Occupational therapy is often introduced at this stage; the occupational therapist will visit the patient and will study his particular case along with other members of the team. If the upper limbs are unaffected, and the patient feels well enough, he may enjoy needlework, leather work, weaving or

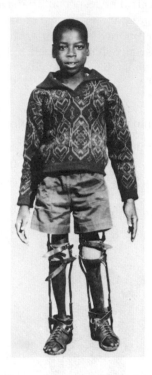

Fig. 18.11   Calipers, and open-toed boots (made in Kenya).

Fig. 18.10   Passive stretching.
   Incorrect—**A.** Forced passive stretching of calf muscles—hyperextending the knee and metatarso-phalangeal joints, straining the intertarsal joints and giving insufficient protection to the bones.
   Correct—**B.** Forced passive stretching of tight calf muscles. **C.** Grasp of physiotherapist on bones of lower limb, and direction of pull of gastrocnemius; (knee must be held in extension because gastrocnemius assists in flexion of this joint). NB Fixation above ankle; pull on calcaneum support of foot as strongly dorsiflexed.

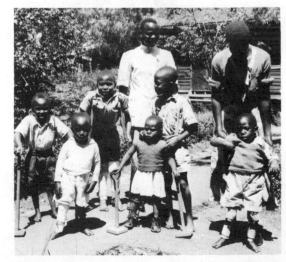

Fig. 18.12   Childrens' walking sticks fixed on to wooden blocks.

toy-making. If they *are* affected, the interest and co-operation of the occupational therapist is even more desirable, for she can play a prominent part firstly in introducing crafts which aid *re-education* of muscle, and secondly, in *rehabilitation* of paralysed upper limbs so that residual handicap can be overcome. The occupational therapist who can devise slings, hand splints, special equipment for the toilet, for reading, eating, and other everyday activities makes a valuable contribution to the patient's recovery.

N.B. *Aids to function described here may also be used for patients handicapped as a result of spinal injury* (Ch. 23).

Muscle recovery may still be expected up to two years from the onset of the disease, but during the convalescent stage it is usually possible to form some idea of the extent of ultimate disability. It should be mentioned here that though most patients show great courage, fortitude and perseverance, there are some who will not accept the situation and who need special consideration. Optimism, unfailing patience and cheerfulness on the part of the nursing and allied teams communicates itself to the patient and is an essential background to treatment.

In cases where the legs and trunk are paralysed but the upper limbs are spared, special exercises are given to over-develop the muscles of the shoulder-girdle and arms; often these become so powerful that the patient is able to lead an almost normal life even if confined to crutches and/or a wheelchair. The patient is first taught to balance while sitting in bed and arm exercises are practised intensively; games such as throwing a ball, and later darts, archery and javelin-throwing are valuable aids to muscular development.

Weight-bearing. If there is widespread paralysis of the trunk and lower limbs so that weight-bearing cannot be achieved, a light wheelchair is ordered and rehabilitation commenced with a view to adopting this as the chief means of locomotion. Even in severely paralysed patients, however, it is well worthwhile to attempt the standing position, even if only occasionally, because the organs of the thorax and abdomen benefit from the change of position, and the patient enjoys it. Moreover, decalcification of the skeleton is prevented to some degree and the standing position helps to prevent

flexion contractures. In the early stages, a 'stander-upper' (tilt-table) is used, when the patient is strapped to a wooden stretcher which can be levered into a vertical position. Otherwise severely paralysed patients require splintage which connects the legs to the trunk, i.e. leg braces (calipers) joined to a pelvic band or spinal support.

In patients who are confined to wheelchairs, special rehabilitation is required with regard to the toilet and other acts of daily living. For example, a housewife must adjust herself to her daily work and many women run a home and care for a family despite the handicap of a wheelchair (Fig. 18.13A, B).

Importance of securing the co-operation of the family and of community health personnel. At the earliest possible moment, the patient's family should be included in the rehabilitation programme and the community health personnel informed of the patient's problems on discharge from hospital. The home conditions will be investigated by the social worker and steps taken to obtain any special equipment necessary, for example, a motor-chair or hand-controlled motor-car (Fig. 18.13C): or the patient may be helped to find ground-floor accommodation; sometimes suspensory apparatus for lifting the patient from bed to chair or into a bath may be required. Needless to say the interest and co-operation of the family is of inestimable value, if only to lead the patient to feel that he is wanted. As soon as possible, the patient is allowed home, say for a week-end, and regular outings such as visits to the theatre are arranged.

Importance of the nurse's part in rehabilitation. It would seem from the foregoing paragraphs that the patient is now out of the nurse's hands—far from it—he needs her as much as ever. The surgeon, the physiotherapist, the occupational therapist, and the social worker (who will be working on the social aspect of the case) all play a major role, but it is the nurse who provides the essential background. Without her active co-operation the efforts of other members of the team cannot succeed. The patient still relies on his nurse to rehabilitate him for the ordinary acts of daily living. It is she who guides his first attempts to feed, wash and dress himself, and who teaches him to use a lavatory and take a bath. *Adaptations* to living conditions are discussed elsewhere.

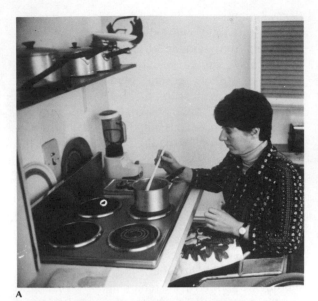

A

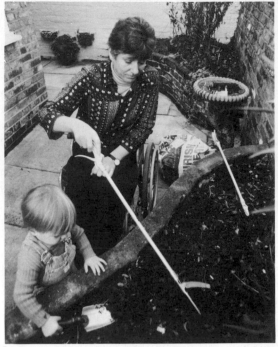

B

Fig. 18.13   (See text.)

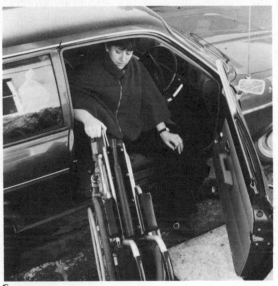

C

Fig. 18.13   (See text.)

Retentive splintage

If there is still residual disability after a long period of convalescence combined with re-education, retentive splintage may be ordered. It should be as light and simple as possible, and it must be remembered that circulatory changes in the skin may predispose the patient to splint sores and that disease atrophy of limbs leads to pathological fracture. Retentive plasters are not as a rule ordered as they are necessarily heavy and tax the patient's

already weakened muscles too heavily. Also, re-education of muscle is well-nigh impossible inside closed plasters. Extensive paralysis may result in shortened, wasted limbs, with slender, rarefied bones and unduly mobile joints. This type of patient often becomes excessively thin, but on the other hand, there may be large deposits of subcutaneous fat due to the restricted activity and inability to take exercise. The last-named type is particularly difficult to manage with regard to splintage. Circulatory changes are almost always present in both types and the affected limbs become cold and blue.

Splintage is very carefully chosen for the individual patient. In cases of widespread paralysis, various appliances or combinations of appliances may be tried out before a satisfactory result is obtained. Even when no further recovery of muscle power is expected, efforts to improve the *functional use* of a limb are not relaxed.

Retentive splintage for different regions

The upper limbs. An abduction splint is occasionally ordered for paralysis of the shoulder muscles and plaster shells, 'working splints' or some device such as the glove shown in Fig. 18.4, are used for the hand. Splintage for the upper limb is discarded as soon as possible, so that *functional use* can be encouraged.

Paralysis of the trunk muscles. Paralysis of the spinal muscles may necessitate a spinal support, which may be combined with an abdominal belt if weakness of the abdominal muscles causes an extreme lordosis. In paralysis of the gluteus maximus, the spinal support may be strapped to two braces (calipers) in order to allow the patient to achieve the upright position. The patient may be taught to walk on crutches, though these may be replaced by sticks if the muscles of the upper limbs are strong. Unequal recovery of the muscles of the trunk may result in scoliosis. A block-leather support or Milwaukee brace may then be ordered. Unfortunately, no splintage has been devised which can overcome the waddling gait associated with paralysis of the gluteus medius and minimus.

Paralysed quadriceps necessitate a brace (caliper) to hold the knee in extension. If two calipers are worn, one ring must be at a higher level than the other to allow the limbs to pass each other comfortably in walking. Plaster shells or light aluminium splints may be worn at night.

Drop-foot is controlled by a plastic splint (Fig. 18.14A, B and C) or by an inside, outside or double iron with posterior stops, or a toe-raising spring, with perhaps a plaster shell for night wear. Anterior stops are ordered if the calf muscles are affected, and in inverted or everted foot would require a T-strap on the opposite side of the deformity.

Operative treatment

This may be ordered in the late stages. Manipulations may be carried out (for example, on the foot) followed by a period of plaster fixation and re-education.

Operations on soft parts. These may be:

1. *Tenotomy* or elongation of tight structures (for example, the tendo-Achilles) followed by plaster fixation and re-education.
2. *Tendon transplants*, which allow a healthy muscle to do the work of a paralysed one, and to correct deformities (for example, the tibialis anticus is transplanted to the outer side of the foot to correct persistent inversion). If a tendon is transplanted, it must be in alignment, strong enough for its new task, comparable in function to its predecessor and dispensable to the part from which it is taken.

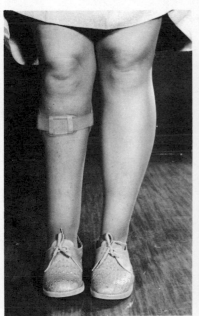
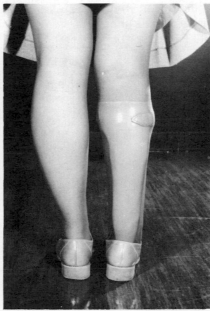
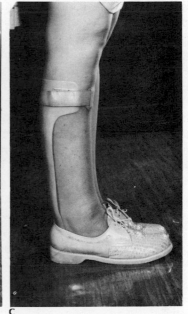

A   B   C

Fig. 18.14   A, B, C. A plastic splint to control drop-foot.

Operations on bone. This is usually stabilisation of a flail joint (for example, the shoulder or foot). It provides a stable joint, function is greatly improved, and splintage may be discarded. *Fusion of the spine* may be advised if there is widespread muscle weakness with progressive scoliosis; *supracondylar osteotomy* of the femur is sometimes indicated for genu-recurvatum. *Operations to equalise the length of* the legs include:

1. *Leg shortening*, either by stapling the epiphyses of the femur and/or tibia, or by some form of osteotomy.
2. *Leg lengthening* is sometimes required (Ch. 15).

Lumbar sympathectomy may be performed if the trophic changes in the lower limbs become troublesome.

After-care continues by means of regular supervision until growth has ceased; a close watch is kept for secondary deformity. Before the patient is discharged from hospital, community health personnel will be made aware of his problems. The nurse must instruct the patient and his relatives with regard to the splintage and the care of the skin. Splints, boots and night splints, if worn, must fit well and be adjusted as growth proceeds and be kept in good repair. Patients with extensive paralysis need suitable living conditions and aids to mobility, e.g. a wheelchair and/or a motor-car. The patients must be warmly clothed because of the poor circulation in the limbs; chilblains must be guarded against and the patient warned against extremes of heat and cold. If deformity of the thorax is present as a result of paralysed muscles, the possibility of intercurrent disease such as bronchitis must be borne in mind. Most important of all is education, vocational training and employment so that even if disabled, the patient can take his place in society.

SUMMARY OF TREATMENT

Acute stage

1. Isolation.
2. Rest, general and local, in a good position; support and perhaps splintage to prevent deformity.
3. Physiotherapy—early passive movements to prevent joint stiffness; active movements as soon as possible.
4. Treatment of complications.

Convalescent stage

1. Intensive re-education, exercise in baths, etc.
2. Retentive splintage, if required.
3. Re-education for home and professional life.
4. Operative procedures.

BIBLIOGRAPHY

Adams J C 1971 Outline of Orthopaedics. Edinburgh: Churchill Livingstone

Apley A G 1977 A System of Orthopaedics and Fractures. London: Butterworths

Crutchley N Y 1983 Post-poliomyelitis assessment. British Association of Orthopaedic Nurses and Association of Orthopaedic Chartered Physiotherapists' New Sheet, December

Fanshawe E et al 1978 Disability without handicap. Nursing Times Supplement, 17 August, 3–20

Guyton A C 1974 Function of the Human Body. London: W B Saunders Co

Hardy G M 1954 Nursing and Treatment of Acute Anterior Poliomyelitis. London: Faber

Huckstep R L 1976 Poliomyelitis. Edinburgh: Churchill Livingstone

Laver G H 1976 Lobar pneumonia necessitating ventilation in a polio victim. Nursing Mirror 142(3), January, 50–52

Stott C P 1955 Management of Acute Poliomyelitis. Edinburgh: Livingstone

Trueta J 1956 Handbook on Poliomyelitis. Oxford: Blackwell Scientific

Turek S L 1977 Orthopaedics: principles and applications. Lippincott, 447

Werner D 1978 Where There is no Doctor. Macmillan Tropical Community Health Manuals

SECTION **THREE**

Care of the injured patient

19

General principles of trauma

INTRODUCTION

A brief description of the commoner injuries of bones and joints is included in this book because the treatment of such lesions is an integral part of an orthopaedic service, and cannot be regarded as a separate entity. The principles of treatment which have already been described in connection with other orthopaedic conditions also apply to the conditions discussed in the ensuing chapters. These include fractures, dislocations and injuries to soft tissues such as tendons and ligaments. The last named may be of equal or even greater importance than injuries of bone, because in the absence of proper treatment the period of disability is likely to be prolonged. In this connection, the nurse will bear in mind the large number of patients treated in the Out-patient or Casualty Department who may never see the inside of a hospital ward but who may very well have suffered an injury which results in prolonged loss of work and earnings and perhaps serious permanent disability, for example, the manual worker who sustains a hand injury.

There are also cases where fractures are accompanied by other injuries which may be even more serious, particularly in multiple injuries resulting from road accidents. Although the aim of treatment is to reduce a fracture at the earliest possible moment, precedence may have to be given to the treatment of other injuries.

An accident, as we all know, can happen to anyone but predisposing causes include carelessness and ignorance of danger, for example, in the young child; loss of mobility or of sight or hearing,

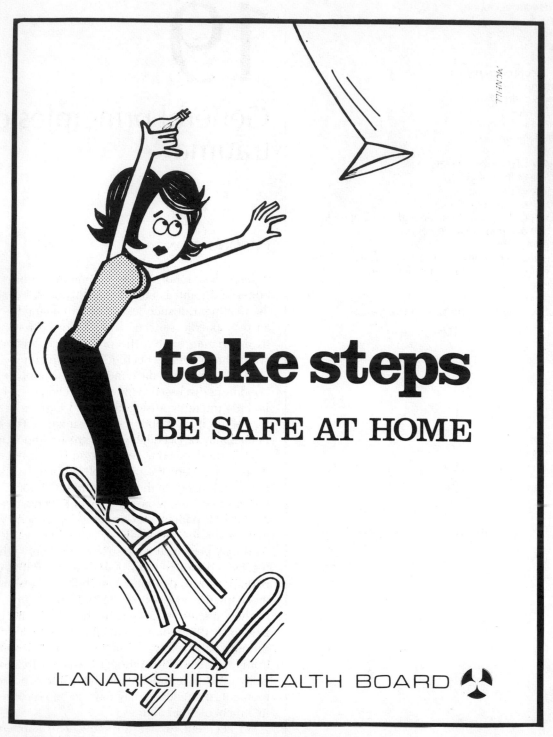

Fig. 19.1 'Take steps—Be safe at home'. (Lanarkshire Health Board.)

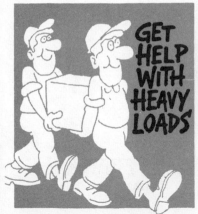

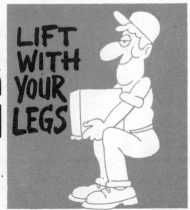

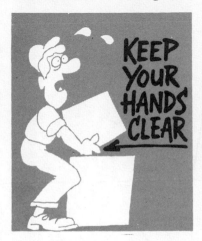

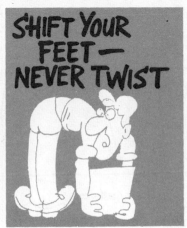

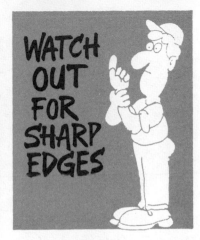

Fig. 19.2 'Manual Handling'. (British Safety Council, London.)

DON'T WAIT....

CLUNK CLICK
EVERY
TRIP

Fig. 19.3 'Clunk Click'. (By courtesy of Royal Society for the Prevention of Accidents.)

as in the elderly; or medical conditions such as epilepsy or cardio-vascular disease; and finally, misuse of drugs or of alcohol.

We tend to think of an accident as a dramatic event occurring on the road or in the air, but in fact many patients sustain their injuries in their homes, their schools, their places of work or recreation (Figs 19.1, 19.2 and 19.5). Housewives, children and the elderly sustain burns, scalds and injuries due to falls. Workers in factories or mines, or on building sites or farms sustain a multiplicity of injuries and the sports field and swimming pool produce their own quota of injured patients (Fig. 19.6). Finally, there are those injured by some form of violence such as civil disturbances or warfare (Skeet, 1977).

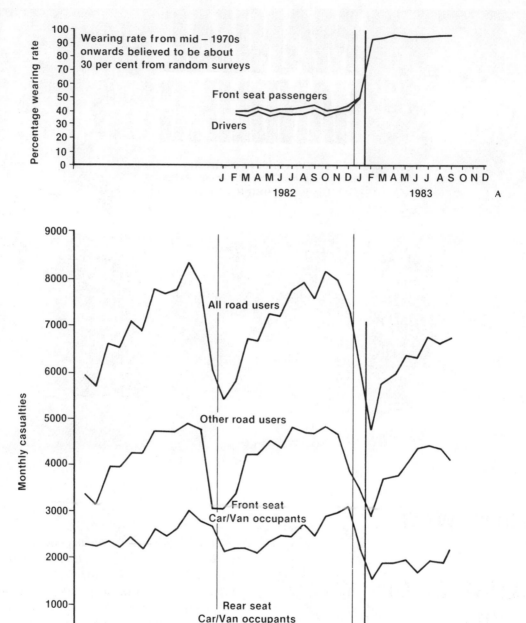

Fig. 19.4 Monitoring of compulsory seat belt wearing (31 January 1983). **A.** Seat belt wearing amongst front seat occupants of cars and light vans: GB. **B.** Fatal or serious injuries: occupants of cars and light vans; other road users; all road users. (By courtesy of West Mercia Police Force.)

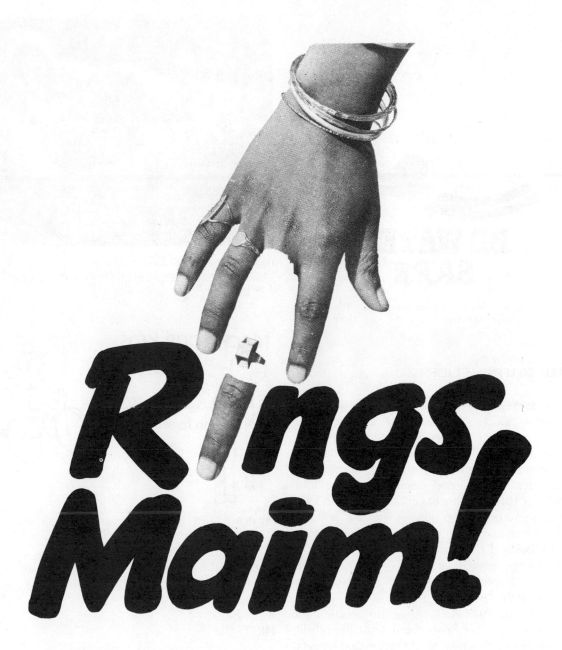

Fig. 19.5 'Rings Maim!' (British Safety Council, London.)

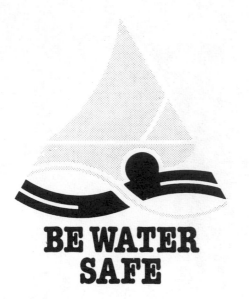

Fig. 19.6 'Be water safe' (By courtesy of the *Royal Society for the Prevention of Accidents*.)

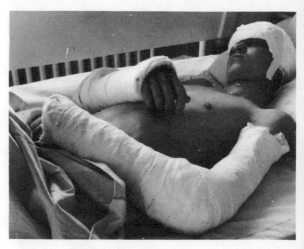

Fig. 19.7 The price that society pays for rapid modern transport. A young road-user lies seriously injured in hospital. (Courtesy of WHO.)

ROAD TRAFFIC ACCIDENTS

On an average day in Britain 18 people are killed in road accidents; (*The Guardian*, 19 June 1978); in the year 1977 injuries in road accidents cost a total of £671 millions without taking into account damage to vehicles or property (*The Guardian*, 22 November 1978). Road casualties in the third quarter of 1983 were 9 per cent lower than in 1982 in the same period because of the seat belt law which came into being in January 1982 (Fig. 19.4): deaths being 1370 and serious injuries 18 600, down 14 per cent (Department of Transport). There were 350 fewer deaths in front seat passengers because of the law.

In the year 1973, over 7 million people were injured in road accidents throughout the world. Among those who died, 90 000 were first hospitalised for periods of up to 30 days. Many were treated in costly intensive care units; great numbers of survivors needed, and go on needing, continuous care (Fig. 19.7). This represents a huge drain on hospital, medical and public health resources, not to speak of the human suffering whose magnitude can only be guessed at (Kaprio, 1975). For this reason, *prevention of accidents* by formulation and enforcement of legislation, by research into

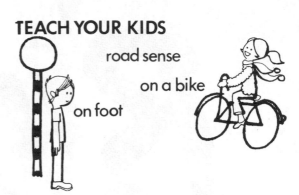

Fig. 19.8 'Teach Your Kids'. (By courtesy of Dr William Thomson and the Lanarkshire Health Board.)

causes and by education of the public is of paramount importance (Figs 19.8 and 19.9).

FIRST AID

The treatment of injured persons begins at the scene of the accident and is only complete on resettlement of the patient at work and in society. *First aid and transport to hospital* is carried out by trained ambulance crews; pending their arrival on the scene the patient must be protected from unnecessary movement (unless he is in danger of further injury), from cold and from meddlesome interference, however well-meant. On the other hand, the

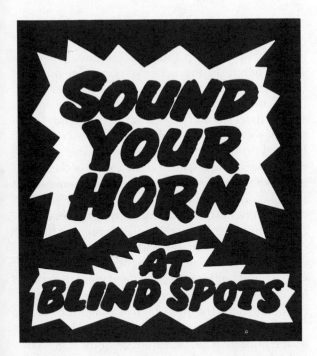

Fig. 19.9 'Sound your Horn'. (By courtesy of the British Safety Council.)

establishment of a *clear airway* is vital, especially in an unconscious patient; secretions or vomit must be removed from the mouth and he must be transported in the semi-prone position. *Exposed haemorrhage* is dealt with by covering wounds with clean material and applying a firm bandage; obvious injuries to the limbs will be dealt with according to their site; a sling or padded wooden splint is suitable for the upper limb, or, it can be bandaged to the trunk, and a lower limb injury can be dealt with by bandaging it to the sound one. A brief note on the transportation of spinal injuries will be found later. *Shock* can be minimised by protection from cold and by careful handling; the patient is rolled gently on to a canvas stretcher (Fig. 19.22) on which he lies continuously until full examination and assessment of his injuries is carried out by the surgeon. If *analgesia* is ordered it should be given intravenously so that it is absorbed quickly; if given by any other route it may not be absorbed, so that further doses given subsequently might have adverse effects; the dosage and time given is recorded for the information of the hospital team.

Nothing is given by mouth; and information is sought (if possible) as to the time and content of the last meal taken.

ACCIDENT CENTRES

Accident centres with special facilities for the prompt reception and immediate resuscitation of casualties, especially those with multiple injuries, are already established in many parts of Britain and are developed or being developed in other countries. In addition 'flying squads' of doctors and nurses may attend the scene of an accident in some areas (Hastings, 1982; Buckles, 1983). Ambulance crews and members of the police force are usually able to warn the hospital of the impending arrival of casualties so that medical and nursing staff are on the alert. It is helpful if the ambulancemen or the police can give the medical team an accurate account of the patient's condition at the scene of the accident and en route to hospital. For example, the position of the patient, whether there was the possibility of inhalation of vomit which may cause pneumonia later (Mendelsohn's Syndrome), or whether there were any sharp objects or other obstacles which the patient may have fallen on. In the case of a road traffic accident, was the patient the driver of a car or was he in the front seat wearing a safety-belt or, alternatively, was he a back seat passenger? This information along with many other observations will help the medical team when making their assessment of the patient in the casualty department. These centres are designed with a special reception area where the patient receives his initial examination and which is equipped not only with splints, plaster bandages, dressings, etc., common to all casualty departments, but with apparatus for suction, intubation, blood-transfusion, and other special items such as tracheostomy sets. There is often a 'shock room' adjacent to the operating theatre where the patient can receive continuous and intensive care until he is fit to proceed to a ward. The unit should include a comfortable room where relatives can wait or even stay overnight. It is the responsibility of the hospital along with the police to notify the patient's next of kin as soon as possible; the fact that the relatives have been informed can be a great relief to hospital staff, especially if the patient's condition deteriorates rapidly or if he requires urgent surgery. If the nurses in the Casualty/Resuscitation Unit are very busy the relatives can be comforted by nursing staff outside the department or by Social Workers who can be a big help if there are any financial problems or other serious difficulties, e.g. involving small children left alone at home. A vivid description of the plight of relatives is given by Turner (1982), himself a social worker, in the *Nursing Times* Patients Page.

ADMISSION AND RESUSCITATION OF A SEVERELY INJURED PATIENT

When the patient arrives, he is examined by the surgeon immediately; the first essential is the establishment of a *clear airway*; secretions in the mouth are removed by suction and an oral or, in an unconscious patient, an endotracheal tube is inserted. When the medical team is confronted with more than one patient with multiple injuries, priorities have to be decided upon by an experienced member of the team (usually the team leader). This is not an easy task; most accident surgeons will place injured patients into four groups, viz. those who require treatment immediately, those who will require it soon, and those that can wait; the fourth group, unfortunately being those that are beyond help. It has been reported that nurses are using the 'triage' system in some centres (Cochrane, 1983; Blything, 1983).

The first examination therefore identifies and deals with any immediate threat to life. The nurse also makes an early examination of the patient and when the airway is assured and any exposed haemorrhage arrested, it is important to record, as a base-line for further reference the patient's pulse, blood pressure, temperature, consciousness level, and pupil reactions. If intra-abdominal injuries are suspected girth measurements are also taken; this is done by placing a tape measure around the patient's abdomen, marking the exact place on the skin where the first measurement was taken so that subsequent measurements can be taken accurately in the identical place. These observations should be continued quarter hourly as long as is thought necessary by the medical team.

A great deal of importance is attached to the observations made by the nursing staff; if they are not carried out at regular and frequent intervals some change in the patient's condition may go unnoticed. For instance, a patient with a head injury may develop intra-cranial pressure which can be detected and treated early if there has been regular recording of pupil reaction, consciousness level, pulse rate and blood pressure. The surgeon then makes an assessment of the extent of the injuries and if they are severe, intra-venous therapy and preparation for *blood transfusion* is commenced at once. In unconscious patients, it may be necessary at this stage to split the clothing carefully for further examination to be made, particularly X-ray examination. An observant, experienced nurse can be very helpful while undressing the patient, by pointing out any bruises, grazes or other signs that may be significant. The hard task of diagnosing fractures, dislocations or internal injury may be helped by the nurse making tactful suggestions, e.g. a pattern of clothing on the abdominal wall will suggest intra-abdominal injury. A bruised or grazed face may lead the doctor to consider an injury to the cervical spine; a limb that the patient does not move may lead to a diagnosis of a fracture. Tyremarks or friction burns may indicate that the patient has at some time been under the wheel of a vehicle, and this may indicate injury to the spine, or to the chest, depending where the marks are in relation to the part. These observations are of particular importance where the patient is unconscious or cannot communicate for some other reason. *Open wounds* are dressed, and chemotherapy is usually ordered. ATS or tetanus toxoid is also indicated where there is an open wound but the surgeon will usually order a test-dose, and the history of previous immunisation is noted, if it is available. Open wounds of the chest must be covered with a simple dressing to reduce the risk of a tension pneumothorax. Sometimes immediate operation is urgently required; the stomach is then emptied by means of a tube, but further preparations, including cleansing of the skin and pre-operative medication is usually carried out in the theatre.

Shock arises after injury as a result of changes in the circulation, primarily designed to maintain the arterial blood pressure at its normal level and to combat the effect of loss of circulating fluid, either as a result of haemorrhage into the tissues or external loss of blood. It also arises when large quantities of extra-cellular fluids are lost through severe vomiting or diarrhoea.

Shock is also seen in cardiopulmonary conditions such as myocardial infarction, cardiac tamponade or pulmonary embolism (cardiogenic shock) or in septacaemia (bacteraemic shock).

Sometimes different causes of shock are seen in the same patient; for example, the severely burned patient may also develop septacaemia. After the injury the individual first goes into a stage of reaction, in which there is intense peripheral vasoconstriction, the pulse rate is increased, and as long as the circulating fluid is sufficient the cardiac output is maintained, so that not infrequently the blood pressure will rise; it may rise as high as 200 mmHg in a fit active young person. The extent of this stage of reaction and how long it lasts will depend on the individual, and on the severity of the injuries. As it passes, the blood pressure gradually falls as a result of loss of circulating fluid, and the patient passes into what is generally recognised as a state of shock—that is, with a thin, rapid pulse; a lowered blood pressure, and cold, perhaps slightly cyanotic extremities; restlessness and irritability may occur as a result of cerebral anoxaemia. If this state of affairs is allowed to continue without restoration of the circulating blood volume, severe injuries will result in death.

This type of shock is known as hypovolaemic or oligemic shock, and bears no relationship to neurogenic or primary shock of the sort that one sees in a fainting attack, though there may be some similarity in the appearance of the unconscious patient. The fainting attack is recognised by the fact that the pulse is always slow and full.

Dehydration also contributes to shock, as when large quantities of fluid are lost from burnt body surfaces; in severe shock there may be insufficient blood passing through the kidneys to maintain renal function and uraemia rapidly develops.

Haemorrhage always gives rise to shock, though shock can occur without haemorrhage; haemorrhage is said to be *primary* when it occurs at the time of injury; *reactionary* when it occurs as the blood pressure returns to normal after it has been abnormally low. *Secondary* haemorrhage occurs when infection invades and erodes blood-clot at

the end of a large vessel, causing it to rupture; since the advent of antibiotics, this type of haemorrhage is rarely seen.

GENERAL MANAGEMENT OF SHOCK

The most important single feature is to restore the circulating blood volume. If the estimated loss is 2 litres, 1–1½ litres may be replaced by plasma expanders; in excess of 2 litres whole blood is required.

Figures of suggested estimated blood losses:

Closed fracture of the femoral shaft	½–1 litre
Open ring fractures of pelvis	2–3 litres
Intra-abdominal haemorrhage	2–3 litres
Haemothorax	1–2 litres

It is also important to relieve pain and to splint and protect any peripheral injuries. These measures should be taken immediately and continued until the general condition of the patient is good enough to permit wound excision and reduction of the fractures and proper immobilisation. It is to be emphasised that the best single estimate of a patient's condition with regard to shock is a series of blood pressure readings, also that the presence of an elevated blood pressure is an indication of shock and requires suitable resuscitation measures to see that the blood pressure does not fall below the normal level. Sometimes the *central venous pressure* is measured by means of a catheter passed through an arm or leg vein until the tip lies in the vena cava near the heart. Pressure recorded here is a guide to the circulating blood volume and acts as a monitor of the extent of shock and the results of treatment.

An observation chart (Fig. 19.10) is commenced at once and the blood pressure recorded every 15 minutes. Blood for grouping and cross-matching in readiness for transfusion may be collected from an open wound, otherwise it is taken from a vein. Haemorrhage is controlled by application of a firm pad and bandage; a tourniquet is rarely necessary, and the foot of the bed is elevated where possible. Maintenance of a clear airway is essential and oxygen therapy, artificial respiration, bronchoscopy or even tracheostomy may be necessary. Accurate measurement of urinary output and body tempera-

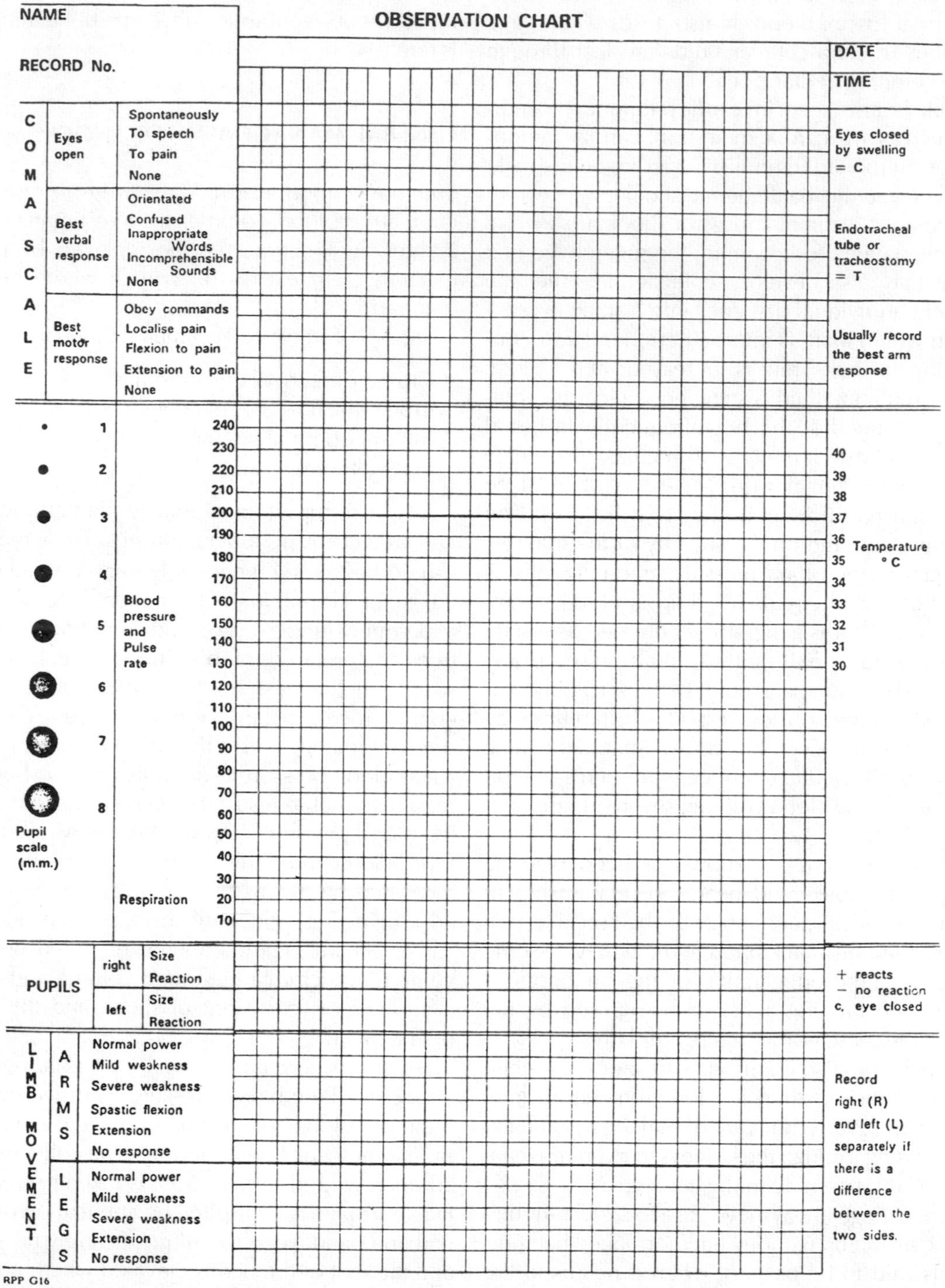

OBSERVATION CHART

NAME		
RECORD No.		

DATE

TIME

C O M A S C A L E	Eyes open	Spontaneously
		To speech
		To pain
		None
	Best verbal response	Orientated
		Confused
		Inappropriate Words
		Incomprehensible Sounds
		None
	Best motor response	Obey commands
		Localise pain
		Flexion to pain
		Extension to pain
		None

Eyes closed by swelling = C

Endotracheal tube or tracheostomy = T

Usually record the best arm response

Pupil scale (m.m.)

1 2 3 4 5 6 7 8

Blood pressure and Pulse rate: 240 230 220 210 200 190 180 170 160 150 140 130 120 110 100 90 80 70 60 50 40 30

Respiration: 20 10

Temperature °C: 40 39 38 37 36 35 34 33 32 31 30

PUPILS	right	Size
		Reaction
	left	Size
		Reaction

+ reacts
− no reaction
c, eye closed

L I M B M O V E M E N T	A R M S	Normal power
		Mild weakness
		Severe weakness
		Spastic flexion
		Extension
		No response
	L E G S	Normal power
		Mild weakness
		Severe weakness
		Extension
		No response

Record right (R) and left (L) separately if there is a difference between the two sides.

RPP G16

Fig. 19.10 Observation chart.

ture is axiomatic. In addition, monitoring of cardiac function by means of an electro-cardiograph. Frequent examination of blood for acid-base state and gas tensions, blood urea, electrolytes, haemoglobin, haematocrit, white cell and platelet counts may also be required.

Synthetic plasma-expanders may be used where blood is not available immediately.

A patient in a state of shock is cold, pale, sweating, restless and if conscious, also frightened. He requires reassurance and protection from noise, fuss and unnecessary commotion. Analgesics are ordered for the relief of pain, and all but essential movement of injured limbs must be avoided. Protect the patient from cold, but do not apply direct artificial heat. NOTHING IS GIVEN BY MOUTH until the surgeon gives permission.

THE METABOLIC RESPONSE TO INJURY

There is a very marked alteration in the chemical processes of the injured patient. For the first 24–48 hours of injury (or indeed, of major operation) the kidneys have difficulty in excreting water and sodium ions. The water effect is stronger than the sodium effect so that the small amount of urine passed tends to have a higher concentration of sodium ions and a higher specific gravity than normal. At the same time, for 3–4 days after injury/operation there is increased elimination of potassium ions in the urine. The breakdown of cells (which normally goes on all the time) is accelerated, and the amount of nitrogeneous products derived from protein, which is discharged in the urine, is greater than the intake, so that the patient is in negative nitrogen balance. This means that there is less protein available in the body for the repair of damaged tissues.

THE UNCONSCIOUS PATIENT

The unconscious patient is a person who has become helpless and no longer aware of his surroundings; functions and reflexes are no longer normal and are reduced in varying degrees. Unconsciousness may be caused by a *medical condition*, such as cerebrovascular accident (Ch. 24) by epilepsy, diabetes mellitus, septicaemia, or by

cerebral infection; cerebral anoxia (lack of oxygen to the brain) may be caused by pulmonary and cerebral tumours, heart failure, inhalations of fumes, severe uraemic, dehydration, or by combinations of *poisons* such as drug over-dose, inhalation of carbon-monoxide, or absorption of lead or mercury.

Trauma as a cause of unconsciousness can be divided as follows:

1. Road traffic accidents and
2. Domestic or industrial accidents, though in both situations the causes of unconsciousness are broadly the same. For example, in either situation one sees head injuries with fractures of the skull; haemorrhage or cerebral oedema; severe loss of blood; injury to the chest causing a low arterial blood oxygen level; plasma loss in severe burns; electric shock; fractures of the long bones; fat embolism, which might give rise to pulmonary oedema; and cerebral and renal damage. In road traffic accidents, however, there is generally more likelihood of multiple injuries than in accidents occurring in other situations.

General anaesthesia is a cause of unconsciousness but in this case its duration can usually be predetermined and complications are rare.

The level of consciousness is recognised by the patient's response to outside stimuli. Voluntary control of responses to sensations are normally under the control of the will; when this control is lost response to stimuli becomes reflex, i.e. automatic in nature, and these reflexes can be used to test the level of consciousness, which may vary between 'confusion' when the patient is unable to answer questions, and complete unconsciousness when there is paralysis of all voluntary muscles and no apparent response to stimuli. In the latter case, however, the deep reflexes may still be present, and though the pain from an injury is not appreciated by the patient it may affect the nervous system and produce shock. In deep coma, the vital centres in the medulla which control the action of the heart and the respiratory mechanism are affected and the outlook is then extremely grave.

Nursing care

The unconscious patient requires unremitting vigilance, constant maintenance of a free airway, a posturally correct but frequently changed position (Fig. 19.11), and scrupulous routine attention to

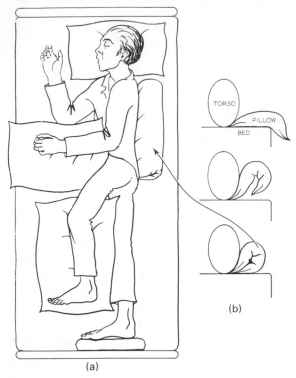

Fig. 19.11 The unconscious patient supported in a lateral position by pillows. B. To show how the supporting back pillow is formed. From *Lifting, handling and helping patients* by Patricia A. Downie and Pat Kennedy. Faber and Faber, London. (By kind permission of the authors and publishers.)

all aspects of personal hygiene. The main points to be observed are *briefly* summarised below.

1. *Vigilance; accurate and regular charting of observations.* These are particularly important in cases of head injury. The pupil-reactions are charted at frequent intervals and any alterations reported promptly. Any change in the level of consciousness, however slight, is also reported. There are many codes used for assessing consciousness level and each nurse will be made familiar with the one used in her hospital at a very early stage in her training. Basically all charts require the same information, viz. the degree of stimulation required to make the patient open his eyes or react in some other way, and the degree of his reaction to verbal commands. In intra-cranial pressure, the pupil on the affected side will constrict due to nerve irritation; the pupil then dilates as the cerebral oedema

increases (Teasdale, 1975). A specimen chart is seen in Fig. 19.10.

Other more general observations are useful in assessing the patient's consciousness level, or to help determine cause of unconsciousness, for example, the colour—has the patient any cyanosis? Is there any smell detected in the breath? What does the skin feel like—is it clammy or dry? Are there any tremors, weakness of limbs, localised involuntary movements, discharge from nose (cerebro-spinal fluid rhinorrhoea) discharge from the ears (cerebro-spinal fluid otorrhoea), incontinence of urine or faeces, or bleeding from any surface? All observations are important and any deviation from normal should be noted and reported immediately to the doctor in charge.

2. *Maintenance of a clear airway.* The tongue is not allowed to slip to the back of the throat and the lateral or semi-prone position is maintained at all times; an airway may be inserted, and oxygen therapy may be ordered; 'bubbly' or irregular respiration is reported immediately and excessive secretions may require the use of nasopharyngeal suction, or bronchoscopy may be indicated; tracheostomy may be required (Fig. 19.12); an endo-

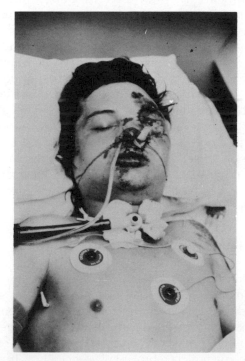

Fig. 19.12 Patient with severe facial injuries and a tracheostomy.

tracheal tube will be passed if the patient cannot maintain his own airway. Dentures should be removed, and a note made of any loose teeth; if there is any danger of inhalation of vomit a Ryle's tube must be passed and the stomach contents aspirated.

3. *Prevention of pressure sores.* These must be prevented *from the first* by frequent turning within the limits of splintage, by eliminating direct pressure on bony points, by movement of the skin and soft tissues, and by keeping the bed and the patient's skin scrupulously clean and *dry*. Even patients who are encumbered by splintage must have their position altered, even if only slightly, every two hours, and others should be turned regularly from side to side, or from the supine to the prone position according to the individual case. Patients in the side-lying position (Fig. 19.11) must have a pillow between the knees and perhaps, under the uppermost arm. The knees, heels, malleoli, greater trochanters, sacrum, anterior and posterior iliac spines, spinous processes, scapulae and elbows should be inspected frequently; even slight reddening of an area of skin must be regarded as a danger signal. It should be remembered that malnutrition, dehydration and anaemia will predispose the patient to pressure-sores.

4. *Care of the eyes, nose, mouth and ears.* The eyes tend to become dry and require gentle swabbing and irrigation; neglect may result in corneal ulceration. The patient who has been unconscious for any length of time or who has required a muscle relaxant to help him accommodate to a ventilator requires pads of vaseline gauze or steri-strips applied to hold the eyelids down and so keep the eyes closed between treatments. The nose must be cleansed and a soothing ointment applied to prevent ulceration of the nostrils, especially if a nasogastric tube is being used. The mouth is prone to infection and ulceration and requires frequent gentle toilet with sodium bicarbonate, glycerine and borax. The ears may also require gentle mopping; in some cases of skull fracture there may be escape of blood or of cerebrospinal fluid.

5. *Care of the bladder and bowel.* There may be incontinence, or an automatic bladder may become established. Urinary output must be measured and charted to assist with correct fluid balance control, and a careful watch must be kept for retention of urine. Intermittent catheterisation, or a self-retaining catheter may be ordered to avoid a wet bed. Urinary antiseptics are frequently ordered. There may be constipation, or faecal incontinence and a twice weekly enema or suppositories on alternate days may be required to prevent soiling. *Scrupulous and thorough daily attention to the toilet of the external genitalia is essential.* Specimens of urine and sputum are sent for culture and sensitivity to the laboratory twice weekly.

6. *Nutrition* is important if unconsciousness lasts for more than a day or two; tube-feeds of high calorie content are introduced as soon as possible (Fig. 19.13A and B) and vitamins are given with feeds. Dehydration may require intravenous infusion, with replacement of chlorides and other electrolytes, though in some cases of head injury fluid may be withheld.

7. *Prevention of contractures, joint stiffness, and venous stagnation.* The limbs are arranged and if necessary supported, in a posturally correct position and all joints are carried through their full range of movement once a day by the physiotherapist. Any change in the limbs such as spasticity or incipient contracture should be reported and full use should be made of pillows, sand-bags and foot-supports, and a cradle supports the weight of the bedclothes. Pressure on the calves should always be avoided and anti-embolic stockings may be applied to prevent deep-venous thrombosis.

Recovery of consciousness. If the patient was unconscious on admission, it is important for the nurse to remember that when consciousness is eventually recovered the patient wakes to unfamiliar faces and in unfamiliar surroundings. He may have no memories, or only confused memories of events prior to his accident. It is also important for the nurse to remember that a patient in a confused or stuporous condition may overhear remarks not meant for his ears, and conduct herself accordingly. The unconscious patient should be spoken to in a reassuring manner and explanations given as if he were conscious. During the period of unconsciousness it is helpful if the nurse tries to remember that she is the patient's 'hands, eyes, ears, and limbs'; this train of thought will help her to identify with the patient's partially or totally absent body functions so that she is better able to

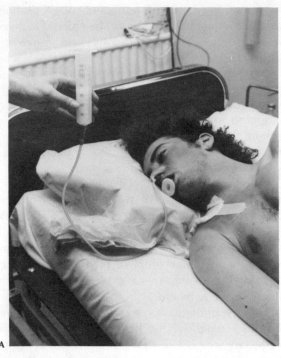
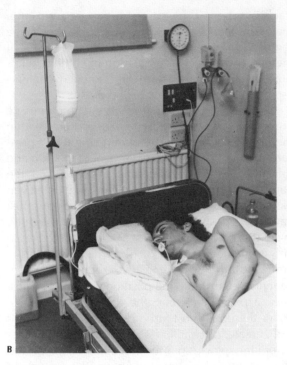

Fig. 19.13 **A.** Intermittent naso-gastric feeding. **B.** Continuous naso-gastric drip-feeding.

fulfil his needs. We would hope that the patient's dependence on others will become less, but such a patient may require help for a very long time—indeed, in some cases for the remainder of his life.

THE PATIENT WITH A HEAD INJURY

Fractures of the skull. As a rule, no surgical treatment is indicated unless the fracture is depressed or open, or both. Depressed fractures are usually in the vault of the skull and are treated by 'pushing up' or decompression. Open fractures require wound excision and toilet and are especially dangerous when they occur in the base of the skull when they may become infected by communication with the cavity of the ear or nose. Escape of blood or of cerebro-spinal fluid from the ear or the nose indicates a fracture of the base of the skull and chemotherapy is ordered to prevent meningitis.

Damage to the brain by jars, jolts or direct blows may produce concussion, cerebral contusion or laceration, leading to cerebral oedema or haemorr-hage either within the brain, on its surface, or one or other side of the dura mater (subdural or extradural haematoma).

These injuries may cause varying degrees of unconsciousness.

The nursing care already outlined for an unconscious patient will also apply in cases of head injury. The most important point in early cases is *constant watchfulness, continuous and accurate recording of observations and prompt reporting of any change*, no matter how trivial it may seem. The importance of the observation chart has already been stressed; the temperature, pulse and respiration rates, the blood pressure and reaction of the pupils to light are recorded every quarter of an hour, at least in the early stages. Dilated pupils, a slow pulse and a rising blood pressure are signs of increasing inter-cranial pressure which may require treatment by lumbar puncture, cranial burr holes or craniotomy.

Assessment of the level of consciousness is another important nursing responsibility. Again, even trivial changes in the patient's behaviour must be accurately recorded and promptly reported.

Maintenance of a clear airway; obstruction of the airway is the commonest cause of death in the unconscious patient; prevention of pressure sores from the first moment, and adequate nutrition are obvious essentials. On the other hand, the patient must not be over-hydrated and in some cases fluid is actually withheld. This will help to reduce any cerebral oedema that might be present; daily assessment of the needs of the individual patient is the guide to the treatment ordered. Examination of specimens of blood and urine are required for the assessment of special requirements such as replacement of chlorides and other electrolytes. Uraemia from renal failure is a dreaded complication and the last resort in treatment is the use of an artificial kidney. It is important that the patient is never over-heated and indeed, hypothermia may be ordered, when the patient is nursed beside an open window and surrounded by ice-bags (Fig. 19.14). This is of prime importance in mid-brain

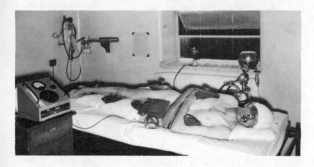

Fig. 19.14 Hypothermia (see text). (Courtesy of Mr Walpole Lewin, the *Nursing Mirror* and the Radcliffe Infirmary, Oxford.)

injuries when the temperature control mechanism may be damaged.

N.B. The temperature of all unconscious patients is taken in the rectum.

Summary

Twelve points listed below summarise the care of a patient with a head injury or one who is unconscious from some other cause:

1. Constant day and night attention and observation.
2. Management of the airway; nurse in the lateral or semi-prone position; keep the airway clear by suction; may have endotracheal tube or tracheostomy tube *in situ*.
3. Suction via an endotracheal tube or tracheostomy tube must be carried out as a sterile procedure.
4. Change of position two hourly, by day and by night.
5. Oral toilet is very important especially if patient is being tube fed.
6. Care of eyes, nose and ears as described earlier. If there is leakage of cerebro-spinal fluid, nose and ears should not be plugged but a sterile pad placed over them.
7. Strict fluid balance chart.
8. Care of the bowels and bladder.
9. Tolerance must be shown by the nursing staff; at some stages of recovery the patient may be very difficult to manage, e.g. restless and noisy, but this actually helps to prevent chest complications and improves muscle tone and joint movement.
10. Restraint should not be used except to prevent further injury. Cot sides should be used and if necessary, padded with pillows. Apply 'boxing glove bandages' to hands to prevent the patient from pulling at equipment.
11. Re-assurance is required by the patient and his relatives.
12. All medication, intravenous fluids, etc. to be given as prescribed, and *adequate fluid balance and nutrition maintained.*

CARE OF THE PATIENT WITH A CHEST INJURY

Fractures of the ribs are the result of direct violence to the thoracic cage and may involve one or more ribs. In young children the ribs are so resilient that fractures are rare, although severe trauma with a 'stove in' chest may have a fatal outcome.

The chest may be injured by penetration, e.g. by stabbing with a weapon or by impalement on sharp objects such as metal railings; or by crushing force, e.g. against a steering wheel; or by blast injuries.

The major problems following chest injuries are:

1. Blood loss—particularly following stab wounds.

2. Pain.
3. Disturbance of the mechanism of respiration.
4. Loss of normal control of bronchial secretions.

Blood loss may be difficult to estimate and apart from that which can be measured in draining bottles, it can be estimated by bruising over the back and loins seen some time after injury; the complications of blood loss associated with other parts of the body become evident along with the ones associated directly with bleeding in the pleural cavity (haemopneumothorax) or cardiac tamponade (bleeding under the pericardium).

Pain. All injuries to the chest are painful; successful management depends upon adequate relief of pain, which is best achieved by injection of local anaesthetic around the fracture site; this relieves the pain but does not make the patient drowsy, so that he can co-operate fully in carrying out frequent deep breathing exercises; early mobilisation is encouraged unless there are other injuries to prevent it.

Disturbance to the mechanism of respiration. This can be disturbed by unstable fractures of the ribs, pneumothorax, haemopneumothorax or rupture of the diaphragm. When multiple ribs are fractured in more than one place the chest wall between the two fractures is unsupported; the elasticity of the lungs pulls the loose segments inwards (paradoxical movement); this generally signifies a severe injury and the patient will require artificial ventilation.

Blood gases. In mild injuries they are usually normal, values of Po_2 and Pco_2: in moderate, there will be a slight rise in the Pco_2 value. In severe injuries the Pco_2 will drop below half its normal value and the Pco_2 rise to compensate for this.

Loss of normal control of bronchial secretions. Uncontrolled pain and a disorder in the mechanism of respiration makes it difficult for the patient to cough effectively; secretions build up and either cause obstruction or pneumonia. Deep breathing exercises are essential along with chest manipulations and assisted coughing usually taught by a physiotherapist.

N.B. A patient nursed on a mechanical ventilator should be turned regularly to drain secretions from the bronchus to the trachea where they can readily be sucked out.

Treatment obviously varies with the severity of the lesion.

Pneumothorax may be due to an open wound of the chest wall, allowing air to be sucked in. The wound requires immediate closure by dressing or suturing. The air must be aspirated to allow the lung to expand, and in an emergency this can be done with a wide bore needle and syringe, though it is best carried out by the insertion of a catheter connected to an underwater seal. In many instances gravity alone will effect satisfactory drainage of fluid. In this case a single receptacle, kept below the level of the patient's chest is all that is necessary. It is, of course, necessary to vent such a system to avoid development of an airlock in the receptacle (Fig. 19.15). Bubbles of air will then

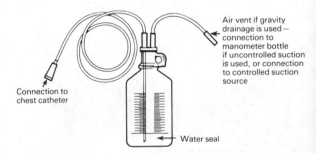

Fig. 19.15 Underwater seal drainage.

appear but as the lung expands these will become fewer and gradually disappear so that after a few days the catheter can be removed.

Haemothorax can be the result of the fracture of a single rib, but is more common in multiple fractures. The treatment is the same as for pneumothorax, but blood must be aspirated or drained; in some cases this can be quite a large amount and may require a change of drainage bottle before the procedure is complete. Bleeding is rarely so profuse as to require surgical intervention, though if a haemothorax is unrecognised it forms a clot around the lung; this obviously prevents re-expansion, and thorocotomy may be necessary to remove the blood clot, and if the patient is to go on to a ventilator then the chest drain is mandatory.

The flail or stove-in chest. As a first aid measure the patient is nursed with the injured side resting on a pillow or rolled blanket, which will act as a splint, diminish chest movements, minimise further damage, and relieve pain so that breathing tends to become easier.

Treatment by artificial ventilation

Once the patient is in hospital he is usually attached to a positure-pressure ventilator via an endotracheal tube; this reduces the fractures by keeping the chest expanded from within and takes over lung ventilation. It also corrects respiratory acidosis, reduces pulmonary oedema and facilitates the use of suction.

The conscious patient may be very difficult to manage because he unwittingly tries to breath against the machine rather than in time with it, and may resist the insertion of the endotracheal tube. A muscle relaxant is required to allow passage of the tube, and a drug such as Phenoperidine is used as a sedative and can be given in fairly large doses (2–4 mg); it may be necessary to repeat this at one-hourly intervals to keep the patient comfortable and breathing in rhythm with the machine. At the commencement of treatment a patient may require a complete muscle relaxant such as Pancuronium to help him accommodate to the ventilator.

Surgical procedures to stabilise the ribs are rarely undertaken, largely because a patient with a severe chest injury often has other injuries as well and the risk of giving an anesthetic which is not strictly necessary is unjustified.

Nursing care

If possible, the patient is nursed in the sitting position propped up by a back-rest and plenty of pillows. During the acute stage, total and intensive nursing care and continuous observation is required, and the patient is never left unattended. London in his book *Nursing Emergencies* (see Bibliography) says 'The prime need is for a clear understanding of what is required, accurate records and careful observation with the danger signs especially in mind'.

Drainage tubes and bottles, if used, are checked frequently and any change reported at once. Observations of the temperature, pulse and blood pressure carried out as for any other acutely ill patient, and particular attention is paid to the patient's *colour* and to the *rate and depth of respiration*. *Cyano-*

sis is reported to the surgeon at once, and the adminstration of oxygen may be ordered.

Intubation or tracheostomy is often required in the presence of serious chest injury, especially in unconscious patients. It ensures a clear airway and lung secretions can be removed by catheter via the tracheostomy tube.

Collapse of the lung is a common complication. If it cannot be treated by physiotherapy, *bronchoscopy* may be required. Humidification may be necessary if bronchial secretions are thick and cannot be aspirated.

NOTES ON THE CARE OF A PATIENT WITH A TRACHEOSTOMY

Indications for tracheostomy are as follows:

1. Obstruction of the upper airway caused by:
   a. Trauma, e.g. from burns, etc.
   b. Infection e.g. diphtheria, bronchitis (especially in infants).
   c. Neoplasm—benign or malignant.
2. Paralysis or extreme weakness of the muscles of respiration, e.g. poliomyelitis, myasthenia gravis, peripheral neuritis, cervical cord injury, etc.
3. Management of the unconscious patient with severe head injury, or in neurosurgery or poisoning, etc.
4. Chest trauma; in this case there is a tendency to intubate immediately, and to consider tracheostomy at a later date.
5. For nursing the patient on a ventilator in the treatment of any of the conditions listed above.

Advantages of a tracheostomy

1. An upper airway obstruction is easily by-passed.
2. The trachea and bronchi can be cleared of secretions by suction.
3. Dead space is reduced, so reducing the effort of respiration and increasing the efficiency of ventilation. Reduction in effort decreases the demand for oxygen, so that this in turn relieves respiratory difficulty.
4. It prevents regurgitation of gastric contents in the unconscious patient.

Disadvantages of a tracheostomy

1. The patient cannot speak—in the later stages a speaking valve may be inserted.
2. There is lack of effective natural humidification.
3. There is grave danger of respiratory infection.
4. Displacement of the tube may occur and it is not as easy to manage as an endotracheal tube.

Psychological care

The tracheostomy patient is dependent upon the nurse and can do little for himself. Initially the alert conscious patient will be frightened and apprehensive but because of the cuffed tube will be unable to speak and communicate his needs; conversely every word and action on the part of the doctors and nurses will be observed. It is essential that an atmosphere of calmness and confidence is created because the patient's emotional state will influence his breathing pattern and the ease with which he accepts mechanical ventilation.

It is important for the patient to be constantly reminded that his inability to speak is only temporary; the patient and family should be re-assured by pointing out the nurse call-button and the fact that suitably trained medical and nursing staff is close at hand continuously. Encouragement and reassurance must be given when attempts are made to swallow fluids or food because the patient may be afraid of choking, because of the short and long-term dysphagia and dysphasia.

Suction

Indications for suction are obvious since it is performed to remove secretions which the patient cannot expel himself; it is carried out as often as necessary. It is an uncomfortable procedure and a very frightening one for the patient until he becomes accustomed to it. Suction must never be carried out for longer than 5–10 seconds at one time, even if there appears to be no visible stress, and not more than two catheters should be passed at one time without re-oxygenating and re-evaluating the condition of the patient. Partial occlusion of the airway by the suction catheter, combined with aspiration of air from the lung while suctioning can result in severe hypoxia and could cause cardiac arrest.

A useful tip for the nurse during suction is to hold one's own breath during the procedure; this gives one an idea of the sensation of breathlessness and is a reminder to stop.

Special note

A tracheostomy is an open surgical wound and strict asepsis is mandatory at all times; moreover, the trachea and bronchi are lined with delicate tissue, so that suction must not take place during actual insertion of the catheter; this is to prevent tearing of the mucosa and collapse of small segments of the lung.

Suction procedure

Note type and amount of secretions obtained. Wash hands before and after procedure.

1. Explain the procedure to patient.
2. Check that suction equipment is working and that there is a y-connection on the end of the tubing. Put on face mask.
3. Select a catheter approximately half the size of the tracheostomy tube gauge.
4. Open the catheter packet and switch the suction on.
5. Put a sterile glove on the hand to be used.
6. Pick up the end of the catheter with that hand and attach it to the y-connection.
7. Remove the catheter from the packet, touching it only with the sterile hand. If the catheter touches anything else it must be discarded and another one used.
8. With the other hand remove the cap from the swivel connector on the tube.
9. Gently pass the catheter down to the carina without suction. The patient will probably cough. If suction is applied on the way down, or if it is too fierce, the tracheal mucosa will be damaged and may become infected.
10. Withdraw the catheter slowly, applying intermittent suction or rolling it between the fingers. Never pass the catheter up and down the tube.
11. Replace the cap on the swivel connector. While this is off the patient is not being ventilated and for this reason the procedure should take no longer than 20 seconds.

12. Discard the catheter and rinse tubing through. If necessary, repeat, using another catheter.

NOTES ON THE CARE OF A PATIENT ON A VENTILATOR

Introduction

The nursing of a patient on a ventilator is becoming a very common experience, not only in Intensive Care Units, but in the surgical and trauma wards of the smaller hospitals. It gives the patient with a chest injury or with pulmonary oedema following fat embolus a more comfortable period of recovery, and the unconscious patient with a head injury is ventilated to give time for full assessment and surgery if required. The patient on a ventilator requires many aspects of nursing care and is totally dependent on the nursing and medical staff; the nurse should make herself familiar with the basic principles of mechanical ventilation not only so as to give care but to convey confidence to the patient; the anaesthetists in charge will always help with explanations.

The care can be divided into two:

1. Nursing care specific to ventilation.
2. General and psychological nursing care.

Nursing care specific to ventilation

The air pressure to the lungs travels via a cuffed endotracheal tube or cuffed tracheostomy tube; in the infant, a non-cuffed naso-tracheal tube is commonly used. Tubes should be firmly secured in place; a conscious patient may need sedation or muscle relaxants to help him accommodate to the tubes and to the machine, and such medication should be given promptly if required. The introduction of a ventilator is usually a resuscitative procedure and the conscious patient will fight against it, but as his condition improves and he becomes more confident the need for medication becomes less.

Suction should be carried out frequently as described for the care of the patient with a tracheostomy; since the introduction of the non-irritant portex tube it is not usually considered necessary to deflate the cuff prior to suction though with the older type of tubes this was required to prevent pressure necrosis and tracheal stenosis; however, the policy in this regard usually depends upon the anaesthetist. If the cuff is deflated, it is important to suck out the naso-pharynx before sucking via the tube; this will lessen the risk of saliva tracking back down into the lungs. The patient should never be left alone while the cuff is deflated. Where there is a deeply unconscious patient or one who has had a muscle relaxant, it is advisable to have a second nurse to hand-ventilate the patient with an Ambu-bag between each passage of the catheter. Humidification is essential in the mechanically-ventilated patient, because air has by-passed the channels usually performing this function; the humidifier is usually incorporated into the machine and is filled with sterile water. During ventilation the level should be checked regularly.

Ventilator recordings are usually made hourly, and include the respiratory rate which can be counted by the chest movement in the usual way; the inflatory pressure is pre-set by the anaesthetist and is read from a gauge on the machine; an increase in pressure usually indicates the need for suction to relieve secretions or an obstruction, whereas a decrease usually indicates a leak in the circuit. Tidal and minute volumes, that is the amount of air taken in in one inspiration, and the air taken in over one minute are read from meters incorporated in the machine, or from a Wright's spirometer which can be fixed in the circuit. Blood-gas analysis is carried out regularly to assess the adequacy of ventilation, and these are measured from sample of arterial blood sent to the laboratory; any change in recordings should be reported. The patient's pulse and blood pressure are usually taken at the same time as the ventilator recordings, and if suction is carried out either routinely at the same hour, or at alternate hours along with the recordings, the patient is then assured of some rest.

Notes on general nursing care

Two hourly turning is carried out not only to prevent pressure sores but also to reduce the risk of chest and urinary complications. *Oral hygiene* is of prime importance, as the patient will probably be fed by intravenous fluids or through a naso-gastric tube, and therefore the mouth will not be kept moist in the natural way. A catheter may be *in situ* in the urinary bladder and catheter toilet and changing of urine bag must be carried out using aseptic technique. Glycerine suppositories may be required to promote normal bowel action.

Notes on psychological care

The conscious patient may have been attached to the ventilator as an emergency with little or no explanation, or, the unconscious patient may wake up and find himself attached to one. In either case, it is a very frightening experience for the patient to find that he is not controlling his own breathing; explanations and a great deal of reassurance are required from the nurse. The patient will be unable to talk because of the tracheal tube but if a muscle relaxant has not been used he must be given pencil and paper for essential communication.

The patient on a ventilator who has been given a relaxant such as Pavulon will appear to be unconscious because he cannot move, but, in fact, he may be very alert mentally and nothing that he is not meant to hear should be said at his bedside.

The patient's relatives also require reassurance and the reason for mechanical ventilation should be explained to them.

Discontinuing ventilation

All sedation should be withheld for at least four hours, so that the patient is alert and able to co-operate in the procedure; the tubes are left *in situ* and oxygen is usually given via a face-mask; the patient then breathes on his own for a short time, commencing with, perhaps, five minutes in one hour before being put back on the machine; the length of time the patient breathes without the aid of the machine will be increased daily until respiration is satisfactory and all equipment will be removed.

THE PATIENT WITH MULTIPLE INJURIES

These cases present complex problems of surgical and nursing management, and it may be helpful to the nurse to read the following brief case-history (Fig. 19.16).

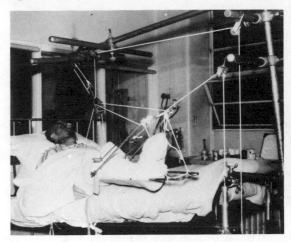

Fig. 19.16 This is the actual patient whose injuries are described in the text. (From the Radcliffe Infirmary, Oxford.)

A man, aged 47, was involved in a road accident and was admitted to hospital in a shocked and unconscious condition, having sustained the following injuries:

1. Compound depressed fracture of the frontal bone of the skull.
2. Compound fracture of mandible.
3. Simple fracture of the left clavicle.
4. Multiple fractures of left radius, carpus and metacarpus.
5. Fracture of upper third of the right femur with gross displacement.
6. Penetrating wound of the right knee joint.
7. Bi-malleolar fracture of the right ankle.
8. Sprain of the left ankle.
9. Multiple fractures of the ribs on the left side, with paradoxical respiration.
10. Lacerations of the skin over the right eye and under the chin.

Treatment

Treatment included the following:

1. Resuscitation, which included blood-transfusion.
2. Operative treatment, as follows:
   a. A tracheostomy was performed to relieve respiratory embarrassment.

b. Débridement of compound compressed fracture of frontal bone.
c. Reduction of fracture of the mandible and fixation by wiring to the maxilla.
d. Reduction of fracture of the right femur and débridement of wound of the right knee. Insertion of a Steinmann pin into the tibial tuberosities and application of Thomas splint and balanced traction to right leg.
e. Suture of soft tissue lacerations.
f. Application of plaster casts to the right ankle and left wrist.

Apart from the specific care of splintage, which is discussed elsewhere, the nursing care required by this patient is now briefly summarised:

1. Vigilance; the patient was observed continuously: An 'observation chart' was commenced on admission. The temperature, pulse and respiration, the blood pressure and pupil-reactions were recorded every quarter of an hour, and level of consciousness noted.
2. Maintenance of a clear airway; chest complications were avoided by moving the patient as much as possible and by early physiotherapy.
3. A fluid intake-and-output chart was maintained continuously.
4. Pressure areas were treated by slight change of position every two hours.
5. Cleansing of the mouth was carried out every two hours.
6. Bathing of the eyes was carried out every four hours.
7. Care of the nose was necessary because a Ryle's tube was passed after 24 hours had elapsed so that high protein feeds could be given.

N.B. During the course of treatment frequent examination of the blood was carried out for estimation of haemoglobin, urea, and electrolytes (sodium, potassium, chloride, bicarbonate and base excess).

BURNS

Burns are discussed briefly here because they may accompany other major injuries and moreover, a moderate or severe burn produces shock and the patient may require resuscitation. Obviously the severity of the burn depends upon the burning agent and the duration of its application; burns are often decribed as *superficial* where the skin only is destroyed or *deep* where the skin and deeper tissues are involved; the latter will require skin grafting and possibly, plastic surgery. Skin contractures are the crippling aftermath of burns, so that passive movements to the part must be carried out as soon as possible.

Burns can be accidental, or deliberately inflicted as suicide, sabotage or non-accidental injury, particularly in children, and it is important to get an accurate history of the accident.

Different types of burns are described as follows, according to the causative agent:

1. Scalds, hot fluid or steam.
2. Dry heat, flame flash or friction.
3. Electric.
4. Chemical.
5. Radiation.

CLASSIFICATION

Superficial

The epidermis only is destroyed; it appears pink and blistered; it is very painful due to exposed nerve endings. The sebaceous glands, sweat glands and hair follicles remain intact; therefore healing is spontaneous.

Deep dermal

Some structures of epithelisation remain; therefore healing is spontaneous but much slower. These burns tend to produce the worst scarring.

Full thickness

No dermis is left; therefore no healing occurs except by surgical intervention (skin graft).

It appears white/charred and does not blanche on pressure. There is very little pain.

It is important to estimate the percentage of the body surface that has been burned in order to treat the patient satisfactorily. This can be done roughly by estimating the patient's hand size as 1 per cent or more accurately by the 'Rule of Nine' as shown in Table 19.1.

Table 19.1

	Per cent
Face and Scalp	9
Back	18
Front	18
Arm	9
Perineum	1
Upper leg	9
Lower leg	9

First-aid measures for treating burns are as follows: Eliminate the cause of the burns as quickly as possible, place the patient in a comfortable safe position, and protect the burned area with clean material; get medical assistance as soon as possible because the patient will become shocked very quickly.

Shock—manifestations and treatment

An adult with an area of 15 per cent or more burns and a child 10 per cent or more are considered 'shock cases'. Shock usually develops after the first few hours until the time the body is compensated for fluid loss by general vaso-constriction, and absorption of fluid from the gut; in less severe cases the shock phase passes after 36–48 hours. In severe burns plasma volume continues to fall rapidly, visceral blood flow is reduced to a dangerously low level, and this affects the kidneys and intestines causing oliguria or anuria. There is failure of absorption in the gut which causes vomiting and eventually, a paralytic ileus. In severe cases red blood cells are destroyed and any deep burn over 10 per cent of body surface will require a blood transfusion. Shock is treated by intravenous infusion of large quantities of plasma and other fluids; oral fluids are also given if permitted. The amount is usually worked out by the doctor who uses one of the formulae calculated and described by experts in this field, the Mount Vernon formula

$$\frac{\% \text{ burn} \times \text{wt in kg}}{2}.$$

This gives the amount of plasma in (ml) to be given in the first 36 hours after injury. But in general terms

it is said that a patient with severe burns can lose body fluid 80 times faster than in normal health; this gives some indication of the amount of fluid required.

The ideal situation in which patients with severe burns are nursed is obviously a special unit, with well equipped shock rooms and with air filters to reduce the risk of infection; the shock room or cubicle should be heated to 90°F (32°C); the nurse wears a gown and mask at all times and visitors can only observe the patient through a glass window in order to avoid heat loss and cross-infection; the commonest cause of death in these patients is infection leading to septicaemia.

An accurate observation chart is essential in order to monitor the patient's condition; it is sometimes impossible to record blood pressure due to the position of the burn, but a pulse can usually be counted from some part of the body; urine is measured hourly along with the fluid intake, and an intake/output chart is essential.

A central venous pressure line should be inserted for the patient with extensive burns; this is the best guide to fluid volume—it also reflects the state of the myocardium and its ability to cope with extra fluids. The pressure is read from a cannula passing into the right atrium or into the superior or inferior venae cava.

Haematocryte readings. This is a means of measuring the proportion of red cells to plasma; (red cells do not usually escape through the capilliaries). A low haematocryte reading means that there are few red cells and a great deal of plasma, i.e. fluid replacement has been excessive or given too fast.

A high haematocryte reading means that there are many red cells and a small amount of plasma, i.e. more fluid is required.

Dressings. Sterile dressings are used, or in some cases of extensive burns the patient is nursed uncovered in a cubicle where the air is filtered, and a cream or lotion such as silver nitrate is applied to the body in aseptic conditions.

Conclusion

It is obviously to the advantage of the seriously burned patient if he is treated in a special 'Burns Unit' with special facilities (e.g. filtered air), where the medical and nursing staff are experienced in this special field and where the most up-to-date treatment can be given. Not the least of the advantages is the fact that when the acute stage is over the patient meets others who, perhaps, are as disfigured by their burns as himself; by this means he may find a 'companion in distress' and so feels less lonely and conspicuous.

FRACTURE OF THE FACE AND JAWS

Fractures of the nose and the mandible are usually obvious because of deformity of the part, but fractures of the zygoma and maxilla are sometimes overlooked and masked by rapid swelling. Fracture of the jaws may cause the tongue to fall back and interfere with respiration, or there may be bleeding into the nose or throat. Where possible, these cases are nursed in the side-lying or prone position and tongue forceps are kept always at hand. Fractures of the maxilla and mandible usually affect 'the bite' of the patient, and should be treated by a facio-maxillary or dental surgeon.

Treatment of facial fractures

The malar or zygoma bones are usually damaged by direct violence; the bone is usually depressed and will require elevation under direct vision, an incision being made above the hair line of the temple; in extreme circumstances wires may be used to hold the bones in the reduced position.

The maxilla is usually injured by direct violence to the front of the face.

1. *Unilateral fractures* are treated by wiring the fractured bone to the sound teeth on either side of the fracture.
2. *Bilateral fractures* are treated by the application of silver capped splints to the teeth, held in position with metal bars and attached to a plaster headband or halo device.

The mandible is usually fractured by direct violence.

1. Unilateral undisplaced fractures usually require no treatment at all; unstable fractures require fixation by wiring the upper and lower teeth together on either side of the fracture.

2. Grossly unstable fractures may require internal fixation with a plate and screw.

Vomiting is extremely dangerous since foreign matter may be inhaled into the lungs. Scrupulous oral hygiene by means of a dental spray is essential; if a semi-solid diet cannot be taken by mouth liquid feeds are given via a Ryles tube passed through the nostril. Wire-cutters and a sucker are kept always at hand.

Fracture of the nose is usually treated by manipulation; the nose is then packed for up to 12 hours with gauze to prevent bleeding; external splintage is occasionally required.

FRACTURES OF THE PELVIS

A fracture of the pelvis is rarely important in itself; it is the associated complications which matter, and in some cases they are a serious threat to life. The two main complications are:

1. Bleeding—several litres of blood can be concealed in the soft tissues around the pelvis without being clinically evident; the first evidence of this will be shown on a well-kept observation chart (Figs 19.10, 19.18 and 19.19).
2. Injury to underlying organs, namely the urinary bladder, the urethra, the blood vessels and the nerves, namely the sacral plexus. A tear of the rectal or vaginal wall is a rare injury.

Types of fractures

1. Fractures not affecting the stability of the pelvic ring; these are relatively minor injuries, and in isolation are not associated with intra-pelvic injury or shock due to severe blood loss. The common ones are:
   a. Fracture of pubic or ischial ramus.
   b. Fracture of the sacrum or coccyx.
   c. Fracture of the blade of the ilium.
   d. Minor fracture of the acetabulum.
   Treatment. Analgesics and mobilisation within the limits of pain; rest in bed is usually limited to a few days.
2. A fracture which disrupts the pelvic ring, when it is broken in two or more places. Blood loss and shock in these fractures may be consider-

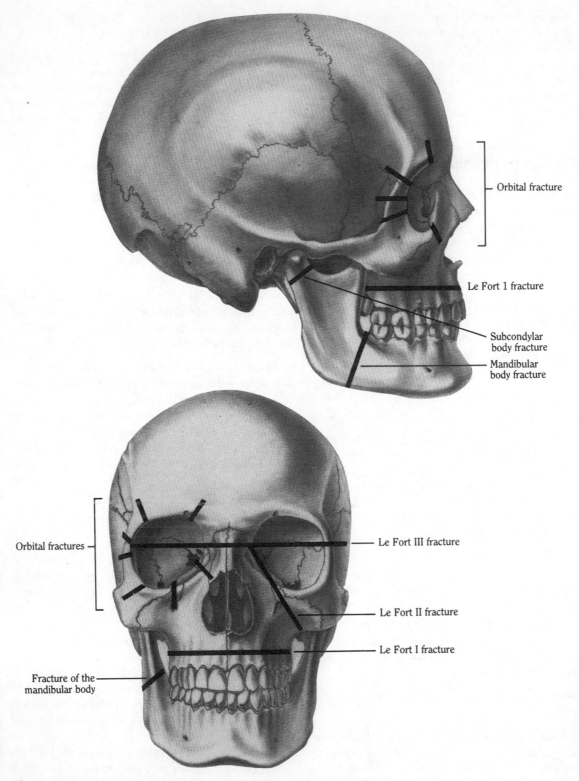

Fig. 19.17 Facial fractures. (Courtesy of Mr Douglas Allan and the *Nursing Times*.)

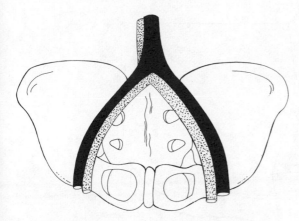

Fig. 19.18 Showing the great blood vessels in relation to the pelvis. When fractures occur haemorrhage is severe and the resulting shock can be fatal.

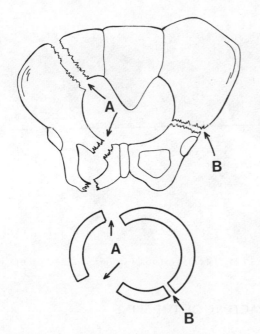

Fig. 19.19 The pelvis forms a ring to protect pelvic organs. When separation occurs in two planes (A) it is important to recognise that damage may have occurred to these organs. Isolated injuries (B) do not have this tendency.

able, and injury to pelvic organs may occur. The common fractures are:

a. Fracture of all four pelvic rami.
b. Hinge separation of the symphysis pubis.
c. Double fracture of the hemi-pelvis (usually with upward displacement) (Malgaines fracture).

d. Major fractures of the acetabulum which involve the lip; this is often associated with dislocation of the hip.
e. Stove-in pelvis, when the head of the femur may be driven through the floor of the acetabulum into the pelvis.

Injuries to the pelvis and abdomen are frequently seen in association with other injuries, particularly in road traffic accidents; injury to another part of the body leads to failure to recognise a pelvic or abdominal injury, e.g. the unconscious patient with a head injury cannot complain of abdominal pain. With this in mind, the importance of the nurse's observations and a well-kept chart with base-line recordings must be stressed.

The pelvis should be examined in all multiple injuries and priority is given to the treatment of damaged internal organs.

Treatment of the fracture follows the usual lines of fracture treatment; i.e. reduction, if required, immobilisation and restoration of function. Separation of the symphysis pubis can often be closed by nursing measures (see Suspensary sling). *Pain* is always a problem and may predispose the patient to chest complications because of reluctance to cough—support for the part and adequate analgesia is required.

Fracture of the pubic rami is not usually displaced and requires little or no manipulation but in these fractures the urethra is likely to be ruptured.

Splintage

1. *A double hip spica.*
2. *Watson-Jones postural reduction and double plaster spica fixation.* This is used for a fracture where there is displacement of fragments or dislocation of the symphysis pubis. An anaesthetic may or may not be given. The upright perineal post is removed from a hip-prop, and the patient is laid on it on the sound side. If greater lateral pressure is required he is laid on the injured side. The body is then covered with a thin layer of wool roll, the iliac crests and sacrum are protected with felt, and a double spica is applied. It must be closely moulded round the pelvis and lumbar spine. When it has set, the hip-prop is cut out, and the hole in the plaster is filled in with padding and covered with a plaster bandage.

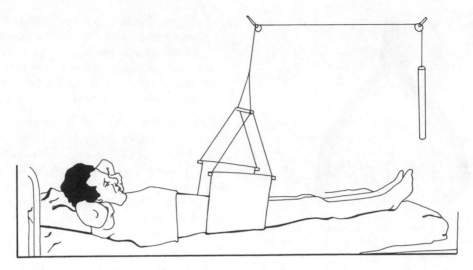

Fig. 19.20 Suspensory sling.

When the plaster is dry, the patient is encouraged to lie on his side. Leg exercises are commenced at once. The plaster is usually changed after about six weeks and is retained for about three months.

3. *Suspensory sling.* A canvas sling is passed beneath the pelvis and attached to cords and weights, in the manner shown in Fig. 19.20. Side-to-side compression of the pelvic girdle is provided and this may correct the deformity. Unfortunately problems occur in the use of bedpans because the condition is so painful, and analgesics will be required.

Mobilisation will begin when pain is relieved and there is no risk of displacement of the fracture.

4. *Continuous skin or skeletal traction.* This is sometimes used in combination with one or other of the aforementioned methods.

5. *The Hoffman external fixation. Double fracture of the hemi-pelvis* is usually caused by falling from a height. The fracture runs through both rami with fracture through or near to the sacro-iliac joint; the hemi-pelvis is usually displaced upwards requiring continuous leg traction via a Steinmann pin driven through the tibial tuberosity with up to 30 lb weight which is then gradually reduced. This may be used in association with an external fixator (Hoffman) (Fig. 19.21).

Treatment is likely to be continued for up to six weeks and weight-bearing is delayed for up to twelve weeks.

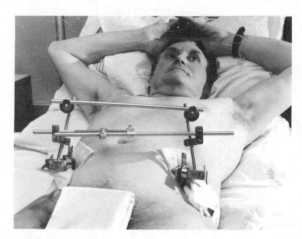

Fig. 19.21 Hoffman external fixation for fracture of the pelvis.

FRACTURE OF THE SPINE

Fracture of the spine may involve the vertebral body. It is a dangerous injury because damage to the spinal cord may result in paraplegia (Ch. 23); this may occur at the time of the accident, *or it may occur from rough handling at a later stage in treatment, even in hospital.* Treatment in hospital is largely determined by whether or not the particular injury is *stable* or *unstable.* It is important for the nurse to remember that an injury can be converted from a stable to an unstable one by rough handling at any stage of treatment. Full neurological examination is essential. This section describes only spinal fractures *without* spinal cord damage.

Every case of spinal injury is treated as unstable until the surgeon pronounces otherwise. At the scene of injury, the patient is rolled on to a canvas stretcher *all in one piece* as shown in Fig. 19.22

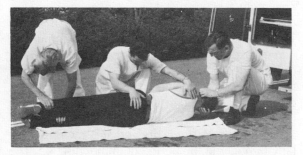

Fig. 19.22 Shows the correct method of rolling a patient, suspected of having spinal injury, onto a stretcher.

and remains on this until he is examined by the surgeon; hard objects in the clothing such as coins and keys in a pocket, are not permitted to press into the body. Other notes on first-aid will be found at the beginning of this chapter.

The treatment of *particular injuries* will now be discussed.

FRACTURE OF A VERTEBRAL BODY

This occurs most commonly in the thoraco-lumbar region, and is due to a flexion injury such as is sustained in falling from a height and landing on the heels, buttocks, head or shoulders. There is generally a small localised kyphos due to prominence of one spinous process. The patient may or may not complain of pain and there may be evidence of damage to the spinal cord.

Treatment

This depends upon the type of fracture. Uncomplicated fractures may be treated by one of the following methods.

1. *Recumbency with early active exercises* is sufficient in some stable types of fracture. The patient is kept in bed until severe pain has subsided (usually 2–4 weeks). Extension exercises are commenced on the lines described later and gradually

increased in strength until full activity is resumed in about 3–4 months.

2. *A plaster jacket, recumbency, and early active exercises.* This may be ordered for more severe injuries. The plaster jacket may be applied in head traction (Fig. 19.23) or in the sitting or standing

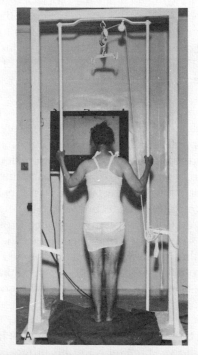

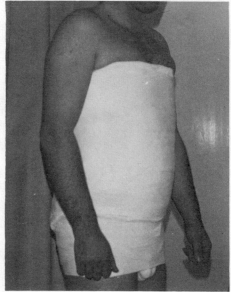

Fig. 19.23 A, B A plaster jacket is applied as the patient stands between two upright supports.

position. *Exercises* are carried out as described later.

3. *Postural reduction and application of plaster jacket by the Watson-Jones method.* As a rule, anaesthesia is unnecessary, though spinal anaesthesia is sometimes employed. Two tables, one about a foot higher than the other, are arranged end to end so that the space between them is a little more than the length of the patient's trunk. All materials for applying the plaster jacket are placed at hand (Ch. 6). A double layer of vesting is applied and stitched between the legs. The patient is then lifted into position, the arms are supported on the higher table, which is clear of the chest; the lower table supports the legs only so far as the upper thighs, so that the trunk sags down between them until the limit of hyperextension of the spine is reached. A loop of bandage tied to the upper table and grasped by the patient sometimes gives a sense of security and aids relaxation. Strips of adhesive felt may be placed around the kyphos, so as to avoid pressure sores. The plaster jacket is then quickly and smoothly applied. It must extend from the symphysis pubis to the suprasternal notch in front, and from the tip of the coccyx to the scapulae behind, so as to prevent the smallest degree of forward flexion of the spine (Fig. 19.24).

When the plaster is hard, the patient is lifted on to the pillows, preferably in the prone position,

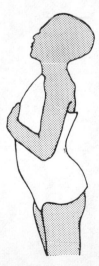

Fig. 19.24 Hyperextension jacket for fracture of the spine. Note that it extends from the symphysis pubis to above the clavicles.

otherwise with several pillows arranged so as to fill in the hollow of the back. The plaster is trimmed at the axillae to allow movement of the arms. Similarly, it can be trimmed over the thighs to allow the patient to sit in a semirecumbent position, but not sufficient to allow him to sit bolt upright. *In no circumstances must it be cut away over the sternum and clavicles or over the symphysis pubis.* The patient can be made comfortable by arranging numerous pillows so that the spine is supported in its arched position and the shoulders and thigh fall away from the jacket in front. Other nursing details are described in Chs 6 and 9.

Exercises for the spinal muscles are commenced as soon as the plaster is dry and are practised regularly throughout the period of immobilisation. The patient lies prone and, whilst an assistant steadies the legs, the head and shoulders are raised from the bed. The patient then raises first one leg and then the other in the air with the knees extended; as his strength increases he raises both legs simultaneously, and finally, the head and shoulders and both legs are hyperextended at the same time. After about four weeks, the position of the fracture may be checked by radiographs and a new plaster applied by the same method. The jacket is worn for about four to six months, depending on the rate of union. When this is assured, mobilising and strengthening exercises are practised until recovery is complete.

4. *Spinal fusion* is sometimes indicated.

SIMPLE CRUSH FRACTURE OF A CERVICAL VERTEBRAL BODY

Treatment

Treatment usually consists of immobilisation in a plaster jacket or collar which holds the neck in extension.

Method of application. With the patient in the sitting or lying position the surgeon supports the head in the position he requires; the neck is extended, but the head is not tilted back on the atlas so far as to prevent the patient seeing the ground in front of him when weight-bearing in plaster is commenced. The arms are abducted out of the way, wool-roll padding is applied in figures-of-eight over the neck, chin, occiput and trunk. The plaster jacket is then quickly and smoothly applied. It must be closely moulded under the occiput and the mandible and extended over the shoulders and down to the iliac crests. The Minerva jacket (Fig. 19.25) encloses the forehead to the eyebrows; in

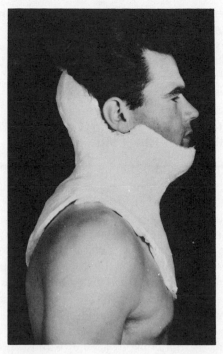

Fig. 19.26 Doll's collar.

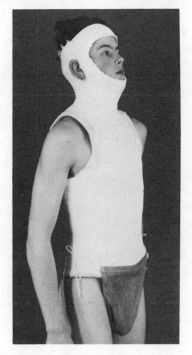

Fig. 19.25 Minerva jacket.

this type of jacket the plaster can be cut away beneath the chin so that the movement of the jaw is permitted. If the forehead is not encircled, the angles of the jaw must be included in the plaster. A window is cut over each ear, and sufficient plaster is cut away at the axillae to allow movement of the arms. The patient is returned to bed and the plaster is supported on pillows as already described; the patient is usually made comfortable lying flat supported on pillows, because in the sitting position the chin-piece may cause some discomfort. It is more comfortable to wear once the patient is allowed up; in spite of its formidable appearance, this type of jacket is surprisingly well tolerated and uncomplicated cases are usually allowed up in a few days. The doll's collar is applied in a similar manner and the same care is needed (Fig. 19.26).

FRACTURE OF A TRANSVERSE PROCESS

Fracture of a transverse process nearly always occurs in the lumbar region, and is usually due to sudden and powerful contraction of the quadratus lumborum. Tearing of this muscle results in avulsion of the transverse process; the accompanying soft tissue damage may be extensive, and is characterised by pain in the flank, which is aggravated by movement of the trunk.

Treatment

A mild degree of injury without separation of the fragments is treated by firm strapping to the lumbar region. Weight-bearing is generally allowed in a few days, and exercises are commenced in three or four weeks.

Severe cases with fracture of several transverse processes and tearing of the lumbar muscles, require fixation in a plaster jacket extending from the nipple line to the lower pelvis. It is generally applied in the standing position, and is retained for about two months. Weight-bearing is allowed in a few days and exercises for the spinal muscles are commenced in about one month; full spinal exercises are gradually introduced when the plaster is removed.

N.B. Fracture of the spine with paraplegia or tetraplegia is discussed in Ch. 23.

TREATMENT AND NURSING CARE IN OPEN (COMPOUND) FRACTURE

A fracture is said to be open or compound when there is a communication between the fracture and the outside air, as, for example, when there is a wound on the skin surface leading to the fracture, or when a fracture of the skull communicates with an air sinus. The shock which accompanies any severe injury may also in this case be accompanied by and accentuated by external haemorrhage. These factors receive primary consideration and treatment as outlined in the foregoing paragraphs, but excision of the wound and reduction of the fracture is undertaken at the earliest possible moment.

On admission it may be necessary to cut away clothing around a wound and apply a sterile dressing or, in the case of haemorrhage, a firm pad and bandage. Suitable analgesics are given for the relief of pain and emergency splintage such as a gutter-splint or plaster shell will be necessary. Anti-tetanus toxoid is usually given, and sometimes, anti-gas-gangrene serum. Since early operation is almost always envisaged, oral fluids are withheld but intra-venous infusion of Dextran, plasma or whole blood is commenced as soon as possible. As in other severe injuries, an observation chart is commenced immediately and the observations already mentioned recorded regularly; any deterioration in the patient's condition is reported to the surgeon at once.

Operative treatment is undertaken at the earliest possible moment and consists of excision of the wound with thorough toilet and reduction of the fracture. Thorough wound toilet is essential to remove all foreign material and ensure a good blood supply. One famous writer says, however (Perkins, 1970) 'remove debris, but avoid dis-arranging the tissues as though turning over goods at a winter sale'. After application of a dressing, appropriate splintage (usually a plaster cast) is applied and the patient is returned to the ward. When possible, the limb is elevated, and the circulation in the extremities is closely watched. Prophylactic chemotherapy is usually ordered.

Skin loss. Sometimes skin-grafting is required, either in the form of a skin flap or a free graft.

Treatment of infected open fractures. Treatment is aimed at *preventing* infection, but if it is already present, or develops after excision of the wound, further excision of tissues to establish free drainage may be necessary. Where possible, a closed plaster is applied and if infection is controlled treatment proceeds as for a closed fracture.

Secondary haemorrhage is rarely seen nowadays, but sudden onset of pain, pallor and faintness should be reported to the surgeon at once. Exploration of the wound and ligation of a bleeding vessel may be necessary.

Later treatment in uncomplicated cases proceeds according to the individual fracture. Infection may cause delayed union, when prolonged immobilisation is often required. Chronic bone infection (osteomyelitis) may lead to formation of sequestra and discharge of pus from a sinus; removal of sequestra may be indicated, and in cases of non-union from any cause some form of bone-grafting operation may eventually be advised.

GENERAL OBSERVATIONS ON THE ADMISSION OF ACCIDENTS TO THE WARD

The mode of admission of the victim of an accident is quite different from that of a routine admission when the patient is fully prepared, arrives at an appointed time, equipped with personal possessions, and often, accompanied by relatives. After an accident, on the other hand, the patient is usually admitted unheralded off the street, in working clothes, accompanied only by an ambulance worker or a police officer and often, in no condition to give an account of himself. Members of the police force and ambulance service give valuable assistance in helping to identify the patient and in informing relatives, and the nurse may be called upon to be particularly tactful in dealing with the alarmed and upset relatives of patients admitted in this way.

In the case of a minor who requires immediate operation, the surgeon and the anaesthetist may take the responsibility of performing it in the absence of formal consent from the parent or guardian.

The patient may be admitted to bed partly or even fully dressed, and removal of the clothing may have to be done gradually as treatment of the general condition and the specific injuries proceeds. On the other hand, the clothing may have been split at the surgeon's initial examination. Similarly, a bed-bath on admission is often contra-indicated and cleansing of the patient's body must be undertaken as and when his treatment and general condition allows. *Personal possessions such as wrist-watches and money must be carefully listed and handed to the proper authority for safe keeping.*

SOME PSYCHOLOGICAL AND SOCIAL CONSIDERATIONS IN INJURY

Apart from the physical shock of an injury, there is also the shock of finding oneself in hospital having suffered an abrupt and totally unexpected disruption of one's daily life and work, not to mention the mutilation of one's body, which, especially in the case of young subjects, may have been hitherto a perfect functioning unit. This may have serious psychological effects because of alteration in body image (Pettitt, 1980). Often the patient must face, without preparation, not only weeks or months of treatment in hospital but perhaps, interruption of studies at a crucial time, or loss of earnings, promotion and opportunities, as well as disruption of family and social life. Macmillan (1980), writing in the *Nursing Times*, quotes a patient as saying 'Well, I am not really keen on all this psychology lark, but you do lose your identity. You know, I am a builder, I have my own business. I am the boss—I have 15 workers and they call me the governor. But that counts for nothing once you put on hospital pyjamas. You just become another patient. You lose that identity, that status, that rôle and you become a nobody'.

The same patient said 'But there's another thing you lose, and that's money. Time is money to me in my business'. Then there is the anxious father or mother of a family, or those with other dependent relatives, and those whose treatment must take place far from their homes and friends so that they cannot receive visitors. Moreover we sometimes see a patient who must face some permanent handicap which may entail learning a whole new way of life.

These circumstances, then, call for mental acceptance and adjustment on the part of the patient; most of them, fortunately, accept their treatment and co-operate with us through thick and thin until final rehabilitation and resettlement is accomplished; but there are some who develop a chip on the shoulder and a few who find in a hospital ward a welcome refuge from work and from the world. From time to time, the surgeon and other members of his team will assess the patient's physical and intellectual status against his social, economic and family background so that plans can be made in readiness for his discharge from hospital. The medico-social worker has a key position in that she can not only deal with financial, family and business matters which are causing immediate anxiety, but can mobilise forces outside the hospital to help the patient on discharge. For example, she can if required contact the Disablement Resettlement Officer, the appropriate housing or welfare authority, or enlist the help of the Medical Officer of Health. Close liaison with community health personnel is axiomatic.

Wright (1981) has drawn attention to the fact that patients who are victims of violence and abuse suffer emotional upheaval as well as physical injury and need special consideration.

These notes are included here merely to remind the nurse that the injured patient, in common with all others, must be viewed as a whole person and treatment includes not only his physical care but a humane, active approach to his individual problems, without which efforts to restore him to society cannot succeed.

FRACTURES

A fracture is a solution in continuity of a bone, usually as a result of external violence, i.e. a break.

Predisposing causes of fracture

These include the following:

Age. Children and old people are prone to fractures, the former because of their unsteady gait, the latter because their bones are osteoporotic and brittle (Ch. 30).

Sex. Up to the age of 50 years, fractures are more frequently sustained by men than by women, because of the hazards of their occupations; after the age of 50 years, they are more commonly sustained by women.

Pathological fractures. These may be due to the following conditions:

1. Disuse atrophy of bone, as seen in the paralysed limb (e.g. in myelomeningocoele or poliomyelitis).
2. General bone diseases, such as Paget's disease, rickets, or osteogenesis imperfecta.
3. Local bone diseases, such as tumours, cysts, or osteomyelitis.

Exciting causes of fracture

Direct violence. In this, the injuring force is applied directly to the bone, and a fracture occurs at the site of impact. A fracture of this type is usually transverse and is liable to be comminuted or compound.

Indirect violence. The force is not applied directly to the bone but is transmitted along some other part of the body; for example, the clavicle may be fractured by a fall on the outstretched hand. The fracture is usually oblique or spiral and is less likely to be comminuted or compound.

Muscular violence. This may be sufficient to produce a fracture, as when the patella is fractured by a violent contraction of the quadriceps in attempting to avoid a fall.

Classification of fractures

A *closed or simple fracture* is one in which the skin is unbroken and there is no communication between the fracture site and the external air.

An *open or compound fracture* is one in which the skin of mucous membrane is lacerated to form a communication between the fracture site and the external air.

An *incomplete fracture* is one in which the continuity of the bone is not entirely interrupted. The commonest example of this is the *greenstick* fracture which occurs in young subjects.

A *complete fracture* is one in which continuity of the bone is entirely interrupted. It is further described according to the direction of the line of fracture, as explained opposite (Fig. 19.27).

A *transverse fracture* is one directly across the bone. It is often due to direct violence.

An *oblique fracture* is one in which the fracture line runs obliquely. It is due to indirect violence.

A *spiral fracture* is one in which the fracture line runs in a spiral. It is due to indirect violence combined with torsional strain.

A *longitudinal fracture* splits the bone lengthwise.

T-shaped and Y-shaped fractures split the bone in the directions signified by the letters. They are most commonly seen at the lower end of the humerus or femur.

An *abduction of adduction fracture* is one in which the distal fragment is abducted or adducted in relation to the proximal fragments.

A *comminuted fracture* is one in which one or both fragments is broken into small pieces.

An *impacted fracture* is one in which one fragment is driven into the other and is thus stable, as in a Colles fracture.

A *multiple fracture* is one in which there is more than one separate fracture in the same bone.

A *complicated fracture* is one which involves some other organ, such as a nerve, blood-vessel, or underlying structures; for example, the bladder may be injured in fracture of the pelvis, or the lung in fractures of the ribs.

Fracture-separation or epiphyses occur in young subjects, when the bone gives way through the epiphyseal cartilage. A metaphyseal fragment is usually detached with the epiphysis.

Clinical diagnosis

The clinical diagnosis of fracture is based on the following findings:

1. *The history of injury.*
2. *Signs of local trauma.* These may include pain, tenderness, swelling, bruising and blistering of the skin.
3. *Loss of function of the part.*
4. *Deformity* may or may not be present. It is caused by the direction of the violence, by the

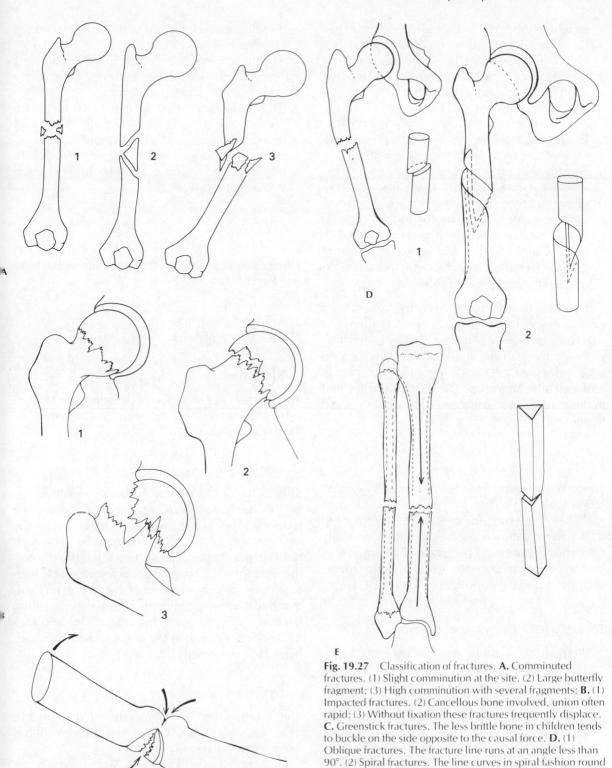

Fig. 19.27 Classification of fractures. **A.** Comminuted fractures. (1) Slight comminution at the site. (2) Large butterfly fragment; (3) High comminution with several fragments; **B.** (1) Impacted fractures. (2) Cancellous bone involved, union often rapid; (3) Without fixation these fractures frequently displace. **C.** Greenstick fractures. The less brittle bone in children tends to buckle on the side opposite to the causal force. **D.** (1) Oblique fractures. The fracture line runs at an angle less than 90°. (2) Spiral fractures. The line curves in spiral fashion round the bone caused mainly by torsional forces. **E.** Transverse fractures. The inherent stability of this type of fracture reduces the risk of shortening and favours union.

weight of the limb, or by muscular contraction. *Displacement of fragments* is described according to their position. There may be angulation, lateral displacement, or longitudinal displacement (over-riding). Rotational displacement may also be present.

5. *Localised bone tenderness.* This is important because it may be the only sign present—for example, in fractures of the carpal navicular.

6. *Soft tissue injuries.* A fracture may be accompanied by damage to skin, to ligaments, blood-vessels, nerves, or to underlying soft structures.

7. *Unnatural mobility* is the abnormal movement at the fracture site which may be elicited by rough handling. This may be accompanied by *crepitus* (grating sounds). which should not occur if the limbs is held securely.

Radiographic examination is carried out in every case of suspected fracture, as none of the above signs may be present. Anterior-posterior and lateral views of the part are required. An oblique view is necessary for the carpal navicular, and may be repeated after an interval. Radiographs with a joint in different positions may be ordered, for example, in injuries to the ankle.

Union of fractures

Union of a fracture in the first instances is by granulation tissues. The haematoma between the bone ends is invaded by living cells and transformed into a form of immature bone called *callus*. Eventually, the callus matures and becomes fully formed bone by the action of the bone cells. Irregular masses disappear, and the bone regains its normal shape.

Factors which influence rate of union

1. *Individual variations* are manifest in the rate of healing of bones as in any other body tissue, so that no arbitrary time limit can be laid down for the rate of healing of a fracture.

2. *The age of the patient.* The younger the patient, the more quickly the fracture unites, and vice versa.

3. *The type of fracture.* Oblique and spiral fractures unite more rapidly than transverse fractures. Impacted fractures unite more rapidly than those in which there is a wide gap between the bone ends.

4. *The presence of infection.* In infected fractures, union is retarded by the associated hyperaemia and decalcification of the bones.

5. *The blood supply of the fragments.* If both fragments have a good blood supply, firm rapid union is expected. If one fragment is deprived of its blood supply, union will be slow. If both fragments are deprived of blood supply, union will be very slow.

THE TREATMENT OF FRACTURES

Three main principles of the treatment of fractures are described:

1. *Reduction.*
2. *Immobilisation.*
3. *Restoration of functional activity.*

1. Reduction

This consists of correction of deformity and restoration of anatomical relationships. It is achieved by the following means:

a. Manipulation

The fracture is reduced by deliberate manipulation by the surgeon's hands. Manual traction is often required. This is the method of reduction in the vast majority of fractures, and may be performed under general or local anaesthesia. It is usually performed forthwith, unless there is severe shock, haemorrhage, or gross swelling of the part; even then, manipulation is attempted as soon as possible, because as time goes by, reduction becomes increasingly difficult as the bone ends become adherent in a deformed position.

b. Operative reduction

This is employed if manipulative reduction has failed or is likely to fail, or if re-displacement has occurred or is likely to occur.

Reduction is confirmed by X-rays, which are repeated from time to time according to the surgeon's orders. In general, some lateral displace-

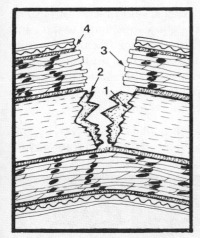

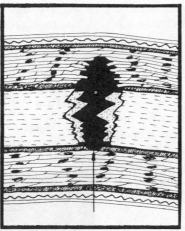

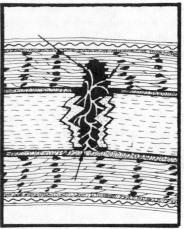

A. As a result of the injury, (1) the periosteum may be completely or partly torn, (2) there is disruption of the Haversian systems with death of adjacent bone cells, (3) there may be tearing of muscle, especially on the convex side of the fracture, and damage to neighbouring nerves and blood vessels, (4) the skin may be broached in compound injuries, with risk of ingress of bacteria.

B. *Fracture haematoma* (i) Bleeding occurs from the bone ends, marrow vessels, and damaged soft tissues, with the formation of a fracture haematoma which clots. (Closed fracture illustrated.)

C. *Fracture haematoma* (ii) The fracture haematoma is rapidly vascularised by the ingrowth of blood vessels from the surrounding tissues, and for some weeks there is rapid cellular activity. Fibrovascular tissue replaces the clot, collagen fibres are laid down, and mineral salts are deposited.

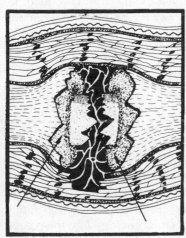

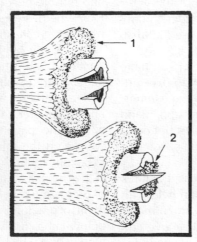

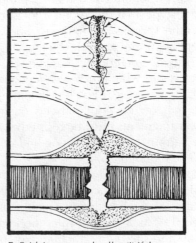

D. *Sub-periosteal bone:* New woven bone is formed beneath the periosteum at the ends of the bone. The cells responsible are derived from the periosteum, which becomes stretched over these collars of new bone. If the blood supply is poor, or if it is disturbed by excessive mobility at the fracture site, cartilage may be formed instead and remain until a better blood supply is established.

E. *This primary callus response* (1) remains active for a *few weeks only*. There is a much less vigorous formation of callus from the medullary cavity (2). Nevertheless, the capacity of the medulla to form new bone remains indefinitely throughout the healing of the fracture.

F. *Bridging external callus* (i) If the periosteum is incompletely torn, and there is no significant loss of bony apposition, the primary callus response may result in establishing external continuity of the fracture ('bridging external callus'). Cells lying in the outer layer of the periosteum itself proliferate to reconstitute the periosteum.

Fig. 19.28 A, B, C, D, E, F These illustrations, with their captions, are taken from *Practical Fracture Treatment*, by Ronald McRae, with kind permission of the author and publisher.

ment in the shaft of the long bones may be considered unimportant, provided that there is no over-riding, angulation, or rotation of the fragments.

2. Immobilisation

This is the means by which reduction is maintained. It must be adequate, uninterrupted, and retained for a sufficient length of time to allow the fracture to unite. Immobilisation is provided by the following means (a) external splintage and (b) internal splintage.

a. External splintage

Plaster of Paris is used in a large number of cases. The application and care of plaster casts has already been described in Ch. 6.

Splints (Ch. 7) are of varying types and in many cases have been superseded by plaster casts. Wooden splints may be used in first aid, and metal back splints, club-foot shoes and cock-ups provide useful pre-operative fixation. Splints of the aeroplane type may be ordered for shoulder injuries and the Thomas bed-splint is widely used in treatment of injuries to the lower limb.

Traction and counter-traction is used in unstable fractures in which there is a tendency to over-riding. For example, in oblique fractures of the femur, the pull of powerful muscles on the upper and lower fragments must be resisted. A description of the various types of traction and counter-traction will be found in Ch. 2.

Extent of splintage. Except for those fractures which can be reduced and the position held with a functional brace the essential joints are immobilised; i.e. as a general rule, the joints above and below the site of the fracture. Notable exceptions to this rule are two of the commonest fractures, i.e. a Colles fracture at the wrist, and a Pott's fracture at the ankle.

Functional bracing

As an aid to the healing of fractures of long bones, i.e. the femur and tibia, the humerus and the radius and ulna, a system of functional bracing has been developed. These braces have the effect of holding a fracture in the reduced and functional position but at the same time allow movement of the joints above and below the site of the fracture. The ones in most common use are (1) the cast-brace for fracture of the femur, and (2) the patella-tendon bearing cast (Sarmiento plaster cast) for fractures of the tibia. Para (3) gives further information.

1. *The cast-brace* is a total contact cast, i.e. has minimal padding around the limb and the plaster

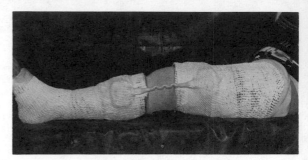

Fig. 19.29 The cast brace for fracture of the femur.

of Paris bandages are moulded into the contours and muscle bulk of the thigh, forming a quadrilateral type of socket, extending from the groin and over the greater trochanter to above the knee by $1-1\frac{1}{2}''$. A pair of hinges of the polycentric type are applied to allow flexion of the knee, these are then attached to a well fitting below-knee plaster cast, either joined to a hinged ankle shoe-insert, or to another plaster cast which includes the foot. This allows the patient to be ambulant and to take weight on the injured limb, but allows the knee to be fully mobile (Fig. 19.29).

2. *The patella tendon bearing cast or Sarmiento plaster* is a total contact cast applied for the treatment of fractures of the tibia; it is a well fitting below-knee cast which is moulded into the patella tendon and which follows the contours of the shaft of the tibia and the malleoli; weight-bearing in the cast is permitted within a few days of injury (Fig. 19.30).

3. *Further information.* The total-contact cast brace converts the normally contoured thigh into a semi-rigid tube, by virtue of the fact that it encloses it in a rigid cast; it is thought that the use of a rigid external support increases the fluid pressure within the thigh, and by this means reduces the weight transmitted through the fracture site;

rather, it passes it through the rigidly held soft tissue at the same time as movement takes place. Despite the movement, the external fixation prevents deformity at the fracture site. It is not proposed that this cast provide rigid immobilisation of the fragments; quite the contrary—it is suspected that since the motion that necessarily takes place at the fracture site during early reparative process is the result of function, it is not detrimental to fracture healing (Sarmiento, 1967).

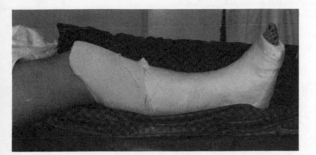

Fig. 19.30 Sarmiento moulded plaster of Paris for fracture of the tibia.

b. Internal splintage

Internal fixation. Internal fixation is indicated:

 (i) Where a fracture cannot be reduced by closed methods (e.g. a fracture of the tibia with soft tissue between the bone ends, or in many fractures of the forearm bones).
 (ii) Where a reduction can be achieved but it cannot be satisfactorily held by closed methods (e.g. fractures of the femoral neck).
(iii) Where a higher quality of reduction and fixation is required than can be obtained by closed methods (e.g. some fractures involving articular surfaces).

In addition, there is a controversial area where the risks of internal fixation in a particular set of circumstances are outweighed, in the experience and opinion of the surgeon in charge, by the advantages. Some of the factors involved may include:

 (i) The possibility of achieving and maintaining a high quality reduction.
 (ii) Earlier mobilisation of joints, with less risk of permanent stiffness, disuse osteoporosis, etc.
(iii) Earlier discharge from hospital, and earlier

return to full function (including work, athletic activities), etc.).

Some of the disadvantages of internal fixation are:

 (i) The possibility of introducing infection. The consequences may be serious (e.g. chronic bone infection with non-union, which may sometimes necessitate amputation).
 (ii) Internal fixation techniques require a degree of mechanical aptitude and experience on the part of the surgeon if the occasional serious failure is to be avoided.
(iii) To cover a wide range of fracture situation, a fairly formidable number of instruments and fixation devices will be required.
(iv) As on the whole the time under anaesthesia is much longer than when conservative measures are employed, the patient's general condition and health is of greater concern: the services of an expert anaesthetist are frequently required.

The method of achieving internal fixation include the use of a wide range of devices (screws, nails, plates, etc.).

External skeletal fixation. With this method the bone fragments are held in alignment by skeletal pins. The central portion of each pin lies in the bone, while the ends protrude from the skin. One to three pins are fixed in each bone fragment. The fracture is reduced with the pins in situ (at open operation, or by using an image intensifier). The pins are then held in proper relation to one another by a rigid external support. Plaster may be used for this purpose, or a rigid mechanical system of clamps and connecting rods.

Such systems are of particular value in the management of compound fractures where the state of the skin and other factors may make the use of internal fixation devices undesirable. They are sometimes followed, even in closed fractures, by pin track infections. The quality of the fixation is also dependent on the pins remaining tight in bone, and there is some risk of non-union.

3. Restoration of functional activity

This means the restoration of full use of the limb. The most perfect union of a fracture in the most perfect position will not benefit the patient if he is afterwards unable to use the limb. Treatment directed towards the restoration of functional activity is commenced as soon as reduction and immobilisation of the fracture has been achieved, and includes not only the injured limb itself, but all other parts of the body whose function may be impaired by the immobilisation necessary for healing of the fracture. For example, a patient whose wrist is immobilised in plaster for a Colles fracture is given exercises not only for the fingers, but for the elbow and shoulder, so that stiffness of these joints will not hinder the function of the limb. A patient confined to bed for fracture of the femur or tibia is given exercises for all joints other than those immobilised. In addition, he is encouraged to move about in bed as much as possible, so that not only is functional activity encouraged, but the complications which attend prolonged rest in bed are prevented (Chs 2 and 5).

Importance of the nurse's part in the restoration of functional activity. Formal exercises may be given by a physiotherapist, but the nurse must encourage her patient in activity of body and mind by her own attitude, and by helping him to do things for himself without detriment to his treatment.

The development of a nice judgement between what must be done for the patient to ensure his comfort and well being, and what in his own interests he must do for himself is an essential part of the orthopaedic nurse's equipment (Chs 2 and 5). Each case is considered individually, and whilst no pains are spared to make the patient comfortable in bed, one must remember that the effort entailed in washing, teeth cleaning, hair brushing, etc. is actually beneficial to the patient, always, provided he is not so young, so old, so feeble or so ill as to be unable to perform these offices for himself.

Summary of treatment directed towards the restoration of functional activity.

1. Active exercises and full use of joints not immobilised. Isometric exercises for affected part.
2. Active exercises for the affected part when immobilisation has ceased.
3. The avoidance of massage and passive stretching.
4. The prevention of oedema throughout the treatment and when splintage is discarded.

THE COMPLICATIONS OF FRACTURES

The complications of fractures include the following:

1. Slow union, non-union, mal-union.
2. Adhesions and joint stiffness.
3. Vascular complications.
4. Myositis ossificans.
5. Nerve injuries.
6. Injuries to vital organs.
7. Skin and soft tissue injuries.
8. Infection.
9. General complications (Chs 2 and 5).

1. Slow union

Slow union is said to be present when the fracture does not unite within the expected time. It may be due to the following:

a. Incomplete reduction.
b. Inadequate or interrupted immobilisation.
c. Excessive traction.
d. Loss of blood-supply to one or both fragments.
e. Infection.
f. Interposition of soft parts, for example, muscle-flaps.

In fractures in which slow union is expected the surgeon will warn the patient to expect a long period of immobilisation. The nurse will refrain from making prophecies as to how long immobilisation will continue, however heartening they may be to the patient. The patient who has been told by a nurse that his fracture will require only a few *weeks'* immobilisation, and finds his limb still immobilised after a *few months* is apt to lose faith in the nurse.

The nurse should take special note of the words *'inadequate or interrupted immobilisation'*. In recent fractures, special care is needed in adjusting splintage and in bi-valving plasters. In lower limb fractures, the patient must not walk in a bi-valved plaster. If he must be moved, he is lifted on to a trolley, moving the body and the affected limb as one unit, avoiding the slightest unguarded movement. If a wheelchair is used, the limb is completely supported on a plank placed on the seat. *In no circumstances will the nurse remove a splint or plaster completely without permission from the surgeon.*

Non-union

Non-union is said to be present when the bone ends are sclerotic, rounded off and the gap between them is filled by dense fibrous tissue. A false joint may be present at the fracture site. Non-union may be due to any of the aforementioned factors.

Treatment is operative and consists of freshening or drilling of fractured bone surfaces, with or without a bone graft. Immobilisation is then continued until union is sound.

Mal-union

Mal-union is said to be present when the fracture has united in a deformed position. Operative treatment may be advised if the deformity interferes with the function of the limb.

2. Adhesions and joint stiffness

These may be due to the following:

a. Failure to exercise joints not immobilised; oedema; neglect of isometric exercises.
b. Inactivity and disuse of joints once immobilisation has ceased.
c. Allowing movements of damaged joints too early, before torn tissues have healed.
d. Passive stretching to a stiff joint.

Preventions of adhesions and joint stiffness

Active exercises. Specific exercises will be enumerated in connection with individual fractures. They are usually supervised by a physiotherapist, but their vital importance must be appreciated by the nurse. She will report to the surgeon any patient who cannot or will not perform his exercises. Exercises not only prevent stiffness of the joints which are not immobilised, they actually help to prevent stiffness of the joint which *is* immobilised. The contraction and relaxation of the muscles maintains their tone, and ensures a free blood supply to the healing bone.

Active use. As soon as possible, active use of the limb is encouraged. This is important, as the patient does not then forget how to use the limb. In upper limb fractures, the hand is used for all ordinary purposes, short of wetting the plaster. In lower limb fractures, the surgeon will order a walking plaster as soon as possible. The patient is taught a normal heel-and-toe gait and encouraged to follow his every-day pursuits. When splintage is discarded, exercises to restore full functional use of the joints which have been immobilised are introduced, and continued until recovery is complete.

Passive stretching is forbidden. Any necessary manipulation will be carried out by the surgeon. Nurses and others must resist the temptation to apply passive stretching to a joint at any stage during the treatment.

Oedema. Oedema of the extremities is not a contra-indication to exercises. Rather, it is an added indication. In addition to active exercises, *the limb should be elevated*, if necessary with the patient in recumbency.

Oedema in the later stages of treatment. As a rule, oedema of the upper limb does not occur after removal of plaster, provided that exercises and functional use have been conscientiously carried out. In the lower limb, however, removal of the rigid support may cause oedema, especially towards the end of the day. This is very likely to occur in middle-aged and elderly patients in whom the tone of the muscle is insufficient to maintain the circulation against the force of gravity. This oedema must be prevented by a supporting bandage which is applied immediately on removal of plaster. If oedema is already present, *the limb must be elevated* until it subsides.

Supporting bandages. These are applied from the web of the toes to just below the knee. There must be no gaps in the bandage, otherwise the tissues will bulge through the gaps when swelling occurs. It is also important that the foot is held at the right angle when the bandage is applied, so that wrinkling in front of the ankle joint is avoided. An Elastoplast or other supporting bandage might be ordered. Many excellent supporting bandages and stockings are sold by manufacturers of surgical equipment.

3. Vascular complications

These include rupture of arteries, traumatic arterial spasm or traumatic aneurism. Partial occlusion of the blood supply to a limb causes ischaemia; complete occlusion causes gangrene.

Volkmann's ischaemic contracture

This is a dreaded complication of injuries to the elbow and forearm. It is most common in supracondylar fracture of the humerus, dislocation of the elbow, or fracture of the forearm in its upper one third. It is due to irritation or injury to the brachial

also inspected at ten minute intervals; they become cold, swollen and either cyanosed or pale. They are held in slight flexion and *cannot be completely extended.* Any attempt to straighten the fingers causes pain in front of the forearm. The patient may complain of severe burning pain in the forearm and hand but the onset is sometimes painless. If arterial spasm is not relieved within six or eight hours, the muscles die, and become matted, fibrosed and contracted; their power is then lost,

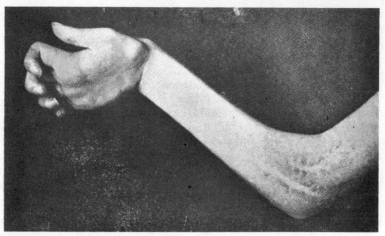

Fig. 19.31　A severe case of Volkmann's ischaemic contracture.

artery; in response to this irritation or injury, there is reflex spasm, not only of the main artery, but of the collateral vessels, so that the blood supply to the muscles is severely diminished. Volkmann's ischaemic contracture may follow slight injuries as well as severe ones and may even be due to constriction by a bandage, splint, plaster or tourniquet, or to compression of the artery by flexion of a swollen elbow. For this reason, cases of injury to the elbow or forearm are frequently detained in hospital for observation until it is certain that the circulation in the limb is unimpaired.

Clinical features

The classical signs of this condition are 4 Ps—pain, pallor, pulselessness, paralysis. The first sign may be absence of the radial pulse. The surgeon will palpate the radial artery before splintage is applied; thereafter, it is palpated at ten minute intervals in cases in which it is not covered. The fingers are

never to be completely regained. The nerves degenerate, even if uninjured at the primary injury, and the fingers become anaesthetic and fixed in a flexed position. Eventually, the typical contractures occur; the picture is one of a combined median and ulnar nerve palsy, with hyperextension of the metacarpophalangeal joints, flexion of the interphalangeal joints, wasting of the intrinsics of the hand and of the muscles of the thenar and hypothenar eminences. This results in severe crippling of the limb (Fig. 19.31).

Importance of immediate measures to prevent this complication

The importance of unceasing vigilance and frequent examination of the fingers after treatment for elbow or forearm injuries cannot be too heavily stressed. Note in particular, pain in the forearm on attempting to extend the fingers; beware the child who cries continually or whose sleep is disturbed. Do not attempt to heat the limb by applying hot-water bottles or by placing the patient near a radiator or fire. Elevate the limb, keep the patient warm, and *if any of the aforementioned signs are noticed, inform the surgeon at once.* DELAY IS DANGEROUS, and may result in permanent crippling of the limb.

Treatment

1. The front half of the plaster or the encircling bandage is removed
2. If the fracture is still unreduced, further manipulation or even open reduction is performed.
3. If the elbow has been flexed, the degree of flexion is reduced, if necessary to below the right-angle.
4. If these measures fail to relieve the symptoms promptly, spasm of the artery may be relieved by blocking the sympathetic nerve-supply to the limb by the injection of novocain. Alternatively, operative exploration of the artery is performed. A damaged portion of the artery may be excised.

Later treatment

If the arterial spasm is relieved, and the symptoms disappear, treatment proceeds as described for individual fractures. In established cases, later treatment is aimed at improving the function of the limb by correction of deformity and re-education of such muscles as are spared.

Correction of deformity. Flexion of the wrist is corrected first either by successive plasters, gaining a little more correction each time, or by wedging the plaster. When about 30 degrees or 40 degrees dorsiflexion of the wrist has been obtained, it is held on an anterior plaster slab, and the fingers are immobilised on wooden spatula splints until extension is obtained. Alternatively, finger-stalls attached to traction loops incorporated in a wrist plaster may be ordered.

Physiotherapy is ordered to restore as much muscle power as is possible and to minimise contracture. Considerable improvement of function may take place over a long period.

Operative treatment. In the late stages, operations on soft tissues, such as muscle-slide of the forearm flexors, or lengthening of tendons in the lower forearm may be performed. Operations on bones include arthrodesis of the wrist or shortening of the forearm bones.

Ischaemic contracture in the lower limb

Damage to the femoral or popliteal artery in injuries of the lower limb may produce arterial spasm and partial occlusion of the blood supply. The changes already described in connection with ischaemia in the upper limb occur, with fibrosis of the muscles and rigid clawing of the toes. Anaesthesia of the foot may be very troublesome and give rise to ulceration of the skin.

Treatment. This proceeds on the same lines as described for ischaemia in the upper limb.

Gangrene

Gangrene due to total obliteration of the blood supply is as a rule more likely to occur in the lower limb than ischaemia. Roaf & Hodkinson (see Bibliography) describe a case of gangrene secondary to the use of a tourniquet.

Treatment. This may consist of amputation of the limb. In any case of incipient gangrene, keep the patient as warm and comfortable as possible, but do not attempt to heat the limb itself. In fact, the surgeon may give orders for it to be exposed to cold air or even encased in ice.

4. Myositis ossificans

Traumatic ossification occurs in injuries in which there is tearing of the periosteum from the bone by avulsion of soft tissue attachments. There is a sub-periosteal haematoma which may be disseminated into surrounding tissue. New bone is laid down in the haematoma so that bony masses are formed which may limit the movement of a joint. Traumatic myositis ossificans is most frequently seen after dislocation of the elbow in childhood, especially if reduction is delayed, or if passive stretching to the joint further tears the periosteum and disturbs and disseminates the haematoma. The ossification is first seen on radiographs as a shadow in the soft tissues in front of the joint, which may then be converted into a block of bone.

Treatment. This complication is avoided by:

a. Prompt reduction of the dislocated joint.
b. Retaining immobility for sufficient time for the periosteum to become firmly adherent to bone and for soft tissue injuries to heal.
c. Allowing the joint movement to recover by the patient's own active exercise, *not by passive stretching.*

Operative treatment. Excision of spurs or blocks of bone may be performed at a later stage of treatment.

5. Nerve injuries

Injuries to nerves may occur at the time of accident or be a later sequel. Peripheral nerve lesions are discussed briefly in Ch. 22.

6. Injuries to vital organs

These may occur as a complication of fracture; for example, the bladder may be damaged in fracture of the pelvis.

7. Skin and soft tissue injuries

Injuries to skin and other soft tissue may require treatment by excision, as mentioned earlier in connection with open fractures. Later it may be necessary to restore skin loss by means of grafting, and other structures such as tendons may require operative repair.

8. Infection

9. General complications

General complications include hypostatic pneumonia, renal calculi, pressure-sores, fat embolism, thrombosis and embolism. Hypostatic pneumonia occurs most commonly in elderly patients. It should be prevented by nursing the patient in the sitting position (when possible) or by frequent change of position in bed. Breathing exercises are always ordered. Renal calculi are also prevented by movement in bed and by the administration of copious fluids.

Visceral complications

Rupture of the urethra or bladder, and perforation of the rectal wall, may complicate fractures of the pelvis.

(i) Rupture of the spleen, kidney or liver may follow severe local trauma, abdominal compression or crushing (such as, for example, run-over injuries).
(ii) Rupture of the intestines or tearing of the mesenteric attachments may also follow abdominal compression.
(iii) Paralytic ileus: ileus is occasionally seen following fractures of the pelvis and lumbar spine, the most likely cause being disturbance of the autonomic control of the bowel from retro-peritoneal haematoma.

Treatment: (a) Naso-gastric suction. (b) Intravenous fluids—the quantity and proportions being determined by the amount of aspirate and other losses, and serum electrolyte estimations. In the majority of cases, bowel sounds return within 36 hours and intravenous fluids and suction may be discontinued shortly afterwards.

Pressure sores are prevented by change of position and by scrupulous care of the skin from the first moment.

Fat embolism

This complication is usually thought to be due to micro-particles of marrow fat escaping into the circulation from the region of the fracture.

It occurs most frequently after fractures of the femoral shaft and pelvis. Commonly, there is an unexplained deterioration in the condition of a patient a few days after sustaining such an injury.

There is a slight pyrexia; petechial haemorrhages appear in the skin; the patient may become confused, aggressive or comatosed.

There may be some evidence of renal insufficiency.

Radiographs of the chest often show mottling of the lung fields; these changes are considered to be due to fat embolisation in the lungs.

Treatment: (a) Heparinisation. (b) Supportive measures such as the administration of oxygen and of intravenous fluids.

INTRODUCTORY NOTE ON NURSING CARE IN FRACTURES

In no branch of surgery is the surgeon's approach so individualistic as in the treatment of fractures. Though the *principles* of treatment already described never alter, variations on the *method of application* will be found, even in patients treated by different surgeons in the same centre. For example, the method of applying traction and splintage in fractures of the femur varies from place to place and from surgeon to surgeon. Having grasped the principles of treatment, it is up to the nurse to discover the particular method of fixation favoured by the surgeon with whom she is working, so that she may anticipate his wishes and carry out his orders.

In ensuing chapters, nursing care is discussed only briefly in connection with individual fractures, because much of the ground has already been covered earlier in this book in connection with other conditions. For example, the application and care of plaster casts is described in Ch. 6 and the application and care of skin-extensions in Ch. 10.

BIBLIOGRAPHY

Adams J C 1978 Outline of Fractures. Edinburgh: Churchill Livingstone

Allan D 1982 Nursing aspects of artificial ventilation. Nursing Times, 16 June

Allan D 1984 Glasgow Coma Scale. Nursing Mirror, 13 June

Allan D 1984 Patients with an endotracheal tube or tracheostomy. Nursing Times, 28 March

Allan D 1984 Patients with facial fractures. Nursing Times, 14 March

Andrews I D 1974 Physiological response following trauma. Nursing Times, 14 March, 387

Apley E G 1977 A System of Orthopaedics and Fractures. London: Butterworths

Blythin P 1983 'Would you like to wait over there please?'. Nursing Mirror, 7 December

Bradley D 1972 Fracture of the pelvis. Nursing Times, 30 March, 376

Bradley D 1975a First aid 1. Main maxims. Nursing Times, 21 August, 1322

Bradley D 1975b First aid 2. Circulatory and respiratory arrest. Nursing Times, 28 August, 1376

Bradley D 1975c First aid 3. Haemorrhage and shock. Nursing Times, 4 September, 1409

Bradley D 1975d First aid 4. Injuries to bones, joints and muscles. Nursing Times, 11 September, 1462

Bradley D 1975e First aid 5. Injuries to bones, joints and muscles 2. Nursing Times, 18 September, 1502

Bradley D 1975f First aid 6. Poisoning, burns and scalds. Nursing Times, 25 September, 1542

Bradley D 1975g First aid 7. Chest Injuries. Nursing Times, 2 October, 1582

Bradley D 1975h First aid 8. Road Accidents. Nursing Times, 9 October, 1622

Bray A P, Thomas J R 1969 Severe fat embolism syndrome following multiple fractures. Nursing Care Study. Nursing Times, 23 January, 109

Brearley J 1973 Crash victim with multiple injuries. Nursing Times, 2 November. Nursing Care Study, 28

Buckles E 1983 A flying squad comes of age. Nursing Times, 2 February, 57–60

Chappell A G 1971 Pulmonary embolism. Nursing Mirror, 8 January, 26

Clarke D B, Barnes A D 1971 Intensive Care for Nurses. Oxford: Blackwell Scientific

Coady T J, Bennett A 1978 Respiratory failure. Nursing Times, 25 May

Cochrane C 1983 Triage is being used in Leicester. Letter. Nursing Mirror, 25 May

Curtis C 1982 Chest Injuries I, II, III. Nursing Mirror, 25 August

Deakin H G, Rann S E 1969 Artificial ventilation. Nursing Times Occasional Papers, 27 March, 49

Devas M B 1971 Stress fractures in athletes. Nursing Times, 25 February, 67, 227

Farrow R 1976 The Nursing of Accidents. Nursing Times, 6 May, 693; 24 February, 231

Goffman E 1979 Stigma—notes on the management of spoiled identity. Hardmondsworth: Penguin

Griffin L 1972 'Jim'—severe head injury. Nursing Times, 24 February, 231

Gunter V 1969 Gas gangrene treated by hyperbaric oxygen. Nursing Times, 24 April

Hardy R H 1978 Accidents and Emergencies. Oxford: Oxford Medical Publications

Hastings C 1982 On an individual basis. Nursing Mirror, 12 May

The Health and Safety at Work Act 1974

High M 1967 Chest and liver. Multiple Injuries. Nursing Times, 24 November, 1580

Hindle J F 1978 The management of multiple injuries. British Journal of Hospital Medicine 19: 219

Hopkins P 1978 Causes and prevention of road accidents. Nursing Times, 28 September, 1594

Huckstep R L 1970 A Simple Guide to Trauma. Edinburgh: Churchill Livingstone

Jamieson K G 1971 A First Notebook of Head Injury. London: Butterworths

Jones G J 1973 Intensive care following multiple fractures. Nursing Care Study. Nursing Mirror, 10 August, 35

Kaprio L A 1975 Death on the road. Geneva. World Health Organisation, 4 October

Knight P N 1973 Rehabilitation of head injuries. Nursing Mirror, 30 March, 14

Lloyd H M 1973 Fat embolism following multiple injuries. Nursing Times, Nursing Care Study, 8 November, 1490

London P S 1961 The reception and treatment of the seriously injured. Nursing Times, 13 October, 1329

London P S et al 1966 Severe injuries that include the head. Nursing Mirror Symposium, 12 August, 1–11

London P S 1967 Nursing Emergencies. Oxford: Blackwell Scientific

London P S 1967 A practical guide to the care of the injured. Edinburgh: Churchill Livingstone

London P S 1969 Head injuries. Nursing Mirror, 16 May, 20

London P S 1971 Nursing in an accident unit. Nursing Mirror, 17 September, 25

Macmillan P 1980 Strange encounter. Nursing Times, 6 November

MacRae R 1976 Clinical Orthopaedic Examination. Edinburgh: Churchill Livingstone

MacRae R 1981 Practical Fracture Treatment. Edinburgh: Churchill Livingstone

Maddocks G et al 1981 Accidents in childhood. Nursing Mirror Clinical Forum, 20 May

Maudsley R H 1973 Gas gangrene and its management. Nursing Times, 15 February, 201

Maxwell M 1983 Everything you need to know about shock. Cover article. Nursing Mirror, 23 March

May A 1974 Internal fixation of fractures. Nursing Times, 14 November, 70, 1777

Moghissi K et al Reprint of 1977 The pleural cavity and injuries of the chest. Nursing Times Publication

Muckle D S 1973 Soft tissue injuries. Nursing Mirror, 9 February, 24

Mountjoy P, Whythe B 1974 Nursing Care and the Unconscious Patient. London: Ballière Tindall and Cassell

Nayman R 1984 Nutritional support of the trauma patient. British Association of Orthopaedic Nurses. News Sheet 7

Norris W, Campbell D 1976 A nurse's guide to anaesthetics, resuscitation and intensive care. 6th edn. Edinburgh: Churchill Livingstone

Nursing Mirror 1977 Stove in Chest. Nursing Mirror Forum, 13 July

Pearson J R, Austin R T 1973 Accident Surgery and Orthopaedics. London: Lloyd-Luke

Perkins G 1970 The Ruminations of an Orthopaedic Surgeon. London: Butterworth

Pettit E 1980 Body image. Nursing, 16

Play it Safe 1983 A guide to preventing children's accidents. Booklet published jointly by the Health Education Council and the Scottish Health Education Group

Ray G 1982 Home accidents. Nursing Times Community Outlook, 11 August

Ring P A 1969 Care of the Injured. Edinburgh: E & S Livingstone

Roaf R, Hodkinson L J 1975 A Textbook of Orthopaedic Nursing. Oxford: Blackwell Scientific

Ross J S, Wilson K J W 1970 Foundations of Nursing and First Aid. Edinburgh: Churchill Livingstone

Rowe N L, Beetham M D 1971 Maxillo facial injuries I. Nursing Times, 26 August, 1957; Fractures of the Mandible, 2 September, 1083; Fractures of the Maxilla, 9 September, 1111

Sarmiento A 1967 A functional below-the-knee cast for tibial fractures. Journal of Bone and Joint Surgery 49A: 855

Skeet M 1977 Manual for Disaster Relief Work. Edinburgh and London: Churchill Livingstone

Smith T et al 1982 The wasted years. Nursing Mirror Cover Article 'Accidents', 12 May

Stoner H B 1977 Measuring the severity of injury. British Medical Journal 2: 1247

Teasdale G 1975 Acute impairment of brain function. 1. Assessing 'conscious level', 2. Observation record chart. Nursing Times, 12 June, 19 June, 17, 94

Thomas S 1969 Fat embolism—a hazard of trauma. Nursing Times, 23 January, 105

Turner D 1982 A long, lonely wait. London. Patients page. Nursing Mirror, 31 March

Whittall K 1970 Intensive care of severe head injury: the role of the nurse. Nursing Times, 30 July, 965

Wishart J 1971 Fat embolism. Nursing Times, 16 September, 1140

Wright B 1981 The victims of violence. London: Nursing Times, 25 November

Young J A 1981 Head Injuries. 1. Advances in care during the past decade. Head Injuries 2. Advances in diagnostic equipment. London: Nursing Times, 30 April, 7 May

Youngman P M E 1972 Chest Injuries. Nursing Mirror, 21 April, 30

20

Injuries of the upper limb

Fractures of the upper limb may be caused by direct violence or, more frequently, by indirect violence, such as a fall on the out-stretched hand.

Aim of treatment

The aim of treatment in injuries to the upper limb is to restore movement of the joints, because this is essential to the function of the limb; conversely, in the lower limb, stability rather than mobility of the joints is the chief functional demand. The treatment of fractures of the upper limb is therefore greatly influenced by the age of the patient. In middle-aged and elderly patients, the immobilisation necessary to ensure union in a perfect position would in many cases result in stiffness of the joints, so that the function of the limb as a whole would be seriously impaired.

It is for this reason that in older patients an imperfect anatomical reduction of a fracture may be accepted, provided that the function of the limb as a whole is regained. For example, in fractures of the clavicle in older patients, movements of the shoulder are commenced within a few days of injury so as to avoid stiffness of that joint; whereas in young patients, movement is rapidly recovered despite several weeks' enforced immobility.

Shoulder stiffness

Stiffness of the shoulder is a complication of injuries to the upper limb. It may be due to adhesions, which may form when movements of the shoulder are neglected during immobilisation of the elbow, forearm or wrist, or it may be due to peri-arthritis.

Peri-arthritis is the name given to degeneration and inflammation of the capsule and soft tissues surrounding the shoulder. It may occur spontaneously or after trivial injury, especially in middle-aged patients. Movements are limited by pain and muscle-spasm, abduction and external rotation being especially limited. Widespread adhesions and gross limitation of movement gives rise to the term 'frozen shoulder'.

Treatment. Rest in a sling is advised during the acute stage. As this subsides, active exercises are gradually introduced, commencing in recumbency and progressing to full swinging movements. Constant encouragement and perseverance is essential; *passive stretching is never employed.*

Shoulder exercises

The movement to be regained first is external rotation.

1. The patient lies on his back with the elbows to the sides and the hands pointing towards the ceiling, gradually turning the hands out until they touch the bed.
2. The hands are clasped behind the head and pressed back until the elbow touches the bed.
3. The shoulders are abducted to the right angle and the patient endeavours to touch the top of the bed with each hand.
4. The patient reaches over his head until he can touch the opposite ear. The same movements are then performed as the patient stands with his back to the wall. He then progresses to 'creeping up the wall', by standing sideways to it and reaching higher and higher with the finger-tips. It is encouraging to mark the level reached each time. Later, internal rotation is regained by placing the hand behind the back, reaching upwards towards the shoulder blades. Later still, swinging exercises are introduced.

Manipulation under anaesthesia may be performed when the shoulder is no longer painful, but the range of movement is not improved by the patient's own efforts. It is performed very gently and is followed by *active exercises only.* Passive movements, as such, are never given.

INJURIES TO THE SHOULDER

'Rotator-cuff' syndrome

Many patients are seen as out-patients with a stiff, painful shoulder which may be the result of minor trauma, or simply to degenerative processes within the musculo-tendinous cuff of the shoulder. Occasionally, pain in the shoulder and arm is referred from the cervical spine.

Treatment. Treatment consists of physiotherapeutic measures, local heat, *active* exercises and the administration of simple analgesics such as codeine; hydro-cortisone injections into tender areas may be advised, and operative repair is sometimes indicated.

Supra-spinatus tendonitis

This is due to degenerative changes in the tendon and in the capsule of the shoulder-joint. It gives rise to no limitation of movement of the shoulder, but there is an acute pain when the tendon impinges on the acromion process during the middle range of abduction of the shoulder; i.e. between 60 degrees and 90 degrees abduction. There may be calcification of the tendon.

Treatment. Novocain and/or hydro-cortisone infiltration followed by radiant heat and exercises. Excision of calcified material may be advised, or, excision of the outer margin of the acromion.

Rupture of the supra-spinatus tendon

This may be partial or complete. Partial rupture gives rise to symptoms similar to supra-spinatus tendonitis. Complete rupture of the supra-spinatus results in loss of abduction of the shoulder, as the humeral head is not then held in contact with the glenoid cavity to allow the deltoid to abduct the arm from the side.

Treatment. Partial rupture of the tendon may be treated by continuous rest in abduction on a Littler-Jones splint or in a plaster spica with removable lid.

Application. Unless otherwise ordered, the splint is worn under the clothes. The patient sits on a stool and an assistant steadies the shoulder throughout; wash the areas of skin which have been covered. Powder the axilla, slide the splint underneath the arm, and fasten the pelvic-band firmly. Gently lower the arm on to the splint and adjust the slings so that it is supported in its entirety. Fasten the webbing band over the unaffected shoulder. Place a pad of splint-wool under the head of the humerus and *be sure that it is supported at all times*. Cover the limb with splint-wool and bandage firmly. See that the splint grips the pelvis firmly.

Nursing care. An abduction splint is reasonably comfortable to wear so long as the patient is up and about; if he is confined to bed, the splinted limb must be supported on pillows.

Pressure sores. These most frequently occur at the point where the pelvis is held by the splint and under the posterior bar, or the internal condyle of the humerus may be pressed against the splint. If a sore occurs under the pelvic-band, the whole of this can be covered with felt and lint, or two pieces of felt can be secured to the bar on either side of a localised sore. Sores under the posterior bar can be prevented by padding the whole bar with felt and lint, or by inserting a strip of sorborubber beneath it. The internal epicondyle can be surrounded by a ring of felt. When the splint is removed for toilet purposes, the arm must be steadied by an assistant. Later, the patient may be allowed to wear the splint over his clothes, until it can be discarded altogether. An axillary wedge is occasionally ordered. *The arm is never allowed to drop to the side.* Abduction exercises are commenced in two or three weeks, and the splint is discarded when the shoulder can be actively abducted well above the right-angle. Operative suture may be advised, and it may be accompanied by excision of the acromion.

Rupture of the biceps tendon

This may occur as a result of degenerative changes in the tendon or in the capsule of the shoulder joint. It may occur spontaneously or as a result of muscular effort. There is a sharp pain in the shoulder which is accompanied by swelling; a hollow appears in the upper arm which is normally filled by the biceps, and the belly of the muscle can be seen to be retracted on movement of the elbow and forearm.

Treatment consists of suture of the biceps tendon.

Fracture of the clavicle

The clavicle is usually fractured in its middle third by a fall on the outstretched hand. There is pain and swelling, and obvious displacement may be present.

Treatment. Reduction and immobilisation is achieved by figure-of-eight bandages, though some authorities regard this as of doubtful value (Huckstep, 1970). A Velpeau bandage might be ordered instead (Fig. 20.2).

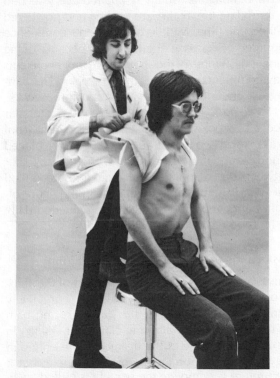

Fig. 20.1 Application of figure-of-eight bandage for fracture of clavicle.

Application of figure-of-eight bandage. Two large pads of splint-wool and at least two 275 cm × 12.5 cm calico bandages are required. Wash and powder the axillae. The patient sits on a stool and the operator stands behind him with one foot on the stool and the knee between the patient's shoulder blades (Fig. 20.1). Place the pads of wool in the axillae and start the bandage in front of the sound shoulder, carrying it across the back, up in front of the affected shoulder, and so on, so that the turns of bandage cross over the scapulae. Each turn of bandage should draw the shoulders upwards and backwards; the bandage must be firmly applied, but not so tightly as to interfere with the circulation of the limb. The end of the bandage is firmly secured, preferably by stitching, and the arm is supported in a sling. Exercises for the fingers, wrist, and elbow are commenced at once. If the arm and hand become swollen, or if the radial pulse cannot be felt, the bandage must be removed and re-applied whilst an assistant maintains traction on the shoulders.

The bandage is usually re-applied every second or third day; the axillae are washed and powdered at the same time. Middle-aged patients commence shoulder exercises after a few days, because of the danger of stiffness of the shoulder. Younger patients may commence exercises in two weeks. The bandage is generally discarded after about three weeks.

'Three-handkerchief' method. Two tubular pieces of stockinette are stuffed with splint-wool so as to form two thick 'sausages'. These are placed round each shoulder and tied tightly together between the scapulae. The shoulders are pulled backwards in the same manner as in the figure-of-eight bandage. The 'sausages' are tightened daily by refastening the ties between them.

Dislocation of the acromio-clavicular joint

This is an injury in which the ligaments of the acromio-clavicular joint are partially or completely torn. There is swelling of the shoulder, and pain is referred to the acromio-clavicular joint. In incomplete rupture of the ligaments, the only sign may be undue prominence of the clavicle, but if the rupture is complete the scapula is pulled away from the clavicle by the weight of the arm, so that the acromion lies below and in front of the clavicle.

Treatment consists of application of a sling, and graduated exercises.

As the patient is generally young and athletic, movement of the shoulder joint is quickly recovered.

Operative treatment consists of fixation of the acromio-clavicular joint by wires or screws, or, excision of the outer end of the clavicle.

Fracture of the scapula

Fracture of the body of the scapula is due to a direct injury which may also cause fracture of the ribs,

or to a fall on the shoulder or the outstretched hand.

Treatment. In middle-aged patients, firm strapping is applied over the affected shoulder from the clavicle to the opposite side of the chest, holding the scapula to the chest wall. The arm is supported in a sling. Finger, wrist and elbow exercises are started at once. Displacement of the fragments is unimportant compared to the danger of stiffness of the shoulder, and shoulder exercises are commenced in about 10 days. In young subjects, the displacement is corrected by means of continuous skin-traction with the shoulder abducted to the right angle.

The Velpeau Bandage. This is a comfortable and effective method of bandaging the upper limb to the trunk, and can be used in the treatment of fracture of surgical neck of humerus, shaft of the humerus, fracture of scapula or following reduction of a dislocated shoulder (Fig. 20.2).

Requirements

Orthopaedic wool rolls 15 cm × 10 cm.
Crêpe or flannel bandages 15 cm × 10 cm.
Pads of non-absorbent wool.
Zinc oxide strapping 2.5 cm.
Plaster of Paris bandage 15 cm.
Soap, water, talcum powder.

Method of application. Two operators are required. The patient is seated on a low table or stool, and the doctor holds the limb in the position required. The axilla on the affected side is washed, dried and powdered; in female patients this procedure is repeated beneath the breasts; one pad of wool is placed in the axilla on the affected side, in the flexure of the elbow, and beneath the breasts in female patients. In humeral shaft fractures, the doctor may place additional pads at the site of the fracture. The arm is laid on the trunk in such a position that the fingers lie just below the shoulder (Fig. 20.2A). Wool-roll bandage is then applied smoothly around the trunk, and in spiral turns over the shoulder (Fig. 20.2A), followed by a crêpe or flannel bandage applied in the same manner and fastened with strips of strapping. The procedure is then repeated twice so that there are six layers of alternating wool and crêpe (or flannel) bandage. The dressing is then encased in a single layer of plaster of Paris bandage, care being taken to see that this does not come into contact with the skin Fig. 20.2B.

If the patient is comfortable the dressing may be left undisturbed for as long as two weeks, when the procedure is repeated. At subsequent changes the bulk of the dressing may be reduced.

lowered until union is sound. Finger, wrist and elbow exercises are begun at once, and shoulder exercises are begun in six or eight weeks. The plaster or splint is not discarded until the patient can actively abduct the arm above the right-angle. Full movements are eventually restored by active exercises.

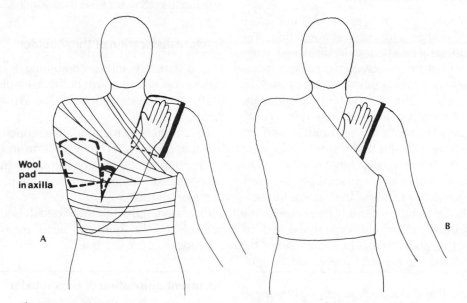

Wool pad in axilla

A

B

Fig. 20.2 **A.** The Velpeau bandage. **B.** Application of a thin layer of plaster completes the dressing.

Fracture of the great tuberosity of the humerus

This may occur as the result of a direct blow or as part of a dislocation of the shoulder. The tuberosity may be comminuted but not displaced, or, there may be avulsion of the tuberosity with or without displacement. There is pain, swelling and bruising, and tenderness referred to the great tuberosity. If the tuberosity has been avulsed, there is loss of abduction as described for rupture of the supraspinatus tendon.

Treatment. In fractures without displacement, the arm is supported in a sling and exercises are commenced in a day or so and practised regularly. The sling is discarded in about a fortnight and full active use of the arm is encouraged. Fractures with displacement require fixation in an abduction splint or plaster spica with removable lid. The arm is abducted, externally rotated and forwardly flexed, so that the avulsed fragment is approximated to the bed from which it is torn. *The arm is never*

Fracture of the neck of the humerus

This may be due to a direct blow on the shoulder, or, due to a fall on the outstretched hand. This causes either an adduction or abduction fracture of the neck of the humerus.

Treatment. A simple crack fracture without displacement is treated by early active exercises to avoid stiffness; immobilisation is unnecessary. Impacted fractures in elderly patients are treated by early active movements. In young patients, adduction fractures are treated by traction and fixation in abduction for about four weeks, followed by active exercises. Abduction fractures, on the other hand, are treated by a sling, and shoulder movements are commenced in about 14 days. Impacted fracture-dislocations of severe type may cause complete disorganisation of the shoulder joint. Elderly patients are treated by the application of an axillary pad or wedge supporting the arm in 30 degrees abduction. Shoulder exercises are commenced in about four weeks. In young patients operative reduction may be advised. Sometimes avascular necrosis of the humeral head supervenes and an arthrodesis of the shoulder is the ultimate fate.

Dislocation of the shoulder joint

Dislocation may occur as a result of a fall which forces the shoulder into extreme abduction. The dislocated humeral head is usually displaced anteriorly and lies beneath the coracoid process (subcoracoid dislocation), and in extreme cases may lie below the clavicle. There is pain in the shoulder, and all movements are limited. There is loss of the normal rounded contour of the shoulder and the elbow cannot be brought to the side. *Dislocation of the shoulder is not infrequently complicated by injury to the branches of the bracial plexus. Every patient is specially examined with this complication in view.* The axillary nerve is most commonly involved, so that the deltoid is paralysed and the power of active abduction is lost. Sometimes the displaced head of the humerus presses on the axillary vessels.

Treatment. The dislocation is reduced by manipulation with or without anaesthesia.

Kocher manipulation. The patient lies on a couch and the surgeon stands at his side. Traction is applied and the arm is very gently and smoothly manipulated first into external rotation, then brought forward across the chest, and finally into internal rotation.

Hippocratic manipulation. The patient lies on a couch and the surgeon grasps the wrist with both hands. He places his unbooted foot close to the axilla between the arm and the chest wall. He then leans back and exerts firm steady traction, and the head of the humerus is levered outwards over his foot and slides back to the glenoid cavity. The patient is then asked to abduct the arm in order to ascertain that there is no rupture of the supraspinatus tendon. If this is so, the shoulder is immobilised in abduction and external rotation as already described. Otherwise, a fairly large pad of wool is placed in the axilla, the arm is supported in a collar and cuff and then bandaged to the trunk. The fingers and wrist are left free and exercises for these joints are commenced at once. The bandage

and sling is discarded in about three weeks and active exercises are commenced.

Dislocation of the shoulder with fracture of the great tuberosity requires the same treatment, unless there is retraction of the fragment by the supraspinatus muscle, when it will be necessary to immobilise the shoulder in abduction, external rotation and forward flexion as already described.

Fracture dislocation of the shoulder

This is a severe injury combining a subcoracoid dislocation with fracture of the neck of the humerus. In severe cases the humeral head may be upside down.

Treatment is by manipulative reduction, traction being applied either with the arm to the sides as in the Hippocratic manipulation, or, by the Robert Jones method when the arm is held in right-angled or hyper-abduction.

Operative reduction may be advised. Avascular necrosis of the humeral head may necessitate arthrodesis of the shoulder.

Recurrent dislocation of the shoulder

In this condition there is repeated dislocation of the shoulder from trivial violence. It usually occurs in young subjects, particularly in athletes and epileptics.

Treatment. Many different operations have been employed for this condition. The Bankart operation consists of a repair of the glenoid fibrocartilage; in the Putti-Platt operation, the subscapularis and anterior capsule are divided and then overlapped to shorten the anterior part of the rotator cuff.

Fracture of the shaft of humerus

Fracture of the shaft of the humerus does not produce over-ridings such as occurs in the femur, because the muscles of the arm are not so powerful as in the leg, and their retraction is prevented by the weight of the limb. Displacement is easily corrected by manipulation and continuous traction is seldom used.

Treatment. Spiral fractures are generally immobilised by a gutter-splint and collar and cuff sling, or by applying a U-shaped slab extending from the axilla, down the inner side of the arm, round the elbow and up the outer side to the shoulder (Fig. 20.3). This is bandaged in position and the arm supported in a sling. Fingers and wrist exercises are begun at once and gentle shoulder exercises in a few days.

Figs. 20.4A and B show alternative methods of immobilising the shoulder joint.

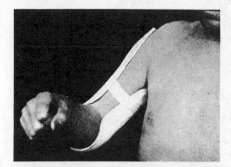

Fig. 20.3 U-shaped slab aplied for fracture of the humerous. The encircling bandage and supporting sling has been omitted.

Horizontal fractures usually unite more slowly and greater immobility is necessary. A plaster spica may be ordered, and the arm is usually held in abduction and forward flexion so that the patient's hand is almost in front of his mouth.

Fractures of the mid-shaft of the humerus may be complicated by radial nerve palsy (Ch. 19).

INJURIES TO THE ELBOW AND FOREARM

Traumatic synovitis of the elbow

This may follow a strain, especially in children. There is swelling, tenderness over the joint, and movements are limited by pain and muscle-spasm.

Treatment. A collar-and-cuff sling is worn for two weeks. A classical collar-and-cuff is shown in Fig. 20.5 and modern versions in Figs. 20.6A, B and C. Movement by the joint is allowed to recover at its own rate; efforts to hasten it by massage, passive stretching, or even *forced* exercises, will be met by increasing stiffness. If these measures are avoided, recovery is generally complete within two months.

Supracondylar fracture of the humerus

This is a common elbow injury in childhood and adolescence. In the great majority, the lower

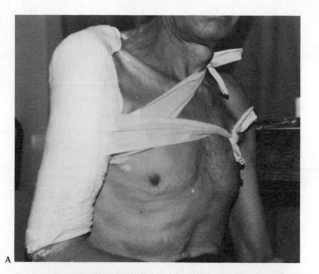

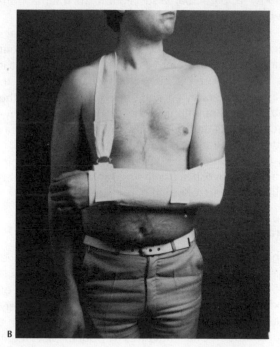

Fig. 20.4 Immobilisation of the shoulder.
A. Plaster of Paris splint.
B. 'Mastersling' universal shoulder immobiliser (Seton Products).

humeral fragment is displaced backwards. In a more rare type, it is displaced forwards.

Treatment. Reduction is obtained by traction and manipulation; in the common type of fracture with backward displacement of the fragment, the elbow is fixed in flexion by a wide posterior slab, which is lightly encircled with a gauze bandage. The limb is then supported in a collar and cuff. The more rare type of forward displacement requires fixation in full extension. Before the plaster slab is applied, the circulation is noted by feeling the radial pulse and by testing the circulation by compression of the fingertips. If there is gross swelling, the elbow must not be so flexed as to compress the vessels in front of the elbow, because of the danger of Volkmann's ischaemic contracture (Ch. 19). Flexion may be increased later when the swelling subsides, and the plaster slab converted into a full plaster. This is generally retained for about three weeks, thereafter a sling is worn for about a week and active exercises are commenced.

PASSIVE STRETCHING IS FORBIDDEN. The elbow is particularly susceptible to trauma from repeated passive stretching.

Movement is recovered by the patient's own active exercises and by no other means. The patient himself, and his relatives, must be warned that it is not only useless but actually harmful to try to hasten matters by carrying heavy weights with the object of straightening the elbow. Nurses, physiotherapists and others must in no circumstances attempt to straighten it.

Complications are Volkmann's ischaemic contracture, myositis ossificans, and lesions of the ulnar, median, or radial nerves.

Fracture of the head of the radius

This is generally due to a fall on the outstretched hand. Pain in the elbow is aggravated by pronation—supination movements, there is limitation of extension, effusion into the joint, and local tenderness over the head of the radius.

Treatment. Crack fractures without displacement are treated by supporting the arm in a comfortable degree of flexion in a collar-and-cuff. Figure 20.5 shows the classical collar-and-cuff, but many commercially-made variations are now on the market (Figs 20.6A, B and C). Finger, wrist and shoulder exercises are begun at once, and cautious elbow movements in a day or two. Marginal fractures with displacement and comminuted fractures of the whole head are treated by excision of the head of the radius, performed within seven to ten days of injury.

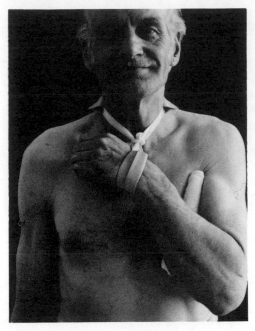

Fig. 20.5 Collar and cuff. The slings round the neck and wrist, are joined by a third piece of bandage.

Fracture of the olecranon

This may be due to direct violence or to muscular violence, when the olecranon is avulsed by the triceps.

Treatment. If there is no displacement, fixation in plaster from the shoulder to the wrist with the elbow in right-angled flexion is generally advised.

In fractures with displacement, operative reduction and suture of the fragment may be performed; tension band wiring with screw fixation is the usual treatment, followed by fixation in full extension until union is firm; a collar-and-cuff is then worn, and active exercises commenced.

An alternative method of treatment which is used in older patients consists of excision of the fragment of the olecranon and suture of the triceps. Immobilisation in a plaster slab is maintained for about three weeks, followed by active exercises.

Displacement of the epiphysis of the external condyle of the humerus

This condition is sustained in childhood. It is treated by manipulative reduction and immobilisation in a posterior plaster slab and collar-and-cuff. Operative reduction may be performed. Failure of

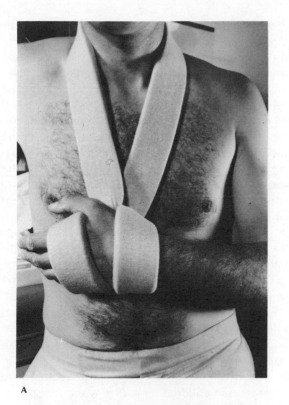

A

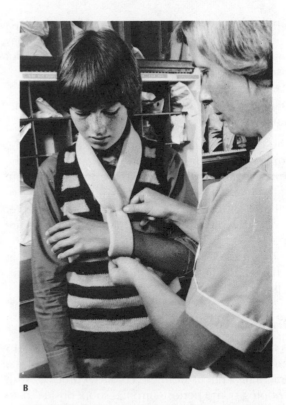

B

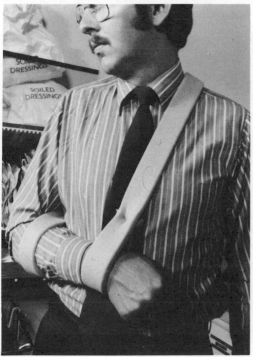

C

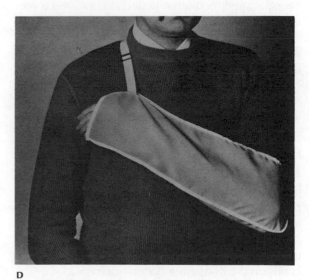

D

Fig. 20.6   A, B. Modern collar and cuff slings. (Seton Products.)
C, D. Arm-slings. (Seton Products and Raymed Division of Thackray).

reduction may cause cubitus valgus. This may be corrected by osteotomy. Ulnar nerve palsy may supervene years later and may necessitate anterior transposition of the nerve (Ch. 22).

Displacement of the internal epicondyle of the humerus

The epicondyle may be torn from its bed by the contraction of the common flexor muscle in the valgus strains of the joint. There may be rupture of the internal lateral ligament with outward dislocation of the elbow, damage to the ulnar nerve, and inclusion of the loose fragment in the joint space.

Treatment. If there is no displacement, rest in a flexed position in a collar-and-cuff is sufficient. Otherwise operative reduction is necessary.

Dislocation of the elbow joint

In dislocation of the elbow joint, the forearm bones are displaced backwards. There is avulsion of the brachialis anticus from the coronoid process, with stripping of the periosteum; the subperiosteal haematoma which is produced may become the seat of ossification if reduction is delayed. There may be associated median or radial paralysis and sometimes, damage to the brachial artery.

Treatment is by manipulative reduction. A plaster slab is applied with the elbow comfortably flexed, and the limb is supported in a collar and cuff. Shoulder and finger exercises are begun at once. Elbow exercises are commenced in three weeks.

Fracture-dislocation of the elbow

This is a serious injury in which dislocation is combined with fracture of one or other of its constituent parts, the olecranon, the head of the radius, or the internal epicondyle.

Treatment consists of reduction of the dislocation. Treatment for individual fractures then proceeds on the lines already described.

FRACTURES OF THE FOREARM

Fractures of the forearm include the following: fracture of one or both bones; fracture of the shaft of the ulna with dislocation of the head of radius (Monteggia fracture), and fracture of the radius with dislocation of the lower end of the ulna (Galeazzi fracture). If there is a fracture of one bone only, angulation and over-riding is prevented by the other; if there is a fracture of one bone only, and its fellow is intact, then over-riding and angulation indicates that there is a dislocation of one of the radio-ulnar joints. The displacement of the fragments depends upon the relationship of site of fracture to the attachments of the pronator and supinator muscles. In fracture of the upper third of the shaft of the radius, the proximal fragment is supinated and the distal pronated. The forearm, wrist and hand is therefore immobilised in full supination so that the lower fragment is in the same axis as the upper one. Fracture of the middle and lower thirds are immobilised with the hand, wrist, and forearm midway between full supination and full pronation. Unless this rule is followed, there will be permanent limitation of supination and pronation movements.

Treatment. Greenstick and crack fractures are often seen in children. Fractures without displacement are immobilised in an unpadded plaster which extends from the upper arm to the metacarpal heads (Fig. 20.7).

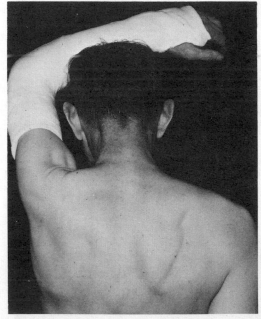

Fig. 20.7 Above-elbow plaster applied for fracture of both bones of forearm. The patient is practising shoulder exercises.

Complete fracture of shaft of radius and ulna

This is treated by manipulative reduction. The patient lies on a table, the elbow is flexed to the right-angle, and counter-traction is applied by passing a calico bandage or piece of ticking over a pad of wool in front of the arm just above the elbow. This is held by an assistant or fastened to a stationary object, such as an upright post. Traction is then applied to the hand, continued until reduction is secured, and maintained whilst a posterior slab is applied. When this has set, the calico sling is cut and the slab is covered by turns of plaster bandage. If angulation is imperfectly corrected, an attempt may be made to obtain further correction by wedging the plaster. A plaster loop may be incorporated in the cast at the level of the fracture; the cast is then suspended by this loop in a collar-and-cuff. Otherwise it is supported in a sling or collar-and-cuff in the ordinary manner.

The plaster must not become loose; fractures of this type are prone to redisplacement; a new plaster is applied as soon as the swelling has subsided, and changed as often as is necessary. It must always include the elbow joint.

Operative reduction may be preferred. A plate and screws are used for internal fixation.

Monteggia fracture

A Monteggia fracture is a fracture of the upper shaft of the ulna with dislocation of the head of the radius.

Treatment. Manipulative reduction may succeed, but open reduction and internal fixation of the ulna is generally necessary. Bone-grafts may later be performed in cases of non-union.

Fracture shaft of radius with inferior radio-ulnar dislocation (Galeazzi)

Fracture of the radial shaft in its middle and lower thirds is usually accompanied by dislocation of the lower end of the ulna. The triangular fibro-cartilage and the tip of the ulnar styloid process is avulsed, and the ligaments of the inferior radio-ulnar joint are torn.

Treatment. Manipulative reduction, with counter-traction by a calico sling and strong traction in the line of the thumb, is followed by plaster fixation from the upper arm to the metacarpal heads. The elbow is flexed to the right-angle, the forearm is held in mid-position and the hand is held in full ulnar deviation. The plaster is closely moulded round the radial side of the wrist. This fracture is prone to redisplacement.

Operative treatment consists of internal fixation with a plate and screws.

Unreduced cases may be treated by excision of the lower end of the ulna.

INJURIES TO THE WRIST AND HAND

Sprain of the wrist

Wrist sprain gives rise to pain, swelling and loss of function of the hand. If this is not quickly relieved by the application of strapping or a cock-up splint, further investigation is required in order to eliminate more serious conditions, for example, a fracture of the navicular.

Colles' fracture of the radius

Colles' fracture is a fracture of the lower end of the radius within 2.5 cm of the wrist-joint. The lower fragment is displaced backwards and tilted to the radial side; there is impaction and, sometimes, comminution of fragments and involvement of the articular surface. Colles' fracture is common in elderly women due to a fall on the outstretched hand. The backward displacement and tilting of the lower fragments gives rise to the typical 'dinner fork' deformity. There is a definite 'step' between the dorsum of the wrist and hand, which is carried to the radial side (Fig. 20.8).

Treatment. This is by manipulative reduction. The fragments are disimpacted by strong traction applied to the fingers and thumb, and the displacement is corrected by direct pressure over the fragments. An unpadded plaster is then applied, extending from the metacarpal heads to just below the elbow, and closely moulded over the radial side of the first metacarpal to the base of the thenar eminence. As the plaster sets, it is moulded by the surgeon so that the carpus and the lower fragment of the radius are pushed inwards and forwards. A thin strip of bandage is taken across the palm of the hand. It must extend over the horizontal creases, and *must not prevent full flexion of the metacarpo-phalangeal joints* (Fig. 6.4).

Finger, elbow and shoulder exercises are commenced *at once*. Delay may result in permanent joint stiffness. A sling such as that shown in Fig. 20.6D is allowed for the first day or two, until swelling has subsided, but it is removed at frequent intervals for shoulder exercises. The hand must not be tucked inside the coat. If swelling is very severe, the patient may remain recumbent with the limb elevated on pillows so that the fingers point towards the ceiling. It may even be necessary to split the plaster down to the skin from the palm to the elbow.

Finger exercises. The more swollen the fingers, the greater the need for finger exercises: no excuse is accepted for their non-performance. The thumb must also be exercised and must be kept out of the way during finger exercises.

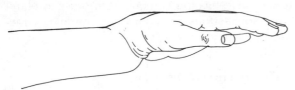

Fig. 20.8 'Dinner fork', deformity in Colles' fracture of the radius.

1. The fingers are fully extended and spread into abduction.
2. The fingers are flexed by touching the palm with the finger-tips.
3. The metacarpo-phalangeal joints are flexed by attempting to touch the front of the wrist.
4. The patient attempts to approximate the tip of the thumb to each finger in turn.

Shoulder exercises. These are especially important in elderly patients; the shoulder is often jarred at the moment of injury and unless movements are begun at once and practised assiduously a 'frozen shoulder' may result.

1. The arm is abducted so that the plaster touches the side of the head.
2. It is externally rotated so that the hand is behind the neck.
3. It is internally rotated and placed behind the back so that the fingers point to the mid-scapular region. As soon as the sling is discarded, the hand is used for all ordinary duties, short of wetting the plaster.

The plaster is retained for about five weeks or until union is sound. A crêpe bandage or other supporting bandage is occasionally ordered for a week or two to control swelling, and wrist exercises and full functional use is commenced.

Fracture of the radial styloid process may be due to a back-fire or to a fall on the outstretched hand.

Treatment is similar to that of a Colles' fracture.

Rupture of the tendon of the extensor longus pollicis

Rupture of this tendon may occur in injuries to the wrist joint. It is subjected to friction as it passes over the radial styloid process and becomes so frayed that it ruptures, sometimes weeks after the original injury.

Treatment consists of a transplantation of the distal end of the tendon into another tendon of the thumb.

Displacement of the lower radial epiphysis

This is an injury of childhood, as a result of a fall on the outstretched hand. The lower radial epiphysis is displaced backwards, or, backwards and outwards. Crushing of the epiphysis may cause premature fusion.

Treatment consists of manipulative reduction and plaster fixation as for Colles' fracture.

Fracture of the carpal navicular (scaphoid)

Fracture of the navicular may be due to a fall on the outstretched hand or to some other injury. Movements of the wrist are limited and painful, there is swelling of the hand, and tenderness on pressure in the anatomical snuff-box. In starting-handle injuries there may be marked swelling as shown in Fig. 20.9. X-rays are taken in three planes, antero-posterior, lateral and oblique. The last-named is often the only one to reveal the fracture. Many cases are diagnosed and treated on clinical grounds alone, as the fracture may not be obvious in X-ray films until two or three weeks after the original injury.

Treatment. Treatment consists of immobilisation in an unpadded plaster cast. The plaster must extend from just below the elbow to the metacarpal heads; it must include the first metacarpal and the thenar eminence, and is closely moulded into the palm as far as the transverse creases. The wrist is

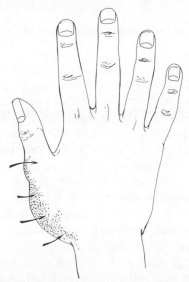

Fig. 20.9 Fractures of the scaphoid. Painful lateral aspect of the wrist following starting-handle injuries. There may be marked swelling as illustrated.

held at 30 degrees dorsiflexion (Fig. 20.10). Finger and shoulder exercises are commenced at once; *the plaster is renewed at once should it become loose, cracked, or damaged in any way.* As the

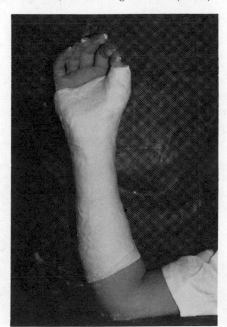

Fig. 20.10 Plaster cast for fracture of the carpal scaphoid.

period of immobilisation is sometimes prolonged, the patient is generally advised to return to light work.

Operative treatment. In fractures of the wrist and proximal pole of the navicular, the blood supply to one fragment is cut off, and aseptic necrosis supervenes. These cases may be treated by excision of the dead fragment. Otherwise treatment may be by drilling or by bone-grafting. In cases in which arthritis of the wrist has developed, arthrodesis may be advised.

Dislocation of the lunate

This may be due to a fall on the dorsiflexed hand. The flexor tendons are compressed by the dislocated bone, the fingers are stiff in semi-flexion, and the wrist is stiff, swollen and painful; there is commonly a median palsy (Chap. 17).

Treatment consists of manipulative reduction and plaster fixation with the wrist in dorsiflexion; the degree of dorsiflexion is later reduced. If this fails, reduction by skeletal traction, or operative excision of the bone may be advised.

INJURIES OF THE FINGERS AND THUMB

The function of the fingers and thumb is of such vital importance that no injury to the hand should be regarded as trivial. Injured fingers are immobilised in the position of flexion; uninjured fingers are left free and actively exercised from the moment of injury; passive stretching of the fingers either by the patient or his friends is strictly forbidden.

Sprains of the finger or thumb

These are treated by the application of strapping for a week or two. Active use is encouraged, but passive stretching is not allowed.

Rupture of ligaments

Rupture of the ligaments of the finger or thumb is treated by plaster fixation for about three weeks. Operative treatment may be necessary. The rate of recovery in ligamentous injuries is often very slow.

Dislocation of the metacarpo-phalangeal joints of the finger or thumb

This is treated by manipulative reduction and plaster fixation in a moderate degree of flexion for about three weeks. Open reduction is sometimes necessary.

Bennett's fracture-dislocation of the thumb

This injury is usually due to a fall or to a blow on the radial side of the hand which forces the thumb across the palm. The fracture involves the carpometacarpal joint; the metacarpal slides down the saddle-shaped trapezium and reduction is difficult to maintain.

Treatment. The fracture-dislocation is reduced by manual traction on the thumb; an unpadded plaster is applied from just below the elbow to the knuckles, including the thumb metacarpal and thenar eminence, and holding the thumb in full opposition to the fingers. The fingers, elbow and shoulder are exercised throughout.

Fracture-dislocations of the finger are treated on the same lines as described for fracture-dislocations of the thumb.

Fracture of the shaft of the metacarpal

Spiral fractures of the metacarpals may be due to a fall on the hand. Displacement is not gross and treatment is by plaster fixation for about four weeks in a posterior plaster slab or complete plaster.

Transverse fractures of the shaft are usually due to a direct injury and generally occur in the first or fifth metacarpal. Over-riding of the fragments is corrected by manipulation. If this fails, open reduction and internal fixation by a bone-peg may be performed.

Fracture of the neck of the metacarpal

This is generally due to direct violence. There is tilting of the metacarpal head towards the palm, and backward angulation at the fracture site.

Treatment is by manipulative reduction. A small strip of thin felt is placed over the finger and a plaster-slab is applied with the metacarpo-phalangeal and interphalangeal joints flexed to a right-angle. The slab is reinforced over the dorsum of the hand and strapped in position. Exercises for all other fingers are commenced at once, and immobilisation is continued for about three weeks.

Fractures of the proximal phalanges of the fingers.

These fractures are generally due to direct injury or to a fall with the finger flexed beneath the body. The majority of fractures are found in the proximal part of the first phalanx, and angulation is produced by the pull of the lumbricals and interrossei, which flex the proximal phalanx and extend the distal. The distal fragment is brought into alignment with the proximal by flexion of the finger.

Treatment is by manipulative reduction and plaster fixation with the metacarpo-phalangeal joint flexed 45 degrees and the proximal interphalangeal joint flexed 90 degrees. A plaster slab is applied to the dorsal surface of the finger and must extend to the elbow. As the finger is flexed, it must lie in its normal relationship to the palm of the hand. Only in the middle finger is the angle of flexion parallel with the long axis of the limb. The index, fourth and fifth fingers converge together in flexion to point towards the navicular, so that they are immobilised in this position. Exercises to the unaffected fingers are practised throughout the period of fixation, which is generally three weeks.

Mallet finger

This condition is due to an avulsion of the extensor tendon from its attachment into the base of the terminal phalanx. It is usually due to forcible flexion of the finger while the tendon is actively contracting, as when the finger is stubbed against an object.

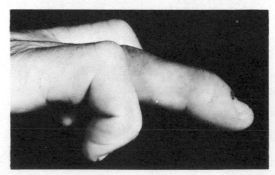

Fig. 20.11 Mallet finger with fracture of the terminal phalanx.

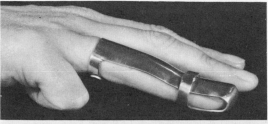

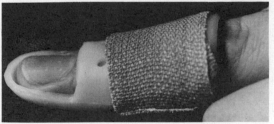

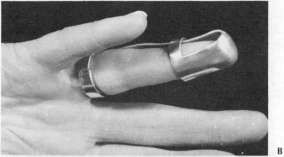

Fig. 20.12 **A, B.** Aluminium splint applied for mallet finger. **C.** Stack type of mallet finger splint (Watson-Jones).

the terminal interphalangeal joint with hyperextension of the distal–the terminal interphalangeal joint cannot be fully extended and the distal interphalangeal joint cannot be fully flexed (Fig. 20.11).

Treatment consists of the application of a splint or a plaster cast holding the terminal interphalangeal joint in hyperextension and the proximal interphalangeal joint in flexion.

Aluminium mallet finger splints of various sizes are kept in stock; the splint is easy to apply and is a convenient method of fixation for housewives since unlike a plaster cast it is not rendered ineffective if it is inadvertently wetted. Figures 20.12A and B show the splint applied. Figure 20.9C shows the stack type of mallet finger splint.

Method of application of plaster cast. A Gypsona bandage is cut to make a little slab six or seven layers thick. Before soaking, it is tried on the finger so as to ensure an accurate fit. It must be long enough to extend from the base of the first phalanx to the tip of the third, and wide enough to extend up the sides of the finger. It is then soaked and applied, the finger being held in the corrected position until it has firmly set. The terminal interphalangeal joint is held in hyperextension between the thumb and finger of one hand while the distal interphalangeal is flexed almost to the right angle by the pressure of the fingers of the other hand (Fig. 20.13). The pressure is not released until the plaster has set firmly. Alternatively, the patient is instructed to press the tip of the injured finger against the tip of the thumb or against the table and hold it in the desired position while the plaster is applied.

The power of active extension of the terminal joint of the finger is lost, though passive extension is normal. Unopposed pull of the long flexor tendon produces the typical 'mallet' deformity–flexion of

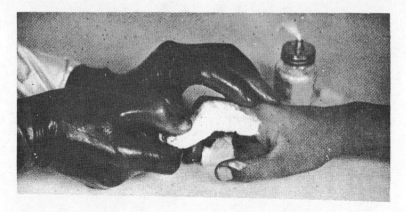

Fig. 20.13 Application of plaster cast for mallet finger. The pressure on the finger is not released until the plaster has set firmly. (Watson-Jones.)

The plaster is worn for six or eight weeks or until recovery takes place.

Operative repair is sometimes required.

Sudeck's atrophy

Sudeck's post-traumatic acute bone atrophy may follow injuries to the wrist, fingers or hand; it is rarely seen in the foot. It is thought to be of nervous origin, but the changes which occur in the limb are typical of those which are due to neglect of exercise during immobilisation. There is persistent pain and loss of function of the limb, and the fingers are stiff, swollen and shiny. X-rays show extreme decalcification of the bones.

Treatment. Pain and swelling of the fingers which persists within a few days of injury must be reported to the surgeon at once, particularly if the overlying skin is shiny. The patient is kept recumbent with the limb elevated, and active exercises at hourly intervals are insisted upon. It may be necessary to change the plaster.

BIBLIOGRAPHY

Adams J C 1978 Outline of Fractures. 7th edn. Edinburgh and London: Churchill Livingstone

Barron J N 1973 Hand Injuries and their treatment. London: Nursing Mirror, 27 April, 37

Charnley J 1970 The closed treatment of common fractures. 3rd edn. Edinburgh: Churchill Livingstone

Chhabra S L 1978 Injuries to the elbow. Nursing Times, 7 September, 1252

Fryer J A 1976 Crush injury to the arm. Nursing Times, 21 October, Theatre nursing supplement 11

Hogan K M, Sawyer J R 1976 Fracture dislocation of the elbow. American Journal of Nursing 76: 1266

Huckstep R L 1978 A simple guide to trauma. 2nd edn. Edinburgh and London: Churchill Livingstone

McRae R 1981 Practical Fracture Treatment. Edinburgh: Churchill Livingstone

Parkinson M 1984 Repair of a comminuted fracture. Nursing Mirror, 18 April

Pearson J R, Austin R T 1973 Accident Surgery and Orthopaedics. London: Lloyd-Luke

Skene K H 1972 Fractures of the shaft of the humerus. Nursing Mirror, 30 June, 26

Smith F M 1972 Surgery of the elbow. 2nd edn. Philadelphia: Saunders

Smith C 1974 Colles' fracture. London: Nursing Mirror, 26 September, 139, 76

Watson M 1978 Hand injuries—1. Primary care. Nursing Times, 16 February, 276

Watson M 1978 Hand injuries—2 amputations. Nursing Times, 23 February, 321

Watson M Hand injuries—3 Principles of the management of complicated injuries. Nursing Times, 2 March, 360

Weeks P M, Wray R C 1978 Management of acute hand injuries: a biological approach. 2nd edn. Saint Louis: Mosby

Wilson J N (ed.) 1976 Watson Jones. Fractures and joint injuries. 5th edn. Edinburgh: Churchill Livingstone

Wilson D 1980. Extending a helping hand. London. Nursing Mirror, 13 November

Winchester I W 1960 The painful stiff shoulder. Nursing Times, 4 March, 281

Wynn, Parry C B 1973 Rehabilitation of the hand. 3rd edn. London: Butterworth

21

Injuries of the lower limb

TRAUMATIC DISLOCATION OF THE HIP JOINT

This injury is usually the result of a powerful thrust applied in the long axis of the thigh, so that the head of the femur is forced out of the acetabulum. It is often referred to as 'the dashboard dislocation', because it occurs in head-on motor collisions, when the knee is forcibly struck by the dashboard. It may be accompanied by a fracture of the margin of the acetabulum. The femoral head may be displaced either behind or in front of the acetabulum. In a more rare type of dislocation, the head of the femur is forced through the floor of the acetabulum.

Clinical features. Traumatic dislocation of the hip joint is a severe injury accompanied by a great deal of shock. There is severe pain and limitation of all hip movements. Posterior dislocation of the femoral head produces internal rotation and adduction deformity with shortening of the limb. Anterior dislocations produce external rotation and abduction deformity, usually with some lengthening of the limb (Fig. 21.1).

It is sometimes accompanied by sciatic nerve palsy (Ch. 22).

Treatment. Manipulative reduction is performed while the patient lies on blankets placed on the floor, and the pelvis is steadied by an assistant. The patient is then lifted on to a hip-prop or orthopaedic table and a plaster spica is applied with the hip in neutral rotation and the knee slightly flexed. Foot exercises and quadriceps drill are commenced as soon as the plaster is dry; immobilisa-

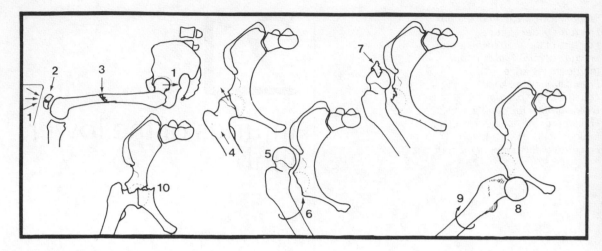

Fig. 21.1 *Traumatic dislocation of the hip:* The hip may dislocate as a result of force being transmitted up the femoral shaft. This most commonly occurs as a result of dashboard impact in road traffic accidents (1). Note that this mechanism may be responsible for simultaneous fracture of the patella (2) or of the femoral shaft (3). Force transmitted up the limbs from falls on the foot, force applied to the lumbar region (e.g. in roof falls on kneeling miners) and rarely force applied directly to the trochanter may also cause the hip to dislocate. If the leg is flexed at the hip and adducted (4) at the time of impact, the femur dislocates posteriorly (5) internally rotating at the same time (6). In some cases, the posterior lip of the acetabulum is fractured (7). If the hip is widely abducted, anterior dislocation may occur—even without any axial transmission of force (8). The femur externally rotates (9). Note that if the femur is on some other part of the abduction/adduction range, that these mechanisms may be responsible for central dislocation type fractures of the pelvis (10). This illustration with caption is taken from *Practical Fracture Treatment* by Ronald McRae, by kind permission of the author and publisher, Churchill Livingstone.

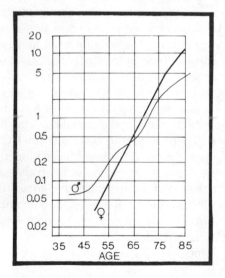

Fig. 21.2 *Incidence:* The Y-axis of the graph represents the yearly incidence per 1000 population and shows that below the age of 60 the fracture occurs most frequently in men, generally from industrial trauma. The incidence increases with age and in later life is three times commoner in women, where hormonal dependent osteoporosis and a degree of osteomalacia are contributory factors. The fracture is seen from time to time in children. This illustration with caption is taken from *Practical Fracture Treatment* by Ronald McRae, by kind permission of author and publisher.

tion is continued for about three months. *Surgery is sometimes required.*

Complications include myositis ossificans and avascular necrosis of the femoral head.

FRACTURES OF THE FEMUR

FRACTURES OF THE UPPER FEMUR

This is a common injury in elderly women and is generally due to a trivial accident such as tripping over a doormat (see Fig. 21.2). The patient complains of pain in the hip, there is a varying degree of external rotation deformity and shortening of the limb. In very old and feeble individuals, the shock produced by the fracture may be sufficient to cause death within a few days. In addition, aged patients are very prone to complications which attend prolonged bed-rest, notably hypostatic pneumonia, pressure sores, uraemia, stiffness of the joints, and mental derangement.

Fracture of the upper femur is divided into two main types:

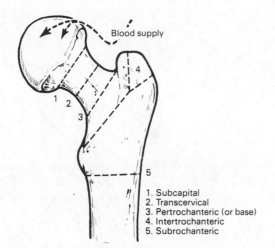

Fig. 21.3 Classification of the levels of fractures of the femoral head. Displaced subcapital fractures or transcervical fractures may rupture the artery and cause avascular necrosis of the femoral head.

1. Subcapital (intracapsular)

This is when the fracture occurs at the junction of the femoral head and neck. In impacted fractures, displacement is slight and union takes place rapidly, but if there is upward displacement of the neck and shaft, interference with the blood supply to the femoral head may result in non-union or even aseptic necrosis (Fig. 21.3).

Treatment. Early operative treatment is recommended, to relieve pain and to allow early mobilisation and so avoidance of the complications of prolonged rest in bed.

Because of the risk of non-union due to unstable reduction, inadequate fixation or avascular necrosis of the femoral head, an operation to replace the femoral head with an Austin Moore or Thompson prosthesis is often performed. The prosthesis itself may cause complications in as much as it may become infected, become dislocated or fail mechanically, nevertheless this form of surgical intervention is commonly used for this type of fracture with better results than the introduction of a Smith Peterson nail. Arthroplasty (Girdlestone) or osteotomy (McMurray) is sometimes advised in extreme circumstances (Ch. 27).

2. Trochanteric (extracapsular)

These fractures occur below the origin of the blood vessels which supply the femoral head; the circulation is maintained and the union is usually uncomplicated.

Treatment usually consists of reduction and fixation by means of a nail-plate. A Smith Peterson nail used without a plate has a tendency to slip out of place and may result in re-displacement of the fracture. Moore's pins may be inserted if the fracture is impacted (these are small pins which hold the fracture quite firmly).

Enders nails (Fig. 21.4C) are long flexible intramedullary pins and have the advantage of being easy to insert; they are therefore favoured in elderly patients, those with an adverse medical history who will require short anaesthetics, or those with multiple injuries. Due to the distance between the insertion site of the pins above the medial condyle and the actual fracture site the danger of infection is practically non-existent.

The patient can bear weight on the limb immediately and this is a great advantage because the complications of prolonged rest in bed are avoided.

Splintage may be ordered prior to operation and various regimes may be adopted operatively as listed below.

a. *Rest in bed* with the limb immobilised between sand-bags.
b. *Simple traction* by means of skin extensions attached to a weight and running over a pulley fixed to the elevated foot-end of the bed.
c. *The patient may wear a slipper nailed to a transverse piece of wood*, or a plaster shell with rotation bar (Figs 21.5 and 21.6); this is to prevent rotation of the limb.
d. *Hamilton Russell traction* (Fig. 21.7A–F). This is a means of immobilising the limb by balanced traction. Traction is applied to the limb both longitudinally and in an upwards direction. Horizontal traction is obtained by skin extensions applied in the usual way (Ch. 10). Commercial extension-packs are generally used. Upward traction is exerted by means of a sling placed under the knee. From the sling, a cord is carried round four pulleys, arranged on a Balkan beam shown in Figs 21.7A–F. The cord runs over a pulley attached to a spreader at the end of the exten-

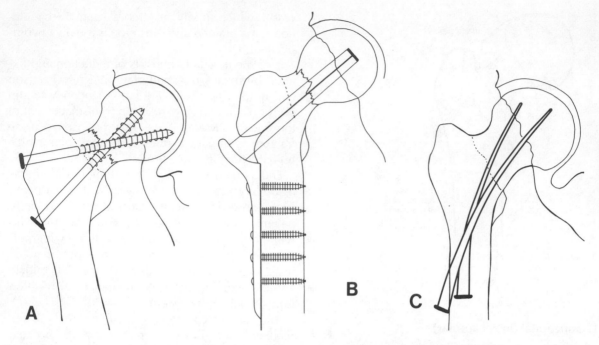

Fig. 21.4 **A.** Crossed Garden screws. Direction of stress forces to resist movements in all planes. **B.** McLaughlin pin and plate. **C.** Enders nails.

sions and carries a weight of about 4.5 kg. The foot of the bed is then elevated to provide counter-traction. A supporting pillow beneath the limb may be ordered, but this must not press on the calf for fear of venous thrombosis.

N.B. The degree of *abduction* ordered must be maintained continuously.

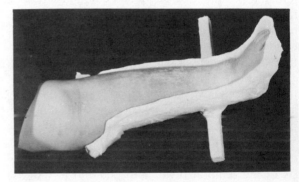

Fig. 21.6 Plaster shell with bar to control rotation.

Nursing care. General care is discussed later. It is essential that the patient does not slip down the bed or the angle of traction is altered. External rotation of the limb must be prevented. The sling under the knee must not become crumpled, or pressure-sores will result. Foot exercises are practised regularly.

The Patrick splint (Fig. 21.8A and B)

An alternative method of treatment is application of a functional brace.

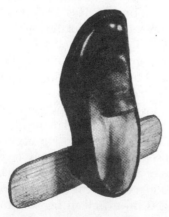

Fig. 21.5 Slipper with wooden cross-bar to prevent external rotation of limb after nailing operation. (Watson-Jones.)

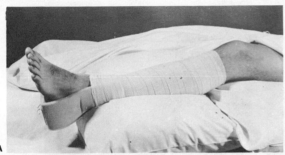
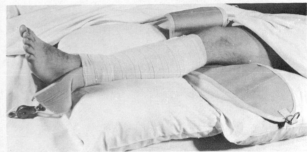
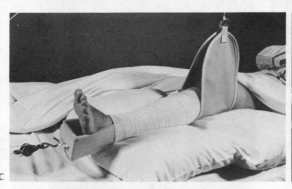
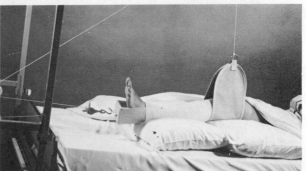
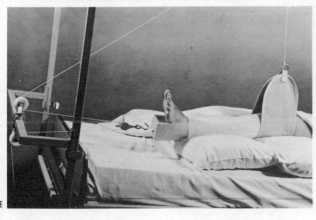
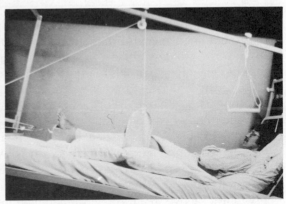

Fig. 21.7   A–F. Hamilton Russell traction. Note the trapeze—an essential part of the apparatus. (Illustration by courtesy of Seton Products.)

This is a lightweight hip spica made of nylon fabric with a supporting beam of nylon rods on the lateral side. It can be adapted to each patient's individual shape or girth by adjusting the lacings and gussets; it is worn only during the day, light traction is applied at night.

It is easily washable and provides the patient with mobility and prevents the complications of prolonged bed rest.

GENERAL NURSING CARE

It should be noted here that contemporary writing on the nursing care of the elderly also applies to these patients (see Bibliography, Chs 1, 2, 3, 5 as well as Ch. 21).

Elderly patients with fracture of the neck of the femur often present a nursing challenge because of their age and because prolonged and continuous

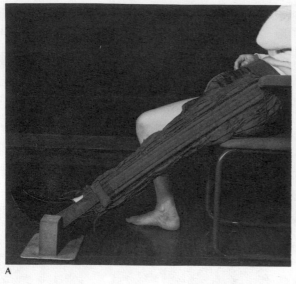

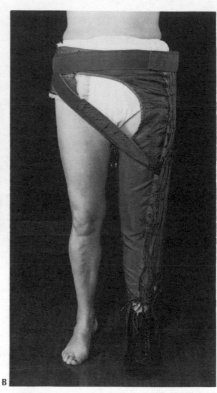

Fig. 21.8 The Patrick splint.

rest in bed exposes the patient to the complications already mentioned, namely hypostatic pneumonia, pressure-sores, stiffness of the joints, uraemia and mental derangement. For this reason the surgeon will frequently order us to get the patient out of bed as soon as possible; indeed, the burning question is often not whether the patient can safely be got up but whether she can safely be left in bed. Moreover, for economic reasons alone, an early discharge from hospital is to be encouraged. It is important to remember that old age in itself is not a deterrent to active treatment and rehabilitation, which is aimed at restoring the patient to her own home and to her place in society. This is not always as easy as it sounds, and requires teamwork of the highest order, not only from the medical staff, the nurse, the physiotherapist, the occupational therapist, the medico-social and other hospital workers, but from the patient's family, the general practitioner and the community health and welfare services. *It must also be remembered that treatment of co-existing disease may be required, and that this may be as important as the local lesion.* Indeed, the elderly patient may already be the victim of

what has been described as the 'giants of geriatrics'—Immobility, instability, incontinence and intellectual impairment (Isaacs, 1976), or the accident which results in a fracture of the upper end of the femur may provide the pathway for the arrival of these giants whose presence compounds the problem of treatment, nursing care and subsequent rehabilitation. The recovery of patients who have sustained fractures of the femoral neck depends on the type of fracture and the patient's physique, general health and social circumstances. It has been noted that patients with caring relatives often recover where the neglected do not (House, 1978).

Members of the family are brought into the picture at an early date; some are quite willing to shift the responsibility of caring for an elderly relative on to the hospital staff, but such people are happily in the minority and it must be remembered that they may have other difficulties and often need advice and help but do not know where to seek it.

The medical social worker holds a key position in the team; it is her job to investigate the social and financial position of the patient and mobilise the forces which exist outside the hospital to help the patient and her family; for example, she may instigate re-housing, or alterations to existing housing, or the provision of home-help. Although strictly speaking the social aspects of the patient's treatment are the province of the medico-social worker, we who have the responsibility of rehabilitating the patient must always be aware of them; all too often, we meet aged patients who are virtually alone in the world and for this reason alone demand our sympathy and care.

On admission

The patient is examined by the surgeon, and the general condition assessed. Operative treatment may be carried out at once or in the course of the next few days. The general condition may be poor at the outset and there may be serious co-existing disease or malnutrition, found all too often in elderly men and women living alone; on the other hand, obesity is not uncommon, and alcoholism is sometimes seen. Dehydration and anaemia may require immediate administration of fluids or of whole blood by the intravenous route, particularly if early operation is contemplated.

Immediate nursing care

Whatever form of splintage is ordered for the affected limb, the patient is usually nursed semi-recumbent, with plenty of pillows and a back-rest. A pulley or 'monkey-pole' (Fig. 21.7F) is fixed to the bed and the patient encouraged from the first to lift herself by grasping the trapeze and flexing the knee on the sound side. It is important that the sound foot is supported at rest by a footboard, or sandbag; this not only prevents foot-drop but prevents the patient from slipping down the bed and exerting shearing-strain on the skin of the sacrum with resultant pressure sores; a cradle is required to support the weight of the bedclothes. At first, the patient may require *intensive and total nursing care* but it must be emphasised that *at the earliest possible moment*, she is encouraged and helped to do things for herself. Only in this way can she finally progress to independence, although it requires imagination and endless patience and expenditure of time and trouble on the part of the nurse. For example it is often easier to wash an aged patient than to help her own fumbling attempts; similarly it is tempting to feed her because her own slow, messy and wasteful attempts tend to interrupt ward routine.

Prevention of hypostatic pneumonia

Posture in bed, movement in bed and early ambulation will be discussed in connection with the prevention of pressure sores and joint stiffness, and these measures are also vital in the prevention of hypostatic pneumonia; *breathing exercises* are given by a physiotherapist, but the nurse must supervise them in her absence; coughing is encouraged and a sputum cup kept always at hand. Signs of chest complications are reported to the surgeon immediately and *chemotherapy* may be ordered. (Ch. 5).

Prevention of pressure sores

In this connection, treatment of *the general condition* is of paramount importance; the patient who is emaciated, dehydrated, anaemic or incontinent of urine and faeces, is heavily at risk (Ch. 5). The patient's position in bed must be altered every two hours, *both by day and by night*. This is the only means by which continuous pressure on one part is prevented; the sacrum, the heels and elbows are inspected at the same time and any flushing of the skin reported to the Ward Sister. It is worth mentioning here that shearing-strain and pressure on the skin of the sacrum during operation often contributes to sores. Moreover, pressure sores may be started by investigations or by surgery, as reported by Dyson (1978) who describes prolonged pressure on a patient's sacral area from an image-intensifier table and further points out that doctors may be unaware of this hazard.

Other studies have shown that an operating table can exert sacral pressure equal to that exerted by lying on a lino-covered floor (Redfern et al, 1973).

The skin is kept immaculately clean and the drawsheet kept taut, smooth and dry at all times. Incontinence of urine and faeces is a potent factor in the formation of pressure sores and will be discussed later; the application of barrier creams or sprays may be useful in these cases. Spirit must not be used and it may be necessary to support the patient on pillows or sorbo-rubber pads in the same manner as that described for a paraplegic patient (Ch. 23), especially in the treatment of established sores. Other aids to nursing are incontinence pads, ripple-beds, sheepskins or water-pillows, and vigilance in preventing the occurrence of pressure sores is required not only while the patient is confined to bed but when she sits in a chair.

Prevention of joint stiffness, contractures and venous stagnation

Turning and change of position in bed has already been referred to; strict attention must be paid to the posture of the patient in bed and later, in a chair. The head is not allowed to poke forward and the spine is comfortably supported by pillows, and the feet by a footboard or by sand-bags as already described.

Active exercises, which may be assisted at first are introduced as soon as possible. Though formal exercises are the prerogative of the physiotherapist, it is the nurse's responsibility to encourage active movement of all joints. *Occupational therapy* is valuable and activities such as writing and knitting (even if only dishcloths) are important, not only for the hands but for the mind.

Incontinence of urine and faeces

Copious fluids are given from the first. The urine must be tested at regular intervals and a fluid intake and output chart commenced at once. Urinary infection is treated by the administration of antibiotics and every effort is made to discover the cause of urinary incontinence. *Wet beds are charted* and reported and in some cases *catheterisation* is necessary in the early stages until control of the bladder is re-established; a fall in urinary output is reported to the surgeon immediately. Bedpans (or, in suitable cases, a urinal) are offered at regular intervals, but *as soon as possible* the patient is helped out of bed on to a commode, or better still, is wheeled to the lavatory on a sani-chair; urinary incontinence often disappears once the patient is up and dressed. Incontinence of faeces is sometimes due to behaviour disorders but it can mean

that in fact there is faecal impaction. As in urinary incontinence, the *cause* should be sought; in patients who have been in bed for some days, faecal impaction readily occurs and a rounded mass of faeces may act as a 'ball-valve' at the anus and prevent the passage of the stool, even though dribbling incontinence is present. *Digital examination* by the insertion of a gloved finger into the rectum will often reveal the cause; olive oil enemata or Dulcolax suppositories are valuable aids, and as in urinary incontinence, access to a bedside commode or a lavatory often solves the problem. It should be remembered that aged patients should not be left on bedpans for long periods; damage to the skin of the sacrum is then inevitable; on the other hand, they must not be hurried; further reference to the care of the bladder and bowel will be made later in connection with restlessness, insomnia and mental confusion.

Nutrition and fluid balance

Nutrition is of vital importance, especially where the nutritional state is already poor, and where starvation of the patient is necessary for surgery to be performed. It has been shown that these patients soon develop negative nitrogen balance and that a diet adequate in protein and calories is essential for their recovery. Unfortunately, the appetite of a feeble old person may not be able to cope with the considerable quantities needed (House, 1978).

Severe malnutrition and dehydration may require naso-gastric feeding or intravenous therapy. *Anorexia* is common, and high-protein foods such as Complan may be ordered for patients unable or unwilling to take solid food, especially in the early stages of treatment. As soon as possible, however, a full mixed diet is offered and again, imagination is needed in placing food before the patient and unremitting vigilance and perseverance in seeing that she eats it. It is important to remember that a feeble old person may have difficulty in coping with certain dishes, such as kippers or boiled eggs, and she may be quite unable to reach a cup of tea placed on her locker. The midday dinner should be cut up, if necessary, at the bedside and large diet cloths or table napkins are required to protect the nightgown and bedclothes. As in all other activities, *getting up* to sit at a table, preferably in the company of others, often shows a marked improvement in the appetite and in the table manners. Sometimes the teeth require attention, or the patient may have soiled, ill-fitting dentures, or no dentures at all; in these circumstances, a dental surgeon is called in. Extra *vitamins* are often ordered for those suffering from obvious nutritional deficiency; in some cases, vitamins may be given by injection in the form of Parentrovite.

Mental changes

These patients are often confused and even noisy on admission, because of shock, pain and fear of the unknown world of 'hospital'. Mental confusion usually improves when these factors are overcome, and it is no excuse for treating the patient in a patronising or over-playful manner; we shall all be old one day and respect for the mind and the personality is something we all demand and must therefore accord to those in our care, however undeserving we may consider them to be; moreover, we would all like to die in harness, in our own homes, so that the patients who are denied this privilege deserve our special consideration.

It is important to discover if the patient has brought with her aids which she uses at home, such as spectacles or a hearing-aid. Deprivation of aids on which the patient is dependent exacerbates mental confusion, and they may well be overlooked when the patient is brought to hospital. Sometimes patients are admitted without so much as a handkerchief and if relatives are not available, the medico-social worker (or substitute) will visit the patient's home to collect articles on her behalf. It is also important to discover whether the patient suffers anxiety regarding, perhaps, a relative left at home, or even a household pet, such as a dog, cat or cage-bird.

Sometimes mental confusion is due to metabolic changes, or to organic disease of the brain, heart or lungs, causing cerebral anoxia; or it may be due to the effect of drugs, e.g. barbiturates or sulphonamides, or to post-operative drugs such as Omnopon.

Sedation

Sedation is given with caution and is carefully chosen for the individual patient. Analgesia may be advised for *pain*, but before giving sedation at night, for example, to the noisy restless patient who is disturbing others in the ward, no stone must be left unturned to discover the cause. Ask yourself, is your patient in pain, agitated, cold, or overheated? Is there a draught round her bed? Is her bed clean, smooth, dry and unwrinkled? Is she hungry or thirsty? Has she a full bladder, a loaded rectum or abdominal distension? An empty bladder and rectum, a hot drink, a warm, smooth, dry, comfortable bed and 'tucking-up' with a few comforting words are firm foundations for a peaceful night. Aged patients on the whole do not tolerate sedatives well, particularly barbiturates, because these may produce a 'hang-over' and drowsiness next day so that when night comes again the patient is simply not ready for sleep. *Activity* during the day must be encouraged and if sedation must be given it is normally in the form of chloral hydrate or Temezepam 10–20 mg. In extreme cases an injection of paraldehyde may be ordered. *Alcohol* is a valuable sedative and 30–45 ml of whisky or brandy with a hot drink is often the answer to the problem. In this connection, Whitley and Smith report an investigation into the night sedation (hypnotics) given to elderly clients in a Part 4 Home, and state that a high-protein sandwich given with a hot drink at 9 pm not only replaced sedation but those clients able to get out of bed to use a commode during the night did so far more easily under the new regime.

Aged patients, and particularly those who are restless require *protection from injury*; hot-water bottles must be well-covered and must not touch the patient. Cot-sides are not used unless absolutely essential; they are often bitterly resented and can exacerbate nervous agitation. When the patient gets up, beware of uncovered radiators and hot-water pipes, and wet or highly polished floors must be forbidden. Care is taken to see that the bath-water or shower is not too hot and a hand-rail near the lavatory seat is essential.

Later treatment

Getting up

This does not mean sitting all day long in a chair wearing a dressing-gown and slippers; it is as bad for the patient as lying in bed, though far less comfortable. As soon as possible, the patient is dressed in her own clothes and shoes and will gradually learn to don these herself. Often *the feet* need special attention, for example, corns or ingrowing toenails may call for the services of a chiropodist. At this stage, the services of the hospital hairdresser will help the patient to take an interest in her appearance and the hospital librarian will offer books and magazines. Again, be sure that aids such as spectacles, if worn, are always within reach. The visiting trolley-shop or Red Cross Shopping Service will supply small needs, and the occupational therapist will intensify her efforts to interest the patient in some art or craft. The patient must not be shut away in a day-room and members of the ward team will never pass her bed or chair without a cheerful word; sometimes the use of a wheelchair is indicated and the patient learns to use it, even to go outdoors. Usually, her first walk is taken with the physiotherapist who will also teach her to negotiate steps and how to use elbow crutches, sticks or other aids to walking. But it is the nurse who takes her on her first walk to the bathroom and lavatory and patiently supervises her activities there until she can manage her own toilet. At this stage too, little tasks may be given since old people like to feel that they are of use; for example, a patient may help another with drinks or a meal, or help in small ways with the ward routine. Activities in the 'daily living unit' of the occupational therapy department are also helpful at this stage. Finally, little walks outdoors in suitable weather are introduced and the patient may be allowed home for a weekend so that her ability to cope with life outside the hospital can be assessed.

Re-settlement

Meantime, the medico-social worker will be working to prepare the home, the family and the community services for her reception. Re-housing has already been mentioned and adaptation of existing housing to meet an old person's needs; for example, if she cannot negotiate stairs, a downstairs lavatory may be required. Thorough investigation of home conditions is necessary before discharge because although the patient who lives alone may insist that she can manage at home, this is often

found to be impracticable, for example, she may be unable to do her own shopping or housecleaning. In this case, the medico-social worker may call on the WVS meals-on-wheels service, or contact the community health authority who will provide a home-help. Other services which may be required are those of the community nurse, the health visitor or the welfare officer; sometimes financial help is imperative (Skeet, 1970). In some hospitals a Health Visitor/Sister liaison is well established, so that the Health Visitor meets the patient in hospital and discusses any problems about her discharge with the ward Sister. Patients who are unable to return to their own homes and have no friend or relative to care for them, may require some form of sheltered housing. Attendance at a Day Centre may be recommended.

Physiotherapy for the elderly orthopaedic patient

The elderly patient rarely presents with a single orthopaedic condition; medical problems are invariably present as well. The gradual process of ageing brings differing disabilities which must be considered—blindness, deafness, urinary and faecal incontinence, contractures, arthritic changes in various joints, diabetes, osteoporosis, to name but a few. When the patient is admitted to hospital, teamwork is essential for the exchange of ideas to establish a baseline for assessment and to work out the rehabilitation programme for the individual patient. Many elderly patients become confused on admission to hospital; this is not surprising when we consider the change of environment, so continuity in the members of the team treating the patient is needed to rebuild the patient's confidence and help his rehabilitation as a whole. Some team members may take a more dominant role than others, depending on the degree of rehabilitation required; the problems concerned with mobility and function to ensure a return to the patient's own environment will mean that the nurse, the physiotherapist, occupational therapist and social worker will all play a large part, reinforced by the other team members.

Physiotherapy here will be dealt with on a general basis to try to give the nurse an insight into what physiotherapy hopes to achieve for the geriatric patient as a whole. Two general facts are to be remembered throughout the treatment:

1. The patient is helped out of bed as soon as possible and as soon as the doctor gives permission; so that some degree of mobility is achieved at the earliest possible moment.
2. Patients in this age category cannot cope with prolonged periods of exercise in any form, so the rehabilitation programme is set at a pace to suit the individual patient.

The patient is assessed from the start of treatment and it is the physiotherapist's aim to motivate the patient so that even while in bed, exercises are taught and explained to encourage a degree of mobility and independence which is helpful not only to the patient but to the nursing staff as well.

Aims of physiotherapy

1. *Prevention of pressure sores* is achieved by:
   a. *Bridging exercise.* The feet are placed firmly on the bed, the knee or knees flexed to a right-angle, with arms either flat on the bed, or using arms to help lift the buttocks off the bed with elbows flexed. Alternatively a trapeze can be used to help the exercise. When the feet are firmly placed and the knee or knees flexed, the patient lifts the buttocks off the bed, as for example in Russell traction (Fig. 21.7F). This position is useful for toilet purposes, also as a preliminary position for teaching bed mobility; with a trapeze the patient can move from side to side in bed, reach personal items from locker or bed table, or move up and down the bed for changing position, e.g. from sitting to lying.
   b. *Rolling.* This is accomplished by turning the head and uppermost arm, with the legs crossed (if possible) so that the pelvis tilts towards the side to which the patient is rolling. This is a useful activity for changing bed linen and for the patient to use on a two-hourly basis for relief of pressure; also if the patient cannot achieve bridging adequately because of the type of injury or because of immobilisation, e.g. in traction to both legs or a heavy plaster cast, or simply because of general weakness and lack of muscle power.

2. *Prevention of chest complications.*
   Deep breathing exercises are taught, both general and localised, but bed mobility as in (a) is a great help as the patient is not in a static position and drainage of the lungs can take place in the various positions of side lying, lying and sitting; this can be reinforced by changing the elevation of the head or foot of the bed at regular intervals.
3. *Maintain circulation.*
4. *Maintain joint range, thereby preventing contractures.*
5. *Maintain muscle tone.*
   A general regime of active movements is taught and a record kept of each individual patient's progress.

The sitting position

When this is allowed an important factor is the bed height and also subsequent height of the chair, be it armchair or wheelchair; the height of the toilet bowl is also important; the thighs should be fully supported and hips and knees flexed to a right-angle so that the feet rest on the floor (or the foot-plates of a wheelchair) with the heels vertically below the knees. Adjustable beds, chairs and raised toilet seats mean that it is possible to adapt to the individual patient's height, so that transfer from wheelchair or from a standing position to bed, chair or toilet is facilitated. Door widths are also checked in the home to make sure the patient can cope with wheelchair or walking aids provided. It is important the team works as a whole to see that this situation is adhered to so that the patient can maintain independence and not require help from a chair that is too low or too high; in the former, the patient would not manage without a struggle (if at all) and the latter could be a danger since falling out of a chair can at worst cause an injury and at best, undermine the patient's confidence.

Balance in the sitting position is first taught with both arms supporting the patient, progressing to single arm support, then free sitting; when this is achieved the patient is encouraged to wash and dress himself. The patient must stand erect as soon as possible, support being provided where necessary so that the patient is in a stable position and balance is checked. Weight-bearing, (be it weight-bearing on only one limb, partial weight-bearing or full weight-bearing, depending on the condition), starts between parallel bars or with other necessary support, e.g. pulpit frame, rollator frame, tripod, forearm support gutter frame, standing frame, crutches or walking sticks, with perhaps a caliper or splint in place.

Treatment programme progress is aimed at;

1. *Increased muscle power.*
2. *Increased joint range.*
3. *Increased mobility for improvement of function.*

Exercises are preceded in many instances by heat treatment and in some cases, by drugs to help reduce pain and swelling and aid relaxation. Group activity is also useful at this stage as the competitiveness of the situation helps stimulate the patient who then becomes more enthusiastic and confident. As mobility increases the patient should be achieving more independence in the ward with a view to his forthcoming discharge. The occupational therapist and social worker will assess the patient's home conditions so that alterations can be made if necessary and any liaison with the community services be made prior to discharge.

When the patient has achieved stability with a wide base and substantial supporting aid, it may be possible to progress to a narrower base and a different, less substantial walking aid. For example, a walking frame (Fig. 21.9) or rollator may be exchanged for two walking sticks; eventually only one walking stick might be required. This progression should be well thought out and discussed with the elderly patient so as not to undermine his confidence or destroy the independence he has already achieved.

The whole team is made aware of the particular aids the patient is using and what degree of help is required, so that he does as much as possible for himself. The patient's maximum potential must now be considered and he should be encouraged in all aspects of his self-care and independence. The appropriate walking aid should be labelled for the patient's own use, and walking distances are increased, keeping in mind the individual home conditions. For instance, if he is unable to walk from lounge to toilet because of breathlessness, pain, etc., it must be seen that a chair is available for rest *en route* or, as an alternative, a commode

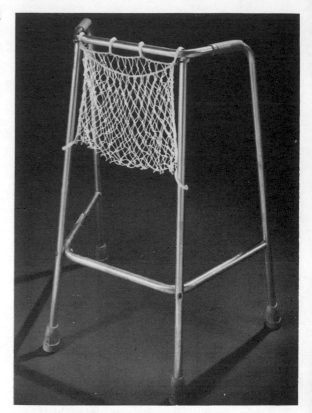

Fig. 21.9 Walking frame. (Zimmer.)

is provided by the Social Services Department. The patient may have to go up a steep flight of stairs to the bedroom or bathroom so that he has to be independent in this, or other arrangements must be made, such as an extra hand rail, the bed brought downstairs, and/or a district nurse calling once a week to help the patient upstairs to the bath. It is also important that the patient's independence is extended to walking, or manipulating a wheelchair, on all types of differing surfaces, linoleum, carpeting, loose rugs, slopes, paving, steps from one level to another, rough ground. Alterations to home conditions should include the removal of loose rugs which are a notorious safety hazard.

A case conference attended by all members of the team involved with the rehabilitation programme of the individual patient is now of great value, especially where problems regarding management and subsequent discharge are to be resolved. The patient's relatives may be invited to such a conference to adjust to the discharge of an elderly patient, when they may be required to offer support or to discuss the functional capacity of the patient. It is important to realise that each person in the team works towards the goal of helping the patient to achieve maximum independence so that the unavailability of any one team member is against the best interests of the patient.

Conclusion

It will be obvious from the foregoing paragraphs that the task of caring for these patients and of re-habilitating them demands exacting work not only from the nurse but from an army of people, both within and without the hospital. A few patients, unfortunately, never recover the physical status that they enjoyed before their injury, but many are restored to surprising activity and survive to enjoy a happy old age.

FRACTURE OF THE SHAFT OF THE FEMUR

Fracture of the shaft of the femur may be due to direct or indirect violence. Deformity and shortening of the limb readily occurs because the action of the powerful muscles of the leg produces over-riding, angulation and rotation of the fragments.

Subtrochanteric fracture of the femur

In this injury, the proximal fracture is abducted by the gluteal muscles, while the distal fragment is adducted by the adductors. The two fragments are therefore brought into alignment by abducting the limb. Continuous traction may also be necessary, to overcome the pull of the adductors. If the fracture is at a lower level the proximal fragment is not only abducted by the gluteal muscles, but flexed by the ilio-psoas tendon. This type of fracture is treated with the hip joint in flexion. *Surgery* may be required.

Treatment. (1) *Plaster spica*. The limb is immobilised in a plaster spica with the limb abducted (Ch. 6). (2) *Balanced traction* by means of Russell traction or by means of skin extensions and a Thomas bed-splint, which is either suspended, or, tied to the elevated foot-end of the bed, and either flexed at the knee or fitted with a Pearson attachment.

(3) *Open reduction and internal fixation*. Internal fixation may be achieved by means of a Kuntscher nail.

FRACTURE OF MID-SHAFT OF FEMUR

In fracture of the femur at this level, continuous traction is necessary in order to maintain full length and normal alignment of the limb. End-to-end opposition of at least one half of the fractured sur-faces is generally considered satisfactory, but over-riding angulation or rotation of the fragments must be corrected. There may be interposition of muscle-flaps between the bone ends, so that reduction is impossible except by operative means.

Treatment: (1) *Manipulative reduction.* (2) *Immobilisation* by one of two methods:

(a) Fixed skin traction in a Thomas bed-splint (Fig. 21.19);
(b) Balanced skin or skeletal traction with suspension (Fig. 21.23).

Requirements:

1. The mattress is supported by a fracture board, and arrangements are made to elevate the foot-end of the bed.

2. A right or left Thomas bed-splint of the correct size (Fig. 21.10); measurements are described later. The ring should fit closely against the ischial tuberosity, but it must not fit so tightly as to cause pressure sores. If the injury is very recent, remember that swelling of the thigh is inevitable.

3. Skin extensions are usually made of strips of 7.5 cm wide 'one way stretch' orthopaedic strapping (Fig. 21.13), or a commercial extension-pack as seen in Fig. 10.1 and 10.3–8.

4. Three metal gutter-splints; one must be long enough to support the limb from the upper thigh to the lower calf. Two shorter ones are required to enclose the thigh. Any grooves in the splints from previous use are 'ironed out' by moulding them over a rounded surface such as a bed rail or hot-water pipe.

Splints which have become very misshapen are best treated by placing them on the floor and treading out the dents. Alternatively, plaster slabs may be used as local splints, or, the surgeon may prefer to apply local pads and bandages.

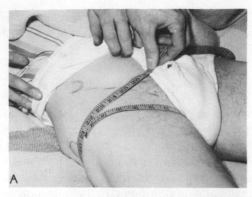

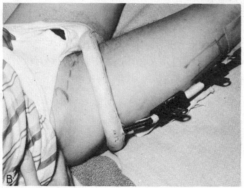

Fig. 21.10 **A.** The correct method of measuring the thigh for a Thomas splint. **B.** Note the snug fit of the ring. (With kind permission of the Accident Hospital, Birmingham.)

5. Other requirements include three strong calico or leather slings for the splint (Fig. 21.11) and paper clips or safety pins to secure them; gauze and calico bandages, splint wool, safety pins, needle and cotton, lampwick extension ties, and tincture of benzoin, if ordered, for painting the skin before extensions are applied (Fig. 21.12).

Reduction of fracture and application of splint. The fracture is reduced by manipulation under general or local anaesthesia. The surgeon supports the limb (Fig. 21.13) and maintains traction while the nurse applies extensions in the manner already

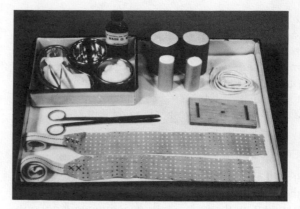

Fig. 21.12 Tray set for application of skin-extension. In this illustration, the strapping extensions are home-made. Commercial traction kits are commonly used instead.

described (Ch. 10). The splint is then gently guided over the limb and pushed firmly against the ischial tuberosity. The slings are placed beneath the limb and the long gutter-splint on top of them. A pad of wool is placed behind the lower end of the femur to help preserve the normal forward curve and to prevent hyperextension of the knee.

The knee joint is held in 5 degrees or 10 degrees flexion at all times. The slings are then adjusted and fastened with the clips. They must be tight enough to allow two-thirds of the thigh to be seen above the lateral bars of the splint and one-third below. One sling supports the femur, one the knee, and the other the calf. The extension tapes or cord are pulled taut and fastened to the end of the splint. The small gutter-splints, if used, are then moulded so that they conform to the shape of the thigh; this is done by grasping a splint at each end and twisting

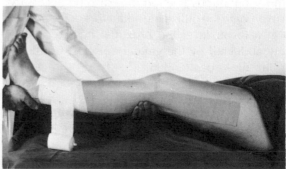

Fig. 21.13 The surgeon supports the limb while the skin-extensions are applied and the splint is guided over the foot and up the limb until the ring reaches the groin.

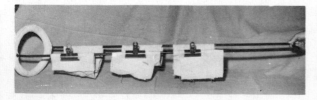

Fig. 21.11 Bed-splint ready for application. (With kind permission of the Accident Hospital, Birmingham.)

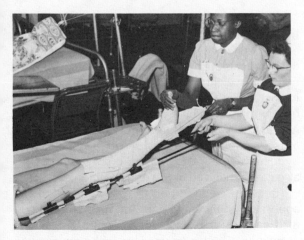

Fig. 21.14 An alternative method of holding the limb and applying the splint. (With kind permission of the Accident Hospital, Birmingham.)

it into a spiral shape so that the upper end lies over the trochanter and the lower end in front of the knee. A smaller one is applied to the inner side of the thigh. Alternatively, plaster slabs or local pads secured by a bandage can be used. The whole splint is then covered by a firm encircling bandage. A gallows may be used to support the foot, but it must not interfere with the traction. The position is checked by radiographs and by measurement of the limb. An illustration of the completed apparatus appears in Figs 21.22 and 21.23.

Sometimes, the splint is tied to the raised foot-end of the bed (Fig. 21.15). Not only is traction

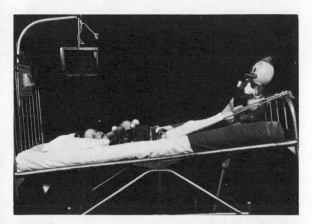

Fig. 21.15 Thomas bed-splint with skin extensions applied for fracture of the shaft of the femur. The splint is then tied to the raised foot-end of the bed. (With kind permission of the *Nursing Mirror*.)

increased, but the pressure of the ring in the groin is relieved.

Suspension of the splint is similar to that shown in Figs 21.19, 21.22 and 21.23. The splint is slung on an overhead beam by weights which are so balanced as to allow the patient to move about the bed for nursing purposes.

Nursing-care. The bed-splint ring requires the same care as described in Ch. 10. A nursing care study in the *Nursing Times* (Richards, 1982) gives a nice description of the care of a little girl such as the one shown in Fig. 21.15. *Pressure sores must not occur* and the patient is taught to move the skin and soft tissue underneath the ring at regular intervals. The extension tapes are kept taut at all times; forward or backward angulation may be corrected by adjustment of the slings; lateral angulation may be corrected by adjustment of the gutter-splints, or by local bandaging over pads of wool. Any such adjustment made by the surgeon must be maintained.

Exercises for the sound limb and for the foot and toes are practised throughout the period of fixation, and quadriceps drill is generally introduced in about four weeks. In uncomplicated fractures, in which immobilisation has been perfect, union of the fracture is expected in about 12 weeks.

Skeletal pin and balanced traction

Requirements

1. A bed elevated at the foot by blocks about 30 cm high, with either a single or double Balkan beam. The mattress is supported by a fracture board.

2. A Thomas splint with Pearson knee-flexion attachment; slings, clips, three gutter-splints, splint-wool and bandages.

3. A Steinmann pin or Kirschner wire and stirrup, or Denham pin and sliding hooks (Figs 21.16 and 21.17).

4. Cords, weights and pulleys.

Method of application. The skin is prepared as for any other operation. A general or local anaesthetic is given, the pin is driven through the upper end of the tibia, and the stirrup is attached. The splint is then guided over the limb until it is in contact with the ischial tuberosity, and the knee

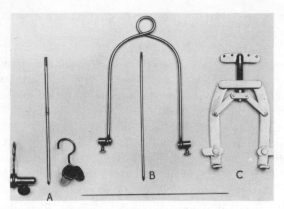

Fig. 21.16 Apparatus for applying skeletal traction. **A.** Denham pin and sliding hooks. **B.** Steinmann pin and stirrup. **C.** Kirschner wire and traction spreader. (With kind permission of the Accident Hospital, Birmingham.)

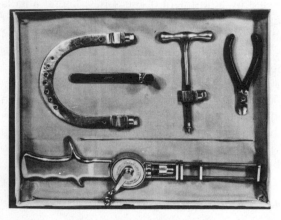

Fig. 21.17 Apparatus for applying skeletal traction. From left to right above: Kirschner stirrup; spanner; tightener; wire cutters, and wire. Below: Zimmer drill with special adaptation to facilitate easy insertion of the Kirschner wire.

flexion attachment is adjusted so that the knee is flexed about 30 degrees. The thigh is sometimes supported by a gutter-splint, and the slings are adjusted as already described. The splint is then slung from the overhead beam from cords at the end, and from just below the ring by cords which pass over the head of the bed, so that it is supported at its four 'corners' (Fig. 21.19A). A weight of from 4.5 to 9 kg is suspended from the stirrup of the pin over a pulley at the foot of the bed (Figs 21.19–21.22). The foot may be supported by a gallows or by a piece of strapping applied to the sole and attached to a cord and small weight at the head of the bed (Fig. 21.23). When over-riding of the fracture is corrected, angulation and rotation

is also corrected by manipulation and controlled by gutter-splints, plaster slabs, wool pads, or adjustment of the slings as already described. If the fragments are in satisfactory end-to-end apposition, the weight is reduced so that they become impacted (Fig. 21.18). Distraction of the fragments by too much weight will cause delayed union or non-union of the fracture. *The fracture is reduced by the traction at its initial application, not gradually by increasing the weight over a long period.* This also causes delayed union or non-union.

Traction is relied upon to maintain end-to-end apposition of the fragments and maintain the correct length of the limb, not to control angulation or rotation. This is corrected by deliberate manipulation and controlled by local splintage.

When reduction is secure and check X-rays show satisfactory position, the whole of the splint may be covered by a bandage.

Nursing-care. The weights are so adjusted by trial and error that while continuous traction is exerted on the fractured limb, the patient and the splinted limb move about the bed as one unit. The patient can raise himself for bedpanning and for treatment of the back. If the patient is uncomfortable and slides up or down the bed, then the weights are not correctly adjusted. The nurse must nor rearrange the weights herself; she must not allow passers-by to bump against them, and there must be no friction between them and the bed or the wall or any other object. They must always hang free. The bed must be moved with the greatest care. Movement of the pin in its track must be guarded against so as to minimise infection.

Later treatment. A caliper is occasionally ordered, but nowadays *cast-bracing* is used for early ambulation (see Ch. 19). An elasticated supporting bandage may be applied from the toes to the upper calf to prevent oedema, with a crêpe bandage to the knee. The caliper is applied as described in Ch. 10. *It must be weight-relieving;* that is, it must be of such a length that the ring is pressed against the tuber ischium and the heel is clear of the boot when the patient stands upright. The caliper or cast-brace is discarded when the fracture is soundly united.

Exercises to recover knee movement are then practised assiduously, and re-education in walking completes the treatment.

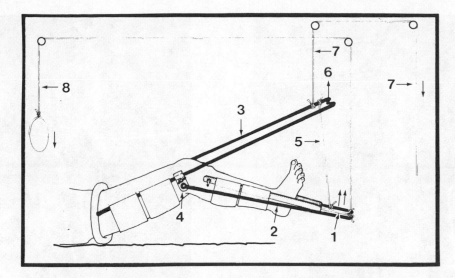

Fig. 21.18 *Early mobilisation techniques:* (i) Where there is abundant callus and the fracture cannot be sprung, splintage may be discarded and the knee mobilised till there is sufficient mature callus to allow weight bearing. (ii) *The Pearson knee-flexion piece:* this may be used as soon as some stabilising callus appears at the fracture site.
Methods: The traction cord (1) is transferred to the Pearson attachment (2) which is fixed to the Thomas splint (3) and hinges at the level of the knee axis (4). An adjustable cord (5) may be used to gradually advance the range of permissable knee flexion. The end of the Thomas splint is raised (6) and supported while a cord (8) may allow the patient to assist his knee extension manually.

Cast-bracing has been devised as a means of allowing early ambulation while healing of a fracture takes place, and of preserving joint movement and muscle strength (see *Journal of Bone and Joint Surgery* 52A: 1563–1578). It has already been discussed in Ch. 19.

Open reduction and internal fixation

If reduction cannot be obtained skeleton traction because of interposition of soft parts, internal fixation is supplied either by a tibial graft, by a stainless steel plate and screws, or, by a Kuntscher nail. A

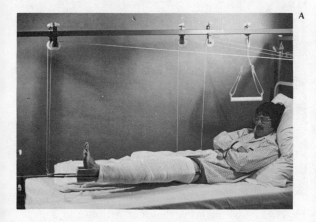

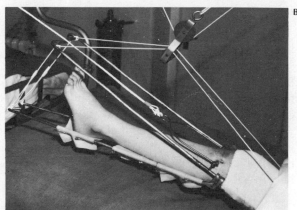

Fig. 21.19 **A.** Shows suspension of the Thomas splint at its four 'corners'. **B.** This illustration shows the skeletal pin and Pearson flexion-piece in position, and with Figs 21.20–22, the arrangement of the cords, pulleys and weights. (With kind permission of the Radcliffe Infirmary, Oxford.)

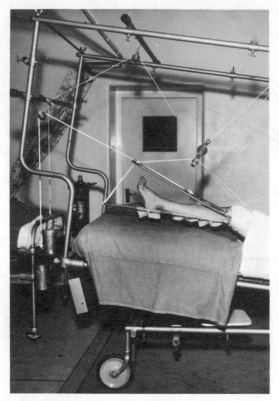

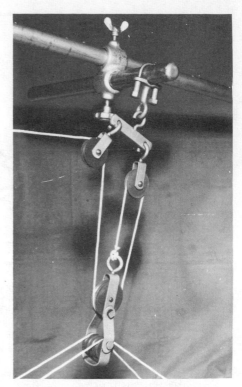

Fig. 21.21 (With kind permission of the Radcliffe Infirmary, Oxford.)

Fig. 21.20 Figs 21.19, 21.21 and 21.22, also show the general arrangement of the cords, weights and pulleys. (With kind permission of the Radcliffe Infirmary, Oxford.)

plaster spica may be applied post-operatively, quadriceps drill is begun within a few days, and the plaster is generally removed in about 12 weeks, when non-weight-bearing exercises are commenced.

SUPRACONDYLAR FRACTURE OF THE FEMUR

Supracondylar fracture of the femur is less common than fracture of the mid-shaft. It may be complicated by pressure on the popliteal artery.

Treatment consists of manipulation and skeletal traction on a Thomas bed-splint with Pearson flexion-piece, or on a Braun splint. The knee is held in about 20 degrees of flexion.

FRACTURES OF THE FEMUR IN CHILDREN

Figure 21.15 shows a child with a fracture of the

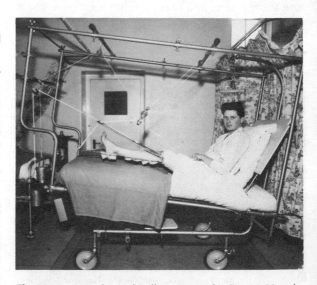

Fig. 21.22 Note that in this illustration and in Figs 21.20 and 21.21, the lower supporting sling has slipped down so that it is resting beneath the head instead of just above it; nevertheless, the patient is obviously quite comfortable. (With kind permission of the Radcliffe Infirmary, Oxford.)

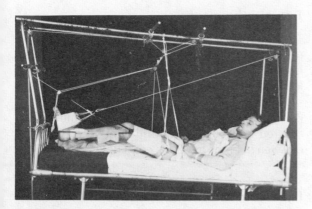

Fig. 21.23 Another illustration of a fracture of the shaft of the femur treated by balanced skeletal traction on a Thomas bed-splint with Pearson knee-flexion attachment. (With kind permission of the *Nursing Mirror*.)

femur immobilised by means of traction in a Thomas splint.

Treatment by balanced traction without a splint

Some authorities believe that this is all that is required. Mr Graham Apley describes this method of treatment and the following extract is taken from his book *A System of Orthopaedics and Fractures* (Reprint of Fourth Edition, 1975) and Fig. 21.24 is reproduced by permission of the author and publisher. 'It is not generally appreciated that the Thomas splint does not really "immobilise" the fracture. Essentially, it is a device for the attachment of slings and strings.

The simplest method of holding reduction is by traction without a splint. Skeletal traction is used for adults and skin traction for children. Weights are attached and hung over pulleys at the foot of the bed, whcih is raised. The leg is merely cradled on pillows, which also serve to prevent backward sag. Activity is started at once and, as soon as the patient can lift his leg, knee-bending exercises are begun.'

An alternative to the conventional gallows traction shown in Fig. 21.24 is the use of a traction hoop similar to that shown in Fig. 14.10.

INJURIES TO THE KNEE

The knee joint depends for its stability on its extensor mechanism, the quadriceps muscle. Any injury to the joint produces rapid and severe wasting of this muscle, which in itself constitutes a severe disability; the knee is deprived of its natural support and is unprotected from the strains of weight-bearing. *It is therefore of vital importance that contraction of the quadriceps is commenced immediately after knee injuries and continued for five minutes of every waking hour.* The only exceptions

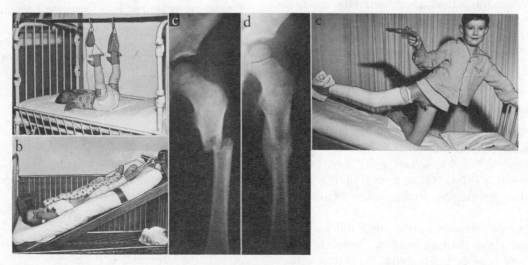

Fig. 21.24 Fractured shaft of femur, **A–D.** Traction without a splint is certainly adequate in children, and skin traction is sufficient. **E.** Clearly this fracture has united (by permission of Mr. A. Graham Apley and Butterworth).

to the rule are cases in which there is an open wound communicating with the joint, or traumatic haemarthrosis; even then, quadriceps drill is commenced as soon as possible.

Quadriceps drill

This is usually taught by a physiologist, but it is such an essential part of the treatment of knee injuries that the nurse should be prepared to supervise the exercise. Vague directions are not enough. The patient should sit or lie in a comfortable position and the exercise is demonstrated on the sound side first; clothing such as tight pyjama trousers must not be allowed to interfere with the exercise. Place a hand behind the knee and instruct the patient to press the knee down against it, to the command, 'tighten—and relax'. A strong contraction of the quadriceps should then be seen; it must be followed by complete relaxation. *Alternate contraction and relaxation of the muscle is performed for five minutes hourly.* Some patients 'cheat' by contracting the gluteus maximus instead, the control of the quadriceps being completely inhibited. This must be overcome at all costs. It may be necessary to demonstrate the exercise on oneself or on some other healthy individual. Massage and electrotherapy is rarely ordered; it cannot take the place of the patient's own efforts and only encourages inertia. When the patient has mastered the technique of quadriceps contractions, he then progresses to straight-leg raising, first against gravity only, then against the resistance of a weight tied to the foot.

Traumatic synovitis

This may follow an injury to the knee, producing pain, swelling and effusion.

Treatment. (1) A few days' rest. (2) A pressure bandage (p. 473). (3) Quadriceps drill. (4) A back-splint may be ordered, applied in almost full extension.

Recurrent synovitis may occur if full control of the quadriceps is lost and wasting allowed to occur. *Treatment* is as outlined above. Weight-bearing is restricted until control of the quadriceps is regained.

Traumatic haemarthrosis

This occurs if a severe strain or twist of the knee ruptures the blood-vessels of the synovial membrane. The knee swells rapidly, with severe pain, local heat, and rise of temperature.

Treatment. (1) Rest. (2) Aspiration of the joint. (3) A pressure bandage. (4) A back-splint may be ordered. (5) Quadriceps drill after 10 or 14 days, or when haemorrhage has ceased.

Injuries of the collateral ligaments

Sprain of the medial ligament is caused by an abduction strain of the extended knee. There is swelling, bruising, local tenderness, and pain when the knee is manipulated into valgus.

Treatment. (1) A pressure bandage. (2) Inside raising to the heel of the shoe. (3) Quadriceps drill.

The external lateral ligament is less often injured. Treatment proceeds on the lines already described.

Rupture of the medial ligament

This is evidenced by pain, swelling, bruising, local tenderness and lateral instability of the joint.

Treatment. (1) A plaster cylinder in almost full extension for about two months. Any lateral deviation is corrected when the plaster is applied. (2) Quadriceps drill.

Operative treatment may consist of a suture or reconstruction of the ligament.

Rupture of the lateral ligament occurs less frequently; it is often accompanied by lateral popliteal nerve palsy (Ch. 22). Treatment proceeds on the same lines.

Rupture of the cruciate ligaments

The cruciate ligaments may be ruptured by an abduction or hyperextension strain of the knee, or by a violent blow on the front of the tibia. There is unnatural antero-posterior movement of the tibia on the femur.

Treatment proceeds on the lines laid down for rupture of the internal lateral ligament.

Operative reconstruction of new ligaments may be undertaken.

Dislocation of the knee

This may be momentary, accompanying rupture of the ligaments; occasionally it persists.

Treatment. (1) Reduction by traction and pressure. (2) Plaster fixation; weight-bearing is allowed in about six weeks. (3) Quadriceps drill.

Operative treatment consists of open reduction. Dislocation of the knee may be complicated by vascular catastrophe or by nerve involvement such as damage to the lateral popliteal nerve (Ch. 22).

Injuries to the semi-lunar cartilages

The medial semi-lunar cartilage (medical meniscus) is more often torn than the lateral, because of its attachment to the medial ligament.

The mechanism of injury is a weight-bearing rotation strain, either when the tibia is forcibly externally rotated on the femur or the femur is internally rotated on the fixed tibia. Tears of the medial semi-lunar cartilage often occur in miners and footballers, whose occupations subject the knee to the forces described.

Clinical features. An accurate and detailed history will reveal the occurrence of a rotation strain. The patient describes a sharp pain on the inner side of the knee, accompanied by a tearing sensation. He may fall to the ground and be unable to rise. The joint may 'lock' in semi-flexion. It can be flexed, but not extended; extension may be restored spontaneously or by manipulation by the patient or his friends. The recurrent case learns to 'unlock' the knee for himself, but complains that the knee feels unstable and 'lets him down'.

The patient is examined lying on a couch; the trousers are removed, and both knees are exposed. There may be swelling and effusion, and local tenderness over the affected cartilage. Wasting of the quadriceps may be marked; manipulation of the knee by the surgeon may elicit a 'click', or movement of the displaced cartilage may actually be felt.

X-rays are generally ordered to exclude loose body formation.

Treatment of torn semi-lunar cartilage

This consists of an operation to remove the affected cartilage (meniscectomy), in order to prevent recurrent trauma to the joint and subsequent osteo-arthritis.

Preparation for operation. Intensive quadriceps drill is introduced at once. In addition to the routine preparation, the skin is prepared from the groin to the toes.

Post-operative treatment. A pressure bandage is applied as soon as the operation is completed; the surgeon usually prefers to do this himself. The limb is then bandaged to a metal back-splint in full extension. The back-splint should be covered with only a thin layer of wool, because thick padding combined with the bulk of the pressure bandage would not allow full extension of the knee. Alternatively, the upper and lower ends of the back-splint may be padded, leaving a gap in the middle in which the pressure bandage will rest. The limb is then supported on a pillow.

Quadriceps drill is resumed as soon as the patient recovers consciousness, and is continued for five minutes of every hour. On the second day, the pressure bandage may be cut, especially if there is swelling of the leg, and a fresh one applied.

Application of a Jones pressure bandage

Wind a thick layer of splint-wool around the knee. Start to bandage directly over the joint. Take three tight firm turns straight round the knee, add another layer of wool, then three more turns of bandage, and so on until all the bandage is used up. Some surgeons prefer to extend the bandage to the top of the supra-patellar pouch, others take it only to the upper border of the patella.

Exercises are continued hourly throughout the day. Young, vigorous patients may be allowed up in a few days according to the surgeon's orders, otherwise the sutures are removed and the back-splint discarded on the eighth or tenth day, and if the quadriceps are powerful and knee movement perfectly controlled, the patient is allowed up. A longer period of non-weight-bearing is advised if there is any effusion in the knee.

Re-education in heel-and-toe walking is essential; the patient is taught to walk without a limp, and the knee must be fully extended at every step.

The external (lateral) semi-lunar cartilage is less often injured than the internal (medial). Treatment proceeds on the same lines.

Cyst of the lateral semi-lunar cartilage

A cyst of the external (lateral) semi-lunar cartilage appears as a localised swelling on the outer side of the knee.

Treatment consists of removal of the cartilage and cyst. After-care proceeds as laid down for removal of a semi-lunar cartilage.

Loose bodies in the knee joint

These are due to the following causes: (1) *Osteo-chondritis dissecans*, a condition in which a small flake of bone becomes detached from the articular surface of the femoral condyle, or more rarely, from other parts of the articular surface. (2) *Osteo-arthritis of the knee* with detachment or fracture of osteophytes (Ch. 27). (3) *Chondromata* of the knee joint.

Loose bodies may produce symptoms similar to those of cartilage lesions, such as recurrent pain, locking, and effusion.

Treatment consists of removal of the loose body. Post-operative treatment proceeds on the lines already described for meniscectomy. Synovectomy may be indicated for multiple chondromata.

Rupture of the quadriceps

This occurs when a violent contraction of the quadriceps is made in attempting to avoid a fall. The patient experiences a painful tearing sensation, the knee joint fills with blood, and active extension of the knee is lost. A gap can usually be felt between the torn muscle fibres.

Treatment consists of operative repair. The limb is immobilised in full extension on a back-splint or in a plaster cylinder for three weeks. Quadriceps drill and exercises are commenced in about 10 days. Thereafter, mobilisation without weight-bearing is commenced and continued until the knee flexes 90 degrees.

Fracture of the patella

This occurs in accidents as described above. *Treatment* is by one of the following methods:

1. Suture of the lateral quadriceps expansion and excision of patella. The after-care is as already described for suture of ruptured quadriceps.

2. Suture of lateral quadriceps expansion and patella, followed by the application of a plaster cast in almost full extension. Quadriceps drill is started at once, and weight-bearing in plaster in a few days. The plaster is worn for about two months, followed by active exercises and re-education in walking.

Stellate fracture of the patella may occur as a result of direct violence, and is often compound. Those with only minor displacement require a guarding plaster for about three weeks. Quadriceps drill and weightbearing starts immediately. Manipulative reduction is sometimes necessary, but if the displacement is such as to preclude the restoration of smooth joint surfaces, operative excision of the patella is the usual method of treatment.

Dislocation of the patella

Lateral mobility of the patella varies greatly in different individuals. It may be dislocated by a strain of the knee or by direct violence, and is accompanied by a traumatic synovitis of the knee.

Treatment. (1) A back-splint or guarding plaster for about two months. (2) Quadriceps drill. (3) Active exercises and re-education in walking when the plaster is discarded.

Recurrent dislocation of the patella

This may be due to a congenital abnormality of the knee joint or may follow a previous injury.

Treatment may consist of transplantation of the tibial tubercle to the inner side of the tibia (Hauser). Patellectomy may be preferred, or, in early cases, lateral release and medial plication. A plaster cylinder is worn for 6–8 weeks.

Fracture of the lateral condyle of the tibia

This injury is due to an abduction strain of the knee, and is usually accompanied by tearing of the medial collateral ligament.

Treatment usually consists of continuous skin-traction in a Thomas bed-splint, with the knee bandaged into varus. This is retained for about six weeks, when non-weight-bearing exercises are commenced. Operative reduction is sometimes required, and gross disturbance of joint surfaces with subsequent osteo-arthritis may necessitate arthrodesis of the knee at a later date.

FRACTURES OF THE TIBIA AND FIBULA

FRACTURE OF THE SHAFT OF THE TIBIA AND FIBULA

This may be due to direct or indirect violence. It is often compound because the tibia lies subcuta-

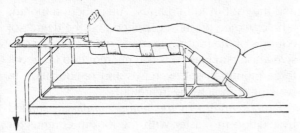

Fig. 21.25 Fracture of the shaft of the tibia treated by skeletal traction and plaster fixation. The limb is supported on a Braun splint.

neously. In oblique and spiral fractures, there is a strong tendency to over-riding of the fragments.

Treatment

Treatment consists of manipulative reduction and plaster fixation. The knee is flexed, sometimes over the end of a table, and after manipulation a posterior slab is applied from the toes to just below the knee. This is quickly enclosed in a plaster bandage, and as the plaster sets, the fragments are moulded by the surgeon's hands. When the plaster has set firmly, the knee is straightened until it is held in a position of 10 degrees or 15 degrees flexion and the plaster is extended up to the groin. During application, a ridge at the junction of the two halves of the plaster must be avoided.

Skeletal traction. This may be ordered if the reduction is unstable. A Steinmann pin or Kirschner wire is driven through the lower end of the shaft of the tibia, and incorporated in a plaster cast. The traction pin is fixed to a stirrup and the limb sup-

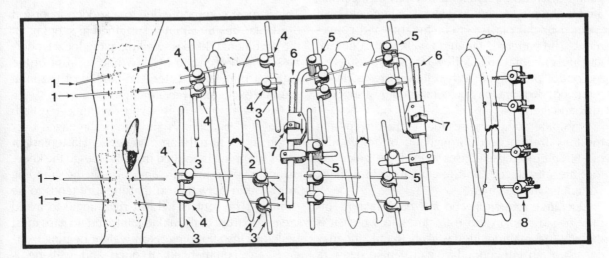

Fig. 21.26 *External fixation systems:* The previous methods do not prevent undesirable movement at the fracture site, nor do they offer provision for local bone absorption; the incidence of non-union tends to be rather high. Nevertheless two-pin fixation will preserve length until sound wound healing is achieved when more radical surgery may be carried out if required.

Better control is possible when two or more pins are inserted into each fragment and linked together mechanically. There are several systems based on these principles (e.g. Hoffman, A. O. External Fixator, Universal Day Frame, etc.). In the Hexcel system illustrated Steinman pins are inserted into each fragment (1). The fracture is reduced (2) and the ends of the pins connected in pairs to rods (3) by split clamps (4). The rods in turn are rigidly connected together by further clamps (5) to square section threaded bars (6) which allow compression of the fragments (7).

Other systems rely on cantilever compression screws—e.g. Oxford system (8).

All these external fixation methods are designed to support the fracture *without* plaster until union, and at the same time to give access to the wound. Their disadvantage is the risk of pin-track infections and loosening.

This illustration, with captions, is taken from *Practical Fracture Treatment* by Ronald McRae, by kind permission of the author and publisher.

ported on a Braun splint (Fig. 21.25) or in a flexed Thomas bedsplint which in turn may be suspended to a Balkan beam. From 2 to 5 kg weight is suspended over a pulley and the foot of the bed is elevated. A new unpadded plaster is applied in a week or two when swelling has subsided, and the traction pin is removed when the plaster has set.

Correction of deformity by wedging the plaster. If alignment is not perfect, it may be corrected by wedging the plaster at a site indicated by the surgeon. Pieces of cork are inserted into a splint in the plaster and the position of the fragments is checked by radiographs.

Treatment by external fixation is shown in Fig. 21.26.

Later treatment

Toe exercises are commenced at once. Clawing of the toes must be prevented. Weight-bearing in a closely moulded unpadded above-knee plaster is usually ordered in about six weeks at the surgeon's discretion. A walking iron may be incorporated in the plaster, but in general, a large old boot worn over the plaster is comfortable and convenient. The patient is taught to walk with a normal gait and encouraged to follow his usual pursuits.

Control of oedema. When the plaster is finally removed, oedema may be controlled by a supporting bandage.

Physiotherapy. Exercises for the quadriceps and the toes are practised throughout; on removal of plaster, mobilising exercises for the knee, ankle and foot are introduced, and re-education in walking completes the treatment.

Operative reduction and internal fixation. This may be advised in those fractures in which it is thought that manipulation is likely to fail, and may consist of an intramedullary nail, single screw, a plate and screws, or a bone graft from the opposite tibia. After-treatment proceeds as already described.

Fracture of the shaft of the fibula

This occurs, as a result of direct violence and is a simple injury which is treated by the application of a supporting bandage. It is, however, often part and parcel of a Pott fracture.

INJURIES OF THE ANKLE AND FOOT

Rupture of the tendo-Achilles

This injury occurs in the middle-aged and elderly, as a result of some unaccustomed strain when the calf-muscles are actively contracting. There is pain, swelling and bruising at the site of rupture, and the patient is unable to walk or rise on the toes. A gap in the tendon may be palpable.

Treatment. Operative repair is usually required, followed by plaster fixation with the knee flexed and the foot in full equinus. After about a month, a below-knee plaster is applied and the degree of equinus of the foot is gradually reduced in successive plasters. Fixation is usually required for about three months. Foot exercises and re-education in walking complete the treatment.

Partial rupture of the tendo-Achilles is treated by fixation in plaster with the foot in equinus for about two months.

Sprain of the ankle joint

This is most commonly due to a sudden inversion or plantar flexion strain is sustained in slipping off the pavement. There is swelling, pain, local tenderness, and bruising just below and in front of the external malleolus. Lateral instability of the joint must be excluded by examination.

Treatment. If there is severe swelling, the limb is elevated on pillows and firmly bandaged over wool. In the usual case, however, Elastoplast or other strapping is applied from the toes to the knee, using firm even pressure and carrying the strapping from within outwards so that the foot tends to be everted. The foot is held at right-angle to avoid creases in front of the ankle joint, and no gaps must be left in the strapping. Non-weight-bearing exercises are commenced at once and walking is allowed in a few days. Full recovery is expected in about three to six months.

Dislocation of the ankle joint

In very severe sprains the lateral ligament is avulsed from the lateral malleolus. In addition to the swelling, bruising, and local tenderness, there is unnatural mobility of the talus when the foot is manipulated into inversion. X-ray examination with the foot held in full inversion will reveal the lateral tilt of this bone; sometimes a flake of bone is avulsed from the lateral malleolus by the ruptured ligament.

Treatment consists of an unpadded plaster cast with the foot at a right-angle and in neutral rotation. Toe exercises are commenced at once and weight-bearing is allowed as soon as the plaster is dry. The plaster is renewed when the swelling subsides and is worn for about ten weeks; thereafter supporting strapping is applied from the toes to the knee for a week or two, and foot exercises and re-education in walking are commenced.

Recurrent dislocation of the ankle joint

This may follow an untreated severe sprain; the ankle 'lets the patient down' when walking on uneven ground.

Treatment may consist of an outside raising to the heel of a shoe with a flat wide heel, or, an inside iron and outside T-strap. Exercises are given to strengthen the peroneal muscles. Operative repair of the lateral ligament may be advised.

Fracture-dislocation of the angle joint—(Pott's fracture)

Various fracture-dislocations of the ankle joint are referred to as 'Pott's fracture'. The essential feature is a fracture of the lower end of the fibula, with rupture of the medial collateral ligament with or without avulsion of the medial malleolus and lateral or posterior dislocation of the ankle joint. The fracture may be further complicated by a posterior marginal fracture of the lower end of the tibia. Pott's fracture of the common type is sustained by abduction, adduction or rotation strains of the ankle joint, often as a result of some simple accident such as slipping off the pavement. It is common amongst elderly women.

Treatment. Treatment of Pott's fracture consists of manipulation and plaster fixation with the foot in right-angled dorsiflexion; inversion or eversion of the foot may be required according to the type of fracture. In cases in which swelling, ecchymosis or blistering is severe, the patient may be kept recumbent with the limb elevated on pillows and immobilised in a posterior plaster shell until the swelling subsides. Otherwise reduction is undertaken as soon as possible. In uncomplicated cases, an unpadded plaster cast is applied immediately after reduction, but if gross reactionary swelling is expected, a padded cast is applied and the patient is confined to bed. The plaster is changed to an unpadded one as soon as the swelling subsides. In cases without gross bone damage and in which reduction is secure, weight-bearing in plaster is allowed in a few days; in more severe cases it is allowed as soon as an unpadded plaster can be applied. The patient either wears a plaster boot or a walking iron is incorporated in the plaster. Toe exercises are practised throughout the period of immobilisation, which in general is not less than eight to ten weeks. Walking in plaster is encouraged as circulation and muscle tone is thereby maintained.

Later treatment. As in all lower leg fractures, a supporting bandage may be required on removal of plaster to prevent swelling. Movement of the joint is recovered by active exercises. Re-education in walking is essential; an inside raising to the heel of the shoe may be ordered. In very heavy patients further protection of the ankle joint by an outside iron and inside T-strap is occasionally advised.

Open reduction and internal fixation by one or more screws may be undertaken in very unstable fractures.

Displacement of the lower tibial epiphysis

Treatment of this injury proceeds on the same lines as for a Pott's fracture. Compression of the epiphysis may very occasionally lead to premature fusion and arrest of growth of the tibia, with late deformity.

FRACTURES OF THE BONES OF THE FOOT

Fracture of the calcaneum (os calcis)

This is usually the result of a fall from a height, when the patient lands heavily on his heels. It is not uncommonly accompanied by a fracture of the spine. The diagnosis is made from the typical history of a fall on the feet, the painful and tender heel, the broadening of the calcaneum and the limitation of inversion—eversion movement when movement of the ankle is relatively free. Radiographs in special positions may be ordered.

Treatment. There are various schools of thought in the treatment of this injury, but the most widely held view at the present moment is that no fixation should be applied. Older methods utilised plaster fixation and mechanical devices to attain and maintain reduction. These methods are credited with causing permanent stiffness and pain in the foot.

The patient is prevented from weight-bearing on the injured limb for 12 weeks, and is taught exercises to develop all muscle groups controlling the foot and ankle. Weight-bearing on crutches is permitted provided the injured foot is not put to the ground, but if both calcanei are fractured, as is often the case, the patient is confined to bed for the full period of twelve weeks.

Fracture of the calcaneum with gross displacement and subsequent avascular necrosis may necessitate arthrodesis of the sub-talar or even the mid-tarsal joints.

Fractures and dislocations of the talus (astragalus)

Fracture of the talus is sustained in dorsiflexion injuries of the foot and may be accompanied by partial or complete dislocation of the bone. Dislocation without fracture is due to a severe inversion strain or to an injury which forces the forefoot into abduction or adduction. In the latter injury there may also be fracture of the navicular or of the metatarsals.

Treatment. Uncomplicated cases are treated by manipulation and the application of a below-knee plaster holding the foot in right-angled flexion. Fracture of the neck of the talus with sub-talar dislocation requires fixation in a position of full equinus and eversion. In some cases, skeletal transfixation or open reduction is necessary to replace the displaced talus. Weight-bearing is not permitted if the blood supply to the bone is in doubt. Avascular necrosis may cause degenerative arthritis and sub-talar arthrodesis is then indicated.

Fracture of the shaft of the metatarsal

This is generally due to a direct injury. Treatment

consists of immobilisation in a walking plaster until union is sound.

March fracture

This is a crack fracture of the shaft or neck of the second, third or fourth metatarsal. It is so named because it is a fatigue fracture sustained by soldiers during route marches, though it may occur during ordinary walking. There is a predisposition to march fracture of the second metatarsal in 'metatarsus atavicus', a congenital abnormality in which the first metatarsal is shorter than normal, so that excessive weight is borne on the second.

The patient complains of pain beneath the affected metatarsal which is tender to pressure. X-rays may show no fracture until two or three weeks after it has in fact occurred, when continued weight-bearing has caused excessive callus formation.

Treatment consists of a walking plaster which is worn until union is sound.

Fracture of the neck of the metatarsal

This is usually due to direct injury. The metatarsal head is displaced into the sole of the foot, so that malunion causes severe pain and disability.

Treatment consists of pulp traction to the toe, fixed to a wire extension which is incorporated in a plaster cast; the cast is well moulded beneath the metatarsal heads to restore the transverse arch. Traction is continued for about four weeks, and a walking plaster is worn for a further period of about three weeks. Operative reduction is sometimes necessary. Malunited fracture of the metatarsal neck is treated by excision of the metatarsal head.

Fractures of the toes

Fracture of the proximal phalanx of the toe is usually due to direct violence; the displacement corresponds to similar fractures of the proximal phalanges of the fingers—flexion of the distal interphalangeal joint and hyperextension of the proximal interphalangeal joint.

Treatment proceeds on the same lines, i.e. the toe is immobilised in flexion until union is sound.

Comminuted fracture of the phalanges of the great toe

This is due to a direct crushing injury, such as a weight dropped on the toe, and may be open.

Treatment consists of a collodion and ribbon-gauze splint. Weight-bearing is allowed in a boot with the toe-cap cut out and fitted with a metatarsal bar to the sole. Drilling of the toenail may be required to relieve the pain of a sub-ungual haematoma.

BIBLIOGRAPHY

Adams G 1983 Girdlestone's operation. Nursing Mirror Clinical Forum, 13 July

Adams J C 1972 Outline of Fractures. Edinburgh: Churchill Livingstone

Anderson Sir F 1976 Practical Management of the Elderly. London: Blackwell Scientific

Beck M E 1975 Nutrition and Dietetics for Nurses. Edinburgh: Churchill Livingstone

Bradley D 1970a Fractures of the upper end of the femur. Part I. Nursing Times, 26 November, 1523

Bradley D 1970b Part II. Nursing Times, 1552

Briscoe S 1983 Fractured femur. Nursing care study. Nursing Mirror, 29 June

Brislen W et al 1981 Risk comes before a fall. Nursing Mirror, 23 September

Bromley D D 1966 The Psychology of Human Ageing. London: Penguin

Brown P 1983 Clinical teaching opportunities (Care of a patient before and after total hip replacement.) Nursing Mirror, 8 June

Brown P 1983 Torn right medial meniscus. Nursing care study. Nursing Times, 13 July

Caird F I, Judge I G 1979 Assessment of the elderly patient. Tunbridge Wells: Pitman Medical

Charnley J 1970 The closed treatment of common fractures. 3rd edn. Edinburgh: Churchill Livingstone

Chartered Society of Physiotherapy 1975 Handling the Handicapped. London: Woodhead-Faulkner

Corkery P 1966 Management of fracture in the ankle region. London: Nursing Mirror, 21 October, 2–4

Crow J 1977 The nursing process. Nursing Times publication.

Cruise V J, Wright, W B 1978 Better geriatric care—making it happen. Nursing Times, 21 September, 1563

Dandy D 1979 Meniscectomy. Nursing Times, 23 August

Davies E M 1975 Let's Get Moving. Mitcham, Surrey: Age Concern

Dyson R 1978 Bed sores—the injuries hospital staff inflict on patients. Nursing Times, 15 June, 30

Flanders J 1984 Potts luck. Nursing Mirror, 18 April

Fleetcroft J P 1983 The musculo-skeletal system. Edinburgh: Churchill Livingstone

Gore I 1976 Physical activity in old age. Nursing Mirror, 19 February, 48

Grant P M 1976 Hospitalisation—and the elderly patient. Nursing Care Study. Nursing Times, 11 March, 379

Hawker M 1976 Keep-fit exercises for geriatric patients. Nursing Mirror, 19 February, 50

House S 1978 Post-traumatic nitrogen metabolism in the elderly. Nursing Times, 31 August, 1457

Huckstep R L 1970 A Simple Guide to Trauma. Edinburgh: Churchill Livingstone

Isaacs B 1976 Giants of geriatrics. Nursing Times, News Feature, 11 March, 362

McRae R 1981 Practical Fracture Treatment. Edinburgh: Churchill Livingstone

Menzies J 1982 The whole team won. Nursing Mirror, 30 June

Norton D, McLaren R, Exton-Smith A N 1975 An Investigation of Geriatric Nursing Problems in Hospital. Edinburgh: Churchill Livingstone

Orpwood J 1981 Two hips for old. Nursing Care Study. Nursing Mirror, 9 August

Pearson J R, Austin R T 1973 Accident Surgery and Orthopaedics. London: Lloyd-Luke

Pinel C 1976 Pressure sores. Nursing Times, 5 February, 172

Powell M 1973 Limb traction—some aspects of nursing management. Nursing Mirror, 27 July, 26

Pusey R 1978 Pott's fracture. Nursing Times, 3 August, 1293

Redfern et al 1973 Local pressures with ten types of patient-support systems. The Lancet, 277–280

Richards H 1982 A child with a fractured femur. Nursing Times, 13 January

Robb B 1967 Sans Everything. London: Nelson

Skeet M 1970 Home from Hospital. London: Dan Mason Research Committee

Smillie I S 1978 Injuries of the knee joint. 5th edn. Edinburgh: Churchill Livingstone

Stewart M C 1970 My brother's keeper? London: Health Horizon

Wainwright H 1978 Feeding problems in elderly disabled patients. Nursing Times 30.3: 543

Wells T 1980 Problems in Geriatric Nursing Care. Edinburgh: Churchill Livingstone

Whitley M W, Smith H 1981. Elderly clients and withdrawal of night hypnotics. Nursing Times, 19 March

Wilson J N (ed.) 1976 Watson-Jones fractures and joint injuries. 5th edn. Edinburgh: Churchill Livingstone

Winkley D 1981 McKee-Arden—Total hip replacement. News-Sheet of the British Association of Orthopaedic Nurses and the Association of Orthopaedic Physiotherapists, March

Wong J 1983 Hip replacement. Nursing Mirror Clinical Forum, 13 July

22

Peripheral nerve lesions

CAUSES

Peripheral nerves arise from the spinal cord and convey nervous impulses arising in the brain and spinal cord to the various structures of the body. We are concerned here only with those which supply the limbs. The structure of a peripheral nerve is shown in Fig. 22.1. Motor fibres pass from the anterior horn cells of the spinal cord to end in conjunction with the muscles which they activate; sensory fibres pass from the skin and other structures to the spinal cord via the posterior root ganglia; in addition, sympathetic fibres arise in the spinal cord and pass to the blood vessels and sweat glands.

Peripheral nerve lesions are caused in many ways. A nerve may be severed by direct violence, such as a laceration; it may be compressed by pressure within the body, as in haemorrhage, or by some outside agency such as a splint or plaster. It may be injured by traction, as when the circumflex nerve is stretched in dislocation of the shoulder joint, or, loss of blood supply may cause death of the axon cylinder, as in Volkmann's ischaemia (Ch. 20). A peripheral nerve is sometimes affected by poisons such as arsenic or lead. *Leprosy* also attacks peripheral nerves (see Bibliography).

Peripheral nerve lesions are classified as follows:

1. Complete division of a nerve and its supporting sheath—neurotmesis.
2. A lesion in continuity, with crushing or compression of axons without rupture of supporting sheath—axonotmesis.
3. Transient nerve block—neuropraxia.

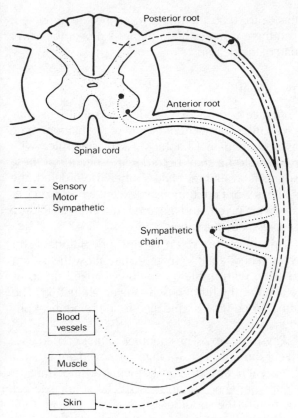

Fig. 22.1 The structure of a peripheral nerve. (With kind permission from Ring, P. A. (1969) *The Care of the Injured.* Edinburgh: Churchill Livingstone.)

CLINICAL FEATURES

The lesion may be partial or complete, depending on the degree of injury to the nerve. As we have seen, peripheral nerves contain both motor, sensory and sympathetic nerve fibres. A lesion of such a nerve will therefore present the following features:

1. *Paralysis* of all muscles supplied by the nerve below the level of injury.
2. *Anaesthesia* of the area of skin supplied by the nerve.
3. *Trophic changes in the skin.*
4. *Loss of certain tendon reflexes.*

Treatment

Treatment is largely determined by the degree of certainty as to whether the lesion is a complete division of the nerve, a lesion in continuity, or a

transient nerve block. In the early days this may be difficult to decide, but in cases in which there is an obvious cause of complete severance of a nerve, such as a deep wound, early operative suture is undertaken. This is done when there is no risk of infection, usually when healing of the wound has taken place. Paralysis due to a lesion in continuity often recovers spontaneously with conservative treatment; if not, exploration is undertaken at a later date. Paralysis due to transient nerve block always recovers with conservative treatment.

Conservative treatment

1. *Splintage.* Splints are applied to prevent overstretching of paralysed muscles and deformity from contracture of healthy ones or from the action of gravity. In the case of the hand, in which mobility of joints is of paramount importance, splints which allow controlled movement are usually ordered.

2. *Physiotherapy.* This is aimed at the re-education of paralysed muscles and the prevention of contractures and joint stiffness. The last-named is of vital importance, because even if treatment is successful and the paralysed muscles recover, the function of the limb will be greatly impaired if the joints have been allowed to become permanently stiff. Joint stiffness and contractures must therefore be prevented by giving passive movements at least once each day. Active exercises are given to re-educate paralysed muscles, and electrical stimulation is sometimes ordered, because it retains muscle bulk and minimises wasting. Some special aspects of physiotherapy are discussed later.

Operative treatment

1. *Nerve suture.* This is followed by immobilisation in a plaster cast in a position which relieves tension on the nerve. For example, suture of the median nerve would require fixation with the elbow and wrist flexed. The joints are gradually straightened as the nerve unites. The rate of regeneration of a nerve is estimated at about 2.5 cm per month.

2. *Nerve grafts.* Grafts may be performed to bridge a gap between the nerve ends when a section of non-essential nerve is taken from some other part of the body.

3. *Tendon transplants*. These are performed in cases of irrecoverable paralysis; for example, some of the flexor tendons of the wrist are transplanted to the extensors in cases of irrecoverable radial palsy.

4. *Operations on bone*. These include bone-block operations and stabilisation of joints. These operations are performed to correct deformity, to provide stable joints, and to improve the function of the limb as a whole.

NURSING CARE IN PERIPHERAL NERVE LESIONS

1. The limb must be kept at an even temperature. Do not apply direct heat for fear of burning the insensitive skin; the patient should be warned against touching hot plates, radiators, etc.; on the other hand, a paralysed limb should never be allowed to become cold and stiff.

2. Splintage must fit comfortably and perform the function for which it is designed, i.e. the prevention of overstretching of paralysed muscles and deformity due to contracture of healthy muscles or the action of gravity.

3. The skin must be kept clean and dry. *Pressure sores from splints or plasters must not occur;* if there are trophic changes in the skin they will heal only very slowly.

4. Avoid swelling by elevation and support, and by preserving full movement of the joints; chronic oedema will result in fibrosis.

5. Never allow a paralysed limb to dangle helplessly. Joints which are deprived of their muscular supports are easily dislocated.

6. Remember the importance of physiotherapy in preventing joint stiffness and in the re-education of paralysed muscles.

LESIONS OF PERIPHERAL NERVES IN THE UPPER LIMB

THE CIRCUMFLEX NERVE

The circumflex nerve lies just below the shoulder joint, and for that reason is liable to be stretched in a fracture of the humerus or dislocation of the shoulder. There is partial or complete paralysis of the deltoid, so that the arm cannot be abducted, and there is anaesthesia of the skin over the lower part of the deltoid.

Treatment

Splintage consists of an abduction splint. This may be a Littler-Jones splint or one of the platform type as described in Chapter 7. A plaster spica with removable lid may be ordered if neither of these splints is available. Unless otherwise ordered, the splint is worn continuously, except when exercises are being given, and the arm is not allowed to drop helplessly by the side.

An abduction splint is very uncomfortable to wear in bed, and the surgeon may allow the patient to sleep with numerous pillows banked up so as to support the limb in right-angled abduction. The arm can be firmly bandaged to the uppermost pillow.

Physiotherapy. The shoulder-joint is carried passively through its full range of movement at least once each day; this is particularly important in elderly patients, and it is essential that full external rotation of the shoulder is preserved. Active exercises and electro-therapy are also given.

THE RADIAL NERVE

The radial nerve may be severed in lacerations of the arm, or compressed in fracture of the humerus. It is also liable to compression from splints and plasters, from crutches in the axilla, or from a chairback in 'Saturday night paralysis'. It is sometimes compressed by a tourniquet, or by the edge of an operating table if the arm is allowed to hang over the side.

N.B. It can also be damaged by an intramuscular injection.

There is complete wrist-drop due to paralysis of all the extensors of the wrist. There is also loss of extension of the thumb and of the metacarpophalangeal joints of the fingers, though the interphalangeal joints can still be extended by the lumbricals and interossei. The grasp is weakened, because the extensors cannot carry out their normal function as 'fixation agents' of the wrist. In the normal hand, the wrist is stabilised by its extensors to allow the

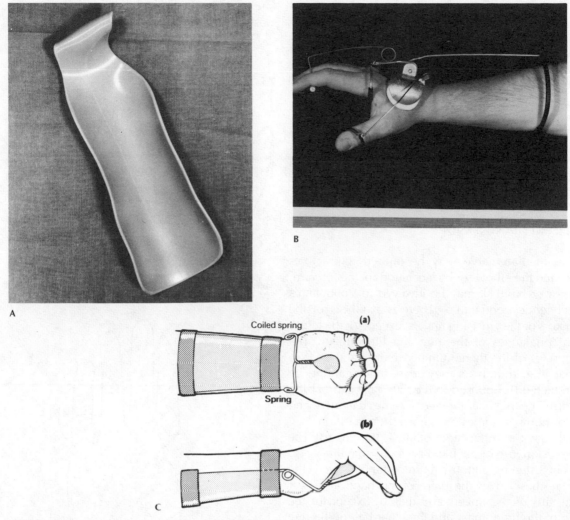

Fig. 22.2 A. Metal cock-up splint for radial paralysis (Watson-Jones). **B.** Brian Thomas working splint for radial nerve paralysis.
C. A lively splint for wrist drop.
   (a) Palmar view. Note how the fingers and thumb are free to move.
   (b) Lateral view.
(After Wyn Parry, *Rehabilitation of the hand.*)

flexors to function in grasping the object. The nerve to the triceps usually escapes, as it is given off in the axilla. Anaesthesia is usually confined to a small area over the dorsum of the web of the thumb. The prognosis is good.

Treatment

Splintage consists of a cock-up splint which must not extend beyond the proximal interphalangeal joints of the fingers. A short metal cock-up splint as shown in Fig. 22.2A may be used as a temporary measure, but a long cock-up is never used, as stiffness of the fingers is more disabling than the paralysis. Other splints allow flexion and extension of the fingers without stretching the wrist extensors such as the splints shown in Fig. 22.2B and C. If these splints are not available an anterior plaster shell may be used to support the limb. A posterior plaster shell may be fitted with traction loops attached to finger-stalls. Active flexion of the fingers and thumb is then possible against the resistance of the traction loops, which take the place of the paralysed extensors.

Physiotherapy. This is instituted at once, and proceeds on the lines already described.

Operative treatment. Nerve suture may be performed, followed by fixation in plaster with the wrist dorsiflexed and the elbow in a moderate degree of flexion, depending upon the site of suture. In irrecoverable cases, tendon transplantation is often employed. The pronator radii teres is stitched to the extensor tendons of the wrist, the flexor carpi ulnaris to the extensor tendon of the fingers, and the flexor carpi radialis to that of the thumb (Robert Jones).

THE MEDIAN NERVE

The median nerve may be injured in fractures around the elbow, or by lacerations of the forearm, wrist or hand. It may be involved in Volkmann's ischaemic contracture. There is paralysis of the flexors of the wrist and fingers, except for the terminal phalanges of the ring and little finger. The muscles of the thenar eminence are paralysed, so that the thumb is powerless and cannot be abducted or opposed to the little finger (precision grip). The thenar eminence becomes flattened, and the thumb assumes a characteristic position as it falls back into the same plane as the fingers. The precision grip of the hand is grossly impaired, e.g. as in fastening buttons. An important feature is the anaesthesia over the palm of the hand and over the tips of the fingers and thumb, except for the tip of the little finger and the ulnar half of the ring finger (Fig. 22.3). This is a serious matter, because the patient is unable to feel objects (for example, in his pockets) and also because it renders him liable to burns from cigarettes, hot plates, etc. Trophic changes in the skin and nails are marked; median palsy is commonly associated with pain, sweating and coldness of the skin of the hand. This is known as 'causalgia'.

Compression of the median nerve in 'carpal tunnel syndrome' is discussed in Chapter 28.

Treatment

Splintage is applied to hold the thumb in opposition to the fingers. This may take the form of a splint such as shown in Fig. 22.4 or an interior plaster

shell holding the fingers and thumb in the optimum position, i.e. in the grasp position.

Physiotherapy is always ordered.

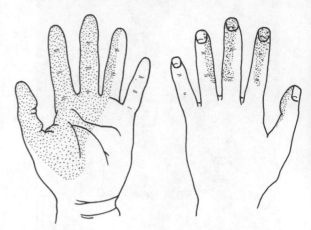

Fig. 22.3 Area of anaesthesia in complete median paralysis (Watson-Jones).

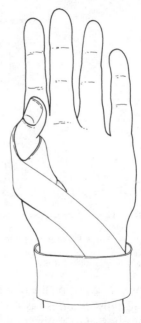

Fig. 22.4 Splint for a median nerve lesion, when active opposition of the thumb is lost. A leather band around the wrist is fastened to a strip of lined rubber material. When the hand is relaxed the thumb rests in a good functional position for opposition. Extension can still be performed against the resistance of the elastic strip. (After Barr, N. *The Hand*, Butterworth.)

Operative treatment. Nerve suture is followed by fixation in a plaster cast holding the wrist and elbow in flexion.

THE ULNAR NERVE

The ulnar nerve may be injured in fractures around the elbow joint or in lacerations of the arm. In common with the median nerve, it may be involved in Volkmann's ischaemic contracture. There is paralysis of the interossei, the inner two lumbricals, the muscles of the hypothenar eminence, part of the flexor brevis pollicis, and the adductor of the thumb. Wasting of the interossei is shown by the characteristic hollows between the metacarpal bones. Paralysis of these muscles, which normally flex the metacarpo-phalangeal joints and extend the interphalangeal joints, causes a claw-hand due to the action of the opposing muscles. The little finger is immobilised and cannot be opposed to the thumb, so that fine movements of the hand are lost. Anaesthesia of the skin is confined to the ulnar side of the hand, the tip of the little finger and the ulnar half of the ring finger (Fig. 22.5). When the patient grasps a piece of cardboard with the two thumbs laid flat, the terminal interphalangeal joint on the affected side cannot be extended because of the paralysis of the thumb adductor and the unopposed action of the flexor longus pollicis.

In comparing lesions of the median and ulnar nerves, it is interesting to note that in the former there is loss of 'precision grip' of the hand, as in holding a needle, but in ulnar palsy, there is loss of 'power grip' as in holding a rod.

Treatment

Splintage may consist of a dorsal plaster shell holding the fingers in flexion at the metacarpo-phalangeal joints and extension at the interphalangeal joints. Splints of the 'knuckle-duster' or 'mouse-trap' type are frequently ordered, to prevent contractures and clawing of the hand (Fig. 22.6).

Physiotherapy is always ordered.

Operative treatment. Nerve suture is followed by fixation in plaster with the wrist and elbow in the flexed position.

Delayed ulnar paralysis

This may follow a fracture of the lateral condyle of the humerus with subsequent cubitus valgus deformity. The nerve becomes stretched in its lengthened course and ulnar palsy develops many years after the original injury.

Treatment is by transposition of the ulnar nerve from its normal bed behind the internal condyle of the humerus to a new position in the muscles

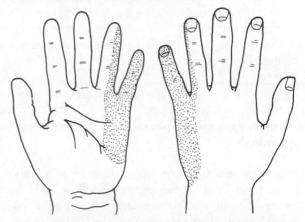

Fig. 22.5 Area of anaesthesia in complete ulnar paralysis (Watson-Jones).

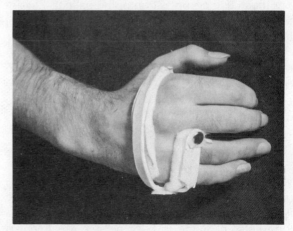

Fig. 22.6 A simple home-made splint for use in claw hand caused by ulnar paralysis. It is made from Orthoplast, a plastic material which softens in hot water and can be moulded to fit the patient. A band of velcro passes down between the middle and ring fingers to the palmar orthoplast strip. The metacarpo-phalangeal joints are thus held in flexion while the long flexors and extensors are able to function.

in front of the elbow joint. This relieves tension and friction on the nerve by shortening its path. See also Chapter 19.

Lesions of the brachial plexus

These are commonly caused by traction on the arm, or by injuries which force the arm or shoulder into abnormal positions. In lesions of the whole plexus, the arm is completely paralysed and anaesthetic and hangs uselessly by the side.

Treatment. Splintage may be ordered, holding all joints in the optimum position. *Physiotherapy* is always ordered. *Operative treatment* may consist of tendon transplants (in cases of partial recovery) or stabilisation of joints. Treatment by arthrodesis of the shoulder and amputation of the arm may be required.

Physiotherapy for peripheral nerve injuries in the upper limb

In serious nerve injuries, the patient must be prepared for a long period of rehabilitation; even in the most favourable circumstances it may be many months before recovery occurs, and moreover the most skilled surgery will not restore function without the active co-operation of the patient. Physiotherapy is aimed at helping and teaching the patient to assist in his own recovery.

The most common nerve lesions encountered are probably those affecting the hand, and restoration of function here is very important because of the complicated mechanism and diversity of delicate movements possible in the normal hand.

The physiotherapy given is adapted to the various stages of treatment.

Treatment before surgery (delayed repair). For various reasons a divided nerve is not always repaired immediately after injury and where there is lack of movement due to paralysis of muscles the joints are liable to become stiff. Treatment is aimed at maintaining joint mobility, good circulation and healthy skin in preparation for surgery.

Passive movements must be given to the joints of the limb at least twice daily to maintain their range of movement; if this is not done consistently, contractures will develop, when intensive treatment including stretching, splintage and wax baths may be required.

Active exercises are given to all uninvolved joints to prevent them from becoming weak and stiff; for example, a patient who has a nerve lesion preventing his using his hand can easily lose full shoulder elevation, and weakness of elbow and shoulder muscles may occur simply from disuse. Sometimes the power in an unaffected group of muscles can best be maintained by dynamic splintage. Weakened muscles should not be kept in a continually overstretched position as this lessens their power when they are innervated once again; a resting or night splint may be fitted to keep them in the shortened position.

As well as the loss of motor power, the sensory deficit must be considered, and the patient warned of the dangers of burning or damaging insensitive areas; at the same time the limb should be kept warm. It is most essential that while awaiting surgery, the patient is taught to keep his limb in the optimum condition and regular checks are made so that appropriate treatment can be given if necessary.

Treatment after nerve repair or grafting. Immediately after operation or injury, it is vitally important to avoid oedema, particularly in the hand. There may also be damage to joints, bones and tendons and the circulatory system is affected. Oedema leads to stasis which can cause deposition of collagen and fibrosis of muscle tissue, resulting in a weak, sluggish hand. For this reason the hand is kept elevated, following the principle of the hand higher than the heart. When the patient lies in bed, an arrangement of slings attached to an overhead beam or to an intravenous drip stand is effective; when he sits, the arm can rest on a table on pillows, and when walking, an efficient sling will keep it in position. Cold packs are often applied; the commercial jelly-type are preferred to crushed ice which may be too cold when the sympathetic nervous system is affected, also the former can be applied over a light dressing without making it wet. Another method of reducing oedema is by the pneumatic sleeve which is placed over the limb and rhythmically inflates and deflates to give a pumping action. When oedema is present the hand is usually rested in a good functional position and will probably require a splint.

After surgical repair, a plaster splint is applied, keeping joined nerves in a short position so that there is no strain on them and they cannot be overstretched. As early as possible, movements are given within the dressing or splint. Active movements keep uninvolved muscles in tone and passive movements maintain joint range; both help the circulation, and are given several times a day.

Sometimes a graft is inserted in a severed nerve, this may be taken from another area, e.g. the sural nerve. In this case note any disturbance of gait.

The patient is taught the regime to follow and may be allowed home a few days after surgery, returning for examination of the wound and removal of sutures at about fourteen days. At three weeks all dressings and splints are usually removed and treatment progressed; at this stage, active exercises are often started in warm water. Passive movements are given, gently at first to avoid stretching the repaired structures too strongly; as we expect recovery to begin, treatment is similar to the pre-operative phase. In the case of repairs commonly carried out at the wrist, some contractures often occur after 6–8 weeks so that steps are taken to correct them; deep massage with oil and lanolin is given as the soft structures are stretched out, and frequently renewed serial plaster of Paris splints are applied to maintain the correction between treatments.

When recovery of muscle power starts, specific active exercises are given to encourage the muscles to contract. 'Trick' movements may become a habit, so the patient must be shown exactly how to use the newly innervated muscles so that he can practice these exercises. Mass movements of the limb and patterns which facilitate the use of the required muscles, games, normal work activities with adaptations to tools all help. There may be a place for electrical stimulation of muscles in the early stages of their re-education.

Re-education of sensory function. As well as exercising the motor functions of the nerves, their sensory function can also be developed as recovery takes place. Retraining is given by means of a system in which the patient learns to identify objects solely by touch, using the part of the hand formerly denervated. These objects are varied as to size, shape and texture and become gradually more difficult as recovery progresses. It is found that by practice not only the sensory, but also the motor function, can be improved. Repaired nerves recover at an average rate of one millimetre per day, so depending on the site of repair or grafting, a long time must elapse before maximum recovery is obtained. If possible, the patient is returned to some form of employment and is reviewed at regular intervals.

LESIONS OF PERIPHERAL NERVES IN THE LOWER LIMB

THE SCIATIC NERVE

The sciatic nerve may be injured in deep lacerations such as gunshot wounds. It may be stretched by posterior dislocation of the hip joint; more rarely, it is injured in fracture of the pelvis.

N.B. It can also be damaged by an intramuscular injection.

In a complete lesion there is paralysis of the hamstrings and of all the muscles below the knee; there is complete anaesthesia of the lower leg and foot, except for an area on the inner side of the leg. Anaesthesia of the sole of the foot is a very troublesome feature and trophic ulcers quickly occur.

Treatment

Nerve suture is followed by fixation in a plaster spica holding the hip extension, the knee in flexion, and the foot in plantar-flexion. Irrecoverable cases may require a caliper or double iron for weight-bearing, and sometimes, amputation of the limb.

THE LATERAL POPLITEAL (COMMON PERONEAL) NERVE

This nerve is very liable to injury as it is superficial where it winds round the neck of the fibula, so that it may be compressed by splints, plasters, or tight bandages. It may be damaged in dislocation of the knee or by strain or rupture of the lateral ligament. There is paralysis of the anterior tibial group of muscles and of the peronei, so that the foot cannot be dorsiflexed or everted, and there is anaesthesia of the outer aspect of the leg and dorsum of the foot. If untreated, an equino-varus deformity of the foot will develop.

Treatment

Splintage consists of a plaster shell or club-foot shoe holding the foot in right-angled dorsiflexion and slight eversion.

Physiotherapy is commenced at once. Weight-bearing splintage may consist of a plastic splint (Fig.

18.14, 22.9) a Rizzoli splint (Fig. 22.7) or toe-raising spring with or without a double iron (Fig. 22.8), or, a double iron with posterior stops (Fig. 7.7). An outside T-strap may be necessary, and a plaster shell is usually ordered for night wear.

Operative treatment may be required to correct deformity and may take the form of a stabilisation of the foot, with or without tendon transplants, or,

some other procedure such as Lambrinudi drop-foot operation.

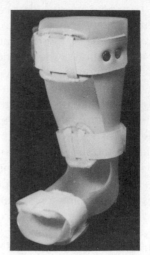

Fig. 22.9 Plastic drop-foot splint (Taylor). (See also Fig. 18.14.)

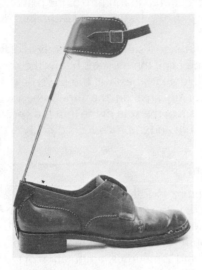

Fig. 22.7 Rizzoli splint.

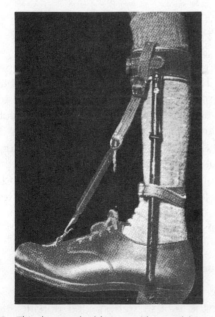

Fig. 22.8 This shows a double iron with toe-raising spring which might be ordered for permanent foot-drop; sometimes the iron is dispensed with, and the spring is then fastened to a leather band encircling the leg below the knee.

Application of a double iron

The heel of the boot is either fitted with square sockets which exactly fit the iron or, tubed and fitted with contrary stops (Fig. 7.7).

Application. The plaster is bi-valved in readiness, and the skin cleaned. An Elastoplast or crêpe bandage may be applied for the first few days to control swelling. Unfasten the strap and apply the iron, put on the boot and fit the lower ends into the tubing.

A T-strap, placed on the opposite side to the deformity may be ordered to control incipient varus or valgus deformity of the foot. The patient is then taught correct walking by a physiotherapist; special exercises, and a plaster shell for night wear are usually ordered.

Daily care. See that the iron fits closely just below the knee. A tendency to pressure sores can be controlled by padding the surface of the ring with felt. The boot must be kept in good repair and if contrary stops are used, they must be constantly inspected as they tend to yield to the pressure of the iron and allow a little movement.

A Rizzoli splint

This is fitted in the same way, but the iron is placed at the back of the limb (Fig. 22.7). It has the advantage of being less noticeable than other splints, particularly beneath trousers. Splints which are even less conspicuous are now being made from plastic materials.

BIBLIOGRAPHY

Peripheral nerve injuries

Seddon H 1975 Surgical disorders of the peripheral nerves. 2nd edn. Edinburgh: Churchill Livingstone
Sunderland S 1978 Nerves and nerve injuries. 2nd edn. Edinburgh: Churchill Livingstone

Radial nerve

Dolenc V 1976 Radial nerve lesions and their treatment. Acta Neurochirurgica 34: 235
Gore R V 1968 A new method of nerve repair: repair of a lesion of the radial nerve with a branch to the triceps muscle. British Journal of Surgery 65: 352

Ulnar nerve

Rychak J S 1977 Injury to the median and ulnar nerves secondary to fracture of the radius. A case report. Journal of Bone and Joint Surgery 59A: 414

Median nerve

Lewis M H 1978 Median nerve decompression after Colles's fracture. Journal of Bone and Joint Surgery 60B: 195

Sciatic nerve

Spiegel P G 1974 Complete sciatic nerve laceration in a closed femoral shaft fracture. Journal of Trauma 14: 617

General

Adams J C 1971 Outline of Orthopaedics. Edinburgh: Churchill Livingstone
Addison H 1981 Brachial plexus injury. Nursing Times, 26 August
Apley E G 1977 A System of Orthopaedics and Fractures. London: Butterworths
Dalton J 1983 Leprosy—a curable disease, and Arogya Agam—place of Health. Nursing Times, 5 and 12 October
MacRae R 1976 Clinical Orthopaedic Examination. Edinburgh: Churchill Livingstone
Pearson J R, Austin R T 1973 Accident Surgery and Orthopaedics. London: Lloyd-Luke
Roaf R, Hodkinson L J 1976 Textbook of Orthopaedic Nursing. London: Blackwell
Smith C 1980 Peripheral nerve lesions 1 & 2. Nursing Times, 20 and 27 November
Yeoman P M 1971 Traction injuries of the brachial plexus. Nursing Mirror, 22 January, 26

SECTION | FOUR

Care of the
paralysed patient

23

Spinal cord injury

INTRODUCTION

The central nervous system consists of the brain, the spinal cord and the peripheral nerves, as shown in simple diagrammatic form in Fig. 23.1. This diagram shows how lesions of the motor system affect muscle tone and reflexes and produce different kinds of paralysis; lesions of the lower motor neurone (Fig. 23.1A) cause flaccid paralysis, as in poliomyelitis (Ch. 18) while those of the upper motor neurone (Fig. 23.1B) produce spastic paralysis as in cerebral palsy (Ch. 14). The word paralysed is usually taken to mean loss of the power to move, with or without loss of skin sensation. In practice

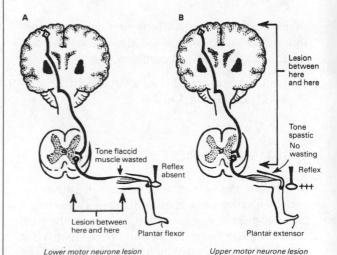

Lower motor neurone lesion   *Upper motor neurone lesion*

Fig. 23.1   A, B. Lower and upper neurone lesions. (By courtesy of Blackerstaff, E. R., *Neurology for Nurses*. Reprint 1970. London: Hodder and Stoughton.)

the word covers a wide range of conditions due to a variety of causes and with an equally wide variation in the degree of disablement. *Paresis* is the word used to describe partial paralysis or weakness of the power to move, and *palsy* is commonly used in combination with some other descriptive term, especially connected with involuntary or shaking movements—notably cerebral palsy (Ch. 14).

It should be noted here that the paralysis referred to above applies to motor loss only; sensory nerves are not affected. On the other hand, lesions which involve both motor and sensory pathways result in loss of sensation and movement, e.g. spinal injury with complete or partial transection of the cord (Ch. 23), or damage to a mixed peripheral nerve (Ch. 22).

Causes of paralysis may be:

1. Congenital anomaly, e.g. spina bifida (Ch. 14).
2. Infection, e.g. tuberculosis (Pott's paraplegia) (Ch. 17), or poliomyelitis (Ch. 18).
3. Degenerative conditions, e.g. motor neurone disease, multiple sclerosis.
4. Cerebro-vascular accident (Ch. 24).
5. Malignancy; tumours of the spinal cord may lead to hemiplegia, paraplegia or tetraplegia (Ch. 31).
6. Injury to the brain or spinal cord, e.g. head injury (Ch. 19), traumatic paraplegia or tetraplegia (Ch. 23).

In this discussion we shall consider only those conditions likely to be encountered by the nurse working in an orthopaedic department, viz.

1. Traumatic paraplegia and tetraplegia (Ch. 23).
2. Adult hemiplegia (Ch. 24).

TRAUMATIC INJURIES OF THE SPINE

These may occur from any number of causes but usually involve some form of high velocity. Among the commonest cause of these injuries is the road traffic accident and it remains to be seen what impact the recent seat belt legislation will have on the numbers. Among the other common accidents are those sustained following a dive into shallow water (cervical injuries), falls from heights and the consequences of a number of recreational pursuits, horse riding, rock climbing, trampolining etc.

The mechanics of the injury have a significant bearing on the amount of damage the spinal cord receives and this, coupled with the immediate and longer term care, dictates the amount of disability the patient suffers. Frequently the nature of the mechanics can only be pieced together from a careful history, the appearances at X-ray and the neurological pattern presented by the patient. However, these must be considered as a whole and serious doubts must be cast on using the X-rays as the only indication of the damage the spinal cord has sustained. Immediate treatment is therefore undertaken in a way which enhances the ability of the spinal cord to retain as much of the function as possible and lays the foundation for the comprehensive care that follows such an approach.

Notes on the transportation of patients with spinal injury are seen in Chapter 19 but Fig. 23.2 is repeated to reinforce the importance of the care required to minimise further injury.

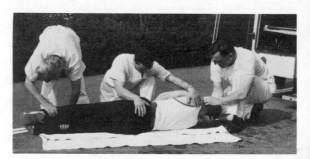

Fig. 23.2 Further injury to the spine must be avoided by moving the patient 'in one piece'.

SPINAL CORD INJURY UNITS

Because of the serious nature of these injuries specialised centres have been developed in many parts of the world. These centres are dedicated to the total care and rehabilitation of paralysed patients and although medical, nursing and paramedic skills and expertise is the first pre-requisite for success, facilities such as those shown in Fig. 23.3A–E are a desirable background for treatment.

The aim of Spinal Injury Units is to receive any newly injured patients as soon as possible post-injury as this enables the total care of the patient

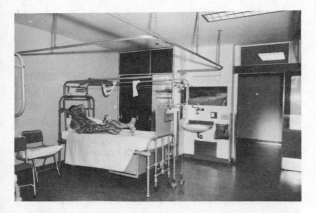

A

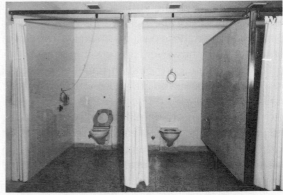

D

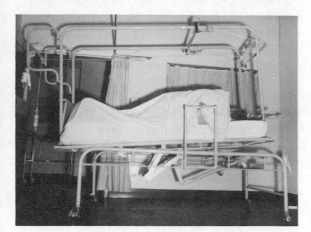

B

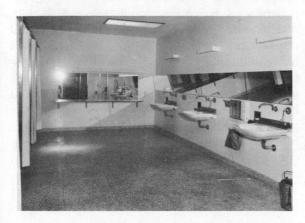

C

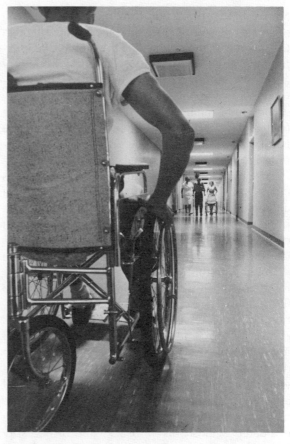

E

Fig. 23.3   Shows some special features of a Spinal Injury Unit. **A.** Wide bed-spaces in the ward; wide doorways; beds with a firm base, soft mattress, and lifting/transfer aids attached. **B.** Special beds where indicated (in this case) for skull traction. **C/D.** Spacious and accessible toilet facilities. **E.** Wide corridors for the passage of wheel-chair. (From the Royal Perth Rehabilitation Hospital, Shenton Park, Western Australia, by courtesy of Sir George Bedbrook.)

to be planned from the earliest stages and ensures that the chances of the horrendous complications that can occur in these patients are at least reduced. It must be said, however, that great improvements in the immediate care of such patients in general hospitals have occurred and lapses are now a rarity, mainly because of the efforts made by those staff and former patients of Spinal Injury Units in making the principles of care known to those involved. Of particular value is the Spinal Injuries Association publication 'Nurse Management in the General Hospital: the first 48 hours following Injury'.

THE PATIENT

Spinal injury does not discriminate either with regard to age or socio-economic group although the patients in the main fall in the eighteen to forty-five age group with a ratio of men to women of about 5:1. Although the flexibility of the spinal column is greatest in youth as is the circumference of the spinal canal, young children are not immune from serious spinal cord injury and the elderly are particularly vulnerable when degenerative conditions are present in the spinal column.

The principles of treatment outlined in this chapter will, of necessity, deal with the care of all such patients but the first and most important principle is that each patient will be unique when considered within his own social and psychological background and the care given has to be planned with this constantly at the forefront of the minds of those who are in a caring role. To do less than this is to condemn the patient to a production-line care which will only partially meet his needs. The treatment of the patient with a spinal injury must be likened to a 'college of life' where the eventual objective is rehabilitation to a level where the patient is using to the full the physical and mental resources which he has left. Success or graduation from this college can therefore be evaluated against this yardstick, and of necessity the patient must be a full participating member of his team of management, eventually becoming managing director with his family, general practitioner, district nurse, social worker as members of the board.

THE CARING TEAM

It is in the care of spinal injuries, perhaps more than any other area that the team concept is seen to best advantage and provides a framework for care which is unique. The only prime carers are the patient and his family but beyond these are the professional carers whose complete interdependence on each others' skills give a structural cohesiveness to the team work concept. The skills of the orthopaedic surgeon, physician, urologist (often now found in the one person, the consultant in spinal injuries) will be complemented by the skills of the nurses, physiotherapists, social workers, occupational therapists, Disablement Resettlement Officers, each having particular skills which will play their part in the eventual rehabilitation of the patient. It is, therefore, a team working with mutual respect for each other, self-motivated and with the highest degree of professional integrity. Any failure in the caring cycle for the patient with spinal injury reveals itself: the forgotten change of position, the bad technique in catheterisation, the inadequate physiotherapy resulting in perhaps a pressure sore, urinary infection or joint contracture which compromises the patient's eventual and final rehabilitation.

Such professionals will have developed the most appropriate approach to the patient, remembering that the over-emotional approach linked with overt sympathy and lush sentimentality is to do the patient a disservice as it is only his courage, self-discipline and perseverence that ensures successful rehabilitation. Because of the special demands made upon him, a degree of 'involvement' in the patient's emotional and psychological needs will, in the right setting, give the patient strength and courage at a time when this is most necessary. This calls for a maturity that has nothing to do with age but with training, experience and common sense coupled with the best instrument for successful treatment and rehabilitation—that is, the inescapable iron hand in the kindest and warmest of velvet gloves.

Definitions

Tetra-plegia (sometimes called quadriplegia) is the term used to describe paralysis to some extent of all four limbs as the result of an injury to the cervical

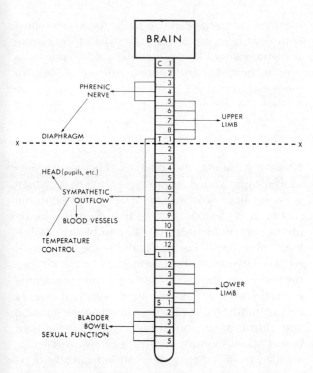

Fig. 23.4 Shows in diagrammatic form loss of function resulting from injuries at different levels of the spinal cord.

spine, and in addition the muscles of respiration will be affected. Paraplegia is used to describe paralysis at any level below the first thoracic vertebra, involving the trunk and lower limbs. Figure 23.4 shows the loss of function suffered from injuries at different levels of the spinal cord but this assumes that the cord damage is complete transection, whereas in practice this is not always the case. Staff caring for these patients need to memorise the level of injury pertaining to each patient together with that patient's physiological abilities as it is only with this knowledge that realistic planning and implementation of care, together with realistic goal setting, can occur. Obviously this knowledge is only a part of the wider consideration of the needs of the patient and overcomes the lumping together of all as 'paras' or 'tetras' for they must never be referred to as such.

IMMEDIATE EFFECTS OF THE INJURY

Clinical picture

As described earlier, injury to the spinal cord can occur in a number of ways with a variety of results

ranging from a temporary bruising of the cord to a complete transection at the level of injury. Initially the presenting signs and symptoms may be similar and the principles of treatment will be consistent irrespective of the eventual expected outcome. It will have been seen that these patients have the most profound injuries as all of the major systems of the body will be affected. There will usually be bony injury involving either a fracture or fracture dislocation which will be stable or unstable, the latter giving rise to the opportunity for more cord injury if not handled well. There may be severe pain from the site of injury. The intercostal muscles will be paralysed with the diaphragm affected in an injury at cervical vertebrae 3, 4 or 5 with a dramatic fall in the patient's respiratory function. In cervical injuries all four limbs will have sensory and motor loss in a complete transection of the cord, or if the lesion is incomplete a variety of different combinations. The skin is therefore vulnerable to damage from excessive pressure and pressure sores can develop in the first few hours following injury.

The sympathetic nervous system will also be affected with a reduction in blood pressure, kidney function and temperature regulation. The patient is therefore hypotensive, will have a reduced urinary output and will be poikilothermic, that is, takes his body temperature from the ambient temperature. There may be very reduced bowel functions and paralytic ileus is a common occurrence. The bladder will be unable to empty with eventual retention of urine.

Bleeding will take place at the level of injury and can continue for some time; there will also be contusion and oedema. This, if extensive, can confuse the neurological picture when it appears that the level of the lesion is extending up the cord with serious repercussions if in the cervical level as it can lead to more diaphragmatic involvement and severe respiratory distress.

In addition, and most importantly if we are to understand the nature of the condition thoroughly, consideration has to be given to the effects on the brain of the severe reduction in sensory and motor activity. This is most marked in the patient with an injury to the cervical spine where the only inputs left are those of sight, smell, hearing and taste. As a rule, therefore, the brain appears to react in a way which is fairly predictable; the level of activity is reduced considerably and patients exhibit the results in sleep, lassitude and a lack of interest in their immediate surroundings. Although this is essentially a physiological response some believe that there is an element of a subconscious psychological response which gives the time necessary for a coping mechanism to be developed.

MEDICAL TREATMENT

This is directed towards making the patient's condition as 'stable' as possible as soon as possible as it is only then that planned care can take place. It is here that effective rehabilitation begins, not as a concept to be injected into the care at a time in the future but from the very beginning.

The priorities of medical intervention will be decided if they are not altogether obvious. For example, the patient with a cervical lesion with sufficient respiratory distress to make his situation life threatening will not need his spinal alignment adjusted as the first priority, although this will need to be attempted later in line with other priorities. Such patients may require intubation or tracheostomy and positive pressure ventilation with regular estimation of blood gas levels. If there are other injuries these may be a greater priority than the spinal injury, for example haemothorax, penetrating wounds of the abdomen, head injury etc., and these are not necessarily uncommon.

Various techniques may be used to make the fracture or fracture-dislocation stable. The whole philosophy varies from one Spinal Injury Centre to the next but in the main the United Kingdom tends to be more conservative, that is, less interventionist than other countries. Reduction of a dislocation is usually therefore attempted by careful positioning and/or traction rather than surgery.

REDUCTION OF OEDEMA

A few centres believe that much of the permanent damage to the spinal cord is the result of bleeding and oedema into the spinal canal and that any reduction to this phenomena will aid cord recovery. Surgery takes place to insert a fine bore cath-eter into the spinal canal to bathe the affected area with very cold sterile fluid as an aid to minimise oedema, rather like the external cold compress as used in First Aid and sports medicine. Results of these trials are as yet inconclusive.

'SPINAL SHOCK'

Following trauma, the spinal cord below the level of the lesion shows an absence of activity which is the result of what has been described as 'spinal shock'. It is this phenomena that gives rise to the immediate problems of bowel and bladder symptoms which will last for perhaps the first initial week. Thereafter the symptoms may change depending on the level of the injury and the degree of cord damage. Paralytic ileus is treated usually by the traditional methods of intravenous infusion and gastric aspiration through a Ryles tube until bowel sounds return. Gastric distension is to be avoided as this can exacerbate an already depleted respiratory function. At this time care of the mouth is particularly important with the use of frequent lip-moistening techniques, lemon juice drops and small sips of fluid being used to retain the balance within the oral mucosa. Once abdominal activity returns then fluids will need to be given liberally as detailed in the section under bladder care.

Within this period of spinal shock, reflex activity in the spinal cord below the level of the lesion is absent although the injury may be an upper motor neurone lesion (usually above the level of the first lumbar vertebra). The recovery from spinal shock is usually heralded by the return of some reflex activity which is harnessed for use in developing the treatment of the bowel and bladder. In lesions below lumbar 1, which are lower motor neurone lesions, reflex activity does not recur and this distinction is of importance and needs to be understood if the right techniques are to be used in the patient's total care as it conditions the care of the bladder and bowel.

It is the return of reflex activity that gives a guide to the respiratory function of the patient as the neurological picture is now clearer after oedema and trauma has been reduced. It may be that assisted respiration can be discontinued although in very high cervical lesions this may have to continue indefinitely. Diaphragm pacing to produce ventilation in a tetraplegic patient with upper motor neurone lesion of the phrenic nerve has been tried. This system is implanted to pace the left and right hemi-diaphragms alternatively and removes the need for positive pressure ventilation.

SKULL TRACTION

This is used in cervical spine injuries with calipers inserted into the temporal bones under local anaesthesia. Crutchfield or Cones' calipers are usually used. The head of the bed is elevated and a 7 or 9 kg weight is suspended over the end of the bed and traction arranged in a way that facilitates reduction, either in flexion, extension or hyper-extension, dependent upon the bony picture at X-ray. Rolls of sorbo rubber will help to support the neck at the cervical curve and a fenestrated sorbo rubber pad covered by a pillow case is used to relieve pressure on the occiput. X-rays are taken at intervals until the reduction is secured and the weight is then reduced to about 5 kg and the neck supported in the position that maintains the reduction. Traction is continued until the bony injury is healed and further damage cannot occur. Exceptionally, an operation may be performed which may involve open reduction and fusion but is usually delayed until the patient is deemed to be fit for a general anaesthetic. Very exceptionally, if there is clear clinical evidence of instability then early operation can take place. The nursing care of patients with skeletal traction is dealt with below.

DORSO-LUMBAR FIXATION

Again practice differs, with various techniques being used ranging from early operation and internal fixation to later operation and either internal fixation or fusion. Most clinicians accept that surgery takes place only in a situation where clear indication of a positive benefit to the patient's neurological or orthopaedic condition is expected to result rather than the criteria of having a good appearance at X-ray.

Most centres use the techniques of positioning in bed, supporting the natural curves by pillows strategically placed and allow the natural forces of gravity to exert their influence on the bony disruption.

NURSING CARE

It is somewhat artificial to separate this from what has been described earlier as the patient will require nursing care throughout a particular medical treatment. However, it is considered that a diary of events as enumerated above will help rather than hinder the process of understanding of what is likely to happen to the patient from the earliest time following admission through to discharge.

These patients will require unremitting care from the first moments; nursing care is the base on which the eventual outcome will hinge. Frequently, as has been described, the patient is gravely ill and will require intensive nursing care as for any other severely injured patient. Needless to say, the patient will need careful monitoring of all of his physiological systems but will also need the constant knowledge of the presence immediately at

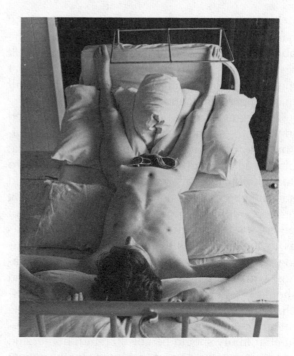

Fig. 23.5 The trunk and limbs are supported on many soft pillows, so that no bony prominence is subjected to pressure.

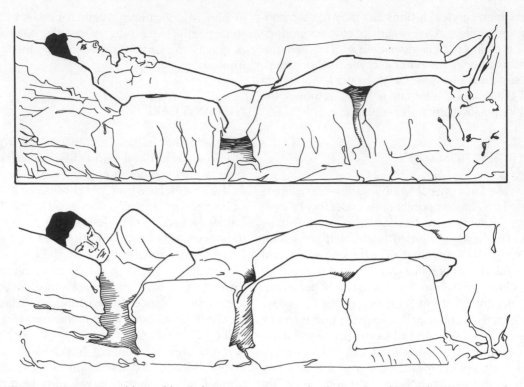

Fig. 23.6 In some parts of the world paraplegic patients are nursed on large sorbo-rubber pads as shown in these illustrations.

hand of a skilled well-trained nurse who will be able to sustain his spirit through the very difficult first few days following his injury. It is here that the seedbed of the relationship occurs which will make final rehabilitation a reality.

The relatives at this time will need to be involved in the care, to understand the nature of the condition, the course of events that are expected to take place and the part they are expected to play. To keep the relatives at arm's length at this time could and sometimes does, compromise the whole caring process. Although the neurological picture may not be complete enough to give a definite prognosis as to the final abilities of the patient and if it is too soon in the first few days to share this information with the family, reasonable targets can and should be set regarding the patient's eventual discharge. It is generally recognised that after a three months' stay in hospital the patient with a thoracolumbar injury should be able to return home, and about six months is a reasonable time for the patient with a cervical injury.

This information shared with the relatives allows them to have a positive approach to the whole care cycle rather than the negative approach which results in the only expectation being one of long-term institutional care.

It is now too that a start can be made on the contact necessary with the patient's general practitioner, district nurse, social worker and health visitor if they are to play their full part in ensuring a 'soft landing' when the patient returns home. Only by following such a system can the 'college of life' approach be sustained.

To say these patients require unremitting care from the first moment is easy enough as it is also easy to discuss the details of nursing care. But it is far from easy to carry it out; in fact it is difficult, arduous and exacting, requiring a relentless discipline and meticulous attention to detail from every member of the caring team and indeed in due course from the patient himself. It is imperative that every member of the nursing team (and again in due course the patient himself) learns the chain

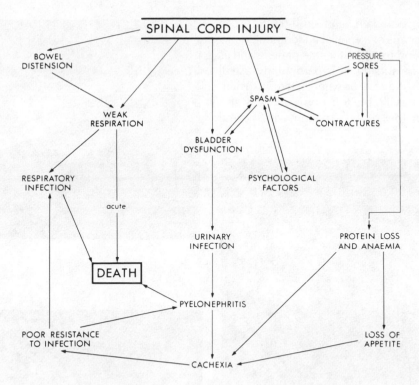

Fig. 23.7 Lack of attention to nursing detail can set up a vicious circle of complications, as shown in this diagram.

of events that can be set up by neglect of nursing detail and the vicious circle of complications that can ensue (see Fig. 23.7).

As has been mentioned earlier, it is imperative that every member of the team realise that in caring for these patients we have no second chance and the quality of care has to be of such a high order that nothing is left to chance, otherwise it will seriously interfere with recovery and rehabilitation or even endanger the patient's life.

TOTAL CARE

Although the typical clinical picture outlined above describes the medical and nursing problems it must be reiterated that no two patients are the same even if the clinical picture is exactly replicated. The method of approach will need to be varied depending on a view of the patient as a 'whole person' in the context of his emotional and social environment.

The patient will be admitted to a prepared area with all the items of equipment that are necessary at hand. He will be placed in either a standard hospital bed with a foam mattress of at least 10 cm thickness or some of the specialised turning beds available will be used. These are detailed below.

THE EGERTON-STOKE MANDEVILLE TILTING AND TURNING BED

This is fitted with a polyester foam mattress divided into three longitudinal hinged sections, controlled by electric motors placed on each side of the bed. Pressure on the appropriate button elevates one section of the mattress so that the patient is tilted gently into the right or left lateral semi-supine position while remaining in the centre of the bed.

Additional support for the trunk and positioning of the limbs by means of pillows is also shown in Fig. 23.8, and the head or foot of the bed is easily tilted by means of a hand-crank or by means of an additional motor; the head and foot rails can be removed when necessary for nursing attention or for X-rays to be taken, and skull-traction can be applied by means of a special attachment.

This bed is comfortable for the patient and is a valuable aid to nursing; it is particularly useful where turning is difficult or where there is insufficient manpower available to carry it out. It is also of great benefit to the paralysed patient who is cared for at home.

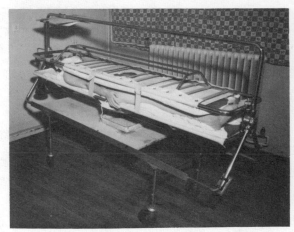

A

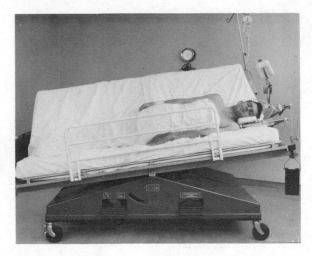

Fig. 23.8 The Egerton-Stoke Mandeville tilting and turning bed—Mark II—provides turning to either side by up to 65 degrees and tilt head up or down by 15 degrees. Accessories include a skull traction unit (devised by Sir Ludwig Guttmann) as shown in this illustration. (With kind permission of Egerton Hospital Equipment Ltd.)

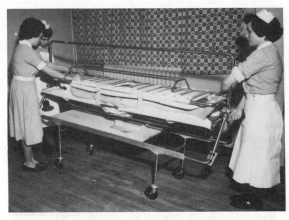

B

STRYKER BED

The Stryker turning bed can be a useful piece of apparatus for treatment and nursing care in cases of fracture of the spine with paraplegia (Allan, 1984), especially in high lesions and in those requiring skull traction (Figs 23.9A, B, C and D). It is not often used in the United Kingdom but a description is included here because it may be the only nursing aid available, e.g. in developing countries. The great advantage is that the patient can be turned quickly, easily and with minimal disturbance as he lies between the two halves of the bed like the filling in a sandwich (Figs 23.9A, B and C). The disadvantage is that the patient may feel very frightened and lonely (Robertson, 1978) and can see only the ceiling in one position and only the floor in the other.

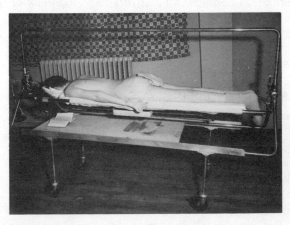

C

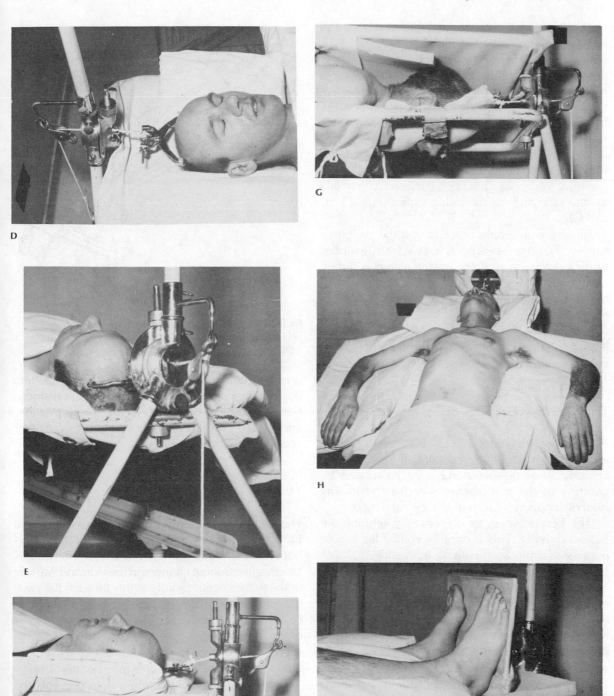

Fig. 23.9 **A.** The upper stretcher is strapped into position before turning. Note: an improved model of this apparatus is now available. **B.** Turning is easily carried out by a nurse standing at each end of the bed. In this illustration a third nurse steadies the patient's head. **C.** The patient is now lying prone for treatment of the skin of the back. **D–G.** Skeletal traction applied. **H–I.** Arm-supports and a footboard are also supplied. Stiffness of the shoulders must be prevented.

The Stryker bed consists of a wheeled trolley of tubular steel to which are attached two stretchers which can be clamped together by a simple screw device. Both stretchers are covered by canvas strips padded with sorbo-rubber on which the patient lies. Pillows can also be used where necessary. In the supine position, the patient lies on the lower stretcher, and the perineal region can be reached for nursing purposes by unfastening the canvas sling under the buttocks (Fig. 23.9B). For the prone position, the upper stretcher is provided with a hole for the face and for the pubic region (Figs 23.9C and G).

Turning is a simple procedure; if the patient is supine, the upper stretcher is screwed into position, turning straps are applied, and the patient is turned as shown in Figs 23.9A, B and C). To return to the prone position, the procedure is simply reversed.

Arm-supports and a footboard are also supplied (Figs 23.9H and I). Stiffness of the shoulders must be prevented.

THE KEANE ROTA-REST BED

This bed was developed in Eire (Keane, 1971) and additional models are continually being developed. The one shown in Fig. 23.10 appears by courtesy of the manufacturers and the following brief description is taken from their catalogue.

'The bed achieves its objective by keeping the patient moving. This is done by rolling the whole mattress frame and patient from side to side (approximately 55 degrees each way). The process is continuous, each complete cycle taking eight minutes. This relieves the nursing staff of the repetitive routine of manually turning the patient every two to three hours. The patient is prevented from sliding sideways off the bed by means of upholstered side supports.

The bed is supplied complete with mattress, pillow and all the necessary upholstery, which is covered in washable PVC cloth.'

These beds are, however, only aids to patient management and not essential pre-requisites.

The position of the patient in bed is a vital nursing responsibility and must be checked following any

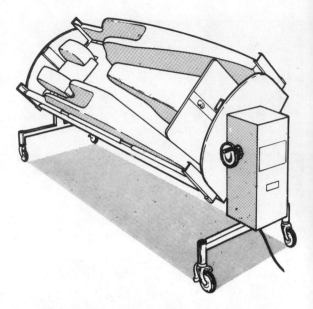

Fig. 23.10   The Keane Rota-rest bed. (With kind permission of Hugh Steeper (Roehampton) Ltd.)

nursing attention the patient receives. Correct positioning contributes to an even weight distribution, reducing the risk of pressure sore formation, and reducing the risk of joint contractures and other conditions such as drop-foot.

TURNING

The patient's position will require to be changed from the very beginning at two-hourly intervals both day and night. Turning is in fact of vital importance, since trophic changes in the skin and wasting of the tissues occur rapidly at this time. In the past, pressure sores in the paraplegic were thought to be inevitable; this is no longer true, but neglect of the turning regime can to this day result in sores such as those seen in the patient depicted in Fig. 23.11; later, four-hourly turns may be sufficient.

The object of regular turning is to prevent sustained pressure on any one part and subsequent pressure sores; during the turning procedure the whole body and in particular the sacrum, ischial tuberosities, trochanters and other bony prominences are inspected carefully; any flushing or discolouration of the skin is noted and that part must be relieved from further pressure at all costs. Once

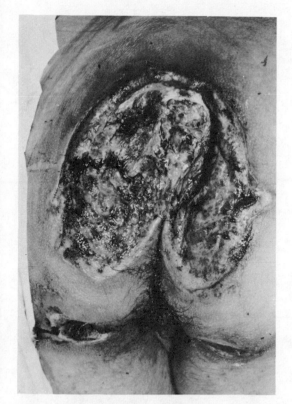

Fig. 23.11 The pressure sores seen in this patient occurred in the first 48 hours following injury.

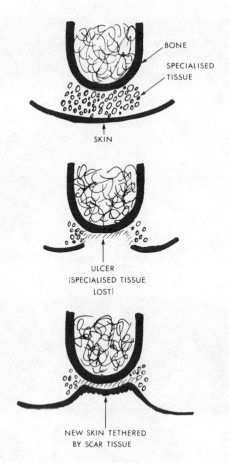

BONE

SPECIALISED TISSUE

SKIN

ULCER (SPECIALISED TISSUE LOST)

NEW SKIN TETHERED BY SCAR TISSUE

Fig. 23.12 Illustration of the vulnerability of the skin in a healed pressure sore (see text).

the skin breaks down, e.g. over the ischial tuberosity, specialised weight-bearing tissue is lost, and an ulcer appears. Even if this heals, the new skin is tethered by scar tissue, and is forever in danger of breaking down again (Fig. 23.12).

Moreover, pressure sores act as an irritant and increase muscle spasm and contractions; further, draining sores lead to dehydration, anaemia and loss of body protein. Eventually the patient may be seen to be in an emaciated, devitalised, exhausted state called cachexia. Sometimes a pressure sore will become so deep as to invade a neighbouring joint, e.g. the hip joint. Treatment of pressure sores by excision of underlying tissues or by skin-grafting operations is sometimes required combined with excellent nursing care to facilitate healing and to prevent further complications.

METHOD OF TURNING

Carefully explain to the patient both the procedure

and the need for it. It is usual to have a system which ensures that everyone knows which position is next: one that has been used successfully is left side, right side, back. This ensures there is no confusion and each skin area is therefore relieved of pressure for two or four hours until the patient is placed in that position again. Sometimes a position has to be omitted if there are contra-indications but this makes the skin especially vulnerable and should be avoided if possible.

Assemble the turning team and reassure the patient; we will assume that he is lying on his left side (Fig. 23.13A).

At least four people are required, working smoothly as a team; the leader stands at the patient's right hand; note that the limb is supported in its entirety as the pillow is removed (Fig. 23.13B). The four members of the team now place their arms

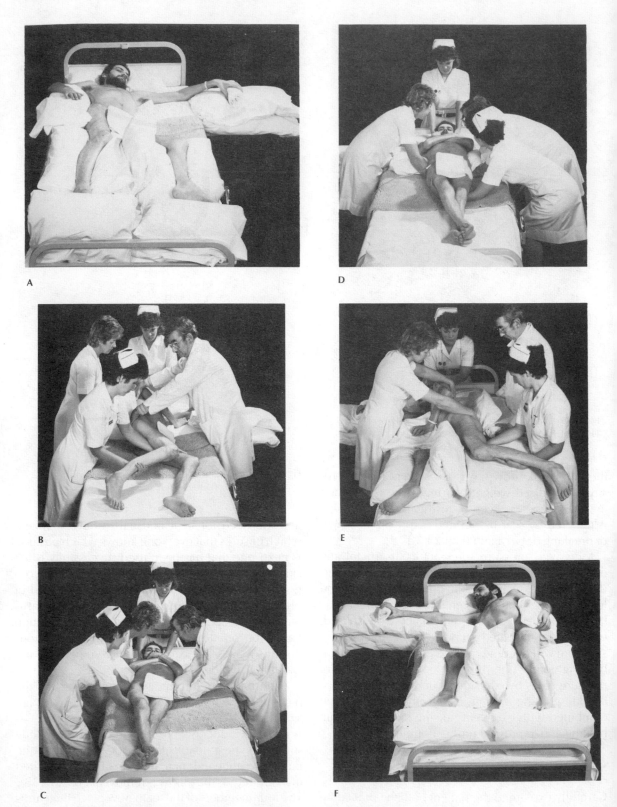

A

B

C

D

E

F

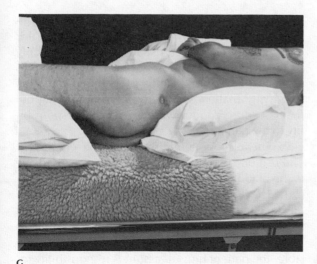

G

Fig. 23.13 A–G. Turning a tetraplegic patient (see text).

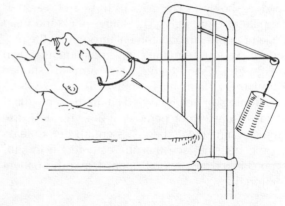

Fig. 23.14 Skeletal traction applied for fracture of the spine in the cervical region.

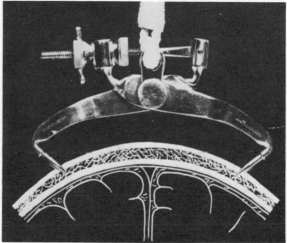

A

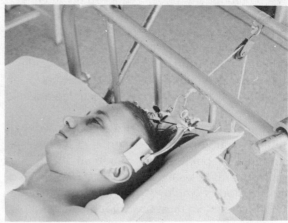

B

Fig. 23.15 A, B. Crutchfield calipers *in situ* in the outer table of the skull.

beneath the patient (Fig. 23.13C); if he is able, he clasps his arms on his chest and holds his head forward, otherwise a fifth person is needed to support the head (Fig. 23.13C). At a command, he is lifted all in one piece to the side of the bed and smoothly rolled on to his side (Fig. 23.12D and E) while the alignment of the spine is not disturbed. The lower leg is then gently flexed at the hip and knee and the upper one is held in extension; both feet are held at right-angles to the leg (Fig. 23.13F). It will be seen from Fig. 23.13C that the patient is nursed naked except for a small towel over the genital area (pyjama jackets and other garments are easily wrinkled, soiled or soaked with sweat), and the draw-sheet and pillows are kept absolutely dry, smooth, and free from crumbs, wrinkles or creases at all times. A cradle is usually required to keep the bedclothes off the feet and before leaving the bedside be sure that the catheter if in situ is not kinked and is not pressing into any part of the body. In some centres the penis is taped to the abdominal wall to avoid penile-scrotal fistula. Finally, leave the patient comfortable with his locker and belongings within reach.

If the patient has skeletal traction the following applies: Figs 23.14 and 23.15A and B show the skull calipers in situ; daily inspection of these is essential. Turning is carried out as a two-hourly ritual as already discussed for paraplegia. The turning team assembles, and the team leader holds the head as shown in Fig. 23.13A to G and reassures the patient constantly. The spine, neck and head are kept in the same alignment throughout the procedure. To turn from the supine position as shown in Figs 23.13C and D the nurses' arms are slipped below the patient as is shown in Fig. 23.13E. 'Positioning' in bed is carried out in the same manner as discussed for paraplegia and again, a dry, smooth, immaculate bed is essential. Before leaving the bedside, see that the catheter, if in situ, is not kinked or pressed upon; leave the patient comfortable.

GENERAL HYGIENE

The daily toilet routine for these patients will not be discussed in detail since so much has been written earlier in this book on this aspect of the care of the helpless and the immobilised patient (Chs 5 and 9). It goes without saying that this applies here; in particular, scrupulous attention to the daily toilet of the genitalia is imperative: it is often helpful in the interests of hygiene to clip the pubic hair, but actual shaving of the part should be avoided.

CARE OF THE BLADDER

For the first 48 hours after injury, the patient is often profoundly shocked and treatment of the paralysed bladder and bowel is not usually attempted at this stage. At first, in 'spinal shock' there is retention of urine, but later there is distension with overflow. Various regimes can be adopted; intermittent catheterisation is the method of choice nowadays; otherwise, continuous drainage by means of an indwelling catheter which is connected to a sealed bag is used.

Sometimes a daily bladder washout is ordered. The technique of catheterisation is described and illustrated in publications named in the Bibliography (Hardy & Elson, 1976; Jones, 1977). Whatever method is employed, permanent damage to the urinary system must be avoided by the following means:

1. Scrupulous, infallible, aseptic technique must be strictly adhered to at all times. Catheterisation procedures are sometimes carried out in a special dressing room, rather than in an open ward. In some centres, catheterisation is carried out only by medical staff; in others, nurses or ward orderlies are specially trained in this procedure. The thing that really matters is that the person carrying out the procedure is fully aware of his or her responsibility to the patient.

2. The utmost gentleness must be employed. The use of force may result in permanent damage to the bladder mucosa.

3. The fluid intake-and-output is measured daily and accurately recorded. The urine is examined frequently. Any abnormality, or fall in output is reported to the surgeon at once. As soon as possible, the patient himself assumes responsibility for his fluid chart.

4. Rise of temperature, rigor or other signs of urinary infection are reported to the surgeon at once. In the tetraplegic patient, the temperature chart may be an unreliable guide due to loss of body temperature control.

Antibiotics are prescribed when required.

It should be mentioned again that once urinary infection has occurred the patient is thereafter always liable to a 'flare-up' of the condition; chronic urinary infection eventually leads to pyelonephritis.

5. Distension of the bladder and stagnation of urine must not occur; the aim of treatment is to establish a modified bladder activity which results in a definite act of micturition; this prevents back-pressure on the kidneys and also prevents precipitate from collecting in the bladder; in the later stages of treatment, micturition can sometimes be initiated manually by gentle compression of the lower abdomen or some other stimulation. Sometimes there is insufficient relaxation of the urethral sphincter and a high residue of stagnant urine is left in the bladder, to form a potent source of infection. Operative treatment is sometimes required, either a trans-urethral resection of the bladder neck or sphincterotomy. Uro-dynamic investigations are of inestimable value in determining the treatment required to ensure the bladder is completely emptied at each act of micturition.

6. A high fluid intake (3000 ml daily) is absolutely imperative to prevent the formation of renal calculi and subsequent infection. From the first,

the patient must fully understand the necessity for this; five pints of fluid in 24 hours is rather more than most people are accustomed to and drinks must be 'spaced out', and given in various forms according to the patient's likes and dislikes. As soon as possible, paraplegics should assume responsibility for their own fluid intake and output and for recording this on their charts. 'A glass of water hourly' is a good maxim. The nurse has a special responsibility with regard to tetraplegic patients, who cannot 'help themselves'; drinks must be palatable, pleasantly served and given by means of a straw or bent glass rod which is kept for the patient's exclusive use. In the event of abdominal complications, with vomiting, when the patient cannot take fluid by mouth, it must be given by the intravenous route.

TYPES OF BLADDER

The condition of the paralysed bladder is described under two main headings, viz.

1. The automatic bladder is found when the reflex arc is intact, i.e. in upper motor neurone lesions, when the bladder can be trained to empty in response to a stimulus such as supra-pubic tapping, stroking the thighs or stimulation of the rectum or of the genital organs; in time the patient learns the stimulus which will evoke the act of micturition. Unfortunately in the male patient such a stimulus can also induce priapism, that is, a penile erection, which interferes with the mechanics of micturition.

2. The autonomous bladder, on the other hand, is found in lower motor neurone lesions where there is no reflex activity, but since the abdominal muscles may have some power the bladder can be emptied by straining and by manual pressure on the lower abdomen.

BLADDER TRAINING

This can be a difficult, arduous, painstaking and exacting exercise, not only for the nurse but for the patient; but since successful re-training of the bladder often spells not only social and economic independence but freedom from urinary complications, it is infinitely worthwhile. If the reflex arc is intact and intermittent catheterisation is being carried out, the first indication that bladder training can commence in earnest will be that the patient voids in between the intermittent catheterisation intervals. Stimulation to capitalise on this situation must then be continued but supplemented by catheterisation. Eventually the need for catheterisation will diminish once the automatic bladder is functioning well. If the patient has an indwelling catheter then the catheter is clipped off and released at 2, 3 or 4 hourly intervals, once 'spinal shock' has resolved.

Later, the catheter is removed for an hour and the patient attempts to pass urine voluntarily. Using manipulations to initiate micturation, the patient is helped and encouraged to find a stimulus which he can use himself to invoke his act of micturition. On re-catheterisation, the amount of residual urine remaining in the bladder is measured, and if this is not more than 100 ml the catheter is removed for longer and longer periods until the patient can remain dry for as long as 4 to 5 hours. At the same time, distension of the bladder with back-pressure and dilatation of the ureters must be avoided at all costs because of the danger of hydro-nephrosis. Urinary investigations such as cystometry or an intravenous pyelogram may be ordered, and general malaise with rise of temperature must call a halt to the proceedings. Any such set-back means a new start and sometimes, several separate attempts over a period of some weeks is required before a satisfactory regime is established. When the catheter is finally discarded altogether, it is usually considered necessary to assess the residual urine at weekly intervals, and any subsequent urinary infection may require treatment by re-insertion of the catheter, bladder wash-outs and administration of antibiotics. In lower motor neurone lesions with an autonomous bladder a more positive approach has to be followed. Urine is not voided reflexly and the patient has therefore to make a conscious effort on a timed basis to empty the bladder. Straining and expression of the bladder is of more value than stimulation but 'training' to empty the bladder is more difficult as the patient has to make a conscious effort on every occasion.

CARE OF THE BLADDER IN A FEMALE PATIENT

During the acute stage, the management of the female bladder is the same as already discussed for the male; once more, infallible aseptic technique and the utmost gentleness are imperative. However, the management of urinary incontinence in the female in the later stages of treatment is not so easy as in the male, in whom it is relatively easy to fit an unobstrusive urinal worn under the trousers (Figs 23.16A–D).

Pratt (1971) reports that bladder training can succeed in 60 to 65 per cent of women and describes a method of expressing the female bladder. In general, however, if bladder re-training fails then the alternatives are as follows:

(a) To continue with intermittent catheterisation, the patient with 'good hands', that is a paraplegic, learns how to undertake this for themselves. Non-sterile techniques may be employed.
(b) To place an indwelling catheter in the bladder, clamped and released at 4 hourly intervals.
(c) An ileal bladder is sometimes formed when the ureters are transplanted into a detached loop of ileum to form a reservoir and the urine drains out into a special bag worn under the clothes. This is rarely used now; The paraplegic patient soon learns to keep the skin and urinal clean herself (Fig. 23.17).

N.B. In some intractable bladder problems implantation of electrodes for the stimulation of the sacral 2, 3 and 4 anterior roots of the cauda equina has been tried in some centres.

RE-TRAINING THE BOWEL

In the paraplegic, the use of mild laxatives, or small, mild enemata may be necessary in the early stages but, as soon as possible, an attempt is made to train the bowel to empty at the same time each day, or even every second day. While the patient is confined to bed, suppositories are inserted at a regular time and the patient is placed on his side on an incontinence pad. Bedpans are never used because they damage insensitive skin; defaecation is often assisted by abdominal massage which the patient learns in time to carry out himself. As soon as possible, the patient is wheeled to the lavatory on a sani-chair fitted with a rubber cushion to protect the skin (Fig. 23.18).

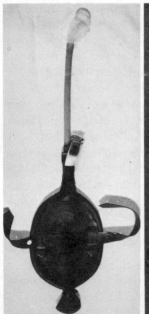 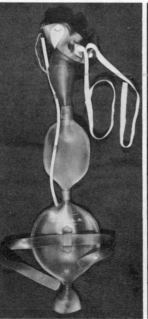 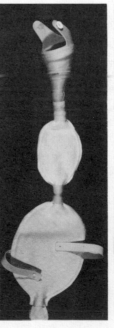 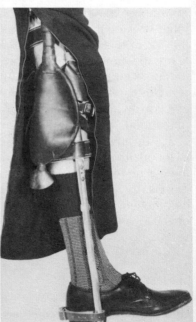

A   B   C   D

Fig. 23.16 A–D. Male urinals of various types.

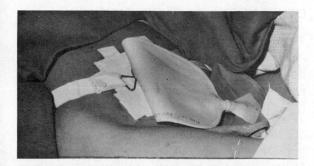

Fig. 23.17 Urinal for use with an ileal bladder.

A definite regime and a 'habit' time, either morning or evening, is essential since it means that the patient is free during the day-time for other activities including, eventually, those directed towards his discharge from hospital. As rehabilitation proceeds, the patient learns to transfer from wheelchair to lavatory himself and, at this stage, should decide for himself at what time of day he wishes his bowels to move and how best this can be fitted in to his routine on return to his home and his job. Many patients prefer an evening session in the lavatory; the important thing is that the paraplegic with useful upper limbs assumes responsibility for his own bowels at the earliest possible moment. The importance of his fluid intake and of his diet cannot be too heavily stressed; dietary indiscretions lead to constipation or diarrhoea.

In the tetraplegic, who cannot help himself, a regular bowel movement into an incontinence pad must be established by the use of suppositories inserted at a regular time (e.g. in the early morning), combined with abdominal massage. Again, the fluid intake and the diet are of vital importance; unfortunately these patients often develop a reluctance to accept fluids and have a fickle appetite. Abdominal distension must be avoided and sometimes the careful use of a flatus tube is indicated.

If possible, routine manual evacuation of faeces is avoided especially in the tetraplegic who is permanently dependent upon another for this service. If bowel training fails however, impacted faeces may be present, with dribbling incontinence and constant soiling, and manual evacuation by insertion of a gloved lubricated finger into the rectum is the only remedy. Patients can be taught to perform manual evacuation with the aid of a mirror (Pratt, 1970). Again it must be stressed that the difference between the nature of the lesion, that is whether it is upper or lower motor neurone has a great deal of bearing on the management.

In the upper motor neurone lesion the insertion of a suppository will, after a short space of time, produce a reflex response which empties the bowel well. Defaecation is, therefore, on the whole a reasonably short procedure even when the patient is lying down. Sitting on a toilet in an upright position aid this process.

However, with a lower motor neurone lesion, in the absence of reflex activity, much more effort is required, including straining and abdominal massage to get the complete bowel evacuation that ensures an 'accident free' day.

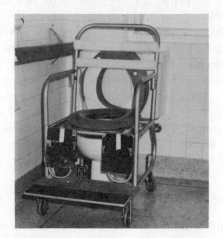

Fig. 23.18 A sani-chair with protective rubber cushion.

SPASM

Spasm is the name given to involuntary contraction of muscle groups which occurs in an upper motor neurone lesion following recovery from spinal shock. Sadly, sometimes patients misunderstand the involuntary movements as some herald of motor recovery, so adequate preparation of the patient to expect 'spasm' and an explanation of the meaning is of particular importance.

Not only is it disagreeable or even painful for the patient, but as in any condition where spastic muscles hold a joint in a deformed position for any length of time, a contracture of that joint is certain to occur, for example, flexion and adduction of the hip or flexion of the knee. Excess spasticity, if noted during nursing attention, should be reported to the surgeon at once. Continuous attention to the correct posture of the patient in bed is vital in the prevention of spasm, particularly the position of the foot at a right-angle to the leg and pressed against a firm support as shown in Fig. 23.19.

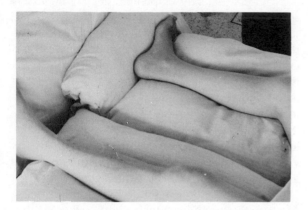

Fig. 23.19   A close-up of the feet supported by firm pillows, without pressure on bony points.

The physiotherapist may employ special measures to reduce the spasm, such as 'brushing' opposing groups of muscles. Sometimes the surgeon will order gentle 'tethering' of a spastic limb by means of a sheet. Early weight-bearing is valuable in the prevention of spasm. In this connection, a tilt-table is a valuable item of equipment.

The presence of pressure sores, distension of the bowel, bladder distension and infection, mental agitation and joint contractures all tend to increase spasm; conversely, spasm also exacerbates these complications, so that the presence of one complication predisposes the unfortunate patient to the others, as shown in Fig. 23.20. The obvious moral is that these vicious circles must never be started.

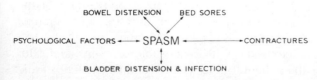

Fig. 23.20   Muscle-spasm is increased by other complications, and other complications increase spasm—another vicious circle.

OTHER NURSING CONSIDERATIONS

The care outlined above deals with the patient as a series of systems which need to be maintained if the complications that can occur are to be avoided. This is perhaps unfortunate but should not detract from the concept of treating the patient as a whole person. The challenge in the nursing of patients with spinal injury is to integrate the care in meaningful ways and to begin the involvement of the patient in his own well-being as soon as he is capable of doing this. Constant vigilance is required to see that the patient is given the support that is required, for this reason visiting must be as flexible as possible to integrate the family into the caring process.

The patient will, for at least the first six to twelve weeks, be confined to bed until the bony injury has healed, and during this time increasing mental stimulation will be required. Here the other members of the team also play their part, especially the occupational therapist and even carefully vetted volunteers. The latter can do much to relieve the inevitable boredom of being in bed provided their input is carefully supervised by the ward sister.

NUTRITION

This deserves special mention because the tetraplegic patient depends upon others for every mouthful of food, and good nutrition is imperative whatever the level of injury. Again, visiting friends and relatives can be very helpful in this connection. In order to receive an adequate intake of food and the vitally important quantity of fluid, the tetraplegic patient must be fed patiently, unhurriedly, cheerfully, with every drink and meal of the day, supplemented by Complan feeds, if ordered. These patients often become extremely fussy about food but the vital importance of a full balanced diet and copious fluid intake must be pointed out. As in other similar cases, inability to accept food or fluid by mouth may necessitate tube-feeding or intravenous therapy.

PSYCHOLOGICAL SUPPORT

Inevitably, many questions will be asked by the patient regarding his condition and the response from all members of the team must be consistent. The doctor has a key role to play in this, sharing with the team the policy that applies and ensuring that everyone understands what information has been given to the patient and what the relatives have been told. Psychological support is very necessary but has to be based on realism rather than the platitudinous mutterings of an inadequate carer. Sometimes professional help from a psychologist or psychiatrist may be necessary but in the author's experience this is the exception rather than the rule, as is the use of large doses of anti-depressant drugs. Rehabilitation is not a concept that applies to only the patient's physical condition but to the whole person and it is, therefore, imperative that the patient is in the mood to tackle the learning of the new physical skills essential to his wellbeing as soon as he is able to get up.

It has been noted (Starrett, 1961, quoted by Wilson-Barnett, 1979) that long-term paraplegic patients sometimes display defences such as denial, hostility and aggression, although the initial onset of the condition was associated with high levels of anxiety caused by disruption of the body image.

It has also been noted that many nurses find working with these patients very stressful and require special consideration and support from their seniors and teachers (Jacobs, 1982).

For the paraplegic patient, total independence is a realistic goal which most feel able to grasp and achieve; for the tetraplegic patient this is much more difficult. In most cases some dependence on others is going to be necessary and the skill lies in convincing the patient that this does not make him unique in any way because all of us have some dependence on others, be it physical, social, emotional or psychological.

SPINAL CORD INJURIES IN DEVELOPING COUNTRIES

It has been pointed out (Bedbrook, 1981) that 'it is unrealistic to expect developing countries to have either the facilities or the staff to look after patients to the usual high standard of a paraplegic centre in a rich country'. It is further pointed out, however, that 'much can be done by having fairly cheap additional equipment in the ordinary surgical wards, or better still, in a special ward or part of a ward for such paralysed patients'.

The nursing care required by these patients is identical to that required by those in rich countries, though as Sir George Bedbrook again points out, there are often added difficulties due to climate, to malnutrition and to lack of even simple facilities such as soap and water and drugs. Despite these difficulties, many patients are restored to a useful life by the devoted efforts of doctors, nurses and paramedical staff, and most important of all, by the patient's relatives.

Physiotherapy in spinal injury. 1. The early stages

This is outlined as follows:

1. Treatment of respiratory complications in cervical cord injury, assisted coughing.
2. Prevention of contractures and joint stiffness; other complications.
3. Later treatment in the gymnasium.
4. Transfers, walking and other activities.
5. Standing transfer in tetraplegia.

The successful rehabilitation of these patients depends on the integrated efforts of all hospital ward staff, and eventually on the patient's own attitude and efforts. The duties of the physiotherapist often overlap those of the nurses and she must form a close liaison and rapport with the ward Sister and her staff.

Physiotherapy treatment starts at once, on the day of the patient's admission. After the initial medical examination, and when nursing preliminaries have been completed, the physiotherapist is usually needed for attention to the limbs and joints and especially to the respiratory tract in cervical injuries.

Cervical cord injury

1. *The respiratory tract.* At the earliest opportunity, it is important to assess the patient's respiratory state by measuring the vital capacity with a spirometer. This information is needed at an early stage, so that subsequent improvement or deterioration of respiratory function can be detected. Skill and understanding are needed in measuring the vital capacity of a newly injured patient; with

experience, the physiotherapist learns to take into consideration the patient's mental state and the degree of his fatigue. Co-operation by the patient may be difficult to obtain if he is heavily sedated or if he is in a state of reduced awareness due to hypoxia. In a high cervical lesion, the vital capacity may be only a fraction of the normal value. The physiotherapist must record the figure daily, along with the position of the patient at the time, i.e. supine, or right or left lateral position.

Paralytic abdominal ileus. This is a common complication in the early stages of a cervical cord lesion. The abdominal distension restricts diaphragmatic movement, and so further reduces the vital capacity. If assisted coughing is applied too vigorously at this time, it may cause regurgitation of the gastric contents.

Expectoration difficulties. The muscles of the thorax and abdomen give the expulsive force to the act of coughing; in the tetraplegic, however, power in these muscles is lost, and if secretions are excessive, assisted coughing will be needed, particularly in the case of a heavy smoker. In these cases it is important to administer this treatment at frequent intervals during the day, and if necessary, at intervals throughout the night as well. Before giving assisted coughing, it is often necessary to percuss and vibrate the chest wall. At times, when secretions are difficult to clear, it may be necessary to put the patient in a head-low-tilt position. In positioning the patient for working on the chest, the assistance of the nursing staff may be required, and if the patient is on skull traction, a senior member of the nursing staff has to hold the head of the patient while the position is changed. The patient may become frightened and upset, as well as fatigued from the assisted coughing. For this reason 'little and often' is a better policy in giving coughing assistance rather than a prolonged and exhaustive period of treatment. It is also good practice to concentrate particularly on assisted coughing just before and just after a patient is turned by the nurses.

Assisted coughing can be given by an experienced nurse, if no physiotherapist is at hand at the moment of need; although it may appear simple to perform, it is in fact, a skill acquired by experience requiring manual dexterity and knack, as well as understanding of the individual patient.

Method. The heel of the one hand is placed on the epigastrium, below the arch of the front ribs and sternum (Fig. 23.21A). A firm thrust upwards and posteriorly, is made to synchronise with the patients attempts to cough. The other hand is placed on the chest wall, or over the sternum, giving further pressure and vibrations at the moment of coughing: in this way, the physiotherapist provides some of the expulsive coughing power which is usually derived from the contraction of the abdominal muscles. In patients where expectoration is difficult, it may be necessary to turn the patient into a semi-prone position when the assistance of several nurses is needed to hold the patient in this position.

Tracheostomy. In dealing with the tracheostomised patient, the physiotherapist must ensure

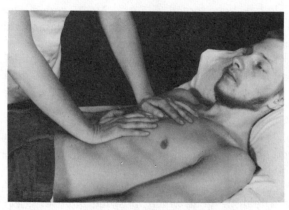

A

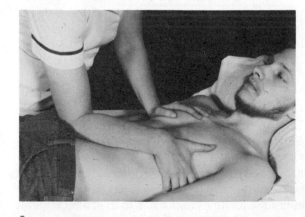

B

Fig. 23.21 A, B. Chest manipulations are essential for adequate ventilation of the lungs.

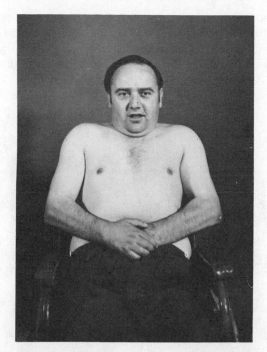

Fig. 23.22 The patient assists coughing by pressing on the upper abdomen.

that her visits to the bedside coincide with the nursing procedure of sucking out secretions. Vibration and percussion of the chest wall in a 'wet' patient will help to rid the bronchial tree and trachea of obstructing secretions; the physiotherapist may be asked to provide humidification.

Diaphragm failure. During the first few days following a very high cervical cord injury, the diaphragm may become weaker as the neurological level rises, so that the physiotherapist must be alert to this possibility. One side of the diaphragm may become paralysed before the other and if the patient is turned onto the side with the most activity this will be lost so that there may be danger of hypoxic collapse.

2. Prevention of contractures and joint stiffness.

Passive movements. The patient who is unfortunate enough to suffer from paralysis of the limb muscles will develop additional disability if contractures are allowed to occur; the physiotherapist has the paramount role in preventing these complications. Each joint of the affected limbs is moved passively through a full range of movement, at least twice a day. Joint range and muscle length are

maintained in this way, and circulation is also stimulated. If the flow of venous blood remains sluggish in the lower limbs, the serious complication of *deep vein thrombosis* may occur; passive movements, however, diminish this danger. When carrying out passive movements, the physiotherapist may be the first to observe the warm swelling of a lower limb which indicates the presence of a deep vein thrombosis. *Peri-articular ossification* causes loss of range of hip or knee movement and will be detected at the time passive movements are given. This is an unusual but important complication of paraplegia, which may substantially add to the disability by reducing the range of hip and knee movement, so that the patient is unable to assume a comfortable sitting position.

In many patients with cervical cord lesions, there is a loss of power in the triceps muscles, while power in biceps is still present. The physiotherapist must give assiduous attention to these elbows, since they are liable to develop severe contractures of the biceps muscles. The arms of these patients should not be allowed to remain flexed at the elbows for long periods. If the hands of a tetraplegic show any signs of oedema and limited range, a 'boxing glove' splint is applied to control the swelling, and the patient should be nursed with the hands in a slightly elevated position to assist venous drainage. The splints are removed at least twice daily, to check the skin and circulation to the fingers, and to perform essential passive movements.

Much can be done to promote improvement in muscles that are only partially paralysed. Active assisted movements are given to these muscles or muscle groups. Resisted exercises, including the use of weights and springs are appropriate when treating unaffected or only slightly weakened muscle (please see later treatment).

REHABILITATION AND RESETTLEMENT

The patient who happily recovers from his spinal injury and is restored to his family, his work and his place in society needs no mention here. But there are those who only partially recover, and those in whom no recovery of function is possible. On the other hand, improvement of function may proceed over a long period, and at no time during the course of treatment will the nurse make prognostications either to the patient or his relatives as to what his ultimate disability is likely to be, except in collaboration with the doctor in charge of the case.

Rehabilitation begins as soon as the general condition allows. It has been pointed out that the first preliminary need for successful rehabilitation is *optimum general health*. 'It is no good talking about rehabilitation to a patient who is febrile, toxic or profoundly anaemic.' (Jones, 1977.) The second preliminary requirement is strong rapport between the patient and members of the orthopaedic team who not only know him well but who also have knowledge of his home situation, family and employment (Jones, 1977). The paraplegic patient will commence exercises aimed at strengthening the muscles of the arms and shoulders. As soon as the sitting position is allowed, balance is taught in that position; transfer to a tilt table may be used to accustom the patient gradually to the upright position. A self-wheeled litter as shown in Fig. 23.23 is invaluable when the use of a wheelchair

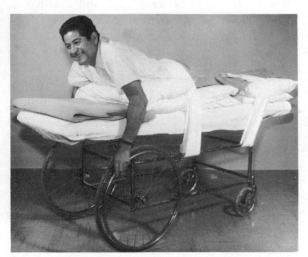

Fig. 23.23 A self-wheeled litter or 'prone gurney' provides mobility when the use of a wheelchair is contra-indicated. (With kind permission of Rancho los Amigos Hospital, Downey, California.)

is contra-indicated, e.g. where there are sacral sores. A special wheel-chair is ordered for each patient and it is important to remember that this is not simply a means of locomotion but an active

splint, as will be obvious to anyone who watches a group of paraplegic patients participating in competitive 'wheelchair sports' (Fig. 23.31). The wheelchair soon becomes an essential part of the

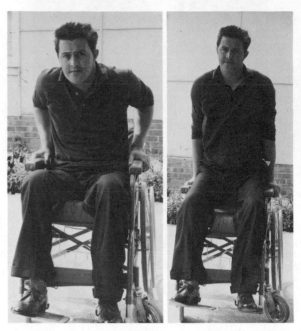

Fig. 23.24 When in a wheelchair, regular change of position is vital to avoid continuous pressure on bony joints. Note the zippered trousers.

patient's life, but it should be mentioned here that in low lesions its use should not rule out attempts at ambulation with or without braces (calipers) and crutches. Figure 23.32 shows a patient learning to manage his own braces. The assumption of the upright position helps to drain the urinary system by gravity and activity of this kind also helps to strengthen the skeleton and lessen the risk of pathological fractures. It also helps to prevent contractures. Moreover the assumption of an upright posture is of psychological benefit to the patient. Figure 23.30 shows a patient in the Oswestry standing frame.

From his first moment in a wheelchair the patient is taught to lift himself at hourly intervals so that the pressure on the sacrum and ischal tuberosities is relieved, as shown in Fig. 23.24. A tetraplegic patients who lacks the power to raise himself fully is taught to lean forward and to 'hitch' as shown in Figs 23.25A and B, otherwise he must be raised by the nurse at regular intervals in the manner

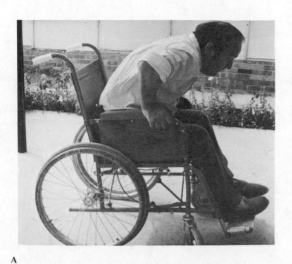

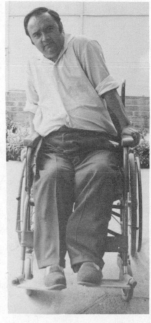

A
B

Fig. 23.25 A, B. The tetraplegic patient who has insufficient power in his limbs to raise himself from his wheelchair learns to lean forward and to 'hitch' the pelvis to relieve pressure on bony points.

shown in Fig. 23.26. At this stage, a rubber urinal may be worn under the clothing and the patient is taught to keep the urinal clean and free from odour: different types of urinal are shown in Figs 23.16A–D and a 'spare' should be available for each patient. As an alternative the successful use of long-term indwelling catheters has been reported (Westling, 1978) as has intermittent self-catheterisation by non-sterile technique (Whitfield, 1976). At this stage, the patient has learned to manage his own bowel and must, in fact, be in complete charge of this and all other aspects of his care before he leaves the hospital. Patients who can strain to some extent and who are able to sit on a lavatory usually respond to Dulcolax suppositories. Again, discipline in the matter of a regular habit, a balanced diet and a full fluid intake cannot be too heavily stressed. On the other hand, obesity must be avoided. Activities are increased each day and provided the bath-tub is accessible he learns to use this himself (Fig. 23.27), but in this connection the patient should be warned against the dangers of

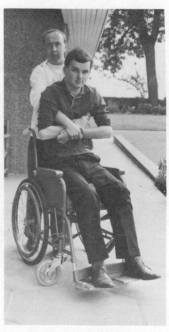

Fig. 23.26 The nurse must lift the tetraplegic patient who is unable to change his position unaided.

Table 23.1 Activities of daily living and the degree of function expected from patients with lesions at different levels of the spinal cord.

Function	Cord level C4	C5	C5–6	C6	C7	C8–T4	T4–S3
Eating	D	WD-1+	WD	1	1	1	1
Bathing	D	D	1+	1	1	1	1
Grooming							
Clean teeth	D	WD-1+	WD	1	1	1	1
Brush and comb hair	D	WD-1+	WD	1	1	1	1
Shave (men)	D	WD-1+	WD	1	1	1	1
Make-up (women)	D	WD-1+	WD	1	1	1	1
Wash	D	WD-1+	WD-1+	1	1	1	1
Dressing							
1. Upper limbs	D	D	WD	1+	1	1	1
2. Lower limbs	D	D	D	WD	1	1	1
Toilet							
Bladder	D	D	D	WD-1+	1+	1	1
Bowel	D	D	D	WD-1+	1+	1	1
Bed							
Sitting	D	D	D	1+	1+	1	1
Positioning	D	D	WD-1+	1+	1+	1	1
Transfer							
Chair/to bed	D	D	D	1+	1+	1	1
to toilet bowl	D	D	D	1+	1+	1	1
to car	D	D	D	1+	1+	1	1
Wheelchair							
Independent indoors	D	WD-1+	WD-1+	1	1	1	1
Independent outdoors	D	D	D	WD-1+	1+	1	1
	(electric chairs)						can walk with crutches and calipers

KEY: D = Completely dependent
     1 = Independent
WD = Performs with difficulty
1+ = Independent with nursing assistance or with device.

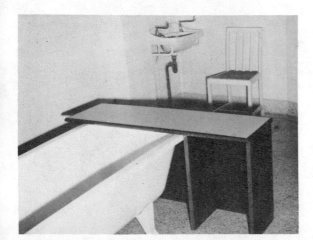

Fig. 23.27 Free access to the bathtub is aided by the wooden seat designed by a nurse and made by a hospital carpenter.

scalding; this also applies in the use of a shower. It is also important that the patient learns to inspect every part of his body *daily*, using a handmirror for inaccessible parts; the penis and scrotum should be inspected carefully, and medical advice sought at once if anything abnormal is noticed; epididymo-orchitis or penile-scrotal fistula is sometimes seen. *Turning* at least once or twice during the night is still necessary; patients whose arms are strong learn to turn themselves but the tetraplegic must be turned by his nurse or by some mechanical means.

Physiotherapy in spinal cord injury. 2. Later treatment in the gymnasium

1. *Sitting balance.* Most paraplegic and tetraplegic patients, especially the latter, may need several days to get accustomed to the upright sitting position. Balance is impaired owing to the paralysis of the trunk muscles. Moreover, after lying in bed for several weeks, the patient suffering from a high level cord lesion will be affected by postural hypo-

tension when he starts to sit up. The physiotherapist may have to use a tilt-table at first, to help a patient with a cervical lesion to make the adjustment by gradual stages, and the patient eventually adapts to vasomotor instability. Once this has occurred, and sitting balance is secure, the more active rehabilitation commences. One of the main objectives of this more strenuous treatment is to develop and maximise the power in the muscles that are not affected by the injury, or are only partially weakened. The physiotherapist, therefore, employs manual resisted exercises, or uses springs and weights. Press-ups are also used, and in the final stages rope-climbing and weight-lifting are among the exercises most often used.

2. *Mat work*, with the patient lying on the floor, is of importance in the treatment of the trunk muscles. All patients are given rolling exercises, and are taught to sit-up unassisted from the lying down position, although this may be beyond the scope of many patients with cervical lesions. Sitting balance and posture can be enhanced by the restoration of tone to the para-vertebral muscles. Treatment times fit in with catheterisation times, when people require intermittent catheterisation or attention on other aspects of bladder training. Control of excess spasticity in the trunk muscles contributes to better functioning of the automatic bladder and bowel.

3. *Further balancing development*. The physiotherapist sits the patient over the side of a low plinth, and also in long sitting on the floor mat, and he learns to balance unsupported; progress is made to throwing and catching a medicine ball in this position. Once secure sitting balance is achieved, the patient proceeds to learn self-dressing and to transfer from bed to chair etc.

4. *Transfers*. Although it will be impossible for some patients with cervical lesions to transfer unassisted from bed to chair etc., this ability should be attained by all patients with thoracic or lumbar lesions provided they are not elderly or overweight. Extra difficulty may be encountered by those who have also sustained upper limb injuries, by patients with short arms, and sometimes by the not-so-young female patients. As a preliminary to learning transfers, the power in the arms, shoulders, and trunk must be developed as fully as possible; regular practice is required in transferring from the

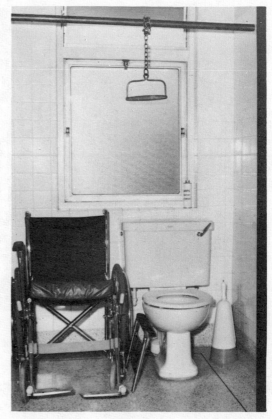

Fig. 23.28 Free access to the lavatory is essential for paralysed patients. This is provided by the 'monkey pole' placed above the lavatory.

wheelchair to the bed, to the bath, w.c. or into a car. There are many practical tips which the physiotherapist can impart, and 'know-how' is as important as muscular strength. Transfers must be achieved without dragging the buttocks along a surface which might cause skin abrasions and subsequent sores.

5. *Wheelchair drill*. The paraplegic patient should soon become well accustomed to his wheelchair; one of the first points in which he is instructed, is how to push up at frequent intervals in order to relieve pressure on the buttocks. Once he is able to manoeuvre the wheelchair easily and confidently indoors, he progresses to instruction in negotiating rough ground, grass, and how to get up and down curbs and slopes. Back-wheel balance is taught to the more athletic patients, and some acquire enough agility and confidence to propel the chair along on the rear wheels only. This

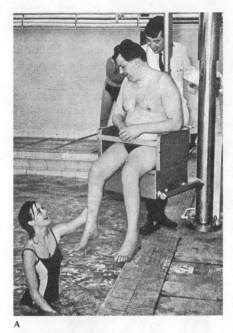 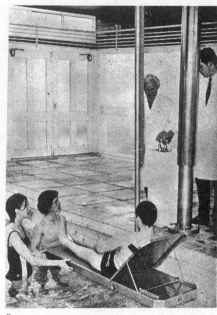

A   B

Fig. 23.29 A. B. Swimming is both enjoyable and therapeutic.

is extremely useful for traversing rough ground or for mounting a pavement.

6. *Swimming pool.* Exercise in the swimming pool is both useful and enjoyable to the paraplegic and tetraplegic patient. This activity can only be carried out when bowel training has succeeded so that function has become regular. Excess spasticity responds well to hydrotherapy. It is important to note that the tetraplegic is liable to become hypothermic, so that the temperature of the water must not be below 86° F.

7. *Sports.* Sporting activities are included in the rehabilitation of these patients, and can stimulate fresh interest and enthusiasm in addition to the therapeutic value obtained. Table-tennis, archery, bowls and basketball are among the most popular sports in which the wheelchair patient can participate.

8. *The standing frame* (Fig. 23.30). It is an important principle in the rehabilitation of both paraplegics and tetraplegics, that the patient must stand regularly. It combats the tendency to develop flexion contractures at the hips, knees and ankles, and it is valuable in moderating and controlling muscle tone. Regular weight-bearing encourages

the tone of bladder and bowel, and osteoporosis, with risk of pathological fractures is also prevented. Patients who use a standing frame, are provided with one for use at home. Patients with lower cervical lesions can usually be left to remain standing on their own, but those with a higher cervical injury will require a steadying hand to prevent them from falling sideways in the frame. The standing frame, is, on the whole, used for patients with cord lesion levels above D.12. Patients with lesions at lower levels than this are likely to gain more from walking exercises, with leg braces or calipers.

9. *Walking.* Although it is possible to train patients with lesions above T.12 to walk in calipers (Fig. 23.32), it has been found that once home, most of them give up doing this exercise, since they find it difficult to move over carpets and around furniture; also, putting on the calipers in order to stand or walk takes too much time. Patients with lesions at T.12 or below, however, are more likely to be able to develop caliper-walking well enough for useful locomotion to be achieved; this is particularly the case if some power is present in the muscles performing hip flexion. A four-point gait may be taught to some patients where one

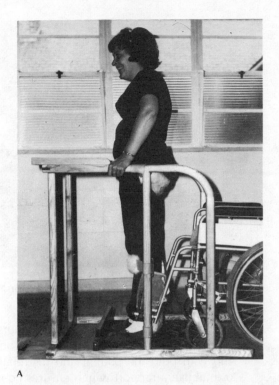

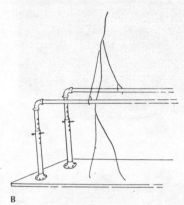

A

B

Fig. 23.30 **A.** The Oswestry standing frame. **B.** Parallel bars are used for practice in walking.

crutch is placed forward, followed by the opposite leg, followed by the second arm and crutch, and then the other leg; the patient then continues forward in this sequence. The alternative method of ambulation, is the 'swing through' gait, where the patient pushes his weight upwards and forward, on his elbow crutches, letting his legs swing forward, so that the feet are planted on the ground just in front of the crutches; when balanced securely in this position, the crutches are brought forward in preparation for the next step.

Much preliminary work is necessary before the patient is allowed to use crutches; standing balance in the parallel bars has to be perfected first; in order to balance, the pelvis is carried forward, while the upper trunk is leant back, so that the hips are held in slight hyperextension. Unless the patient has some power in the gluteal muscles, he will 'jack-knife' forward if he allows the trunk to move forward too far. It is possible for this standing posture to be maintained without holding onto the bars and when standing and walking have become assured,

the swing-through gait may be taught, using one crutch and one bar at first progressing later to two crutches.

10. *Standing transfers in tetraplegia.* Some tetraplegics are able to transfer from chair to bed and toilet independently, but mid-cervical and high cervical lesions usually require assistance; one method is shown in Fig. 23.33 by which one helper may assist the patient to transfer. All other methods of lifting usually require at least two people, so that the method shown is particularly useful for transfers from chair to bed, toilet, easy chair and car, provided there is the right combination of weight, height, age etc., between patient and helper. One point to stress, when performing a standing transfer, is to avoid pulling the patient into the upright position by his clothing, since the trouser seams can cut into the skin in the natal cleft area and cause a sore. Hand should ideally be placed under the ischial tuberosities; in this way, one is able to lift the patient into the upright position.

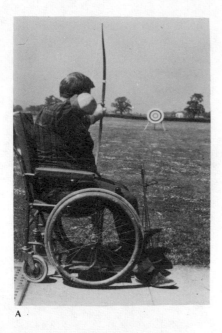

A

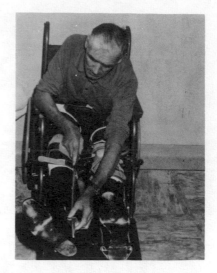

Fig. 23.32   Patient learning to manage his calipers.

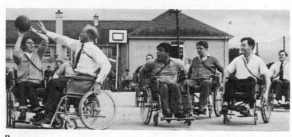

B

Fig. 23.31   A. Archery is a popular pastime. **B.** Which are the patients and which are the doctors? This photograph was taken at a basketball match between a group of paraplegic patients and members of the medical staff; on this occasion the patients won.

Occupational therapy in spinal injury

A good working relationship with the nursing staff is essential for the Occupational Therapist working on a Spinal Injuries Unit. She is continually encouraging patients to become independent and to do as much as possible for themselves. For the tetraplegic patient in particular, this is often a considerable struggle and much difficulty is experienced. On a busy ward where there is a routine to be followed, it is only too easy for staff to 'do' things for patients rather than follow time-consuming 'do-it-yourself' techniques.

Occupational Therapy begins at the moment the patient emerges from the intensive nursing care situation. It is important to establish a good relationship with both the patient and his relatives, and to establish a rapport which ensures co-operation leading to and success in later rehabilitation programmes.

Early stage of treatment. While the patient is confined to bed the provision of a reading aid can do much to dispel the boredom and apathy which may occur with enforced, prolonged bed rest. This may be an electrical appliance, e.g. the 'Talking Book', using cassettes, or may be made in the Occupational Therapy Department for example, a bookstand which holds a book or paper in position over the horizontal patient. Prismatic glasses and the provision of a bed-mirror are also very helpful in widening a patient's vision and increasing his knowledge of his surroundings. Where useful muscle function is present, the patient should be encouraged to use this constructively in the form of some suitable activity while in bed; the therapist gives advice on this, and also encourages relatives and friends to assist her in guiding the patient's activities; relatives and friends often appreciate being involved in this way.

Wheelchair activities. When the patient gets up in a wheelchair the rehabilitation programme can get under way in earnest. Adjustments to the chair may be needed to ensure a satisfactory sitting and working position, for example, the footplates may

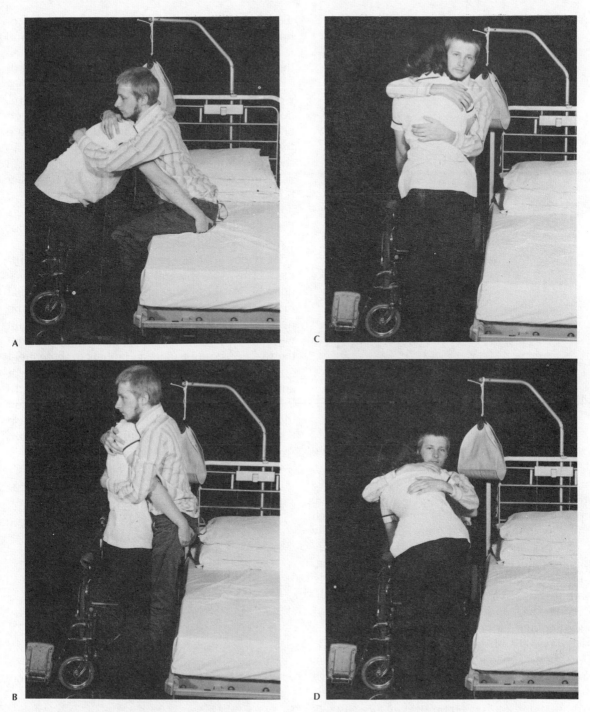

Fig. 23.33   A. *Standing transfer from bed to wheelchair*; the patient sits over the side of the bed, with feet flat on the floor, heels directly in line with knees. His arms are placed around the shoulders of the helper, while her hands are placed under each ischial tuberosity; her knees are just to the side of the patient's knees. The patient then leans forward. **B.** The helper pushes up under the ischial tuberosities, and stands up, at the same time, bringing the patient into the standing position; the helper's knees slip forward to lock the patient's knees. **C.** Maintaining this position, the patient is then swivelled around to the wheelchair. **D.** The patient's trunk is then brought forward, and he is guided into a sitting position in the wheelchair by controlled release of assistance at ischial areas and knees.

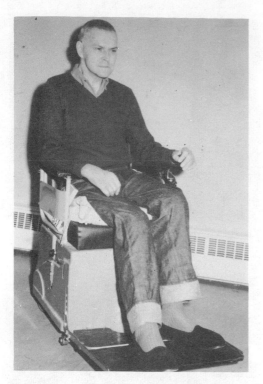

Fig. 23.34 Electrically-propelled chair activated by finger control. Models operated by means of a mouth-stick are also available.

need adjustment, the brake levers extended and a leather heel strap is sometimes required.

Activities of daily living (ADL). The patient's independence in these activities is always of prime importance so that any aids or adaptations which enable them to be carried out as easily and safely as possible are provided at the earliest possible moment, directed toward independence in eating, drinking, personal toilet such as cleaning the teeth, combing hair, shaving, applying make-up, washing hands, face and body front. Learning new ways of writing and typing, managing coins and using a telephone are all included in this section.

Dressing. The paraplegic patient should soon learn to become independent in dressing; though advanced age, excess body weight, lack of perseverance and the presence of pain or spasticity may be limiting factors to the achievement of this, despite instruction and supervised practice. Some tetraplegic patients can be taught to dress independently, but this is an exhausting process and must be realistically related to the rest of the day's activi-

ties. Velcro fastenings instead of small buttons or hooks, loops on zip tags, modified styles and fashions and choice of suitable fabrics are often the solution to many of the difficulties encountered.

Transfer activities. The Occupational Therapist works closely with the Physiotherapist in this activity and the attainment of transfer from wheelchair to bed, toilet, bath, car and easy-chair are those most commonly required. Many patients gain sufficient strength to perform these transfers without assistance. For others the provision of a transfer board, or the use of a lifting pole with chain, or advice and encouragement to relatives or others caring for the patient may be the additional factor required to make transfers possible.

Activities in the occupational therapy department. This is an integral part of the treatment programme for these patients. It is the start of social interaction with patients from other wards in the hospital, with the staff of the department and with visitors. It is the beginning of learning to accept the reactions of outsiders and others to the patient confined to a wheelchair, and from a resettlement angle it is the start of working to and adhering to a timetable. Activities are chosen to strengthen innervated muscles and to teach the patient to use them to their maximum; to teach the development

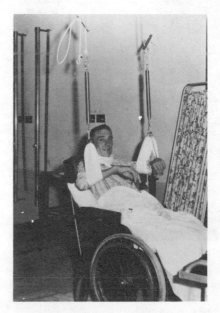

Fig. 23.35 Overhead slings help the tetraplegic patient to use his hands.

of 'trick movements', and to increase independence to the full; to provide mental stimulation in the form of concentration and a sense of achievement. Activities in this group include—craftwork, remedial games, graded strengthening activities, sport, and within the heavy workshop, woodwork, metalwork, and industrial type work. Cooking, together with general kitchen work and home planning and other housecraft activities are practised with the disabled housewife in relation to her own home; male patients are also encouraged to practise kitchen skills with safety.

Hobbies and interests. Apart from their very real therapeutic value within the treatment programme many of the above mentioned activities can form the basis of absorbing interest or hobbies to be followed up at home after discharge from hospital. These not only play a part in alleviating dangerous boredom and its inevitable consequence, but also encourages participation alongside able-bodied people, for example in clubs devoted to archery, table tennis, chess etc.

Home resettlement. A visit to the patient's home is essential; there must be close liaison between the hospital, Community Nursing and Social Services Department, the patient and his family. The house must be assessed as to its suitability for a wheelchair-bound person to cope with relative ease, and any necessary alterations planned and decided upon. Usual difficulties include steps at access, narrow doorways, restricted turning areas and inaccessible bathrooms and w.c.s. Existing facilities may only require minor alteration, or the addition of a lift may make the facilities upstairs accessible; an extension may need to be built on at the side or rear of the property, or if none of these is feasible complete rehousing may be required. Various nursing aids may be necessary, e.g. hospital type bed, hoist, and other aids may increase independence about the house, e.g. POSSUM equipment.

Work resettlement. In this sphere the Occupational Therapist works closely with the Disablement Resettlement Officer (DRO) who in turn will link with his counterpart in the patient's home area. The previous job with its requirements must be considered together with the patient's disability, its implications and the safety aspect. Alterations may be necessary at the factory or office and the interest

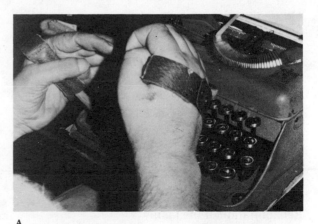

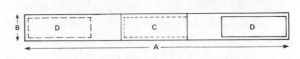

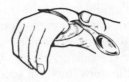

Fig. 23.36 A. Learning to use a typewriter by means of pegs attached to leather cuffs. **B.** A simple but effective aid is a narrow leather strap with velcro-fastening which fits around the hand of the tetraplegic patient, and has a palmar pocket which can hold a spoon, toothbrush, comb, etc.
Details of fabrication: (A) width around hand with a 3 in overlap fastening (standard size is 12 in). (B) 1 in wide. (C) Pocket stitched on three sides. Pocket size is the palm-width—at 3 in. (D) Two pieces of velcro (3 in) stitched to overlap material; use soft, but strong leather; care should be taken that it does not damage insensitive skin.

and co-operation of the employers are essential. The Occupational Therapy staff have the opportunity to assess work potential, interests, aptitudes etc. and together with this information and the services of the DRO a suitable job, or re-training programme can often be instituted.

Transport. It is essential that whenever possible a patient becomes independent on the road; information on choice of car, car conversions, insurance and licence requirements and regulations should be readily available from the Occupational Therapist. She should also make her patient aware of the other benefits and allowances available, often through the Social Work Department of the

Hospital, e.g. Mobility Allowance, Motability Scheme, Orange Badge Scheme.

The Occupational Therapist working in this field has a varied and interesting role to play in the contribution she can make towards the successful rehabilitation of the patient who not only has to adapt to a severe disability but to the reactions of people around him. Despite this it is possible for the paralysed patient to achieve independence and a satisfactory and satisfying quality of life, as illustrated in Figs 23.37A, B, C, D and E.

Rehabilitation of the family

From the first, the patient's family is included in the rehabilitation programme and this may entail some of its members spending many hours in the ward at different times of the day, or at night and at the weekend. Nothing is more disheartening for the patient, his family and for the hospital staff than the patient who, after discharge home, is readmitted with pressure sores, urinary infection and other complications. The doctor, nurse, physiotherapist, occupational therapist, medical social worker and community nursing staff must all work together in teaching and training the family; the nature of the patient's disabilities are explained to the relatives in simple terms, stressing the signs, symptoms and dangers of the complications aforementioned, and at the same time urging them to seek advice immediately if any adverse signs arise. In this connection, the support of the family doctor and of the community nurse and health visitor is imperative. In at least one centre, a nurse attached to the Spinal Unit acts as liaison officer with community personnel and visits patients in their homes and/or places of work; in one area, members of the public were recruited and trained as 'Care Attendants' to assist in the management of these patients (Osborne, 1975); this plan is now being developed on a national basis. An example of team-work between hospital and community health services.

In the case of irrecoverable tetraplegia, the patient's family must fully appreciate the extent of the task to which they are committed, and for this reason, a 'trial trip' is often instituted when the patient is allowed home for a week-end; it is quite another matter to undertake his care day in, day out, and to submit to the discipline which the patient has already learned and which in turn must be accepted by his family. Some families are quite unable to cope with the situation but others tackle it with courage and common sense and are able not only to maintain the patient in physical health, but to give him his place in his own home.

Social resettlement. Physical rehabilitation of the patient is of little avail if his social resettlement is neglected.

Advice on social problems, as we have seen, is available from many sources which can be tapped by the patient through the medical social worker or, in her absence, through doctor, nurse or other member of the health team, or from one of the many organisations which now exist to help handicapped people. The book *Paraplegia—A Handbook of Practical Care and Advice,* named in the Bibliography is written from first-hand knowledge and not only lives up to its title but includes lists of useful addresses where information and help can be obtained on a wide variety of subjects (Rogers, 1978).

Rehousing and alteration to existing housing (Figs 23.27 and 23.28) to suit the needs of a paraplegic patient is vital and negotiations with the appropriate housing authority should be begun as soon as the surgeon allows; on the other hand, accurate assessment of the patient's needs is essential so that time and money is not spent needlessly. The patient's employers are approached with a view to his return to work either at his old job or an alternative one suited to his ability; sometimes a new trade must be chosen and learned; then there is the problem of transport to work, and a hand-controlled motor-car or other vehicle must be supplied. Tetraplegics may be supplied with an electrically-propelled chair controlled by the hand (Fig. 23.34), or the mouth and with electronic aids such as the 'Possum' device, which operates different gadgets in response to 'blowing'. The patients own general practitioner will have been kept informed of the rehabilitation programme; and the services of community nurses are especially valuable in the case of tetraplegics.

Sex and marriage. It is quite understandable that married persons who become paralysed will worry about the stability of their unions and perhaps, about their acceptability to and ability to satisfy their marriage partners; similarly the unattached

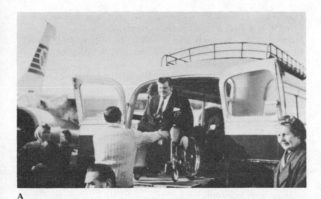

A

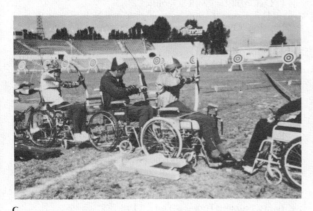

B

Fig. 23.37 A. Transport via specially adapted bus with hydraulic tail lift. (At Heathrow Airport en route to Israel 1968.) **B.** New Zealand 1974—Commonwealth Games. Unloading the aircraft carrying U.K. teams at Dunedin. **C.** Archery for tetraplegics—Israel. **D.** Discus throwing for a paraplegia (Heidelberg Olympics, 1972). This illustration demonstrates the extension of the body swing. The wheelchair is anchored to a concrete ring sunk into the field. **E.** Social life—relaxing with friends at Heidelberg.

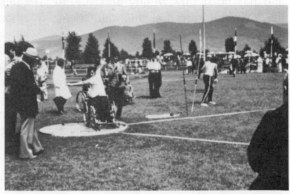

D

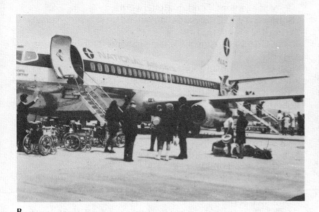

C

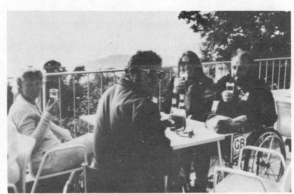

E

will ponder about their chances of marriage and parenthood. Statistical findings show that about 40 per cent of single people marry after spinal cord injury and that the divorce rate among the paralysed is only slightly higher than that among normal couples (Jones, 1977).

Sex counselling and marital guidance is made available to any patient who seeks it; further reading is suggested in the Bibliography.

Pregnancy does not, as a rule, present problems and with adequate rehabilitation and ante-natal care paraplegic women can bear and raise normal healthy children.

Later supervision. In most centres, the paraplegic

patient is readmitted to hospital for review at regular six-monthly intervals when a comprehensive examination is carried out to ensure that complications such as urinary infection do not occur. In some centres, past patients form their own Social Club and meet periodically for sporting and/or social occasions.

Most difficult of all from the point of view of rehabilitation and resettlement is the tetraplegic with a high lesion; if he has no use or only very limited use of his upper limbs he cannot even cope with his own basic toilet needs and is reduced to the physical status of a baby; if he cannot work and has no family willing and able to give him the love and care that this status demands, then permanent institutional care of some kind is often the only solution to the problem. We must all remember however, that the physical status of a baby does not mean a corresponding reduction in the mental status; patients who look to us not only for physical care but for the respect and recognition which brings happiness to every human being are our special responsibility.

BIBLIOGRAPHY

Allan D 1984 Care of the patient in a wedge-turning frame. Nursing Times, 15 August
Bedbrook Sir G 1981 The Care and Management of Spinal Cord Injuries. New York: Springer-Verlag
Blannin J P, Hobden J 1980 The catheter of choice. Nursing Times, 27 November
Bromley I 1976 Tetraplegia and Paraplegia. A guide for physiotherapists. Edinburgh and London: Churchill Livingstone
Burke D C, Murray D D 1975 Handbook of Spinal Cord Medicine. London: Macmillan Press
Comarr A E 1957 The practical management of spinal cord injuries. Journal of the Indian Medical Profession. Bombay, India, 4 April, 1560
Fallon B 1978 So You're Paralysed. London: Spinal Injuries Association
Goodwood J 1984 A day in a wheelchair. Nursing Mirror, 20 June
Guttman Sir L 1976 Sport for the Disabled. Aylesbury: H M & M Publishers
Guttman Sir L 1964 The married life of the paraplegics and tetraplegics. Paraplegia, 1–11, 182–188

Hardy A C, Elson R 1976 Practical Management of Spinal Injuries. Edinburgh: Churchill Livingstone
Jacobs R 1982 Nurses matter too. Nursing Mirror, 10 January
Keane F X 1971 Mechnical aids to nursing paraplegics. Nursing Times, 23 December, 1603
Lamber J 1978 A lousy, rotten deal. Nursing Mirror, 23 November
Larabee J H et al 1977 The person with a spinal cord injury. American Journal of Nursing, 1319
McRae R 1981 Practical Fracture Treatment. Edinburgh: Churchill Livingstone
Manual of Nursing Policies and Procedures 1984. Urinary catheterisation. Lippincott Nursing Series. For the Royal Marsden Hospital.
Marshall J, Mair J 1967 Neurological Nursing. London: Blackwell Scientific
Nicholls P R J 1971 Rehabilitation of the Severely Disabled: 2, Management. London: Butterworths
Osborne P 1975 Crossroads care attendant scheme. Nursing Times, 23 January, 149
Pellatt G 1984 Nursing tetraplegic patients. Nursing Mirror, 18 April
Pinel C 1976 Pressure sores. Nursing Times, 5 February, 172
Pratt R 1971 Nursing care of paraplegic patients. Nursing Times publication
Robertson C 1978 Life on a Stryker bed. Nursing Times, 4 May, 752
Roaf R, Hodkinson L J 1977 The Paralysed Patient. Oxford: Blackwell Scientific
Rogers M A 1978 Paraplegia. A Handbook of Practical Care and Advice. London: Faber and Faber
Rossiter A 1964 Rehabilitation of the Spinal Cord Injury Patient. Basle: Switzerland. Documenta Geigy. No. 3. North America Series
Rowe J, Dyer L 1977 Care of the Orthopaedic Patient. Jones F. Oxford: Blackwell Scientific
Scott D F, Dodd B 1966 Neurological and Neurosurgical Nursing. Oxford: Pergamon Press
Scott J 1984 Learning to live with paralysis. Nursing Mirror, 18 April
Smith M, Ali N 1980 Long-term catheters—questions nurses ask. Nursing Times, Community Outlook, 10 April
Spinal Injuries Association 1980 People with spinal injuries: treatment and care. Nursing management in the general hospital: the first 48 hours following injury
Starrett D 1861 Psychiatric mechanisms in severe disability. Rocky Mountain Medical Journal 58: 42 (quoted by Wilson-Barnett, 1979).
Stewart W F R 1975 Sex and the Physically Handicapped. Horsham, Sussex: National Fund for Research into Crippling Diseases
Tam G et al 1978 A cost-effectiveness trial of incontinence pants. Nursing Times, 20 July, 1198
Wastling G 1978 Long-term indwelling catheters. Nursing Times, 13 July, 1176
Whitfield H N 1976 Non-sterile intermittent catheterisation. Nursing Times, 16 December, 1961
Wilson-Barnett J 1979 Stress in Hospital. Edinburgh: Churchill Livingstone

24

Adult hemiplegia— the 'stroke' patient

A stroke is the result of interference with the blood supply to some part of the brain, from one of the following causes:

1. Rupture of a blood vessel—*cerebral haemorrhage*;
2. Blockage of a vessel by a clot of blood—*cerebral thrombosis*;
3. *Cerebral embolism*—occurs when a clot becomes detached from a diseased valve in the heart and is carried to the vessels of the brain by the blood stream.
4. *Cardiovascular degeneration* causes narrowing of the walls of blood vessels so that a part of the brain becomes deficient in blood supply.

Strokes vary enormously in severity, depending upon the location and extent of damage to brain tissues; a patient may suffer a major single stroke or a series of smaller episodes.

COMMON RESULTS OF A STROKE

The most common results of a stroke are listed below:

1. Loss of consciousness;
2. Hemiplegia, ranging from severe to slight (hemipareses);
3. Paralysis or weakness of one side of the face with corresponding difficulty in speech and in chewing food, in coughing and swallowing and sometimes, with drooling of saliva from the weak side of the mouth;

4. Impairment of sensation; loss of awareness of the affected side of the body;
5. Impairment of vision; for example in a left-sided stroke there may be difficulty in seeing out of the left side of each eye;
6. Mental confusion; impairment of understanding, for example, the patient may not fully understand what is said to him;
7. Impairment of control of bladder and bowel;
8. Emotional instability, or personality changes resulting in hostile or bizarre behaviour such as sudden outbursts of weeping, obscene language, uncontrolled laughter or other uncharacteristic episodes.

Recovery after stroke may take place in a few days, weeks, months or even years. Some patients recover completely, others are left with some permanent disability and those with very severe involvement of brain tissue may not survive.

TREATMENT AND NURSING CARE

Care of the unconscious patient has already been outlined in Chapter 19, and will not be repeated here.

In general, patients who have suffered a stroke are presented to the orthopaedic service only when the condition of hemiplegia is established. What follows, therefore, is a very brief resumé of nursing care, because many of the guidelines for the nurse are described later in this chapter, particularly with regard to prevention of deformity and recovery of function. The nurse in hospital, however, has a most important role because, in one form or another, she is with the patient twenty-four hours of every day, and it is her essential duty to prevent complications which might retard recovery of function, e.g. pressure sores, contractures or urinary tract infection. She provides the essential background against which improvement of function takes place, including emotional support for the patient who may find his stroke a devastating experience and who, perhaps, may be perfectly well aware of his surroundings but has difficulty in communication.

The nurse not only has an important role in hospital in the prevention of complications but is a link between the patient, his relatives and his home background; *early discharge home* is an important aim of treatment, and at this point the family doctor, the community nurse and the patient's relatives emerge as key figures. Indeed, reports have shown that community care and rehabilitation of the stroke patient can be very successful (Chivers, 1968; Warren, 1969).

General treatment may be required, for example, medication to control hypertension, or dietary measures for obesity. When the patient is admitted to hospital one should make sure he has with him any aids he uses such as spectacles, a hearing-aid, or dentures. A nursing history with assessment of nursing needs and a nursing care plan provides a base-line for delivery of care. A patient with problems of comprehension and communication is helped by having the same nurse or nurses assigned to him regularly, so as to build up a stable relationship which also includes his family. The patient needs reassurance, sympathy and an explanation of what has happened to him and what measures will be taken to aid his recovery. The aim is to give him hope and strong motivation for the task of rehabilitation which lies ahead. If he has some understanding of the possibility of recovery of function and of what is expected of him, his motivation will be strengthened. However, the strongest motivation is soon lost if complications are not prevented; skin breakdown, constipation, urinary infection, poor nutrition due to eating difficulties, and deformity due to joint contractures are the deadly enemies of the stroke patient.

Loss of speech is particularly unnerving for the stroke patient and is usually associated with a lesion in the left cerebral hemisphere. It produces fear and frustration and the patient feels lonely and isolated. If a speech therapist is available, an assessment of the patient's disability will be made and a programme of therapy mapped out. Unfortunately, such services are not widely available, so much of the work devolves upon the nurse; one with whom the patient can identify and who understands his difficulties will be of the utmost value to him.

Firstly, it must be determined whether the patient can communicate verbally or in writing, whether he understands what is said and whether his comprehension is limited to short phrases or to single words. Rudimentary communication is usually not difficult and should be accepted during the early phase, but reliance on such signals will limit the patient's ability to regain a more comprehensive vocabulary later on. Normal conversation in an ordinary setting is a valuable stimulant for the aphasic patient, even if he cannot reply clearly. The nurse should never treat the patient as a child or discuss him with others within his ear-shot. IT MUST BE REMEMBERED THAT INTELLIGENCE, HEARING AND COMPREHENSION ARE NOT USUALLY IMPAIRED. When speaking to the patient the nurse must speak slowly and clearly, and limit herself to a simple functional level at first, using questions that require a simple yes or no in response; using words in association with the objects that they represent aids recovery. Vocabulary is gradually extended, giving the patient plenty of time to respond; it must be remembered that the stroke patient tires easily and he must not be rushed for his replies.

Positioning in bed/chair is of vital importance and is dealt with later in the section on physiotherapy. The physiotherapist and nurse will work together very closely in this area. It is pointed out that the supine position is avoided as far as possible because it encourages spasticity.

Note the importance of preventing contracture of the structures between the ribs and pelvis (Figs 24.1 and 24.2).

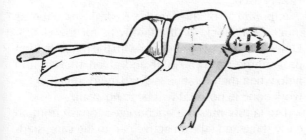

Fig. 24.1 Patient lying on unaffected side. Nothing is placed in the hand or under the sole of the foot. A pillow is placed under the flexed affected leg and foot. A pillow is placed behind the back keeping the patient well on to his side (not shown here). The affected arm is placed on a pillow with the shoulder girdle well forward.

When the patient is in this position, the physiotherapist will carry out passive movements to the affected side; the patient will also be rolled on to his back for these movements, but lying on the back is avoided if possible because reflex activity is strongest in this position resulting in the greatest increase in abnormal tone. **Note** that it is important to align the trunk so that the rib-cage and pelvis are kept as far apart as possible in order to prevent contractures.

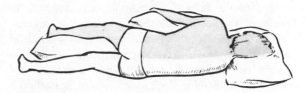

Fig. 24.2 Patient lying on affected side. Nothing is placed in the hand or under the sole of the foot. A pillow is placed under the flexed unaffected leg and foot. A pillow is placed behind the patient's back keeping him well over on his side. The affected arm is extended at the elbow, supinated at the forearm, and the shoulder girdle again brought forward.

Turning. At first, the patient is helpless and must be turned at two-hourly intervals by day and by night and it is mandatory that the bed is completely dry and smooth at all times. As soon as possible, the patient learns to assist by rolling the whole body from side to side; *note that great care is exercised when handling* the affected limbs; the shoulder in particular is a sensitive joint, easily damaged by rough handling.

Passive movements are given regularly to prevent stiffness of joints and contractures and to maintain circulation and nutrition in the paralysed limb. It should be noted that though giving passive movements is generally regarded as the prerogative of the physiotherapist there may be circumstances when a physiotherapist is not available and the nurse must be prepared to give them. As soon as possible the patient is taught to carry out his own passive movements using the sound hand. *It should be stressed again however that careless, rough handling of the joints of paralysed limbs must be avoided.*

Care of the bladder. In the early stages, continuous drainage of the bladder by means of a catheter may be required in order to keep the patient dry, but it is discontinued as soon as possible because of the danger of urinary tract infection. An adequate fluid intake is essential and an intake/output chart is maintained until the condition becomes stable. *Bladder training* by offering a bedpan or urinal at regular intervals is started as soon as possible, progressing to regular visits to the lavatory by means of a sani-chair; in this connection however it should be noted that *accurate observation* is required to ensure that the patient does in fact pass urine and/or stool and that constipation does not occur unnoticed.

Care of the bowel. Constipation is a common problem so that it is essential to keep a regular check on the patient's bowel habits. Constipation can cause many distressing symptoms and must always be suspected if the patient complains of increased spasticity, lethargy, loss of appetite or a general feeling of being 'off colour'. The condition can often be prevented by offering bran products for breakfast or by sprinkling a little bran over the food at meal times. Increasing activity will also encourage peristalsis and reduce the risk of constipation. Sometimes simple aperients, e.g. Senokot, may be prescribed and as a last resort the use of suppositories or enemata might be required.

Learning to eat may be a problem. If the dominant side is paralysed, the patient will have difficulty in manipulating his cutlery and he may dribble, because of his partially paralysed face; in this connection, food may be retained in the mouth on the side of the paralysed cheek so that measures to maintain *oral hygiene* are essential and a mouth wash is given after each meal. Often, elderly people have poorly-fitting dentures, which may be adequate in normal circumstances but not after a stroke; the nurse will appreciate such a problem and seek dental help. In the early stages, the nurse assists by cutting up food so that the patient can manipulate it. The patient's clothes should be protected and he must not be scolded for 'making a mess'. The occupational therapist will be able to supply such aids as non-slip mats, plate curbs and adaptation to cutlery (Fig. 25.19).

Dressing is introduced at an early stage. It is discussed in the next paragraph. The occupational therapist will advise on suitable clothes, fastenings and appropriate dressing techniques.

Other activities. Normal activities which we all take for granted are difficult for the stroke patient and must be built up slowly by re-establishing good patterns of movement starting from teaching the patient how to turn over in bed. The basis of normal movement is established by correct positioning of the patient in the early stages of his illness. The nurse, in consultation with the physiotherapist, endeavours to stimulate the paralysed side by encouraging the patient to use it as much as possible, because the patient will tend to use only the sound side. While the use of the affected side might not be regained fully, over-dependence on the sound side results in the 'one-sided person' whose independence is severely limited. The patient should be encouraged to do as much as possible for himself, but allowing him to struggle on for a long time without help will cause frustration and be counter-productive. Activity is gradually increased as the patient gains more confidence and skill. Some people, for example, find it easier to use the 'bedpan bridge position' to wriggle into their trousers, while others prefer to put them on in a sitting position and hitch them up when standing. For vests or pullovers the affected arm can be put into its sleeve first, followed by the sound one. The sleeves are pushed as far up the arm as possible, then the garment is put over the head. A stroke can cause perceptual difficulties, so the patient may be unaware of his affected limb. Therefore several attempts to get into the garment may be needed. Sometimes difficulties in distinguishing between left and right are experienced, and appropriate labelling or colour-coding may help. Generally speaking, clothes should be fairly loose and front-opening and skirts and trousers should have elasticated waist bands, making toilet visits much easier. Buttons are not easy to manage and should be replaced by velcro fastenings. Elasticated cuff-links or buttons sewn to a piece of elastic through a sleeve buttonhole make this part of dressing independent; neck-ties can be left knotted or the clip-on variety used.

Importance of the family. A stroke is often as much of a shock for the family as for the victim. Unless the family is involved with the rehabilitation programme from the start and given support and help when their relative is discharged, much of the work done in hospital will be to no avail.

The family must be encouraged to visit from an early stage and take an active part in the care, starting to care for their relative in a small way and gradually building up to, perhaps, a weekend visit. This gives relatives an opportunity to see what is involved and a chance to iron out problems as they arise, and when any necessary house modifications have been carried out, the patient can start spending weekends at home. The therapeutic team can then remain in contact with the patient and his family, while gradually letting all parties adjust to the new situation.

To provide realistic goals for the patient and

members of his family, the therapeutic team must visit the patient's home at an early date (Ch. 35) to assess its suitability. Can the home be made to match the patient's capabilities? Would hand rails or ramps be useful? Would moving the bedroom or installing a shower help? The availability of local facilities like day hospitals, out-patient physiotherapy, sheltered work-shops, community nursing services, meals on wheels etc. will influence the time of discharge.

After final discharge, contact with the patient and his family is maintained through members of the community nursing services who are on the spot to give support, iron out difficulties and keep the rest of the therapeutic team involved and informed.

PHYSIOTHERAPY IN ADULT HEMIPLEGIA

The main problems of the stroke patient are:

1. Sensory loss.
2. Loss of balance.
3. Loss of movement.
4. General and spatial disorientation.
5. Developing spasticity.
6. Depression.
7. Aphasia (if it is present).
8. Hemianopia (if it is present).

The aims of the treatment are:

1. To prevent the development of spasticity by the careful positioning of the patient at all times.
2. To make the patient aware of both sides of his body.
3. To restore weight transference using both sides of the body.
4. A return to as near normal function as possible.

The doctor, nurse, speech therapist, occupational therapist and physiotherapist are all members of a team who work closely together in the treatment of the stroke patient. Everyone who comes in contact with the patient, *including relatives and friends*, should be made aware of the aims of the treatment, so that they all make the same approach and reinforce each other.

Each patient's disabilities are different, and each patient's treatment is tailored to meet his individual needs; no two patients have the same disabilities.

It is somewhat difficult to realise in the early flaccid, floppy stage that the limbs will later become spastic, but most patients with a stroke develop some spasticity even though it may be very slight, and correct positioning is very important to reduce this to a minimum. Strong spasticity will prevent rehabilitation and re-education, and the patient will always be very dependent on other people. Spasticity usually starts distally in the fingers and toes and spreads proximally, whilst contractures of soft tissue begin proximally at the shoulder and hip. If the spasticity is not marked the patient will be able to move his limbs more easily in the direction he wishes. The stroke patient's problem is not the lack of individual muscle power but the inability to move the arm or leg in the desired patterns of movement required for normal activities; he cannot control isolated movements at individual joints.

The nurse is a very important member of the team, and even during routine nursing procedures she is helping to re-educate the patient's movements. For example, when the patient is taught to roll over from side to side for bed-making, he is doing some of the movements which will be part of his programme of rehabilitation exercises. When rolling towards the unaffected side, care must be taken to see that the affected arm is brought forward across the body and that the affected leg is also flexed forward so as to prevent contracture of the shoulder girdle and pelvic girdle. Note that it is much easier for a patient to roll from side to side if the head pillows are removed.

When the patient 'bridges' for the positioning of a bed-pan, this movement will also assist his re-education, and eventual recovery. The nurse bends the affected leg and holds it in position with the foot flat on the bed; he 'makes a bridge' by lifting his hips off the bed; the bed-pan is then easily placed in position. During this exercise the patient learns to take weight through both legs.

It is very important that the unaffected arm of the hemiplegic patient is not pulled, and careful handling of the patient's limbs cannot be stressed too strongly. A painful, contracted shoulder can be caused by incorrect handling, and this will hold back the patient's treatment and rehabilitation.

Positioning

It is most important during the treatment of all the stages of hemiplegia that the patient is positioned carefully in bed or chair at all times to minimise the development of contracture of spastic muscles (Figs 24.1, 24.2, 24.3 and 24.4).

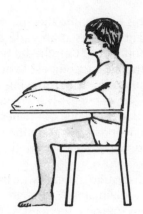

Fig. 24.4 Patient sitting in a chair. Nothing is placed in the hand, but the arm is placed forward on a pillow. The shoulder girdle is brought forward into a relaxed position. The feet are flat on the ground and the heel is held down. The hips are flexed to a right angle and the thighs are well supported. The back is well supported, and the patient sits with weight equal on both buttocks.

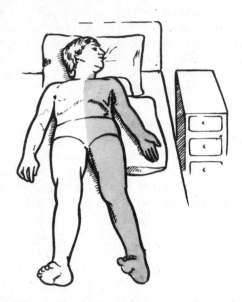

Fig. 24.3 Patient lying on the back (supine). As already stated, this position is avoided as much as possible. Nothing is placed in the hand or under the sole of the foot. A pillow is placed under the arm, shoulder girdle and pelvic girdle of the affected side, keeping the shoulder and pelvic girdle forward, and preventing lateral rotation of the leg. The head is turned towards the affected side, and flexed towards the good side. The locker is placed on the affected side. Note that the position of the head is important in order to prevent contractures.

Careful full range passive movements are carried out at least twice a day at first, and the patient is taught to move his affected arm by using the good arm. He clasps the affected hand with the good hand and raises both arms together. He is encouraged to be aware of his affected side and use it for support, and to turn his head towards that side. If the locker is placed on the affected side and all contact with the patient by staff and visitors is made at that side, it will help him to do this. All positioning and activity is directed towards the affected side.

The nurses will encourage the patient to move his affected arm using the sound one during turning and will tell him when and how they are moving the affected limbs so that the patient is reminded and made aware of the affected side at frequent intervals.

The patient is sat up very early in treatment, and he should be encouraged to rock from side to side, and shuffle forwards and backwards without using his hands. When sitting up in bed, he should try to reach towards his feet whilst holding his hands together and maintaining his balance. It is important that the patient sits as upright as possible in bed as there is a great risk of pressure sores if the half-lying position is used.

Transfer from bed to chair

When transferring the patient from bed to chair, the chair is placed on the patient's affected side, parallel to the head of the bed, and the procedure is explained to the patient. The easiest way to get a stroke patient sitting up over the side of the bed is for the nurse to put her arm under the patient's affected shoulder, and swing the patient's legs over the side of the bed using her other arm. The patient's weight is taken by him on to his affected elbow. After the patient has sat up and put on his dressing gown, putting the sleeves on the affected side first, he can shuffle nearer the side of the bed and let his feet down to the ground. The nurse stands facing the patient, her feet being used to prevent him from slipping forwards on to the floor. She puts her hands around the patient's back, and he rests both his arms on the nurse's shoulders. The patient can easily be raised into the standing position and pivoted around to sit in the chair, whilst the weight is taken through his own legs. Great care is taken in handling the arm, and in preventing the knee from flexing during the sequence of the movement.

The chair should be placed in such a position in the ward as to encourage the patient to turn his head towards the affected side. When the patient stands up from sitting, he puts the good foot forward a little, leans forward from the hips but keeps his back straight and head up, raises his buttocks off the chair, straightens his knees, brings his hip forwards and thus stands up. If there is difficulty in getting up at first, it is sometimes useful to teach him to clasp his hands and push his arms forwards and then stand up. Suitable footwear is very necessary, comfortable low-heeled shoes in good repair being ideal. As soon as possible the patient starts mat exercises and balance exercises in the physiotherapy department, and so that the physiotherapist is the person most likely to know when he is ready to progress to attempts to walk.

Standing and walking

The patient does not stand until his sitting balance is established, and he does not walk until his standing balance is established. He learns to transfer weight from one foot to the other when standing, with his feet apart and also with one foot in front of the other in preparation for walking (see Figs 24.5A and B). Walking is not encouraged until the patient can take his body weight through the affected leg. Ideally, the patient should not walk until the physiotherapist has decided that he is ready to do so, and she will show the nurses the best method of walking for that particular patient.

An important aim for the stroke patient is to walk without a hand-held aid, because it will restrict his independence and freedom. Sometimes this cannot be achieved and a compromise is made by using a walking frame with two wheels at the front, which can be pushed along using both arms; progressing to walking without this aid might be made later.

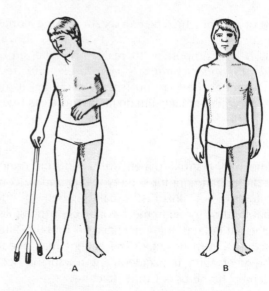

Fig. 24.5 **A.** Patient standing. This figure shows that the patient's body weight is not being taken through both legs. The affected leg has only a small amount of body weight through it, and spasticity is increased. The patient is leaning towards the unaffected side. The head is rotated towards the unaffected side. The shoulder is retracted and the arm is flexed. The pelvis is drawn back and the affected leg is laterally rotated. **B.** This is the posture which should be aimed at, the body weight is equally distributed through both legs, and the body is symmetrical.

Dressing practice with the occupational therapist is commenced very early in the rehabilitation programme, firstly when the patient is in bed, and then, when his balance is satisfactory he is taught to dress himself standing. The affected arm is always put into the sleeve first and removed last. The patient is encouraged to do as much as possible for himself as soon as possible, even though this is time-consuming.

Most patients are taught to negotiate stairs, and if they can manage to climb them by the normal reciprocal method, further instruction is unnecessary. The patient who cannot achieve this is usually taught to lead with the good leg up the stairs followed by the affected one, and with the affected leg followed by the sound leg when coming down. Again, care must be taken not to pull on the affected arm and it is best to remain on the stair below the patient.

The nurse should be aware of the problem of hemianopia if it is present in a stroke patient, as it will often explain some of the patient's difficulties, such as walking into doors, only eating that part of a meal which he can see, or leaving a drink untouched.

It is very important to realise that *the stroke patient's understanding is very rarely impaired*, even though he may not speak; shouting at the patient will not make him do things more easily.

Complications

Sometimes a stroke patient will attend the orthopaedic department for surgery for secondary contractures, but this is usually when a full rehabilitation programme has not been possible, or the patient has not maintained his mobility after discharge from hospital. The patient may attend if he meets with an accident, e.g. fracture of neck of femur, humerus or Colles' fracture.

BIBLIOGRAPHY

Atkinson H W 1974 ed. Joan Cash. Neurology for Physiotherapists. London: Faber and Faber

Bannister A et al 1984 A loss of power. Nursing Mirror, Nursing care study, 18 January

Bickerstaff E R 1971 Neurology for Nurses. London: Oxford University Press

Bobath B 1970 Adult Hemiplegia: Evaluation and Treatment. London: Heinemann

Brocklehurst J C 1969 A new look at strokes. Nursing Mirror, 17 October, 37

Bullock E A 1974 Later stages of Rehabilitation in Hemiplegia. Physiotherapy, December

Chivers R J 1968 Patients with hemiplegia in the care of district nurses. Nursing Times, 22 November, 1604

Clyde N P R 1961 'Stroke' illness—help for patient and family. London: The Chest and Heart Association

Hawker M 1978 Exercises for stroke patients. London: The Chest, Heart and Stroke Association

Howorth I, Prosser J 1976 Cerebro-vascular Accident. Nursing Care Supplement No. 3. Nursing Mirror, 23: 142

Isaacs B 1977 Stroke Research and the Physiotherapist. Physiotherapy, November, 366

Johnstone M 1976 The Stroke Patient. Principles of Rehabilitation. Edinburgh: Churchill Livingstone

Johnstone M 1978a The Stroke Patient. Edinburgh: Churchill Livingstone

Johnstone M 1978b Restoration of Motor Function in the Stroke Patient. Edinburgh: Churchill Livingstone

Lane R E J 1978 Facilitation of weight transference in the Stroke Patient. Physiotherapy, September, 260

Mulley G 1978 Stroke—A handbook for the patient's family. London: The Chest, Heart and Stroke Association

Parry A, Eales C (1976) Hemiplegia 1, 2, 3 and 4. Nursing Times, 14 October–4 November, pages: 1590–1592, 1640–1641, 1680–1683, 1726–1730, 1763–1765

Parry A, Earles C 1976 Hemiplegia 1. Nursing Times, 72: 1590–1592

Parry A, Earles C 1976 Hemiplegia 2. Nursing Times, 72: 1640–1641

Parry A, Earles C 1976 Hemiplegia 3. Nursing Times, 72:1680–1681

Parry A, Earles C 1976 Hemiplegia 4. Nursing Times, 72: 1726–1730

Parry A, Earles C 1976 Hemiplegia 5. Nursing Times, 72: 1763–1765

Roaf R, Hodkinson L J (1977) The Paralysed Patient. London: Blackwell Scientific

Rubin S 1967 Home Care of the Stroke Patient. Nursing Times, 6 October, 1339

Scott D, Dodd B 1966 Neurological and Neurosurgical Nursing. Oxford: Pergamon

Stewart M C 1968 My brother's keeper? London: Health Horizon Ltd. for the Chest, Heart and Stroke Association.

Stickland et al 1978 Stroke. Nursing Times Community Outlook, 9 November, 323–351

Todd J M 1974 Physiotherapy in the Early Stages of Hemiplegia. Physiotherapy, November, 336

Warren Faith C 1969 Home Care of a Hemiplegic patient. Nursing Mirror, 19 December, 28

Watson J E 1972 Medical Surgical Nursing and Related Physiology. New York: W B Saunders, Ch. 22

SECTION | **FIVE**

Care of the patient with non-specific and degenerative bone and joint disease

25

Rheumatoid arthritis

The word 'rheumatism' is in common use by the general public to mean almost any pain occurring in the musculo-skeletal system. The use of this word should be avoided, for it signifies no specific disease and is only of interest because of its derivation from the Greek word *rheumatismos*.

It is true that many of the rheumatic diseases involve tissues outside joints and in this sense are 'non-articular'. In this context, muscles, tendons, tendon sheaths and bursae may be involved.

Arthritis means inflammation involving joints. There are many different types of arthritis but in this section, only those manifesting obvious inflammatory change will be discussed. In this group signs of inflammation are evident particularly in the early stages of disease, e.g. synovitis and joint effusion. The synovial membrane increases in thickness to become an oedematous, highly vascular and richly cellular tissue. The increased amount of joint fluid (effusion) is characterised by having a high protein content and many polymorphonuclear white cells.

The most common member of this group is rheumatoid arthritis. Others which may be encountered with reasonable frequency include psoriatic arthritis, ankylosing spondylitis, the arthritis associated with diseases of the bowel (ulcerative colitis and regional ileitis) and Reiter's syndrome. In other chapters, some of the rare diseases of connective tissue will be mentioned and the degenerative arthropathies (osteoarthritis, intervertebral disc lesions), arthritis resulting from infection, gout etc. are dealt with separately. Arthritis may also occur in association with many diseases which are outside the scope of this book.

RHEUMATOID ARTHRITIS

Definition

A chronic or sub-acute non-suppurative inflammatory disease affecting joints. It is usually polyarticular and of symmetrical distribution. The joints are swollen and deformity will ultimately occur. The patient complains of pain and stiffness, especially first thing in the morning. The disease runs a prolonged course of varying severity with exacerbations and remissions and may result in severe disability. Although the target organ is thought to be the synovial membrane, other systems in the body may be involved. Systemic disturbances are common, e.g. weakness, anaemia, anorexia and loss of weight.

Occasionally many tissues and organs in the body may be involved as well as joints, usually as a result of nodule formation or vasculitis, and there has been a tendency to describe such cases as having 'rheumatoid disease'.

Women are more frequently affected than men (2.5:1) and the common sites involved are hands, wrists, feet, knees and neck although any synovial joint may be affected. Rheumatoid arthritis is common and occurs throughout the world. In this country the overall prevalence is 6.0 per cent in women and 2.5 per cent in men. Over the age of 65 the prevalence increases to 16 per cent in females and 5 per cent in males (Fig. 25.1). This, therefore, is a significant disease.

Aetiology and pathogenesis

The cause of rheumatoid arthritis is still unknown. Early this century, infection was thought to be the cause. Subsequently, allergy, stress, and autoimmunity have been implicated. None of these factors has been shown to be causative and a role for infection has again been suggested. It is postulated that an infective agent (as yet unidentified) may trigger off a series of immunological changes which we know do occur, especially in genetically susceptible individuals.

Several complex mechanisms are involved in these immunological changes. Briefly, two aspects may be considered:

1. An alteration in some of the body's own proteins may occur (or be induced by the causative agent) so that the body's defence mechanisms no longer recognise these proteins as 'self'. The body then reacts as it would to 'foreign' proteins (cf. wrongly cross-matched blood) by forming antibodies against the altered proteins. One of these antibodies is known as 'rheumatoid factor' and is demonstrated in the blood of patients by the sheep cell agglutination test (SCAT), the Rose-Waller, latex fixation, rheumaton, and other similar tests. The SCAT is positive in approximately 70 per cent of patients who have rheumatoid arthritis.

2. On the other hand, the body's ability ('tolerance') to differentiate between 'self' and 'foreign' may fail and antibodies may form against one's own protein even when it has not been altered.

The above is a simplified resumé. Despite intensive research, the many immunological abnormalities that are known to occur in rheumatoid arthritis have not been shown to be causative. In other words there have to be other factors to initiate the situation in which the chain of immunological changes will occur. One such factor may be an infective agent (e.g. a 'slow virus'). It has not been possible to demonstrate such an agent by conventional methods but newer techniques may change this picture.

It is possible that in a suitable or susceptible individual a particular agent may precipitate immunological phenomena and result in the disease we know as rheumatoid arthritis.

Pathology

In normal people the synovium consists of a single layer of lining cells with loose connective tissue underneath and few cells or blood vessels in the stroma. In rheumatoid arthritis, the lining cells multiply to become several layers deep. The synovium becomes oedematous and very vascular. Later there is an increase in chronic inflammatory cells (plasma cells and lymphocytes). The synovium becomes much thicker, very vascular and the site of massive cellular infiltration. The chronic inflammatory cells can be shown to produce rheumatoid factor. The thickened tissue is often called 'granulation tissue' and as such it spreads as a 'pannus' over the articular cartilage. The end result of the inflammatory immunological process is the production of enzymes which are destructive to carti-

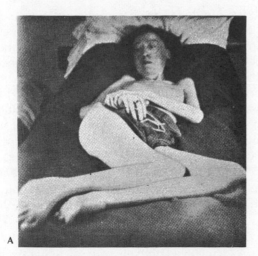

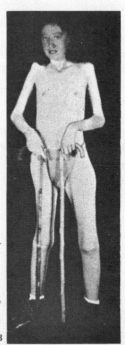

Fig. 25.1   A. Rheumatoid arthritis affecting almost every joint. Note the deformities of hips, knees and ankles. **B.** The same patient after treatment. Note that these illustrations are taken from old photographs. Nevertheless, the gross deformities shown can still occur in cases where treatment is neglected or has proved unsuccessful. **C.** This illustration shows the ratio of the disease between male & female patients (By permission of Dr A. K. Clarke, Royal National Hospital for Rheumatic Diseases, Bath.)

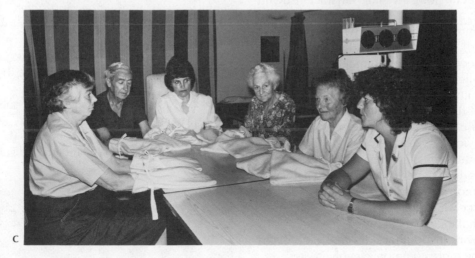

lage and bone. In time this produces erosions and joint destruction with resultant limitation, deformity, subluxation, secondary degenerative change and sometimes fibrous or bony ankylosis.

As with the lining of joints, the lining of tendon sheaths may also be involved and replaced by exuberant granulation tissue, especially in the hand. Tendon rupture can result.

Apart from the changes in joints and tendon sheaths, other tissues may be involved. There is commonly muscle wasting and osteoporosis. Two other features occurring in some patients with rheumatoid arthritis are important, namely nodule formation and vasculitis.

Nodules are most commonly subcutaneous and are seen particularly along the extensor aspect of the forearm. They may also occur in many other sites such as the lung, heart and eye. Vasculitis is the infiltration of the walls of the small arteries with chronic inflammatory cells (plasma cells and lymphocytes) such that the lumen of the vessel may be occluded. The end result of such a process depends upon the vessels involved but may affect almost any organ in the body. Peripheral nerves are especially likely to be affected by vasculitis giving rise to neuropathy. It is therefore possible for many structures other than joints to be involved in rheumatoid arthritis. Nodule formation and vasculitis are more likely to occur in the presence of a high titre of rheumatoid factor. It must be emphasised however that joint involvement is the hallmark of the disease.

Clinical features

The disease can start at any age but the peak incidence is between 35 and 55 years.

Rheumatoid arthritis usually begins with symptoms referable to the joints and stiffness. The onset is most often insidious and slowly progressive. Occasionally it may be episodic and rarely fulminating with acute joint swelling. Characteristically several joints are involved in a symmetrical fashion (i.e. it is common to have both wrists, both knees etc. involved). The patient complains of pain and stiffness especially in the morning and the joints will be swollen. Function is impaired and eventually deformity occurs. Swelling is due to proliferative synovial tissue and to effusion into the joints. Nearby muscles atrophy and muscle wasting becomes obvious.

All synovial joints may be involved but the hands, feet, and knees are commonly the early site. It is uncommon to find involvement of the spine (except the cervical spine), sacro-iliac joints and distal interphalangeal joints.

The following list outlines in brief some of the features of the more commonly involved sites:

1. *Cervical spine.* Pain is often present and associated with limitation. As the disease advances root pressure may occur giving rise to pain and paraesthesiae down the arms. The most important features occur when subluxation occurs either at atlanto-axial level (C1–2) or sub-axial level (usually between the upper fourth or fifth cervical vertebrae). In these cases pressure on the spinal cord, or interference with its blood supply, may result in tetra- or paraplegia or even sudden death. Temporary obstruction of the vertebro-basilar artery system with movement of the neck can result in transient vertigo, ocular disturbances and hemiparesis.

2. *Shoulders.* The gleno-humeral joints are often affected giving rise to limitation with the end result that simple hygiene and toilet may be impossible (brushing hair, washing neck and in severe cases, feeding).

3. *Elbows.* Again pain, stiffness and joint deformity will limit function. Subcutaneous nodules and bursae commonly form around the extensor aspects of the elbows.

4. *Wrists.* The wrists are very commonly involved, initially with soft tissue swelling and later with subluxation (especially in ulnar and palmar directions). A special and common occurrence is subluxation such that the lower end of ulna becomes prominent dorsally. The extensor tendons of the little, ring and middle fingers ride over the roughened lower end of ulna and due to attrition may rupture (Fig. 25.5). With a weak, subluxed, painful wrist, hand function must suffer.

Carpal tunnel syndrome is common, with compression of the median nerve and subsequent paraesthesiae in the hand occurring especially at night and wasting of the muscles of the thenar eminence.

5. *Hands.* In the early stages, soft tissue swelling of the proximal interphalangeal joints and metacarpophalangeal joints is common (Fig. 25.2). Later, ulnar drift (Fig. 25.3) and palmar subluxation

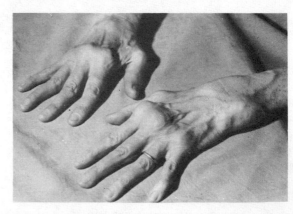

Fig. 25.2 Soft tissue swelling of the metacarpophalangeal joints of the index and middle fingers of both hands and early deformities at the proximal interphalangeal joints.

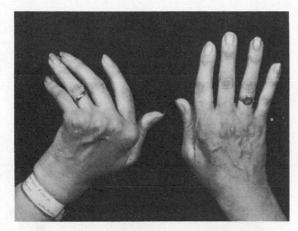

Fig. 25.3 Ulnar drift or deviation of the fingers to the ulnar side.

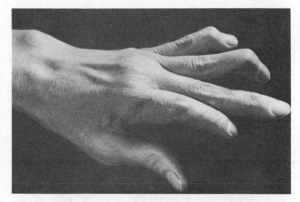

Fig. 25.4 Swan neck deformity of the fingers. (With kind permission of the *Nursing Mirror*.)

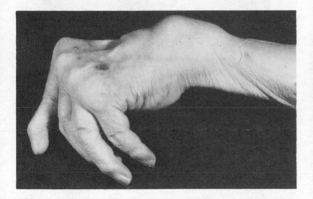

Fig. 25.5 Rheumatoid arthritis. Swelling of the dorsum of the wrist due to tenosynovitis of the extensor tendon sheaths. Note also the swan neck deformity of the index finger and dropping of the middle, ring and little fingers due to rupture of extensor tendons.

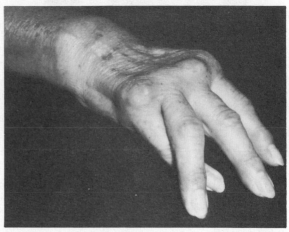

Fig. 25.6 Over-ride of the fingers in rheumatoid arthritis.

are very common at metacarpophalangeal level. 'Swan neck' and 'buttonhole' deformities, are seen in late stages (Figs 25.4 and 25.5). Over-ride of the fingers may occur, as in Fig. 25.6.

The flexor sheaths are often involved giving rise to swollen fingers and poor flexion. Nodules may occur in the tendons and triggering results.

6. *Hips*. These joints are involved in approximately 40 per cent of patients. Their importance with regard to walking, standing, climbing and transferring from chairs and bed etc. is obvious but interference with hygiene and sexual function must not be forgotten. It must be remembered that pain from the hips is often referred to the knees.

7. *Knees*. The knees are very commonly involved. Initially there is synovial thickening and effusion. In later stages, there is deformity (flexion, valgus or less commonly varus). Lateral and cruciate instability add to the deformity (Fig. 25.7). Eventually degenerative changes occur.

Not uncommonly patients with knee involvement have popliteal cysts or 'Baker's cysts' (Fig. 25.8). Apart from causing tightness behind the knee, these cysts may rupture and give signs identical to those of deep vein thrombosis. An arthrogram of the knee usually differentiates the two conditions.

8. *Ankles*. The sub-talar joints are more commonly involved than the ankles but the symptoms are still referred to the hind foot. In late stages the

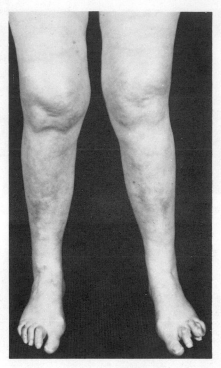

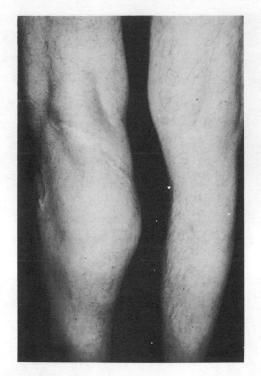

Fig. 25.7   Rheumatoid arthritis affecting both knees and both feet.

Fig. 25.8   'Baker's' cyst.

most obvious finding is that of a painful, valgoid foot.

9. *Metatarsophalangeal joints.* Disease at these joints is common and early (so that it is important to X-ray the feet in the early stages). Symptoms are often disabling and patients complain of pain as if they were walking 'barefoot on cobbles'. Subluxation occurs with clawing of the toes and pressure lesions develop. Hallux valgus deformity is often seen.

Extra-articular features

Weakness and malaise are common complaints. Anaemia is usually found. Vascular lesions, if they occur, may involve many tissues. In the hands, they present as nail fold haemorrhages or as recurrent crops of small painful nodules in the fingers. Rarely a digit may become ischaemic. If peripheral nerves are affected, neuropathy results. This is usually sensory, bilateral and in the lower limbs. In the legs, multiple ulceration can be present. Other manifestations of vasculitis will depend upon the tissue or organ involved.

Nodules are usually subcutaneous and located around the elbows or along the forearms. Less frequently they may be found in other sites such as the lungs or heart.

Pleural effusion is the most common lung finding but nodules (single or multiple) and fibrosing alveolitis are well described.

In the heart, pericarditis occurs in 40 per cent of patients but this is usually asymptomatic. Granulomatous tissue may involve the conduction system or interfere with valve function.

The most common finding in the eyes is dryness due to diminished secretion of tears (following inflammation in the lachrymal glands). This is part of Sjögren syndrome and the patient complains of sore, itching dry eyes. Other lesions of the eye include episcleritis and nodule formation.

These are just some of the extra-articular features occurring in some patients who suffer from rheumatoid arthritis. There are others. It must be emphasised that the disease primarily affects joints and that arthritis is the dominant feature.

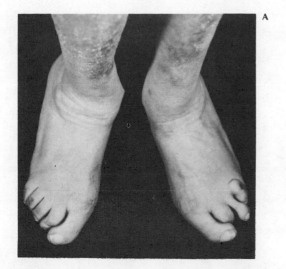

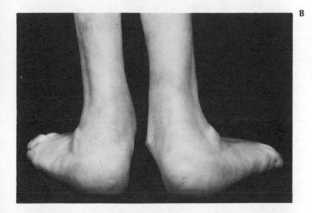

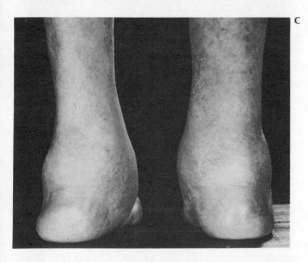

Fig. 25.9 A–C. Rheumatoid arthritis affecting the ankles and sub-talar joints with valgus deformity of the feet. Note also the deformity of the toes.

In this section it is worth mentioning that the side effects of drugs can also affect the clinical picture.

A variant of rheumatoid arthritis has been named Felty's syndrome. In this condition, apart from the arthritis, enlargement of the spleen is found and a low white cell count is present in the blood. Leg ulceration completes the picture.

Blood and synovial fluid changes

Investigations are as follows:

Haemoglobin. Anaemia is common, the haemoglobin level often falling to about 10 gm/100 ml. Levels of less than 8.5 gm/100 ml usually signify the presence of an additional factor such as iron deficiency due to a different cause. The anaemia of rheumatoid arthritis itself is not one of iron deficiency.

ESR. The sedimentation rate is commonly raised but the actual level does not necessarily parallel severity. Measurement of plasma viscosity has replaced the ESR in a number of laboratories.

Plasma proteins. Electrophoresis of plasma proteins shows an increase in gamma globulins — a reflection of the immunological changes taking place.

SCAT. The sheep cell agglutination test is positive in approximately 70 per cent of patients with rheumatoid arthritis. Other tests for rheumatoid factors (rheumaton, latex tests etc.) may be positive more frequently but are less specific.

ANA. The anti-nuclear antibody test has more significance in a disease called systemic lupus erythematosus but is positive in some cases of rheumatoid arthritis.

Synovial fluid. It is useful to examine this fluid. The white cell count is raised with a predominant leucocytosis. The count may be as high as 50 000 per mm^3 or more, giving rise to a suspicion of infection but without the fluid revealing evidence of infection by routine cultural methods. The protein content is also raised, above 3 g/100 ml. The SCAT may be positive. Other tests on the fluid may be helpful (such as the finding of a low complement level).

It must be stressed that although the above tests may help in the diagnosis of rheumatoid arthritis, they are not specific and do not make a diagnosis.

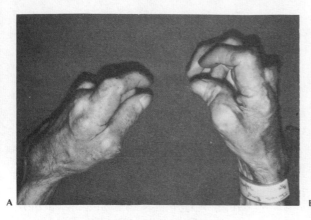

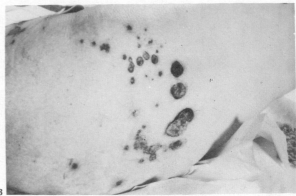

Fig. 25.10   A, B. Rheumatoid arthritis, showing skin changes due to arteritis.

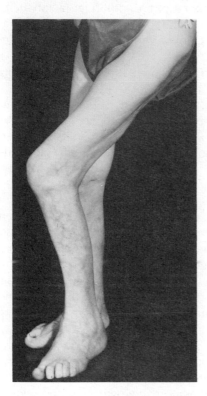

Fig. 25.11   Flexion deformity of the left knee due to rheumatoid arthritis.

Radiological changes

In the early stages, soft tissue swelling and peri-articular osteoporosis are common. Later, erosions appear in the bones at the reflection of the synovial membrane and eventually subluxation and deformity become apparent. Ankylosis may occur.

Generally speaking, X-rays are of most value in assessing the progress of the disease, but apart from this, are of particular importance in such sites as the neck to establish the existence of subluxation. In the early stages of the disease, an X-ray of the feet may show changes in the metatarsophalangeal joints before other sites even though symptoms are absent or minimal.

Special techniques may be applied in certain circumstances. Arteriography can be used to demonstrate the presence of vasculitis. Arthrography can readily show the presence of a popliteal cyst ('Baker's cyst') (Fig. 25.8) behind the knee, and this is especially important when the difficult situation arises of differentiating between a deep vein thrombosis and a ruptured Baker's cyst. Myelography may be necessary to establish the precise role of a cervical spine lesion in producing tetraplegia or paraplegia. More advanced arteriography may help in determining the vascular involvement in rheumatoid disease of the neck.

Additional techniques such as isotope scanning e.g. using radio-active technetium and thermography may be employed in research projects.

Course and prognosis

The course of the disease varies greatly from one patient to another. Even the onset is variable. Although the onset is usually insidious in some cases it is acute and may be precipitated by stress (emotional or physical). One such stressful situation arises after pregnancy and it is not uncommon

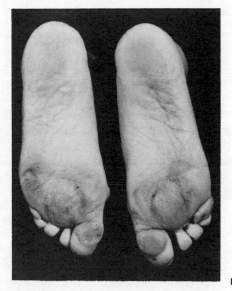

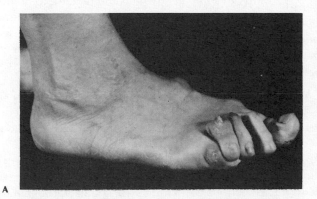

Fig. 25.12   A, B. Rheumatoid arthritis affecting the feet, with dislocation of lesser toes and callosities on the plantar aspect of the feet.

to find the disease either starting or being exacerbated a few weeks post-partum. Occasionally the onset of the disease is episodic with intervals of normality between acute phases. Some cases remit completely within 6 or 12 months of onset, especially if the disease is sero negative (SCAT negative).

Once the disease is established, most cases pursue a downhill course with exacerbations and remissions occurring over a period of many years. Some cases remain mild, affecting relatively few joints. Others can, rarely, have a fulminating course leading to deformity and infirmity over a short period of time ('malignant rheumatoid disease').

Rheumatoid arthritis rarely kills. The patient may expect to live a normal lifespan but this can be cut short by intercurrent infection, amyloid disease (occurring in up to 5 per cent of patients and especially manifested by the nephrotic syndrome), neck involvement with cord compression or ischaemia, or from unsuspected joint infection, especially of the hips.

Unfavourable features as far as prognosis is concerned are as follows:

1. Arthritis of more than a year's duration (some patients improve within the first 12 months).

2. A positive rheumatoid factor test.
3. The presence of nodules or vasculitis (usually associated with a positive rheumatoid factor test).
4. Female sex.

In time, even though after many years the disease may become quiescent, it leaves behind permanent deformity and disability and the possibility of secondary degenerative changes.

TREATMENT

Treatment is complex. Rheumatoid arthritis is one of the many diseases that cannot, at the present time, be 'cured'. Despite this, much can be done to improve the patient. In general the objectives are:

1. to relieve pain and stiffness;
2. to halt the progress of the disease as much as possible;
3. to prevent or correct deformity;
4. to preserve the independence of the patient.

Management depends on the stage and type of disease. Subsequent paragraphs will deal with the 'average' patient. Important factors in management are as follows:

The psychological integrity of the patient

It is essential to obtain the patient's trust and co-operation. He or she must accept the existence of the disease and avoid spending time and money searching for a miraculous 'cure'. Regression to dependency takes time and it is unreasonable to expect that this can be reversed quickly. Dependency and passivity may well inhibit rehabilitation. The patient's will to improve must equal that of those who are treating her.

Functional management

Physiotherapy and occupational therapy must be aimed at rehabilitating the patient to his or her environment. Most commonly this applies to the female patient who has to exist in 'home' situations. It is quite useless to achieve maximum function in a joint if this is not related to the functional needs of the patient. If it is not possible to train a patient to cope with her environment then an attempt should also be made to modify the environment. For example, if a patient has to climb two steps to get to the toilet but can only be trained to climb one, then attempts must be made to remove the second step.

This type of management is not always required but when it is, community facilities may be required. Important factors arise such as proper co-ordination with outside services and proper assessment of a particular patient's requirements.

In a disease with such a prolonged course and with the possibility of constant change these requirements often change as well so that regular reappraisal of the situation is necessary.

Medical management

Pain and stiffness must be relieved. Muscle power has to be maintained. Deformities must be prevented or corrected. If possible the disease process must be halted. The extra-articular features must be recognised and treated appropriately. Constant watch has to be kept for the side effects of treatment (iatrogenic disease).

Rest

It is well-established that resting an inflamed joint will result in a lessening of the inflammation. Rest can be divided into two sections—rest of the body and rest of a particular joint. It is wise to rest the body as a whole for this will lessen active synovial disease. On the other hand, disuse will result in stiffness, muscle wasting, osteoporosis and immobility. In some centres it is the practise to immobilise the body totally for a period of up to a maximum of three weeks in an attempt to lessen disease activity. An alternative approach is to have rest periods of one hour twice a day. In these periods, the patient will rest the whole and parts of the body (with resting splints). Splintage i.e. rest of a particular joint will reduce disease activity, reduce pain and help to prevent deformity. Too much immobility is not good (stiffness, wasting etc.). Too much use is bad (exacerbation of synovitis). A compromise is essential and is best achieved by having rest periods (with the use of splints) throughout the day. Rest splints are commonly made of plaster of Paris but there are newer materials coming on to the market which can be used, e.g. Plastozote, Orthoplast (Fig. 25.14A and B). Resting splints may also be used at night.

DRUGS

Drugs will not cure disease. In using drugs one must always be aware of the following points:

1. The objective to be attained.
2. The regimen should be as safe as possible i.e. the use of the least toxic drug and in the smallest dose necessary to achieve the objective.
3. The anti-rheumatic drugs cause more iatrogenic disease than any other group of drugs.
4. If it is necessary to use the more potent (and more toxic) drugs then they should only be used when constant monitoring is employed.

It is common practice to divide drugs into three groups.

Group A: First-line drugs. Generally speaking these are given to relieve the symptoms of pain and stiffness.

There is an ever-growing number of such drugs. Examples are as follows:

Aspirin
Indomethacin (Indocid)
Mefenamic acid (Ponstan)

Flufenaminic acid (Arlef)
Ibuprofen (Brufen)
Flurbiprofen (Froben)
Fenoprofen (Fenopron)
Ketoprofen (Orudis: Alrheumat)
Naproxen (Naprosyn)
Sulindac (Clinoril)
Azapropazone (Rheumox)
Diclofenac (Voltarol)
Fenclofenac (Flenac)
Piroxicam (Feldene)
Fenbufen (Lederfen)

There is an individual variation with regard to both effectiveness and side effects. It is necessary to find the preparation which gives most relief without adverse effect. Thus it may be that several have to be tried. In such an event each one must be given separately and for an adequate period of time (2 or 3 weeks unless side effects intervene). Adverse reactions (commonly involving the gastro-intestinal tract or skin) are usually not dangerous and are reversible on withdrawal of the drug. Aspirin, and its derivatives, still has a place. Individual drugs have their own peculiar disadvantages apart from the commonly encountered indigestion or rash but on the whole, they are well tolerated and form an acceptable means of treatment. The adverse effect of many years of therapy raises a question which cannot be adequately answered at this time.

The first-line drugs are often supplemented by analgesic drugs taken 'on demand' e.g. low dose aspirin, paracetamol, Distalgesic (dextropropoxyphene).

Group B. Second-line drugs. First-line drugs may not control the disease and it may be necessary to add in more effective, but more toxic agents.

Such drugs include:

Antimalarials
Gold
D-Penicillamine
Cytotoxic drugs

Features of this group include greater toxicity and delayed onset of clinical effect. Because of the toxicity it is essential that these drugs should be monitored. The doctor must see the patient regularly.

Antimalarials. The effect of treatment will not be seen for about 2 months. Generally speaking this is the least effective of this group, but also the least toxic. The chief disadvantage is the possibility of retinal, and in particular macular, degeneration which may be irreversible and may result in blindness if too large a dose is used. A standard regimen is to give 400 mg daily of hydroxychloroquine for three months and then 200 mg daily from then.

Gold. This is commonly given as myocrisin (sodium aurothiomalate) intra-muscularly. After a test dose of 10 mg, 50 mg doses are given weekly until benefit is seen, usually at 400 to 600 mg, when it is cut to 50 mg fortnightly. Subsequently monthly maintenance injections of 50 mg may be given. During the course, blood tests to include white cells and platelets are carried out at fortnightly intervals and the urine tested for albumin weekly. Apart from bone marrow and renal toxicity, rashes, usually preceded by itching, are common. Any trend towards thrombocytopoenia, the presence of albuminuria or the development of a rash are all indications for discontinuing gold. Other side effects may occur but are less common.

D-Penicillamine. This is given as a tablet and it is important to start with small doses e.g. 125 mg a day. This can be increased by 125 mg at intervals of 4 to 6 weeks, building up to a dose usually not in excess of 500 mg per day. Again, clinical effect is not usually obvious for 2 or 3 months.

Monitoring must be carried out, as for gold and the most frequent side effects are very similar. In addition, however, gastro-intestinal symptoms are common, ranging from loss of taste, to severe nausea and vomiting. The indication for the use of penicillamine is as for gold, namely the presence of severe progressive disease which has not been controlled by first line drugs. There is a variation in opinion as to which should be used first but penicillamine tends to give rise to more side effects. It may have a particular advantage when nodules and vascular lesions are a predominant feature of the disease.

Cytotoxic drugs. Azathioprine, cyclophosphamide, and others have been used in the treatment of rheumatoid arthritis, usually for the more rapidly progressive type of disease. They are potentially very toxic, especially on the bone marrow, and must only be used under the closest supervision.

Group C. Corticosteroids. There is no doubt that this group is more likely to give relief of symptoms than any of the others. Unfortunately there are very many side effects associated with their use and after a number of years a price has to be paid. As a rule, the incidence of side effects is related to the amount given. It is important, therefore to give the smallest dose possible to achieve a response. The drug of choice is prednisolone and every attempt should be made to keep the dose at 5 mg per day or less except for a temporary increase during an exacerbation.

The use of corticosteroids in rheumatoid arthritis should be restricted to those patients who have progressive disease despite the use of first and second line drugs and whose quality of life is obviously very poor. They may also be considered for socio-economic reasons and in the elderly. Every attempt should be made to withdraw the drug if it seems appropriate.

Short term corticosteroid therapy (e.g. over a 2 month period) with a gradually reducing dose may be used with less apprehension. Indications for such a course include an acute exacerbation and, sometimes, at the time of introduction of second-line drug therapy to cover the period taken for the latter to be effective. In the latter case, the use of large intravenous dosage is being increasingly used.

Intra-articular therapy

Intra-articular corticosteroids are commonly employed. Various preparations are available. Indications include:

1. Involvement of few joints.
2. An acute exacerbation of disease in a joint.
3. As an adjunct to physiotherapy (e.g. in attempting to correct a flexion deformity or when physiotherapy has failed to achieve sufficient improvement in any one joint).

As with any other invasive technique, care must be taken not to introduce infection. Repetitive injections at frequent intervals into a joint should be avoided and an alternative form of treatment sought. There is a place for the use of local steroid into joints, tendon sheaths and sometimes soft tissues, but it must be used with great care. As a rule the effect of intra-articular corticosteroids is short lived and various other substances have been used

in an attempt to ablate the synovial granulation tissue. Radio-active materials (e.g. radio-active yttrium for knees, radio-active erbium for smaller joints), thiotepa, osmic acid and various others have been, and still are, used with some success but none has so far proved to be entirely satisfactory. Still the search goes on to find a more suitable agent to use for 'medical' synovectomy.

Self-help devices

It is pointless to persevere with an activity of daily living which is painful and difficult for a patient if a simple alternative method can be found. Many aids, such as long-handled combs, special cutlery, etc., are available, and should be selected with the needs of the individual patient in mind. This task is usually undertaken by the occupational therapist but the nurse must be aware of the possibilities. Often the correct selection can only take place in the patient's own home.

Appliances

Splints, working splints and surgical shoes are of obvious importance. Of equal importance is that they fit and are used properly.

Social, economic and vocational factors

Family relationships and attitudes are important. In general we are dealing with a middle-aged or elderly group of the community and the same applies to relatives. Is the family able or willing to help? In the absence of relatives, are neighbours able or willing to help? It is important to have an awareness of living and working conditions. An assessment must be made of housing, stairs, doorway widths, chair and bed heights, working benches, plugs, proximity of services (shopping etc.), toilet facilities etc. In other words, a patient cannot be rehabilitated without knowledge of his or her total home environment.

The community services, including general practitioners, social services, voluntary organisations, works doctors and employers may all be involved. A patient is not just treated in hospital. He or she is prepared for an existence outside hospital and to achieve this end result the hospital and community services must be co-ordinated. What is essential, in a disease of such variation, is the continued need for up to date assessment and the co-operation and integration of all available services.

Corrective or preventive orthopaedic surgery

As with the other facets of management, surgery has a role to play. Prevention consists essentially of removal of the noxious synovial tissue which we know will cause joint damage. Synovectomy is the term applied to removal of the proliferative synovial membrane in joints and tendon sheaths. If the synovial membrane contains enzymes which destroy cartilage and eventually bone, then it is sensible to remove such tissue. Synovectomy is most commonly applied to the knees but may be used anywhere in the body where synovitis occurs. Not only may it delay destructive changes, it also relieves pain and stiffness. Adequate physiotherapy is required to regain and preserve function subsequently.

In the later stages, reconstructive surgery may be required. This is best applied to the hips where total replacement has revolutionised the management of long standing rheumatoid disease. Elsewhere, reconstructive surgery has yet to establish its role. Intensive research is being applied to total knee, shoulder and elbow replacements, but these procedures are not as satisfactory as replacement surgery for the hip. Despite this, many successful arthroplasties are being performed in the knee. Prosthetic replacements may be used in the hands, especially at the metacarpophalangeal level where silastic implants are used. This procedure may be carried out when erosive change has taken place but ideally should not be used as a salvage operation.

Apart from total joint replacements there are many other procedures available as follows:

Cervical spine. Less serious involvement of the neck may be treated by means of a collar. Although this is not sufficient to prevent subluxation it will often relieve pain and symptoms due to root pressure.

Cervical fusion may be life saving and important in terms of preventing further neurological damage in the presence of subluxation. Generally it is best to consider fusion of the whole of the neck other-

wise the fused segment might sublux on lower cervical vertebrae. The total stay in hospital is usually about three months.

Shoulders. Until a suitable prosthesis has been designed, surgery has little to offer here. With a very painful and fixed joint, however, formal arthrodesis may be worthwhile.

Elbows. Excision of the head of radius is a good technique in many cases if there is pain and tenderness at this site associated with painful and limited rotational movements. It would not be expected to improve flexion and extension. When the joint is grossly disorganised the ulnar nerve may be compressed and will need to be transplanted.

Wrists. The wrist must be kept in a good functional position by the appropriate use of splints. Resting splints will relieve pain and swelling and help to prevent deformity. During the day a working splint of plastic or leather will improve hand function if this has been impaired due to a painful, weak wrist. Resting splints should hold the wrist in slight dorsiflexion. Occasionally the application of a plaster cylinder for two or three weeks may help to settle an exacerbation in the wrist.

If the lower end of ulna is prominent and rotational movements are painful, excision of the distal end of the bone is a valuable procedure. This is particularly so if there is rupture of the extensor tendons overriding it.

Carpal tunnel decompression is necessary where there is median nerve involvement.

In the case of a severely disorganised and painful wrist arthrodesis can be expected to give a good result. The position of fixation must be carefully considered in the light of the patients needs. The optimal position may be assessed pre-operatively by using plaster cylinders to immobilise the wrist.

Hands. Extensor tendon rupture can also result from involvement by granulation tissue on the dorsum of the hand. In such cases, synovectomy and tendon repair are carried out. It is also useful at the same time to re-route the tendons on the dorsum of the extensor retinaculum.

Synovectomy and silastic prostheses have already been mentioned. Intrinsic release may improve swan neck deformities if there is tightness of the intrinsic muscles. Buttonhole deformities can be corrected. When there is loss of flexion at proximal interphalangeal joint level, arthrodesis in flexion will improve function, especially power grip, providing metacarpophalangeal joint flexion is good.

Arthrodesis is sometimes required for the joints of the thumb, especially the metacarpophalangeal joint. Flexor tendon involvement (e.g. nodular thickening) may require surgery, but triggering may resolve spontaneously or with the help of local steroid injections.

Hips. Total hip replacement is now a well established procedure. Initially it was performed only in the more elderly patient the idea being that revision was unlikely to prove necessary in the life-time of most patients. Over the years there has been a tendency to operate on younger patients with a result that a second replacement is becoming more common (e.g. after 10–15 years). This is not as satisfactory as was anticipated and as a result, new forms of prosthesis are being developed for use in the younger patient, involving a less major procedure in the hope that at a later date, if necessary a standard prosthesis may be inserted more easily.

Knee. Conservative regimens should be applied to flexion deformities (Fig. 25.11). Serial plasters may have to be used. There are a number of techniques for obtaining greater extension using plaster splints. One such technique is to apply a cylinder after hydrotherapy and the use of an analgesic with the patient lying prone (Fig. 25.18). Forty-eight hours later the plaster is bivalved, and active physiotherapy commenced. For 48 hours the shell of the old splint is used for resting when physiotherapy is not being applied. The procedure is repeated until maximum gain has been obtained.

Serial wedge plasters may be used, the knee being straightened by degrees, either by putting wedges in posteriorly, or by using an attached turnbuckle, but there is some disadvantage in the loss of active physiotherapy that this method entails. Additional methods for correcting a flexion deformity of the knee include: serial plasters under pethidine, or a general anaesthetic; reversed slings on a Thomas bed-knee splint using skin traction; by means of a bent bed-splint. Rarely a posterior release operation and skeletal traction are needed to aid the correction. In all methods care must be taken to guard against subluxation of the knee and inducing fractures in osteoporotic bones.

Synovectomy and total knee replacements have been mentioned. In some cases when the disease has progressed beyond the stage of being helped by synovectomy but has not reached the stage of requiring a total replacement, hemiarthroplasty (MacIntosh) may be useful. New prostheses are being developed (Ch. 8).

Severe valgus or varus deformity is an indication for osteotomy, with or without knee replacement.

It may be necessary to remove a tense Baker's cyst.

Ankle and foot. The valgus foot cannot always be controlled by insoles, supports or wedges. In such cases they require the provision of an outside iron and inside T-strap. For the painful subtalar joint a double below-knee iron is sometimes more effective.

Rarely, arthrodesis of the subtalar joint is performed.

Disabling symptoms and deformities of the forefoot are helped by the provision of surgical shoes, metatarsal insoles or bars.

Painful dislocation of the metatarsophalangeal joints is often treated surgically by trimming the heads of the metatarsals and excising the bases of the proximal phalanges (modified Fowler operation and others). Hallus valgus deformities have to be corrected (e.g. by a Keller's operation).

Special note. Patients with rheumatoid arthritis affecting the cervical spine risk subluxation of the atlanto-axoid joint and subsequent paralysis when under an anaesthetic.

Summary of treatment

There are many surgical procedures available to the rheumatoid patient. The correct timing of any operation is very important. Synovectomy and total replacement will obviously be applicable at different stages of the disease. The state of disease in other joints could have a bearing on what is done (e.g. both hips and both knees must be assessed if one of them is to be approached surgically). One must remember that surgery is not always successful and there are some inherent dangers (such as sepsis occurring in relation to a prosthesis). In many cases, as we are dealing with a relatively old age group, the patient's general health may not permit operation. Unfortunately a number of patients are still receiving corticosteroids and adequate cortisone cover must be provided for any general anaesthetic.

Although surgery has much to offer it will not provide the eventual cure for rheumatoid arthritis. It must be used as part of the total programme for the patient. Combined clinics held by the rheumatologist and the orthopaedic surgeon have much to offer in determining the best method of approach.

It is essential that treatment should be appropriate to the particular type and stage of arthritis in an individual. Many disciplines are involved in the management of every patient.

NURSING CARE IN RHEUMATOID ARTHRITIS

The principles of treatment of patients suffering from rheumatoid arthritis are described in preceding pages; nursing care will now be discussed; it is important to remember that rheumatoid arthritis is essentially a disease of ups and downs so that symptoms may require treatment as they arise, and day to day modifications of nursing programmes are often required to meet the changing demands of the individual patient.

General management

General management requires a comfortable bed and a comfortable chair; bright, cheerful surroundings; ready access to out-doors, to fresh air and sunshine, and an outlook on to some scene of activity is ideal. Freedom from tension, anxiety and emotional stress is essential, as is a happy atmosphere and a cheerful optimistic attitude on the part of the staff. As in other conditions, *the patient's family* receives due consideration and the physician will include relatives in his explanations and directions as to rest, activity, medication and other aspects of treatment. Liaison with the general practitioner and other community health personnel is axiomatic.

Assessment of degree of dependency

In a ward devoted to the treatment of these patients, we might see a wide range of dependency amongst them, varying from one with minimal involvement of a few joints, to one with many joints involved

and a high degree of systemic disturbance, as well as the elderly one with established deformities and disabilities. In general, patients are not kept in bed for a moment longer than is absolutely necessary; but this in itself demands a special attitude on the part of the nurse; when a patient is confined to bed her physical care falls into a recognisable pattern, but in dealing with patients whose care is based on a delicate balance between rest and activity, a large part of the nurse's duty lies in *helping the patient to do things for herself*, particularly with regard to the toilet and to feeding. This often requires more patience and imagination and moreover is often more time-consuming than traditional nursing procedures.

Daily nursing care

On waking, the temperature, pulse and respiration are charted, the general condition is noted and recorded. Medications are given. A cup of tea is then offered; the patient may need help in drinking this and may require an aid such as an angled drinking straw.

The morning toilet. This may commence with the removal of night-splints; if the patient can get out of bed and use the ward lavatory and bathroom, so much the better; on the other hand, she may need help in walking to the bathroom, or she may be wheeled to the lavatory in a sani-chair. A shower-bath, under which a sani-chair can be wheeled, or a hand-shower, is a useful piece of equipment in this connection. If the patient can get up during the day, but cannot rise before breakfast, a bedpan or urinal must be offered. Patients who cannot use the ward bathroom are given a wash bowl, tooth-mug and receiver; the patient may or may not be able to wash herself; in any case she may not be able to attend to her own genital and anal toilet, so that this is a daily nursing responsibility. If the patient is able to carry out her own toilet in bed, make sure that all toilet articles, towel, talcum powder, etc. are placed ready to her hand; together with hair brushes, face make-up and fresh clothing, if required.

Breakfast. Again, the patient may be able to feed herself but it may be necessary to cut up solid food, e.g. bacon, and to place the table napkin, plate, etc. where they are readily accessible.

Bed-making. If the patient is allowed up during part of the day, it may be as well to postpone making her bed until she leaves it, otherwise it is made according to the accepted method, and the patient is left comfortable; patients who have had a poor night or are feeling unwell or are suffering from pain and discomfort often enjoy a nap when the toilet is complete and the bed is made. Patients able to get up may need help with dressing.

During the morning, the routine includes administration of medicaments as ordered, a mid-morning drink, the physicians visit, and physio-therapeutic sessions; the patient may also be visited by other members of the hospital team, e.g. the laboratory technician or the occupational therapist. Co-operation between the nursing team and our co-workers is essential; we are not expected to understand the techniques of their specialised work but unless we take an intelligent interest in it and cultivate a sound appreciation of their rôle in rela-tion to the patient we cannot fulfil our own; to take a simple example, if we know that the patient will be undergoing a morning session of physio-therapy, we will see to it that other aspects of the patient's treatment are completed before the physiotherapeutic session begins. This co-ope-ration must cut both ways in that the physiothera-pist will also play her part in dove-tailing treatment into the patient's routine, including rest periods.

Careful handling of the affected joints is vital at all times and at all stages of treatment, not only because of the pain but because of the grave danger of subluxation, dislocation, or even fractures of osteoporotic bones.

Rest periods are an essential part of the treatment. Half-an-hour at mid-morning, an hour after lunch and an hour after afternoon tea are the usual periods chosen, and splintage may be worn during this time. Pillows under the knees are forbidden at all stages of treatment.

Occupational therapy is mentioned here because the occupational therapist has a special rôle in relation to patients with impairment of func-tion of the upper limbs. It is discussed fully later.

The mid-day dinner is usually the main meal of the day. Again, patients who cannot eat it unaided will require appropriate assistance perhaps in cut-ting up food, or in arranging it in a readily acces-sible fashion. It is important that meals are taken unhurriedly. The importance of *nutrition* in rheu-matoid arthritis, especially if there are vasculitic lesions, is highlighted in an article in the *Nursing Times* (Stephenson, 1984). After the post-luncheon drink and toilet procedures an hour's rest is usually ordered. Patients who are fully dressed may need help in removing foot-wear before resting on their beds, covered with a blanket if required. Rest-splints may be worn during this period. Medica-tions are given as ordered.

Administration of drugs

It goes without saying that administration of drugs ordered by the physician and which have been de-scribed in foregoing pages must be given *at the time prescribed* and in the dosage ordered (Fig. 25.13). It is the responsibility of the nurse not only

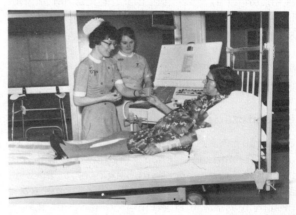

Fig. 25.13 Administration of drugs. Note the variable height (King's fund) bed, the resting splint and walking aid. (With kind permission of the *Nursing Mirror.*)

to administer a drug but to observe its effect on the patient, and in particular, to acquaint herself with the possible side effects already described and to report any sign of these to the physician without delay. This entails unremitting observation of the patient during nursing procedures; the physician relies on the nurse to report to him not only the effect of drugs but on the day to day condition of the patient with regard both to the general state of health and the state of the joints.

This has been described as 'clinical metrology' (Bird et al, 1981).

Some special aspects of nursing care

It has been emphasised that in general, the patient is helped and encouraged to get up, but *rest in bed* may be ordered in the early stages, especially if there is marked systemic disturbance and the joints are very painful. The principles of *rest in bed* and related nursing care are discussed fully in Chapters 2, 3 and 5, as is the *control of rest* and maintenance of a *balance between rest and activity*; this is a most important aspect of nursing care in rheumatoid arthritis since although fatigue must be avoided at all costs, activity *at the correct time*, and *within the correct limits* is vital for the preservation or restoration of functional use of the limb and because of the danger of ankylosis. The extent of activity is controlled by the physician and determined by the degree of systemic disturbance and of pain, swelling and tendency to subluxation or dislocation of the affected joints, and by the age and general condition of the patient.

Position in bed. In patients confined to bed for all or part of the day, and especially where splintage to prevent deformity is not ordered, pay strict attention to posture in bed; bear in mind the possibility of stiffness and ankylosis of joints. If possible, patients confined to bed without splintage should spend part of the day lying in the prone position, if this can be tolerated, with the feet placed over the end of the bed. This position prevents flexion contracture of the hip and knee and equinus deformity at the ankle; if the patient is made comfortable with a pillow under the chest, movement of the shoulders and elbows is encouraged and the tone of the extensor muscles of the back and hips is preserved. Gentle exercises to all joints and muscle groups may be given in this position.

The patient ordered continuous rest in bed, with painful swollen joints, with lassitude, anorexia and general malaise demands intelligent and imaginative exercise of all the arts in the nurse's repertoire to ensure her maximum comfort, outlined as follows: a warm, clean, smooth bed, placed out of draughts yet with a pleasant view; a head mirror is sometimes indicated; privacy for nursing procedures; scrupulous attention to cleanliness of the skin and prevention of pressure sores with care of the mouth, hair, feet, and nails; regular change of position and positioning of the limbs where

necessary; comfortable, unwrinkled night wear, with protection from pressure of bedclothes; light, comfortable splintage, where ordered; a light but liberal diet; well-made appropriate drinks to ensure an adequate fluid intake, and regulation of the bowels. In common with all our female patients, *the use of a urinal* at times other than when the bowels are opened is a valuable aid in preventing fatigue, strain, and undue disturbance, particularly to the ill, exhausted patient with painful joints and severe general malaise.

Splintage

Splints described elsewhere in this book are sometimes ordered, and the principles of their application and care are described in Chapters 6, 7, 9 and 10 in relation to the part for which they are ordered. In rheumatoid arthritis, splints are ordered for the following purposes:

1. To rest and protect a painful, swollen, inflamed joint; e.g. a plaster of Paris splint to maintain dorsiflexion of the wrist. Plastozote (polyethylene foam splinting material) is widely used. Figure 25.14 shows a spinal support made from this material.
2. To prevent deformity.
3. To correct deformity, e.g. a wedged plaster cast for the knee (Ch. 10).
4. As an aid to function, e.g. a walking brace (caliper) (Ch. 7).
5. To ascertain the optimum position of a joint in relation to the patient's functional needs before the operation of arthrodesis (e.g. of the wrist). Chapters 6, 7, 9 and 10 describe the application and care of various plaster casts and splints; in rheumatoid arthritis, the same rules apply, but particular care is required with regard to the following:

1. *Splintage must be comfortable.* These patients have enough to bear without the added discomfort of ill-fitting splints or plasters.
2. *Exercise great care in handling the limbs.* Not only are the joints painful, but very prone to subluxation or even dislocation, and fractures from trivial violence readily occur. In patients on steroids, the skin may be fragile.
3. *Keep an open mind.* Though the principles of

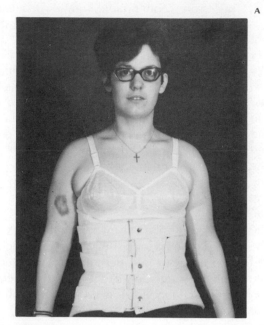

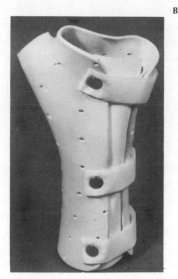

Fig. 25.14 **A.** Patient wearing a spinal support made from Plastozote. (With kind permission of the *Nursing Mirror*.) **B.** Plastic wrist splint (Taylor).

the application and care of splints and plasters do not change, treatment of these patients is highly individualistic and specialised so that experimentation and modification within the limits of these principles is often required.

Nursing management after operation

Operations commonly advised have been described in a previous section; pre-operative and post-operative nursing management has also been discussed at length on various pages of this book. Post-operative treatment in hip operations is discussed in Chapter 27.

Cortisone is sometimes ordered to tide the patient over the critical stage of the operation; the importance of unremitting vigilance with a view to the recognition of untoward reactions, such as collapse due to inadequate dosage, is emphasised once more.

Post-operative period. Nursing care proceeds as described for any surgical procedure, with special reference to the use of drugs, as mentioned above.

REHABILITATION

As stated earlier, this begins whilst the patient is in hospital and not as an after-thought on discharge. The aim of treatment is to render the patient as independent of aid as possible. The nurse has a special responsibility in finding means of teaching the patient to use a normal lavatory and bathroom; to be self-supporting in this respect is surely the basis of independence and therefore a vital part of every rehabilitative programme.

PHYSIOTHERAPY IN RHEUMATOID ARTHRITIS

Physiotherapy for rheumatoid arthritis and kindred conditions varies according to the individual needs of each patient, as does drug therapy, since what helps one patient may not suit another; it may be necessary to try different forms of treatment to find out which will achieve the best results. Before starting treatment, the patient's notes are read and the X-rays examined; the physiotherapist talks to the patient to try to find out as much as possible about home conditions, not only to learn the type of

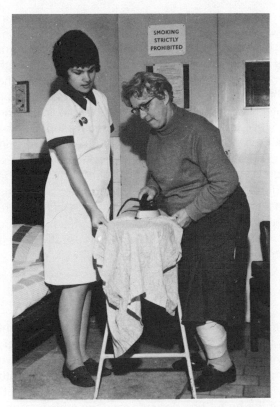

Fig. 25.15 Re-education in activities of daily living is an essential part of the treatment. (With kind permission of the *Nursing Mirror*.)

accommodation, but also the amount of work the patient does, the employment, if any, and the help afforded by friends, relations or social services. All this will give a picture of what we hope to achieve; it is also necessary to confer with the occupational therapist, who will be able to supply added helpful information.

Having established a friendly relationship with the patient, the individual treatments can be discussed with the aim in view. The aim throughout is, to relieve pain, to increase the range of joint movement, to improve muscle power, and so promote greater independence and a more acceptable way of living. For in-patients, it is very necessary for the physiotherapist to work in co-operation at all times with the medical and nursing staff and other members of the team; liaison with the community physiotherapist and others who will care for the patient at home is also essential.

The following list of treatments are those sup-plied in our hospital, and the most suitable treatments are chosen for each individual patient.

1. Damp heat

a. *Hydrotherapy* (Fig. 25.16). This seems to be the most beneficial treatment for nearly all patients.

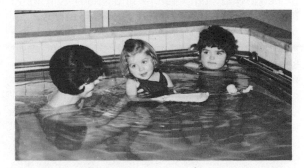

Fig. 25.16 Hydrotherapy.

The contra-indications are: sores or open wounds, a rash which is aggravated by the chlorine in the water, or the patient's real fear of water. The patient is immersed in water in a small pool, the temperature being about 97° F. If it is too difficult for the patient to climb over the side of the pool, he or she is lifted in, or when very heavy and/or handi-capped, a hoist is brought into use. The physio-therapist supports the patient in a floating position (Fig. 26.3), so that a full range of movement in all joints may be carried out. The great advantage of exercising in water is that the patient has a sensation of weightlessness, the warmth produces relaxation and reduction of pain, so that a greater range of movement is achieved; the water can also be used as a resistance to help develop poor muscles. The length of treatment is about 20 minutes, and should be given daily. It has been found that although some people at first regard the pool with some degree of apprehension, after the first treatment most patients cannot wait for the next one.

b. *Hydropacks.* These packs are pre-heated in a boiler, then wrapped in blankets and applied to painful joints over the patients individual towels, in particular to knee, back and shoulder. The packs are kept in position with mackintosh or plastic sheets which help retain the heat; the length of treatment is about 20 minutes. Before applying hydropacks, it is necessary to test skin sensation and to insist that if there is any discomfort the patient attracts attention immediately. These packs are very popular and seem to give great relief from pain; on removal, active exercises are carried out for all the involved joints.

c. *Warm Wax*. In this treatment, paraffin wax is heated to body temperature, and while it is in liquid form, the hands or feet are dipped into the container repeatedly until about five layers are achieved; the whole extremity is then wrapped in paper or in towels to conserve heat. When the wax cools, the paper is removed and the wax is removed like a glove or sock and can then be used to mould into shapes to exercise the hands. Alternatively, the warm wax is poured over the hands as they rest on a metal, plastic or wooden tray; the patient then exercises the hands so that as the wax cools and gradually solidifies it is moulded into different shapes. *Active exercises* are always performed after wax treatment.

2. Dry heat

a. *Infra-red irradiation*. This treatment is given with an Infra-red lamp; the heat is directed towards the painful area, for example the neck, shoulder or back. It may be used instead of hydropacks for a small, frail patient who cannot tolerate the weight of a hydropack. Skin testing prior to treatment is necessary (as with hydropacks) and the patient should not be left unattended. After 15–20 minutes of heat application, massage may be given to the affected part and is found most beneficial; the whole treatment is concluded with active or active-assisted exercises.

b. *Short-wave diathermy*. Many hospitals use this form of treatment for rheumatoid arthritis, but we have found that it is not much appreciated so that it is little used, and will not be described here.

3. Cold application

a. *Crushed ice* in a pack may be used as an alternative to heat, applied to the affected part for about 10 minutes; a plastic sheet covered with a towel should be placed below the joint involved. Skin tests are very necessary to avoid burns and an application of oil may be used; the pack should be damp on the outside to be effective.

Ice may also be used to massage the skin surrounding a sore or ulcer, to improve the circulation.

b. *Flowtronaire*. This can be applied in the form of boots or gloves; the boots are either knee-length or hip-length and the gloves are full-length to the shoulder. These appliances are placed on the affected limbs with the leads attached to an electric control box connected to the mains supply. The purpose of flowtronaire is to reduce oedema and to improve circulation by exerting alternative pressure and relaxation; the control box may be adjusted to give more or less pressure according to the degree of oedema. Great care is taken where there is gross oedema because too much pressure can produce bruising. Treatment is usually carried out for about half an hour.

4. Ultra-violet light

This is used in the treatment of psoriasis; the patient is first immersed in a coal tar bath of warm water, where the affected areas are scrubbed to remove loose tissue. Thereafter the patient lies on a plinth with a theractin lamp at a distance of 36 in irradiating the body, first one side then the other, starting at 2 or 3 minutes according to the type and sensitivity of the skin, and increasing by a minute daily for a month. Following irradiation, the psoriatic areas are annointed with dithranol ointment.

5. Exercises (Active, or active assisted exercises)

In addition to exercises performed under water, after hydropacks and after wax baths, patients should be encouraged to follow their own exercise plan frequently through the day; 'little and often' is better than one long session, and exercises in a class with others can be enjoyable as well as effective. Each joint should be moved to its fullest possible extent with the emphasis on retaining or restoring function. Muscle power can be improved by resisted exercises using sand-bags.

a. *Walking*. Many patients arrive in hospital having spent long periods in bed or in a wheelchair, and whenever possible, they are encouraged to walk with the help of different walking aids. Similarly, following an operation, patients are given assistance and re-education in walking.

6. *Splintage*

Splintage is a very important item in the treatment of rheumatoid arthritis, especially where joints are deformed and unstable, muscle power is inadequate and where there is persistent pain. Supports for the foot, ankle, knee, back, wrist or neck can all be obtained from commercial suppliers. However, resting splints for hands and knees are made from plaster of Paris by physiotherapists, who also make wrist cylinders, knee cylinders, walking plasters and back supports (Figs 25.17 and 25.18). Knee flexion deformity is a very common condition and to correct this, we use serial splints; the patient

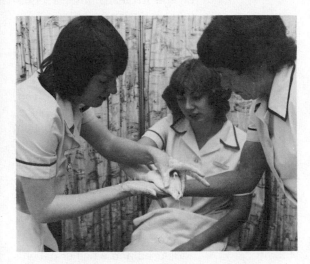

Fig. 25.17 Physiotherapy students making resting plaster of Paris splint for the wrist, under supervision.

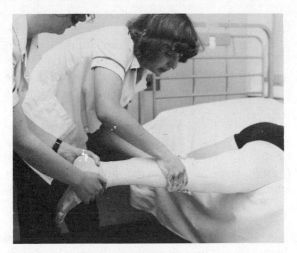

Fig. 25.18 Physiotherapy students applying a serial plaster for correction of flexion deformity of the knee.

is first treated in the hydrotherapy pool in an attempt to achieve as much knee extension as possible; immediately after he is given a relaxing drug and helped to lie prone on a bed, where the knee is encased in a plaster cylinder whilst traction is exerted by a second member of staff. After 48 hours the plaster is bi-valved and the patient is encouraged to exercise the knee whilst still using the plaster back-splint bandaged on for walking and resting. This process is usually repeated twice to achieve full extension of the knee.

OCCUPATIONAL THERAPY IN RHEUMATOID ARTHRITIS

The treatment of the patient suffering from rheumatoid arthritis is essentially that of a team, whose ultimate goals are set by the physician. The occupational therapist has an important role to play not only in giving specific treatment but by increasing the patient's motivation to overcome his difficulties and retain as much personal independence as possible.

Initial contact with the patient can be made by one of two means:

1. *Pre-admission Visit*—to meet the patient in his own environment; this will give the therapist an opportunity to assess the suitability of the dwelling; note any problems; observe attitude of any relatives and their supportiveness; give the patient some idea of what to expect once admitted to hospital.

2. *Initial Interview*—this should be done once the patient has settled into the ward. The following points should be queried and taken into consideration when assessing initially.

Table 25.1

Housing	Privately owned, rented (council or private landlord) tied cottage.
Type of Dwelling	Detached, semi-detached, flat, bungalow, cottage, maisonette, warden controlled, and number of bedrooms.
Position of Toilet and/or Bath	If toilet is outside, establish how far from house it is, and whether flush type or Elsan. In some

cases there is no toilet so alternative sanitary arrangements must be made, e.g. provision of a commode, but even then one must establish who empties it and where.

Steps   Number of steps inside and outside the house; whether there are any handrails.

Stairs   If straight flight or turn, position of bannister.

Type of Heating   If coal fire, establish who brings coal in.

Door Openings   Knobs, handles.
Type of key

Proximity of house to road, and where it is in relation to rest of community—council estate, town centre, isolated.

Path   To house and its condition.
Telephone
Social   Married, widowed, single, divorced. If wage earner, take a brief job description.
If spouse out at work, find out when they leave the house and return.
Number of children and where they live.
Establish the amount of help that they are giving.
Help available outside the house, friends, neighbours, Home Help, District Nurse, Health Visitor, Social Services or Meals on Wheels.

Benefits   It is as well to check that the patient is aware of any benefits they are entitled to: Mobility Allowance, Non-contributory Allowance for Married Women, Attendance Allowance and Sickness and Invalidity Benefit.

The occupational therapist makes a detailed assessment of the patient's ability to cope with their disability in their home environment, and the problems they have with activities of daily living.

Feeding   Common difficulties are in holding cutlery and crockery, and in cutting food.

Dressing   All clothing can present problems according to joints affected. Usual problems are getting clothes over head, reaching down to feet, and fastenings.

Comb Hair/Hygiene   If shoulder and elbow movement is restricted, this will lead to difficulty in reaching to back of the body. The patient may not be able to clean himself adequately after using the toilet.

Picking up objects   May be difficult.

Hand Activities   Such as turning taps, handling keys, manipulating door knobs, handles, switches and plugs.

Transfers   If hips and knees are involved, the height of the various pieces of furniture used by the patient must be examined.
Bed   can either be too high, too low or too soft.
Chair   find out type of chair and whether suitable.
Toilet   may be too low.
Bath or Shower

Mobility   Aids used and whether patients can cope with stairs or steps at home, whether they have a wheelchair or access to a car.

Cooking   Usual difficulties here are peeling vegetables, lifting saucepans and kettles, straining vegetables, moving items around the kitchen, using the oven, turning cooker knobs.

Housework
Shopping   All of these will present problems in the different stages of the disease.
Laundry

Hobbies and Interests   Discover whether the patient is able to cope with previous hobbies.

When assessing the patient, the occupational therapist must try and establish the degree of motivation that the patient has to gain or retain independence and to manage within their own environment—this may range from wishing to feed themselves independently, to a desire to be more competent in the kitchen.

Difficulties with all activities of daily living may occur due to a variety of physical reasons such as joint pain, stiffness, loss of muscle power, limitation of range of movement, deformity.

The aim of the treatment team is initially to relieve the above problems by medication, general care and remedial treatments.

Summary of occupational therapy activities

1. Assessment of patients problems and needs.
2. Liaison with other members of treatment team regarding patients problems and needs.
3. Advice to patients on joint preservation—easier ways to perform activities, therefore applying less stress upon affected joints, supply of possible gadgets and aids to help this.
4. Advice to patients on labour saving ideas and gadgets to enable them to perform activities more simply.
5. Providing aids and adaptations, to equipment, cutlery, clothes and furniture so that the patient can be more independent when he returns home.
6. Liaison with District Councils, Housing Authorities and Social Services for provision of alterations to the patient's home, possibility of rehousing if home is unsuitable, or for the supply of aids and adaptations to the home and its access.
7. Home visits with the patient prior to discharge to find out how the patient copes in the home. This will also give the therapist an opportunity to make suggestions about removal of loose mats, or reorganisation of furniture and to meet the patient's friends and relatives at home.
8. Taking patients shopping for food and clothing prior to discharge if they have no-one to do this for them.
9. Demonstration of patient's abilities to spouse, so that the patient is allowed maximum independence; education of members of the family in what the patient can and should do for himself is important. This can be done more easily with the co-operation of the nurse because she

usually has more contact with the patient's visitors than does the therapist.

10. Work assessment (see the section on occupational therapy in Chapter 35) to assess suitability of work and patient's possible return to it. Liaison with Disablement Resettlement Officer where necessary.
11. Activities to improve muscle strength as already outlined.
12. Encouraging patient to resume hobby activities and join the local branches of Arthritis Care who provide social evenings, advice on aids, and information on holidays at their specialised hotels and self-catering accommodation. There are many other clubs and centres that the person with rheumatoid arthritis can attend, such as Darby and Joan Clubs, Over Sixties Lunch Clubs, Red Cross Clubs, Local Authority Day Centres, Day Hospitals, all of which can provide a social outing for the patient along with specific treatments.
13. Follow-up visit to the patient after discharge to provide a continuity of service and a link for the patient with the hospital. This also affords an opportunity to check that any aids provided are suitable, or that all community services, District Nurses, Home Help are functioning correctly.

Table 25.2

Common aids supplied by the Occupational Therapist. (For other aids see illustrations in Chapters 5, 34 and 35).

Feeding	Padded handles for cutlery. Angled cutlery. Lightweight cups. Sharp serrated knives.
Dressing	Long reach aids, e.g. stocking gutter, long shoe horns, dressing sticks, knicker sticks, velcro fastenings, rings on slippers.
Picking up objects	Helping Hand and Cee Vee Reacher.
Hand Activities	Padded pen, yale lock and key adaptations, cooker knob extensions, provision of lever taps and handles.

Transfers	Bed	raise bed, suggest firm mattress.
	Chair	raise chair, provide new chair, provide ejector seat or powered chairs.
	Toilet	raised toilet seat, or rails or a 'bottom wiper' if the patient has difficulty reaching around to clean himself after using the toilet. This can either be a pair of tongs to hold the toilet tissue, or a specially made toilet tissue holder.
	Bath	non-slip mat, tap rails, bath board or seat, provide shower.
Mobility		Trolley for kitchen, provision of hand rails, second banister and resurfacing pathways in conjunction with Social Services.
Kitchen		Kettle and teapot tipper, vegetable peelers, can openers, cooking vegetables in chip baskets.
Laundry		Rotary clothes line, one handed pegs, light-weight irons.

This brief survey outlines the part that occupational therapy plays in the total rehabilitation of the rheumatoid patient.

Summary of management

The problems of composing an acceptable programme for each individual are as follows:

1. The early diagnosis and institution of a total programme.
2. The nature of the disease with its variable course and the presence of nodules, vasculitis etc. This entails the need for modifications in management and proper assessment.
3. The awareness that one is dealing with a predominantly middle-aged population. Other diseases may influence treatment (e.g. cardiovascular disease) not only in the patient but also in relatives.
4. The relationship between hospital and home. The hospital programme must be based on a total knowledge of all the circumstances and this means continuous assessment.
5. Co-ordination of services. This involves modification of the patient (by treatment) and/or modification of the environment.
6. Adequate provision of aids and appliances. When these are assessed in hospital, their speedy provision must be ensured for the patient to cope with his/her domestic environment.
7. In the case of male patients, employment is important. The type of work and the age-group of the patient have to be considered.

In the total care of the rheumatoid patient we must remember the importance of:

Total and constant vigilance and reappraisal
Proper assessment
Proper co-ordination of services.

In this way only can we hope to rehabilitate the patient to his/her maximum capacity.

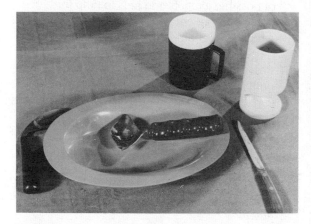

Fig. 25.19 Feeding aids suitable for the rheumatoid patient with loss of normal hand function.

OTHER TYPES OF INFLAMMATORY POLYARTHRITIS

These will be dealt with briefly but it is important to realise that they are to be differentiated from rheumatoid arthritis, on clinical, prognostic and sometimes therapeutic grounds.

1. Associated with psoriasis

This type of arthritis usually begins after the psoriasis (Fig. 25.20) has become apparent, but this is

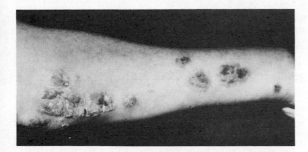

Fig. 25.20 Psoriasis of the skin of the forearm.

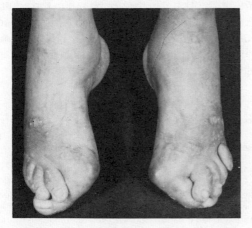

Fig. 25.21 Inflammatory polyarthritis affecting the feet associated with psoriasis. Note the skin lesions, the hallux valgus deformity and dislocation of the lesser toes.

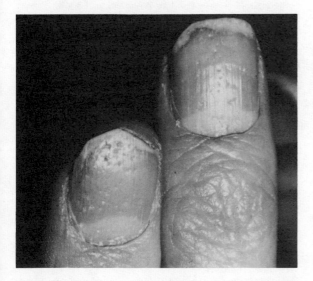

Fig. 25.22 Inflammatory polyarthritis associated with psoriasis showing pitting of the nails.

not always the case. Often the evidence for psoriasis is minimal and nail changes may be the only manifestation of the disease. (Typically, the nails are pitted like a thimble, Fig. 25.22.)

Psoriatic arthropathy is usually a milder form of joint disease than rheumatoid arthritis but is occasionally very severe. The distal interphalangeal and sacro-iliac joints are commonly involved, as are also tendon sheaths. The rheumatoid factor test is negative.

Treatment is similar to that outlined for the rheumatoid arthritis except that antimalarial drugs are contra-indicated. Anti-folic acid drugs such as Methotrexate may be used if the disease is severe.

2. Associated with ulcerative colitis

There is evidence to suggest that a form of arthritis differing from rheumatoid arthritis occurs in ulcerative colitis. Knees and ankles are commonly involved and spondylitis may develop. The small joints of hands and feet are less commonly affected than in rheumatoid arthritis and the distribution of joint involvement is not as symmetrical. Joint signs and symptoms may be transient with no residual damage. Improvement in the peripheral arthritis often follows treatment of the colitis but the spondylitic element does not appear to be influenced in the same proportion.

3. Reiter's syndrome

This is a polyarthritis affecting mainly the joints of the lower limbs and the sacro-iliac joints; it is associated with non-specific urethritis and, in over 50 per cent of patients, there are ocular lesions (usually in the form of conjunctivitis or anterior uveitis). Skin lesions are common. Sometimes the illness follows one of the dysenteries. The symptoms and signs settle but may recur, especially arthritis which could become chronic. A picture of atypical spondylitis may develop. Treatment is symptomatic but the urethritis is usually treated with a tetracycline.

There is an increased incidence of HLA B27 antigen when spondylitis features as part of the arthropathy in the last three disease entities (see Ch. 26).

4. Juvenile chronic arthritis

This disease is an arthritis occurring under the age of 16.

Clinical features. The disease may present in a number of different ways.

1. *Mono or oligoarticular.* In this group it is common to find that the disease remains restricted to just one or two joints. The incidence of eye disease is common as is also the finding of a positive antinuclear antibody test.
2. *Polyarthritis.* Multiple joint involvement without systemic upset.
3. *Polyarthritis with systemic upset.* Systemic features include:
   a. Pyrexia. Typically the temperature rises in the evening (often as high as 40°C) and is down to normal the next morning.
   b. Rash. This is evanescent and takes the form of a salmon pink erythema or maculo-papular rash. It often appears when the temperature is raised.
   c. Lymph node enlargement and splenomegaly.
   d. Pericarditis and pleural effusions.
   e. Iridocyclitis. This is very important because it is usually subacute or chronic and is usually not recognised by the child or his parents. It can eventually lead to blindness and regular ophthalmological examination is essential in all children with juvenile arthritis.

The systemic features may occur with the arthritis, follow the arthritis or even precede it. In the latter case, the children may be extensively investigated for their systemic disease and the diagnosis may not be apparent until arthritis develops.

4. *Iridocyclitis.* Rarely the onset is with iridocyclitis which can precede the arthritis by many years.

Any synovial joint may be affected but knees (especially in the monarticular cases) and cervical spine are common sites. Growth defects are common. Generally growth is retarded. Local growth defects may also occur due to premature closing of epiphyses (for example one digit or one limb may be shorter than its partner).

The patients are seronegative for rheumatoid factor.

The disease is relatively uncommon but it is important because of the disablement it causes for a young person and because of the possibility of iridocyclitis. However, the overall prognosis is good.

Considerable interest has arisen lately in the genetic coding of these children. By means of a process called tissue typing it is possible to detect antigens on cells. One particular antigen thought to be associated with the disease is known as the HL-A Antigen. This is an interesting field of study which might give us more insight into the cause of arthritis not only in the young but in the adult.

Treatment. This is similar to that for adult rheumatoid arthritis and includes physiotherapy, the use of splints, analgesic and anti-inflammatory drugs and occasionally, operative treatment.

BIBLIOGRAPHY

Adams John Crawford 1971 Outline of orthopaedics. Edinburgh: Churchill Livingstone

Ansell Barbara, Lawton Sheila 1978 Your home and your rheumatism. London: Arthritis and Rheumatism Council

Apley A Graham 1977 A system of orthopaedics and fractures. London: Butterworths

Arthritis and Rheumatism Council 1965 Rheumatoid Arthritis. A handbook for patients. London: Faraday House

Bird et al 1981 Clinical metrology. Nursing Times, 4 November

Boyle A C 1974 A colour atlas of rheumatology. London: Wolfe Medical Books

Brattstrom M 1977 Principles of joint protection in chronic rheumatoid disease. London: Wolfe Medical Books

Buchanan W, Watson Dick W, Carson 1976 Recent Advances in Rheumatology, Pt 1. Edinburgh: Churchill Livingstone

Chartered Society of Physiotherapy 1975 Handling the Handicapped. London: Woodhead Faulkner

Chilman A M, Thomas N (eds) 1978 Understanding Nursing Care. Edinburgh: Churchill Livingstone

Copeman W S C 1970 Textbook of the Rheumatic Diseases. Edinburgh: E & S Livingstone

Dixon Allan St J 1965 Progress in clinical rheumatology. London: J & A Churchill

Duthie R B, Ferguson A B Jnr 1973 Mercer's Orthopaedic Surgery. London: Arnold

Fanshawe E et al 1978 Disability without handicap. Nursing Times Supplement, 17 August, 3–20

Farrell J 1977 Illustrated Guide to Orthopaedic Nursing. Oxford: Blackwell Scientific

Kennedy J M 1974 Orthopaedic Splints and Appliances. London: Ballière Tindall

Muller W, Harweth H G, Kehr K 1971 Rheumatoid Arthritis. London: Academic Press

MacFarlane I I B 1970 Arthritis: Help in your own hands. London: Thorsons

Office of Health Economics 1973 Rheumatism and arthritis in Britain

Panayi G S 1980 Essential Rheumatology for Nurses and Therapists. London: Ballière Tindall

Platt A E 1974 The care of the rheumatoid hand. London: Kimpton

Rheumatology—Clinical Forum 1981 Nursing Mirror, 11 November

Roaf R, Hodkinson L J 1975 A Textbook of Orthopaedic Nursing. Oxford: Blackwell Scientific

Rowe J W, Dyer L (eds) 1977 Care of the Orthopaedic Patient. London: Blackwell Scientific

Rudinger E (ed.) 1974 Coping with disablement. London: Consumer's Association—publishers of Which?

Scott J T 1982 Arthritis and Rheumatism. The Facts. Oxford: Oxford University Press

Shiers L G P 1973 Total replacement of knee joint. London Nursing Times, 8 November, 1477

Stephenson V 1984 Leg ulcers I. An alternative treatment. Nursing Times, 4 July

Stone E, Pinney E 1978 Orthopaedics for Nurses. London: Ballière Tindall

Swinson D R, Swinburn W R W 1980 Rheumatology. London: Hodder and Stoughton

Vaughan-Jackson O D 1970 The rheumatoid hand. Nursing Mirror, 9 October, 26

Wilmot A 1973 Total knee joint replacement. London: Nursing Times, 17 May, 626

Wright V, Haslock J 1977 Rheumatism for nurses and remedial therapists. London: Heinemann

26

Ankylosing spondylitis

(SPONDYLITIS ANKYLOPOIETICA, MARIE-STRÜMPELL DISEASE)

Ankylosing spondylitis is an inflammatory arthritis of the spine which always involves the sacro-iliac joints and sometimes, the peripheral joints as well. It has always been regarded as a disease of young men but recently it has been stressed that the incidence is probably just as high in women so that it has been called one of the most under-diagnosed arthropathies.

Causation

The cause is unknown. There is a similarity of ankylosing spondylitis to the arthritis of Reiter's syndrome, ulcerative colitis and some cases of juvenile chronic arthritis.

The finding of HLA B27 antigen in over 90 per cent of patients with ankylosing spondylitis and in many patients having spondylitis associated with inflammatory bowel disease (regional ileitis and ulcerative colitis), Reiter's syndrome and psoriatic arthritis has aroused increasing interest in the influence of genetic factors. This antigen is found on cell surfaces and is determined by genes present in a small segment of one chromosome. The high incidence of this genetic marker in ankylosing spondylitis compared with an incidence of only 7 per cent in the general population must be of considerable importance and its recognition has opened up a new field of research which is now being applied to many diseases other than ankylosing spondylitis. More and more genetic markers are being discovered and have importance relating to aetiology, response to drugs, prognosis etc.

Pathology

In the spine, involvement of the discs is an important feature. The annulus fibrosus, nucleus pulposus, and the longitudinal ligaments become ossified, producing the bony bridging so characteristic of the disease. In the synovial joints of the spine, changes similar to those seen in rheumatoid arthritis occur. The joints between the ribs and the vertebrae may be the seat of a fibrous or bony ankylosis limiting the respiratory excursion of the chest. The sacro-iliac joints undergo bony ankylosis. The hip joints may be involved and ultimately become ankylosed.

Clinical features

The presenting symptoms are usually pain and stiffness in the lower part of the back and around the hips; less commonly, pain begins elsewhere in the spine. Physical signs develop later and consist of loss of movement of the lumbar spine, flattening of the lumbar lordosis and reduction of chest expansion. Eventually the whole spine may become rigid, but this process usually takes several years. The most common peripheral joints to be involved are the hips and the severity of disease at this site may be the factor most concerned in determining functional capacity. Other peripheral joints may be affected and this is particularly so when the disease starts at an early age. It is this type of case that often resembles some cases of juvenile chronic arthritis. There is an increased incidence of disease of the aortic valve in ankylosing spondylitis, and this is manifested by aortic incompetence; ocular inflammation (iritis) is not uncommon. Systemic upset is less marked than in rheumatoid arthritis.

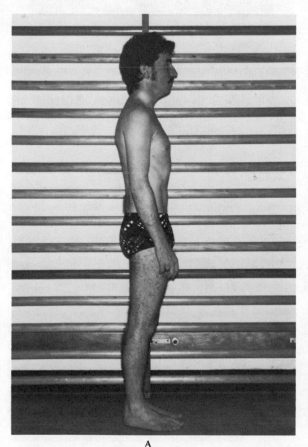
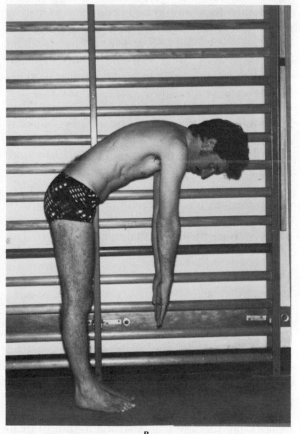

A **B**

Fig. 26.1   The patient's appearance is within normal limits (**A**) until the spine is flexed (**B**).

Radiological changes

Involvement of the sacro-iliac joints is often the earliest radiological sign and this finding may in fact precede other manifestations. Later there is squaring of the vertebrae, ossification of disc margins, and ligamentous calcification giving rise to the typical appearance of 'bamboo spine'.

Blood changes

Some degree of anaemia may be present, and, in early cases, the ESR is usually raised. The rheumatoid factor test is negative. Tissue typing has already been mentioned.

TREATMENT

1. General management

In general, rest and immobilisation, unless strictly controlled, are bad for patients with ankylosing spondylitis; they should be encouraged to lead as normal a life as possible. Few patients become completely disabled and at least 60 per cent can continue to work. Suitable exercises are taught and special attention is paid to posture during working and sleeping hours. Spinal extension exercises are of great importance, so much so that special classes have been established in many physiotherapy departments. If the spine is in danger of becoming fixed then it should at least be possible to ensure that it does so in a functionally good position. It is unfortunate that one sees too many cases in whom fixation has occurred in too great a degree of flexion; this will undoubtedly be accentuated by any hip involvement that may be present (Fig. 26.2).

2. Drug therapy

This consists of many of the non-steroid anti-inflammatory drugs. Phenylbutazone is usually very effective but if possible one of the many alternatives should be used (see first line drug therapy in rheumatoid arthritis (Ch. 25)). Occasionally it may be necessary to use steroid therapy and a course of ACTH would seem satisfactory in a few instances. Deep X-ray therapy was a standard form of treatment at one time and there is no doubt that it is

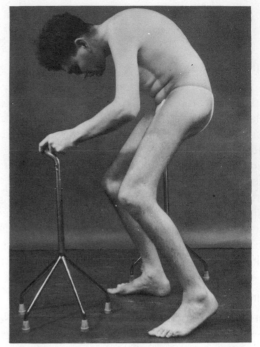
Fig. 26.2 Ankylosing spondylitis in an advanced state.

effective in relieving pain. Unfortunately there is an increased incidence of leukaemia and aplastic anaemia following its use and clinical enthusiasm for this form of therapy has waned. If used at all, a second course should not be contemplated in view of the attendant dangers.

3. Physiotherapy

Physiotherapy, including hydrotherapy (Fig. 26.3), is essential in maintaining movement in joints, in improving posture and muscle tone, and in improving the chest expansion; this should be measured

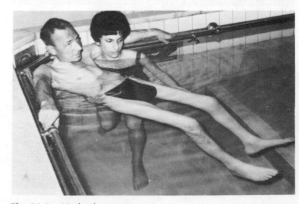
Fig. 26.3 Hydrotherapy.

regularly, and if none can be gained, at least none should be lost.

4. Surgical treatment

The aims of treatment are:

1. the prevention of deformity so that if ankylosis occurs, the affected joints are held in the optimum position for function;
2. the correction of deformity by conservative or operative means; and
3. the re-establishment of mobility in stiffened hip joints by arthroplasty.

THE SPINE

Early cases

It is essential that the patient sleeps on a firm non-sagging mattress, with only one small pillow.

Later cases

Although rarely contemplated now, correction of deformity by conservative means may be indicated if ankylosis has not occurred:

1. CORRECTION OF DEFORMITY BY CONSERVATIVE MEANS USING A SPLIT PLASTER BED (Ch. 9)

The plaster bed is made in the usual way while the patient lies in as good a position as can be obtained. A headpiece is usually included. When it is almost completed, two or three pieces of strip-aluminium are incorporated down the length of the bed. It is then mounted on blocks in the usual way, except that the block beneath the shoulders is so constructed as to enable it to be gradually lowered. The patient is placed in the bed, and nursed as already described in Ch. 9. A day or so is allowed for the patient to become reconciled to fixation, and hyperextension is commenced.

Method. The patient is lifted out of the bed on to pillows. The bed is then split at the site of maximal deformity. It can be hyperextended the desired amount, whilst its original form is still maintained

by the aluminium strips. The block beneath the kyphos is lowered, and the patient is replaced on the bed. Successive beds can be made until full correction is obtained. During the correction, the possibility of complete ankylosis must be borne in mind, and the aim should be *restoration of the normal spinal curves*. It may be necessary to split the bed in two or more places (e.g. in both the lumbar and dorsal regions) in order to produce normal alignment of the spine. *Traction* may be ordered if the hips are becoming involved.

Nursing care

This proceeds on the same lines as described in Ch. 9, including preparation for fixation. As correction proceeds, be on guard against abdominal distension; as a rule, this does not occur as the patient is removed from the plaster bed each day for exercises in the prone position. Constipation must be prevented by regulation of the bowels from the first and vomiting or abdominal pain must be reported promptly. Abdominal upsets may slow down the corrective process.

Physiotherapy

During the process of correction, the patient is usually removed from the bed daily for exercises for the spinal muscles so that any correction gained is controlled and can be maintained. Lying in the prone position for part of each day also helps to prevent abdominal complications. *Breathing exercises* are practised intensively, and *general exercises* to improve the general musculature and to retain joint movement are also given. *Hydrotherapy* is very beneficial (Fig. 26.3).

Later treatment

Splintage. Rarely, when correction is achieved, some form of support for the spine may be ordered to prevent relapse, such as a plaster jacket (Ch. 6), a Jones spinal support (Ch. 9), or some other type of spinal brace. The best form of support however is the patient's own musculature, and continuation of breathing and spinal exercises, and strict attention to posture at home, in bed and at work is an essential feature of later treatment.

2. CORRECTION OF DEFORMITY BY OPERATIVE MEANS

This is achieved by osteotomy of the lumbar and/or of the cervical spine, followed by the immediate application of a plaster bed in the corrected position (Law).

Preparation for operation. General preparation proceeds on the same lines as described elsewhere (Ch. 9). It is essential that the patient is fully reconciled to fixation in his plaster bed before operation.

Post-operative care. This has already been discussed in Ch. 9, but osteotomy of the spine presents special hazards because correction of spinal deformity affects the position and function of internal organs.

Later treatment

When full correction has been achieved, fixation is continued for about three months. Thereafter the patient is fitted with a spinal support and when the legs are fully mobilised, is allowed up. Exercises are continued and the support is gradually discarded.

THE HIPS

CONSERVATIVE TREATMENT

Physiotherapy and hydrotherapy are used to keep the hips mobile. An early flexion contracture of the hips may be corrected by the patient lying in the prone position with the feet over the bed end. Pugh's traction may be ordered to correct an early flexion contracture of the hip (Ch. 10).

Correction by means of Dame Agnes Hunt plaster is described in Ch. 10.

OPERATIVE TREATMENT

Operative treatment may consist of an excision arthroplasty (Girdlestone); or a total hip replacement (Charnley, McKee-Farrar) or some other type of arthroplasty (Ch. 27).

BIBLIOGRAPHY

Adams J Crawford 1969 Flexion deformity of the spine in ankylosing spondylitis. Nursing Times, 17 July, 917
Buchanan W, Watson Dick, Carson W 1976 Recent Advances in Rheumatology, Pt. 1. Edinburgh: Churchill Livingstone
Copeman W S C 1970 Textbook of the Rheumatic Diseases. Edinburgh: E & S Livingstone
Davies Jane B 1969 Spinal Osteotomy for a patient with ankylosing spondylitis. Nursing Times nursing care study, 17 July, 914
MacRae Ronald 1976 Clinical Orthopaedic Examination. Edinburgh: Churchill Livingstone

27

Osteoarthritis

The most common type of arthritis is called 'degenerative joint disease', or, more commonly 'osteoarthritis'. The concept that this is merely a degenerative condition is now being questioned. There is no doubt however, that the florid synovial change seen in rheumatoid arthritis is not found in this disease.

Osteoarthritis is a slowly progressive arthritis. The first detectable change is a degeneration of the articular cartilage of a joint, leading to proliferation of the underlying bone and to the formation of peripheral outgrowths of bone, known as osteophytes. Contracture of the capsule of the joint and spasm of the muscles surrounding it together lead to deformity.

CAUSES

Osteoarthritis most commonly arises without known cause, when it is known as *primary osteoarthritis*. *Secondary osteoarthritis* is due to increased 'wear and tear' consequent upon incongruity of joint surfaces following previous disease or injury. Conditions which may predispose to secondary osteoarthritis include trauma (Chs 19, 20 and 21), infection (Ch. 16), rheumatoid arthritis (Ch. 25), gout (Ch. 29), congenital anomalies (Ch. 14) (e.g. of the hip), growth disorders (e.g. Perthe's disease, slipped upper femoral epiphysis, genu valgum and varum) (Ch. 15) and Paget's disease (Ch. 29).

In addition, denervation of a joint (as in tabes dorsalis and syringomyelia) predisposes to the development of a hypertrophic degenerative arthritis known as a Charcot joint.

Primary osteoarthritis may involve one or at the most a few joints, e.g. the hip or knee; or it may involve many joints forming the so-called *generalised osteoarthritis*. The latter is a condition commonly seen in women after the menopause and affects the distal inter-phalangeal joints of the fingers (causing Heberden nodes) (Fig. 27.1), the

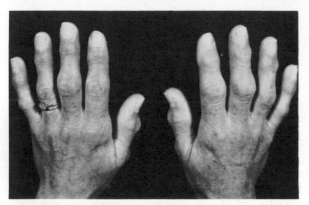

Fig. 27.1 Generalised osteoarthritis affecting the hands showing Heberden and Bouchard nodes.

carpo-metacarpal of the thumb, the cervical and lumbar spines, the hips, knees and metatarsophalangeal joints of the great toes. The cause of primary osteoarthritis is unknown, but it appears that genetic factors, age and occupation are important.

Secondary osteoarthritis is confined to the joints previously affected by the disease process.

PATHOLOGY

There are changes in the articular cartilage, the bone and the capsule of the joint. Localised areas of softening of the cartilage are associated with flaking of the surface and this disruption may extend deeply into the cartilage (fibrillation). Gradually the cartilage is lost and the denuded bone becomes markedly thickened, polished and shiny (eburnation); beneath the eburnated bone cysts form. At the same time new bone formation is taking place peripherally, giving rise to outgrowths of bone (osteophytes) at the margins of the articular cartilage. The 'cast-off' flakes of cartilage are removed from the joint cavity by the synovial membrane which at first proliferates and then becomes fibrotic. Subsequently the capsule too undergoes fibrotic shortening which causes contracture and deformity of the joint.

Why these changes should occur with advancing age is unknown. The relative importance of mechanical factors, cartilage degeneration and low grade inflammatory reactions within the joint is, as yet, incompletely understood.

Clinical features

The patient most commonly complains of pain, stiffness and deformity. Pain is worse after using the joint and relieved by rest; conversely, stiffness is worse after rest; in time there will be limitation of joint movement and deformity, but ankylosis does not occur. Grating sounds (crepitus) are occasionally felt and sometimes heard. Effusions are occasionally seen in the knees. Constitutional upsets do not occur.

Radiological changes

These consist of narrowing of the joint space, sclerosis of the articular ends of the bone, osteophytic lipping, cyst formation and deformation of the joint.

Treatment

Since the cause of primary osteoarthritis is unknown, treatment of the condition is largely symptomatic and empirical. But the aims of treatment are: the relief of pain; the prevention or correction of deformity; and the preservation or restoration of function of the joint. *Prevention* is the best treatment of secondary osteoarthritis.

General treatment. In the early stages the patient must be reassured that the illness is more of a nuisance than a crippling arthritis. Patients must be advised to live within the limits set by their joints. The more a joint is used, the greater the progression of the degenerative change, and therefore rest is important in the treatment of the disease. When weight-bearing joints are involved, periods of rest during the day are helpful, but these should not be too prolonged or there may be some residual stiffness. Obese patients should be dieted. Sometimes a lot of persuasion and education is required in this connection (Fig. 27.2A, B). Palliative treatment (see section on physiotherapy), will often tide

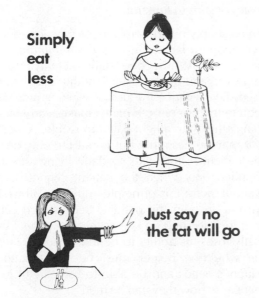

Simply eat less

Just say no the fat will go

Fig. 27.2 A, B. (With kind permission of Dr William Thomson, the Lanarkshire Health Board, and the *Nursing Times*.)

a patient over many years and enable him to carry on with his normal work, though a change of occupation is sometimes necessary.

Drug therapy. Salicylates may be ordered for the relief of pain, but indomethacin may sometimes be more helpful; the side effects of these drugs must be carefully weighed against their possible advantages.

Intra-articular injections of steroids may occasionally be helpful in acute joint flare-ups but the results are usually disappointing. Systemic steroids should never be used in osteoarthritis.

Physiotherapy in conservative treatment of osteoarthritis

Since degenerative joint changes may progress over a number of years it is not always possible or practicable for the patient or the therapist to continue treatment throughout the whole period.

The physiotherapist should try to teach the patient how to live with his condition in such a way as to minimise pain/discomfort and prevent the deformities and secondary adaptive changes

which are liable to occur. To succeed in this the faithful co-operation of the patient is required and although treatment may not be continuous, intermittent encouragement and advice will be needed, the more so as the pathological changes progress and the clinical picture changes.

The condition can affect more than one joint or articular region although as a rule one large joint is affected. It is not uncommon for more than one site to be involved (e.g. the hip and the spine) either at the same time or serially since pain and deformity in one joint can upset the mechanics, balance and posture of the whole body. In this way abnormal stress may be put upon other regions.

The physiotherapist must have a knowledge of normal body mechanics and the effects of degenerative joint disease. Before the therapist can help the patient she must observe and carefully analyse the secondary causes of the patient's disability. The primary cause of osteoarthritis is unknown and there is no known remedy. However, the sequelae can be, if not prevented, at least held at bay, and their eventual adverse effects made less disabling.

Relief of pain, as in any condition, is of prime importance; the patient's active participation cannot be expected in the presence of distracting pain. Drugs may be prescribed by the doctor and may help as long as there are no unpleasant or harmful side effects. Mild, superficial or deep heat gives temporary comfort to some patients. But if there is a low grade inflammation and effusion in the joint the application of crushed ice is usually more effective; such measures can be carried out at home; a *warm*—not hot—hot-water bottle, or tub bath, or hammered ice cubes from the refrigerator and wrapped in towelling could be used. Since any of these measures can be misused, they should only be suggested to patients who are capable of understanding their dangers.

Uses of exercise therapy

An explanation is given to the patient of the importance of correct use, and not overuse, of the affected joint. Simple exercises and positioning are taught. These aim at (1) preventing contractures of soft structures which would lead to deformity, and (2) maintaining good tone in the opposing muscles. For example, the typical deformity in the hip in this condition is adduction, lateral rotation and flexion. The opposite movements are therefore taught—abduction, medial rotation and extension—and the muscles producing those movements are worked strongly. In addition, the hip abductor muscles (which also produce medial rotation) are important in stabilising the pelvis when weight is taken on the leg of the same side. So these muscles must be trained to perform this function adequately. If they do not do so a waddling gait results, the trunk swinging over to the affected side on weight transference; this is not necessarily a true Trendelenberg gait which is present only in a mobile hip; often in osteoarthrosis, some degree of loss of joint movement of the hip is almost always present.

Corrective positioning

If possible, the patient should spend a short period (30–60 min) during the day in a corrective position rather than attempting to adopt this on retiring for the night, because if contractures are present the position will cause pain or discomfort and disturbed sleep. With reference to the hip, the patient should lie supine or prone with the legs in moderate and equal abduction, hips extended and medially rotated. If this routine is adhered to from an early stage after the onset of the arthrosis it will help to prevent or minimise deformity.

Many patients do not seek remedial help until irreversible changes have occurred, so that some degree of deformity will have developed and will interfere with function. The typical position of the hip joint has been described. The knee, which is also commonly affected, is likely to be held in semi-flexion together with varus or valgus. These positions lead to unequal leg lengths, and gait will be difficult and abnormal. To counteract this, when actual correction cannot be gained, an appropriate raising is applied to the shoe. Further improvement may be effected by giving the patient a walking stick which is used in the opposite hand to the affected side—two walking sticks if the condition is bilateral. A 'normal' reciprocal arm-swing gait is taught unless extreme discomfort is causing an antalgic limp. In this case, the sticks (or elbow crutches) are used in such a way that some of the weight is taken through them and the arms; not only will the limp and the pain be reduced but the joint will suffer less trauma.

Notes on aids to function

When supplying artificial aids to function, or compensation for lack of it, only the *minimum* should be issued. Whilst one daily activity may be improved and made easier, another may be penalised. For instance the use of walking aids which require the use of both hands makes carrying anything other than a light bag impossible. A 'normal' gait may be desirable but is not the only need of the patient. Other aids to daily living should be supplied only when the patient cannot manage without them; this principle applies to all workers wishing to help the patient, because aid can be overdone to such an extent that the patient eventually loses his ability to be independent; clearly, the would-be helper must be sensitive to the patient's needs and be able to use careful judgement as to how they can be met.

Various adaptations in the patient's home can make life easier for the sufferer and for the next of kin or relatives who may be giving moral and physical support. Assessment of what is needed is often carried out by the physiotherapist and/or the occupational therapist, and recommendations made to the appropriate authorities. This particular area of reference is in what may be called an 'overlap area'; it is more usually the responsibility of the occupational therapist but can also be undertaken by the physiotherapist.

In time, the patient can become severely disabled; at this point some form of surgery may be considered if the patient is physically and psychologically suitable for this form of treatment.

OSTEOARTHRITIS OF THE HIP JOINT

This deserves special mention and is dealt with first because it is so common, and because it produces greater disability than osteoarthritis of any other joint (see Figs 27.3, 27.4).

Mechanics of the hip-joint. It may not be fully appreciated that the force acting on the head of the femur is much more than the weight of the body. This is because the hip joint acts on a lever

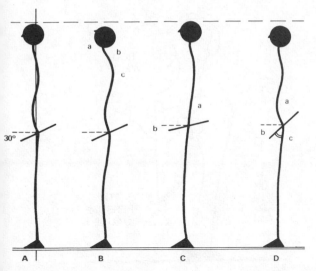

to at least double that of body weight. The patient with an osteoarthritic hip reduces the pull required of the gluteal muscles by limping to the side of the arthritic hip (antalgic hip gait).

Clinical features. There is a constant nagging

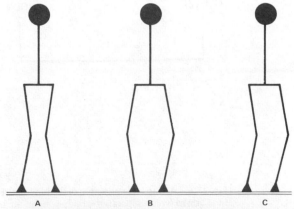

Fig. 27.3   Diagrams to illustrate the typical deformities which may develop in osteoarthritis of the spine and their effects on pelvic tilt. **A.** Normal anterior-posterior curves of the spine and angle of the pelvic tilt. Line of gravity passes through the vertex of the head, the hip and knee, just in front of the ankle joints, between the feet. **B.** (a) Poking chin. (b) Cervical extension. (c) Kyphosis. **C.** (a) Flattened lumbar spine. (b) Decreased angle of pelvic tilt, i.e. backward tilting. **D.** (a) Lumbar lordosis. (b) Increased angle of pelvic tilt, i.e. forward tilting. (c) Flexion of the hip.

principle (Fig. 27.6), the weight of the body at one end of the lever being counterbalanced by the pull of the abductor (gluteal) muscles at the other end. The head of the femur being the fulcrum, is subjected to a summation of these forces amounting

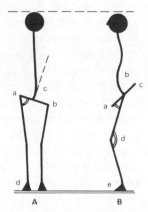

Fig. 27.4   Diagrams to show typical deformities which occur in osteoarthritis of the hip. **A.** (Right hip affected.) (a) Adduction and lateral rotation of the hip. (b) Lateral tilting of the pelvis. (c) Lateral lumbar curve to obtain an upright trunk position. (d) Apparent shortening of the affected leg. **B.** (a) Hip flexion contracture. (b) Lordosis. (c) Forward tilt of the pelvis. (d) Knee flexion. (e) Ankle dorsiflexion.

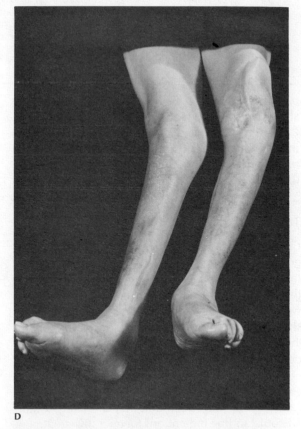

Fig. 27.5   Typical deformities of the knees in osteoarthritis. **A.** Valgus deformity. **B.** Varus deformity. **C.** Right valgus, left varus deformities ('windswept' deformity). **D.** 'Windswept' deformity.

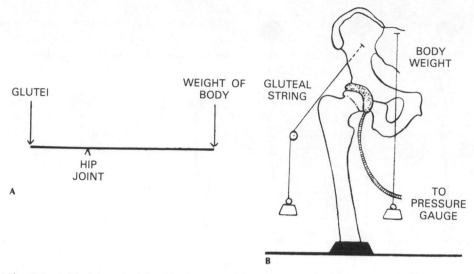

Fig. 27.6 **A.** The lever principle of the hip joint. The joint acts as a fulcrum of a lever, the long arm of which supports the body-weight: the short arm is controlled by the gluteal muscles. **B.** This illustration shows the construction of an experiment performed to determine the distribution of body weight passing through the hip joint. When the patient stands on the leg shown on the diagram and the opposite leg is off the ground, the gluteal muscles, represented as 'gluteal string', contract to hold the pelvis level. Hence the force transmitted through the hip joint shown on the diagram is equal to the body weight plus the pull of the gluteal muscles. (With kind permission of Osborne and Fahrni, *Journal of Bone and Joint Surgery*, May 1950.)

pain aggravated by walking and often disturbing sleep. Stiffness is a marked feature, though the flexion-extension range is often preserved. Eventually there may be a flexion-adduction and external rotation deformity causing apparent shortening of the limb.

Treatment

Conservative. Early cases require treatment by general measures, by analgesics and physiotherapy. Additional conservative measures include the use of a stick or crutch (to reduce the body weight transmitted through the hip), a raise to the shoe, and occasionally some form of support for the hip. A plaster or block leather spica, or a strong corset with a leg piece may be ordered.

Operative treatment. Surgery is considered when conservative measures have failed or when the disease is so far advanced that they are likely to fail. The outstanding indications for operative treatment are (1) *pain* (especially pain which keeps the patient awake at night) and (2) *deformity*.

Before embarking on operative treatment consideration must be given to the patient's age, general health and environment at home and at work, and the nature of his work. For example, will he be able to return to work, or must some alternative employment be sought? Does his home environment include stairs to be climbed? Another important assessment is that of the patient's mental and emotional status, since operative treatment may be only the prelude to a long period of rehabilitation. Each patient requires individual consideration, and the success of the operation often lies as much in his own hands as in those of the surgeon.

Preparation for operation therefore includes explanations to the patient not only of the procedure, but of the subsequent nursing and rehabilitation programme. The patient is admitted to the ward at least a few days prior to operation. During this time he may be allowed up during part of the day and in addition to the routine examinations of chest, urine, blood, etc. the physiotherapist will teach breathing exercises, exercises for the sound limbs and make a pre-operative assessment of the condition of the affected joint and its range of movement. Any splintage which will be used post-operatively is prepared and its use explained to the patient; prior to operation, *a female patient is taught to use a urinal*; this avoids strain on the hip resulting from the frequent use of a bedpan.

Skin preparation includes a daily bath, preferably in the bathroom, and detailed inspection of the skin for scars and blemishes. It is not unusual to find superficial scarring where hot water bottles have been applied in an effort to relieve pain.

Hip operations will now be described briefly, together with the after treatment which is commonly ordered. New operations and new prostheses continue to be devised; only a few will be mentioned here; for information on the most modern prostheses, please see Ch. 8. Since nursing care following these operations is very similar no matter what the procedure, it will be discussed later under one heading.

1. Osteotomy

Intertrochanteric osteotomy (McMurray) with medial displacement of the distal fragment (Figs 27.7 and 27.8) is performed far less commonly than formerly since the introduction of reliable total hip replacements and better methods of fixation. Nevertheless, the operation may still be performed occasionally, particularly in the younger patient in whom there is a greater chance of eventual loosen-

ing of a prosthesis. The exact way in which osteotomy relieves pain is unknown but it may alter the mechanics of weight-bearing through the joint and increase local vascularity. In some cases the rate of progression of the disease may slow and the radiological changes may even improve (Nissen).

Internal fixation of the osteotomy allows earlier mobilisation of the patient and includes:

1. *Nail plate or Wainwright spline* (Fig. 27.7A). This is followed by three weeks' bed rest usually in traction, e.g. Hamilton Russell traction (Fig. 27.13). Partial weight-bearing on elbow crutches is allowed after six weeks and full weight-bearing after twelve weeks.

2. *Harris-Muller compression plate* (Fig. 27.7B). This allows earlier mobilisation and does not usually require traction.

3. *Osborn-Ball compression plate* (Fig. 27.8). This is less liable to angular strains than other devices and allows the patient out of bed within 24 hours. The patient may gradually be allowed to weight-bear after six days and rehabilitation is correspondingly quicker.

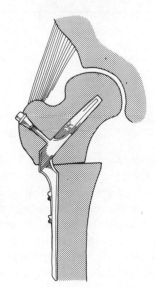

Fig. 27.8   Osborne-Ball compression plate.

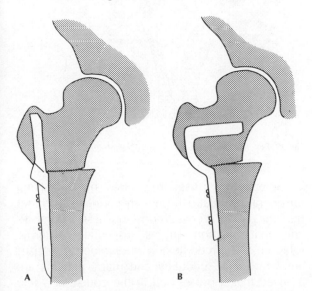

Fig. 27.7   **A.** Wainwright spline. **B.** Harris-Müller compression plate.

2. Arthroplasty

Arthroplasty of the hip is now the treatment of choice for osteoarthritis of the hip which has not responded to conservative measures. The development of durable materials for the manufacture of reliable prostheses and quick setting methymethacrylate cement for strong internal fixation of the prostheses has transformed total hip replacement from, perhaps, somewhat hazardous beginnings to being the single most important contribution of orthopaedic surgery to medicine. Other types of arthroplasty are now rarely performed and do not offer the same prospects of success. They include:

1. *Cup arthroplasty* (Fig. 27.9). This is most likely to be seen now as an historical relic when a patient previously treated by this form of arthroplasty undergoes revision surgery.

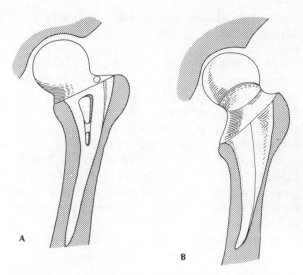

Fig. 27.10   **A.** Moore's prosthesis. **B.** Thompson's prosthesis.

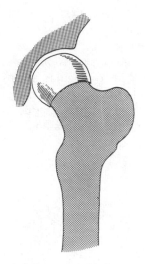

Fig. 27.9   Cup arthroplasty.

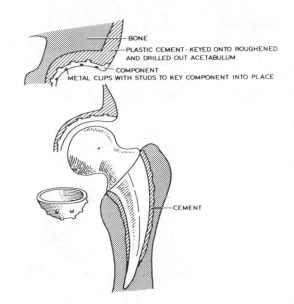

BONE
PLASTIC CEMENT - KEYED ONTO ROUGHENED AND DRILLED OUT ACETABULUM
COMPONENT
METAL CLIPS WITH STUDS TO KEY COMPONENT INTO PLACE

CEMENT

Fig. 27.11   McKee-Farrar total hip replacement.

2. *Prosthetic replacement of the femoral head* (hemiarthroplasty). The Moore's (Fig. 27.10A) is a metallic self-locking prosthesis while the Thompson's prosthesis is cemented into position. Neither should be used in the treatment of osteoarthritis since they cause accelerated damage to the pelvic acetabulum, sometimes eroding right through into the pelvis. However, they remain useful in the treatment of fractures of the femoral neck.

3. *Total hip replacement*. This is a replacement of both the femoral head and the acetabulum by prostheses to form a fully artificial joint. The *McKee-Farrar total hip replacement* uses a modified Thompson prosthesis for the femoral head which articulates with a studded cup cemented into the deepened acetabulum (Fig. 27.11).

The patient is nursed free in bed, but on leaving the operating theatre the legs are bandaged together until the patient recovers consciousness. It is important that rotation strains (especially external rotation) and forced flexion are avoided. Exercises are introduced gradually and many patients are allowed to get out of bed in the course of a few days. Weight-bearing, perhaps with the aid of a stick, is gradually introduced and the patient is dis-

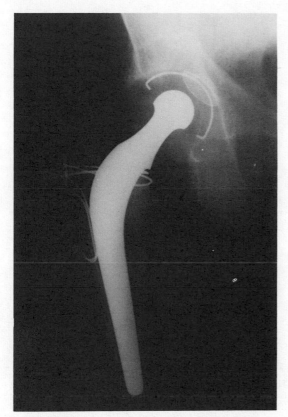

Fig. 27.12 The Charnley total hip replacement.

This splint is comfortable for the patient and makes nursing easier. (With acknowledgement to the *Nursing Times* and Miss M. Williams.)

4. *Excision of the femoral head and neck* (excision arthroplasty) (Girdlestone) uses the upper end of the femoral shaft as a weight-bearing surface in a pseudarthrosis. It is uncommon to use this as the first-line of surgical treatment of the osteoarthritic hip since the total hip replacement has proved itself so effective. It is most commonly used as a salvage procedure following loosening or infection of a total hip replacement. Hamilton-Russell traction with about 6.5 kg of weight is usually ordered (Fig. 27.13), or skeletal traction with a Nissen splint, as shown in Fig. 27.16. Exercises are commenced in about six weeks, and sitting over the side of the bed is gradually introduced. A bucket top caliper (brace with ischial seat) is sometimes ordered, weight-bearing with elbow crutches commenced at about the ninth week, until these can be discarded in favour of one or two walking sticks. One stick may be needed permanently for walking outdoors.

3. Arthrodesis

Arthrodesis may rarely be the operation of choice if there is severe involvement of one hip but a full range of movement in the contralateral hip and lumbar spine. Young patients or those with a history of severe infection of the joint are more likely to be considered for this procedure. It provides a stiff but stable and painless joint. Movement which to the patient apparently occurs at the hip joint, occurs in the lumbar spine allowing the patient to walk normally, sit almost normally and to drive a car. Methods used to fuse an osteoarthritic hip include; intra-articular arthrodesis with nailing and bone grafting (Watson-Jones); or partial excision of the femoral head and acetabulum combined with nailing, bone grafting and a high femoral osteotomy to reduce movement at site of arthrodesis (Pyrford arthrodesis); fixation of the joint by a nail combined with an ischio-femoral bone graft (V-arthrodesis). A one and one-half hip spica is applied post-operatively and is worn for 6 to 12 weeks. Nursing care is discussed in Chs 5, 6 and 10.

charged home in about two or three weeks.

The Charnley total hip replacement (Fig. 27.12) utilises a small metallic femoral head articulating with an acetabular component composed of a plastic material (high density polyethylene) giving a low-friction arthroplasty. The surgical approach to the hip for this operation involves removing the greater trochanter and re-attaching it to the femur with strong wire. Because it used to be thought that this produced a significant mechanical weakness patients were frequently nursed in bed for up to three weeks with the hip in abduction (Fig. 27.14). Although this position is still encouraged post-operatively, early mobilisation is now routine and most patients take their first steps after one week. *The Williams splint* (Fig. 27.15) was devised by a nurse as post-operative fixation to maintain abduction of the hip, to control rotation, and to maintain the pumping action which assists venous return and helps to prevent deep vein thrombosis.

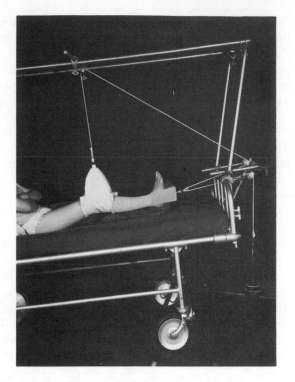

Fig. 27.13A   Hamilton-Russell traction.

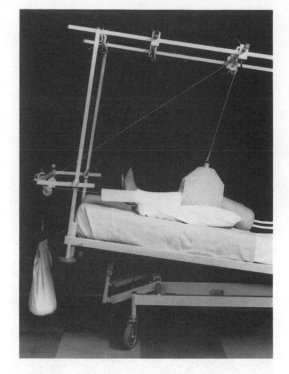

Fig. 27.13B   This shows Hamilton-Russell traction applied using a King's Fund bed. *Note.* The essential overhead pulley is not shown.

4. Muscle release operations

Rarely, release of muscles is used in the treatment of the osteo-arthritic hip. Such releases include: adductor tenotomy; psoas release (O'Malley); or a more extensive release involving the abductors, flexors and adductors (the hanging hip operation of Voss).

NURSING MANAGEMENT IN SURGERY OF THE HIP

It is convenient to discuss this under three separate headings:

1. *Pre-operative assessment.*
2. *General management.*
3. *Management of splintage.*

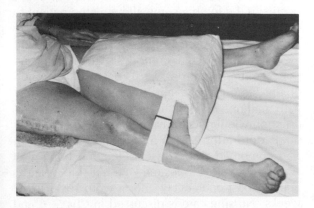

Fig. 27.14   (see text.)

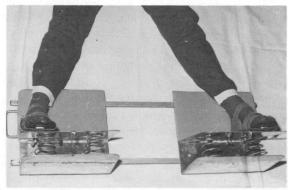

Fig. 27.15   (see text.)

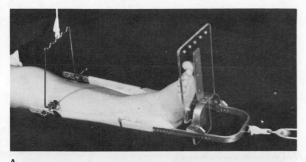

A

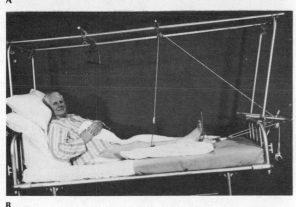

B

Fig. 27.16 A, B. Nissen splint.

These items are inseparable and in practice are carried out simultaneously.

Pre-operative medical and nursing assessment has already been discussed in connection with spinal surgery (Ch. 9) and the same criteria are applied.

General management

The nursing care of patients who have undergone hip surgery calls for a sound grasp not only of the nature of the operation but of the principles of after-treatment, including the prevention of complications. Though programmes of treatment, nursing care, physiotherapy and rehabilitation can be laid down in broad outline, these will vary with the operation performed, the individual surgeon and even more important, with the individual patient. Each patient, therefore, requires individual study, but at the same time the nurse must familiarise herself with the basic requirements favoured by the particular surgeon with whom she is working. It is also helpful if nursing procedures such as the application of traction are practised in the classroom. 'Case studies' of the total care of individual patients are also helpful.

Outline of nursing management. The patients under discussion are often female, middle-aged or elderly, and not infrequently, of substantial build. In general, patients suffering from osteoarthritis are otherwise healthy, though intercurrent disease may be present. But even if otherwise healthy, they are often weary from pain and frustrated from coping with a disability. Once over the post-operative period, however, the patient usually 'settles down', and in the absence of co-existing disease and of complications, looks forward to each new stage of her treatment; she then falls into a category mentioned in Ch. 3, i.e. perhaps not ill in a medical sense but likely to be very uncomfortable. As a general rule, and unless there are serious emotional or social problems, she is usually cheerful, sociable and co-operative. In common with all our patients, she requires respect as an individual and additionally as a mature member of society; a happy atmosphere and a cheerful, hopeful attitude on the part of the staff, together with amenities mentioned in a previous chapter are the essential background to successful treatment.

Post-operative nursing care. On return from the theatre, in addition to the routine observation, treatment and medication required in all major surgery, particular care is taken to maintain the position of the limb in whatever splintage or form of traction has been ordered. Where splintage or traction is not ordered, the limbs are held in a moderate degree of abduction by means of a firm pillow placed between the malleoli. The patient is nursed flat in bed until she has recovered consciousness but is raised to the semi-recumbent position by means of pillows within 24 hours. If, as previously advised, she has been taught to use a urinal before operation, this will avoid lifting her on to a bedpan during the time when the hip is most painful, i.e. during the first 24 hours, and is a valuable nursing aid. *Continuous suction drainage of the wound* is frequently used to prevent the formation of a haematoma. At the conclusion of the operation, the surgeon inserts a narrow plastic drainage tube attached to a 20 cm stainless steel needle into the wound and out through the skin 5 to 8 cm away from the incision. The main wound is then closed and a dressing applied. The needle is detached from the drain which is connected by larger plastic tubing to a *sterile blood-collecting vacuum bottle* (Fig. 27.17A, B, C) when suction immediately commences. The vacuum bottle is placed at the bedside in such a postion that it is below the level of the wound so that suction is aided by gravity, but at the same time there is no tension on the tubing. During nursing procedures, the bottle must be supported at all times so that the drain is not pulled out of the patient; it is also important to see that the tubing does not become twisted or kinked.

The negative pressure (usually $-25\,mm\,Hg$) inside the vacuum bottle will need to be maintained when necessary by using an electric suction pump. To do this:

1. disconnect the large plastic tubing from the bottle;
2. open the clip on the rubber tubing and hence break the vacuum;
3. inject 1 ml of a coloured dye (e.g. Collut. Thymol Co) into the small opening in the glass tube;
4. apply suction to the rubber tubing and, as the vacuum increases in the bottle, the level of coloured dye in the glass tube will fall;
5. close the clip on the rubber tubing, and re-attach the large plastic tubing to the rubber tubing;
6. open the clip and blood from the patient's wound will be seen to flow again down the drainage tube.

Drainage is usually required for between 24 and 48 hours after operation, or occasionally for an even longer period.

Removal of the drainage tube is carried out with full aseptic precautions; a corner of the dressing is lifted and the drain removed by gentle traction without disturbing the wound itself. A sterile pack is placed over the site and the upper dressing replaced.

The volume of blood drained from the wound is recorded in the patient's notes.

On the morning following operation, the patient is washed, the mouth cleansed, the hair combed and arranged and the nightwear and bed linen changed. At this stage, the hip is likely to be painful so that nursing procedures must be carried out unhurriedly, smoothly and gently. *As soon as possible*, the patient uses a pulley placed over her bed or, if more convenient, the bar of her Balkan beam (Fig. 27.18), to raise herself for inspection of and treatment of the skin of the buttocks, but in the early stages she may require help in this procedure, which must be carried out as two nurses raise the

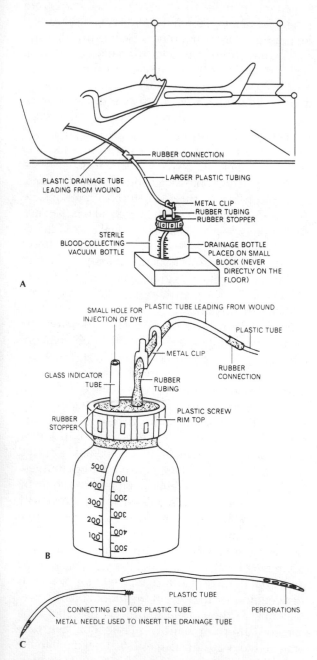

Fig. 27.17 **A–C.** Apparaus for continuous suction drainage of wound.

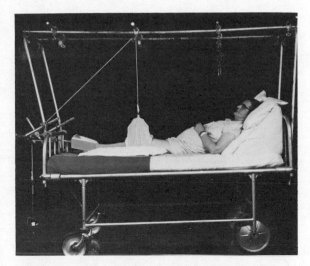

Fig. 27.18 Modified Hamilton-Russel traction. (With kind permission of the *Nursing Times*.) N.B. Raising the foot-end of the bed is omitted in this illustration.

patient gently while a third carries out the treatment, changes the draw sheet and straightens the bottom sheet. When the patient is able to help herself by grasping a pulley, it is advisable to steady the affected limb so that its correct alignment in relation to the trunk is not lost; as already stated, forced flexion or rotation must be prevented.

Daily nursing care. Patients vary in their reactions to operative treatment; some are quite happy to return to an open ward at an early stage, while others benefit from a few days 'peace and quiet', protection from noise and from a surfeit of visitors. Similarly one patient may be totally dependent for several days, while another may be quite ready to attend to part of her own toilet within 24 hours of operation; it is then permissible to allow her to wash her hands and face, clean her teeth and apply make-up, but imagination is required in order to anticipate the patients needs so that toilet materials are placed ready to hand. Any action, such as leaning forwards or sideways to gain access to a locker is forbidden for the first 7 to 10 days. On the other hand, the serious complications of immobility must be borne in mind and it is a mistake to limit the patient's activity to the extent that she becomes an easy prey to pneumonia, pressure sores and deep vein thrombosis. It is essential that the patient spends at least one hour per day lying flat on the back to prevent flexion contracture of the hip. As

soon as possible, careful turning so that the patient lies on the sound side for a few hours each day is usually permitted, provided the correct alignment of the affected limb with the trunk is not lost; if necessary, the affected limb is supported by pillows. The object of turning, however limited by splintage, is the prevention of pressure sores and other complications.

As soon as the general condition allows, and as the pain in the hip subsides, the patient gradually assumes responsibility for her own personal toilet. She may wash her trunk herself within two to three days and undertake her own vulval toilet, provided materials are placed near at hand, but washing the back, the buttocks and anal region and the unaffected limb remains the responsibility of the nurse for so long as the patient is confined to bed.

Bedpans are given with great care; as soon as possible the patient raises herself by means of a pulley, flexes the sound knee while the affected limb is steadied by one nurse and another places the bedpan in position; the anal toilet is carried out in the same manner. An aperient or suppository is sometimes required in the post-operative period. The importance of the use of a urinal in the prevention of undue strain on both patient and nurse has already been stressed.

Physiotherapy in hip replacement surgery

Patients requiring total hip replacement are admitted into hospital 2–3 days prior to surgery in order that various tests may be carried out and assessments made; it is the latter which particularly concern the physiotherapist and it is assumed here that medical and nursing assessments have already been made.

The patient may have had pain and stiffness in one or both hips for many years with consequent decrease in functional ability and mobility. A limp may develop caused initially by pain and discomfort in the joint leading to weakness and wasting of the gluteus medius and the development of deformity.

Pre-operative assessment. Assessment will reveal the ability of the patient to run a household, hold down a job, do the shopping, get into and out of a car, on and off a bus or train; it will also indicate the patient's ability to carry out simple everyday

Table 27.1 Physiotherapy assessment and progress form

CONSULTANT: DATE:

NAME:

DIAGNOSIS:

CHIEF COMPLAINT:

PRE-OPERATIVE COMPLICATIONS:

RANGE OF MOVEMENT		Pre-operative Lt. Rt.	Post-operative Lt. Rt.
Flexion	–		
Extension	–		
Abduction	–		
Adduction	–		NB Adduction is not tested.
Medial Rot.	–		
Lat. Rot.	–		
Shortening	– Real Apparent		
Inter-malleolar separation –			

GAIT PRIOR TO SURGERY:

DATE OF SURGERY:

Post-operative Complications:

FUNCTIONAL ACTIVITY:

  Date patient stood

  Date patient walked
    With frame
    With crutches
    With sticks

  Date removal sutures

  Date patient sat in chair

  Date patient tried stairs

GAIT PRIOR TO DISCHARGE:

Date of Discharge

Comments:

activities such as dressing, bathing, sitting, rising from a chair and negotiating stairs. In the physical assessment the range of movement of both hips, the presence of deformity and degree of muscle wasting should be observed and true and apparent shortening measured and recorded. Movement of the lumbar spine should be examined and any increase in the normal lumbar curve observed. This is particularly relevant to the nursing care as many patients complain of low back pain when the supine position has to be maintained for any length of time. A small lumbar pillow to support the spine may help to alleviate some of the discomfort. An analysis of gait prior to surgery will facilitate re-education of walking following operation and the use of crutches can be taught at this time. In conjunction with the nursing staff the post-operative management and the necessity to *maintain abduction and avoid adduction* is explained to the patient. *Prior to surgery* the patient is instructed in:

1. Deep breathing exercises, including lateral, costal and diaphragmatic breathing, to prevent hypostatic pneumonia and assist venous return.
2. Bilateral foot exercises, particularly strong dorsiflexion and plantar flexion of the ankle to prevent deep venous thrombosis.
3. Bilateral isometric quadriceps and gluteal exercises to maintain function and aid circulation.
4. Active exercises to the sound limb.
5. The use of a monkey pole, (trapeze, patient-helper device) to aid movement in bed, to facilitate nursing care and help to prevent the complications of immobility.

A post-operative regime

Day 1. The exercises already enumerated are supervised by the physiotherapist and the patient encouraged by nursing and physiotherapy staff to practice them frequently.

Day 2–5. Active and active-assisted hip and knee flexion and hip abduction exercises in a small range are added to the routine exercises and the patient encouraged to flex knee and hip actively at regular intervals. The patient's posture is checked to see the pelvis is level, that weight is evenly distributed; and that both lower limbs are maintained in abduction and neutral rotation.

When the drainage tubes have been removed and the patient's general condition is satisfactory, weight-bearing may commence. The Charnley wedge (Fig. 27.14) is removed and with the affected limb supported by the physiotherapist the patient moves to the side of the bed towards the affected side, thus maintaining the limb in the abducted position. The patient may rest on the side of the bed with both feet supported on the floor to adjust to the vertical position, *avoiding extreme flexion* at the hip and knee on the affected side; the patient then stands up with the aid of a walking frame, taking weight on both feet. Deep breathing is encouraged to prevent dizziness. Weight transference from one foot to the other, taking some weight through the hands, is practised, progressing to 'marking time'. After 3–4 minutes the patient is helped back into bed, the limb being supported in the abducted position and the Charnley wedge is replaced. Depending upon the patient's general mobility and the height of the bed, this procedure may require the assistance of two people.

On the third or fourth day if all is satisfactory the patient may sit out of bed to use a commode; abduction and flexion of the hip and knee must be carefully controlled to avoid dislocation of the hip and to minimise pain and discomfort in the muscles of the thigh. The same procedure as that for sitting in an armchair, described later in the text, is followed but considerable help will be required at this stage.

Day 5–10. By this time, the patient may be supported in bed by a back-rest in the half-lying position. The back-rest is removed at night and for an hour in the afternoon and the patient lies flat to avoid any tendency to hip flexion deformity occurring.

Active and active assisted movements to the affected limb are continued, and the range of hip flexion and abduction gradually increased. Quadriceps exercises and foot movements are continued vigourously. Pain or discomfort in the calf muscles, restriction in dorsiflexion of the ankle or the presence of swelling in the limb must be reported to the Ward Sister at once. Leg lengthening exercises, to further strengthen gluteus medius are now additional to isometric quadriceps and gluteal contractions. This is done by alternately thrusting each heel towards the foot of the bed. Graduated weight-bearing continues, and walking commences using elbow crutches and a three-point gait in the sequence set out below:

1. Stand with weight equal on both feet. Place elbow crutches outer side of each foot.
2. Place crutches forward.
3. Place affected limb to level of crutches taking weight through the limb and crutches.
4. Step through with second limb. The feet should point forward, an equal stride taken with each step and a good general posture encouraged.

Sitting

The patient may sit out of bed for a short time in an armchair with the feet supported on a footstool, the length of time being increased daily. The chair should be of an appropriate height making sitting and rising from it easy and comfortable. On sitting, the patient:

1. Places crutches at the side of the chair.
2. Stands against the seat of the chair.
3. Places the affected limb forward and the opposite hand on the arm of the chair.
4. Sits down and back, avoiding too sudden flexion at the hip and knee.

To rise, the patient:

1. Places the sound foot firmly on the floor, with the knee bent and the foot tucked slightly under the chair.
2. Places hands on the arms of the chair.
3. Pushes up on sound limb and hands and stands up.
4. Reaches for the elbow crutches.

Sitting posture should be checked periodically to ensure that the pelvis is level and equal weight is transmitted through the buttocks. As soon as possible the patient should dress in his own clothes and if necessary, the occupational therapist may advise on suitable aids and adaptations (Ch. 35). Sensible comfortable footwear should be worn. Leg lengths are checked for any discrepancy and if there is shortening the appropriate shoe must be raised.

Day 10. By this time, the patient is up and about, able to get out of and into bed, sit in and rise from a suitable armchair, walk to the bathroom and negotiate stairs.

Stair drill. Hold the banister rail with one hand and an elbow crutch in the other, carrying the second crutch horizontally in this hand.

To negotiate stairs

To ascend: (1) Grasp banister rail, place sound limb up on to step. (2) Bring affected limb and then elbow crutch up to it.

To descend: (1) Grasp banister rail, place affected limb and elbow crutch on step below. (2) Bring sound limb down to it.

Progression

When the sutures have been removed (between 10–12th day) and wound healing has occurred, a bath in the bath-tub is a welcome event. Minimal help into and out of the bath will be required at first.

As confidence and competence increase, more weight is taken through the affected limb, and at the discretion of the surgeon elbow crutches are discarded in favour of walking sticks.

On being discharged home between 12–14th day, the patient is instructed as follows:

1. to rest for an hour every afternoon either in the supine or prone position;
2. to progress to taking equal weight through both limbs;
3. to walk 'little and often', taking equal strides with each step;
4. to maintain an upright posture;
5. to avoid full flexion of the affected hip for the first two months;
6. to avoid crossing one knee over the other— because of the danger of dislocation.

The patient is reviewed by the surgeon in 4–6 weeks.

As the days go by, *physiotherapeutic sessions* are increased in length and in range, and usually occupy a large part of the patient's time and energy; excessive fatigue must be avoided.

Occupational therapy. This may be introduced in the early stages while the patient is confined to bed, and activities in the 'daily living unit' may form part of the rehabilitation programme to prepare the patient for discharge.

Management of splintage

Many surgeons now feel that a foam gutter splint to hold the leg in a position of abduction is perfectly adequate without the need for traction. For the purposes of this discussion we will assume that a Thomas bed-splint with Pearson flexion attachment has been ordered as post-operative fixation. A Hodgen splint (Fig. 27.20) is sometimes used instead.

Preparation. When measuring the thigh, and preparing the splint, make allowance for a large dressing over the hip. Below-knee extensions are applied and covered with a towel; extensions extending from the upper thigh to just above the knee and having long ties will be required at the time of operation. The bed is fitted with a Balkan beam and is taken to the operating theatre ante-room, together with a tray containing the extensions already mentioned; slings, cord, clips, pulleys and weights.

Application of traction. At the conclusion of the operation, the splint is guided over the leg until the ring rests against the ischial tuberosity. Slings are placed beneath the limb and fastened with paper-clips. A pad is placed below the head of the tibia and the limb is laid gently on to the slings. The below-knee skin extensions are now fastened to the flexion piece; the above-knee extensions with long ties are then applied and fastened to the end of the splint (Fig. 27.20). *Fixed traction* has now been applied to the limb; heavier traction can

be exerted by raising the foot-end of the bed (*balanced traction*). Two cords are now knotted on either side of the top of the bed-splint and passed over the double pulley A shown in Fig. 27.19 and fastened to the end of the splint, holding it at the angle of flexion required. Another cord is knotted around pulley B, passed back over pulley C, over pulley D and finally over pulley E at the foot of the bed. Sufficient weight is applied to allow the patient to lift the splinted limb easily—usually 0.5, 1.0 or 1.5 kg, depending on the weight of the patient. The weighted cord attached to the end of the splint and passing over pulley F is simply to ease the pressure of the splint in the groin.

The splinted limb is now suspended from the Balkan beam in the degree of flexion and abduction desired by the surgeon. A sling or bandage to maintain internal rotation may also be ordered (Fig. 27.19B).

Daily nursing care. The area of skin beneath the ring of the bed-splint requires treatment as described in Ch. 10. Frequent movement of the skin and soft tissues so that continuous pressure does not fall on one area is imperative, and as soon as possible the patient is taught to do this. The extensions and bandages are inspected daily; pay special attention to the point where the extensions may press into the ankle or foot; often quite small adjustments are all that is required to make the patient comfortable. See that the foot is warm, of normal colour, and moving freely. The weights are also

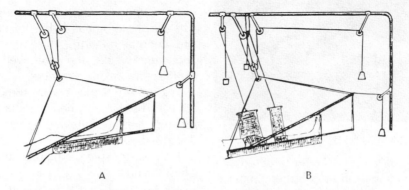

A   B

Fig. 27.19 **A.** Shows the method of arranging the cords, pulleys and weights. **B.** Shows the method of applying internal rotation bandages, which may be ordered after an arthroplasty of the hip. A crêpe bandage is applied to the limb either above or below the knee (or, as in this case, in both situations) passing from without inwards. The end is then rolled round a piece of wood of suitable size, and to this is attached a paper clip. A weighted cord is then tied to the paper clip and arranged over a pulley, as shown.

inspected daily; friction between the cords, weights and other objects must be prevented. Observe the patient closely; if the weights are correctly balanced between the traction force, the body weight and the degree of elevation of the foot of the bed, the patient will both look and feel comfortable, and will be able to raise herself quite easily for nursing purposes while the body and limb move as one unit. For example, if the patient depicted in Fig. 27.13 persistently slides down the bed and has difficulty in raising herself and in maintaining the semi-recumbent position, then it is likely that the traction weight at the foot of the bed is not countered by sufficient weight at the head of it, and more must be added at this point. On no account must the weight which supplies the traction force be reduced without instructions from the surgeon. Correct balance can only be achieved by adjustment of the counter-weights for each individual patient.

Correct balance is also important from the point of view of prevention of pressure sores since in the absence of proper control shearing strains are exerted on the skin of the buttocks and the heels.

A Hodgen splint is shown in Fig. 27.20. Application and care proceeds on the lines already described. It may be used after cup arthroplasty (Law).

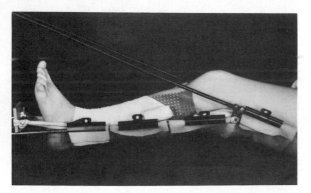

Fig. 27.20 Hodgen splint with flexion attachment (see text).

Hamilton-Russell traction is often ordered after osteotomy with spline fixation, prosthetic replacement of the femoral head and Girdlestone excision arthroplasty. The method is shown in Fig. 27.13 and modified in Fig. 27.18. About 6.5 kg of weight is usually ordered and the foot of the bed is raised enough to prevent the patient from sliding downwards.

Nursing care and observations proceed on the lines described above and it is important to see that the sling behind the knee is kept smooth at all times.

Bucket-top caliper (brace with ischial seat). This splint is used in some centres following the Girdlestone operation. A cast is taken of the patient's thigh, as described in Ch. 6. The caliper is fitted eight weeks after the operation, and is worn continuously, even in bed. Some patients find this a great ordeal, but some surgeons regard it as an essential part of the after-care in order to maintain length of the leg and prevent flexion contracture at the hip. Daily nursing care is described in Ch. 9. Weight-bearing in the caliper is gradually introduced at about the eighth or twelfth week following operation and a raising to the shoe is always necessary to compensate for shortening (Figs 7.2A and 10.16). The caliper is worn continuously for about six months but non-weight-bearing knee exercises are practised assiduously and when flexion of the knee and some degree of stability of the hip has been regained the caliper is gradually discarded.

Alternative methods of after-treatment

1. About four weeks after operation, traction apparatus may be replaced by a plaster shell holding the limb in internal rotation. Sometimes the plaster shell is fitted with a roller-skate and this is worn for abduction-adduction exercises on a sloping board.

2. In some cases, post-operative fixation consists of a plaster spica holding the limb in abduction and internal rotation. This may be retained for about three weeks, and is followed by roller-skating exercises as already described.

3. Broomstick plasters are sometimes used (Fig. 15.10). These are applied in abduction and internal rotation, and are followed by exercises as already described.

4. A plaster spica. Nursing care is described in Chs 5, 6 and 10.

On discharge, the patient will be walking, perhaps with the aid of crutches or sticks; or sometimes, a caliper; *the social worker* will get in touch with community health personnel, and will satisfy herself that the home and work conditions are suitable for the patient's reception and it is usual for her to report to the hospital or to an after-care clinic for review and assessment after about three months.

OSTEOARTHRITIS OF THE KNEE JOINT

Osteoarthritis of the knee joint is frequently seen in obese women following the menopause when it may be associated with the development of generalised osteoarthritis. It may be associated with genu valgum or varum (Fig. 27.21). An obvious

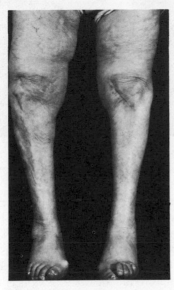

Fig. 27.21 Bilateral osteoarthritis of knees, associated with genu varum.

pre-existing cause such as previous meniscal damage or surgery or osteochondral fracture may be present (Ch. 21) but in the majority of cases no cause is found.

In early cases, treatment consists of general measures, such as weight reduction, physiotherapy, the use of a stick, analgesics and intra-articular injections. In later cases, conservative treatment consists of some form of splintage, such as a plaster cylinder; a knee-cage or a caliper (Chs 7 and 10). Manipulation under anaesthesia may be advised.

Operative treatment may be: (1) Removal of loose bodies. (2) Patellectomy. (3) Upper tibial osteotomy. (4) Joint débridement and drilling of the articular surface (Pridie). (5) Total knee replacement. (6) Arthrodesis of the knee joint.

Total knee replacement

Total knee replacement has become an effective and much more reliable procedure for the treatment of osteoarthritis but still falls short of the standards set by total hip replacement. The bewildering array of prostheses available bears witness to the fact that none can be said to be completely reliable. It is possible to divide them into three broad categories.

1. *Resurfacing* of the femoral and tibial condyles (Fig. 27.22A).
2. *Semi-constrained prostheses* replacing the femoral and tibial articular surfaces, allowing flexion, extension and anterior/posterior glide but limiting rotation.
3. *Hinge prosthesis* (Fig. 27.22B).

Physiotherapy in total knee replacement

Total knee replacement is indicated where there is severe pain and stiffness in the joint associated with deformity and instability caused by gross degeneration of the joint surfaces. In some cases several joints may be affected causing increased handicap and disability. It is particularly important that a careful functional assessment, as discussed in a previous chapter, is carried out to ascertain the patient's capabilities and motivation. At this time the post-operative procedure can be explained and the value and importance of co-operation and perseverance emphasised.

In the physical assessment the physiotherapist should note and record:

1. The range of movement in the joint and degree of limitation of flexion and extension.
2. The quality and power of movement through the range.
3. The presence of deformity and instability of the joint.
4. The quality of quadriceps contraction and degree of muscle wasting.
5. The mobility of the patella.
6. Any associated weakness of the calf muscles and hip extensor muscles.

An analysis of gait, the type of walking aid used and the distance the patient can walk prior to surgery will give some indication of the re-education and gait training required after operation. The

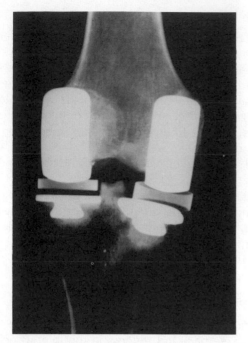

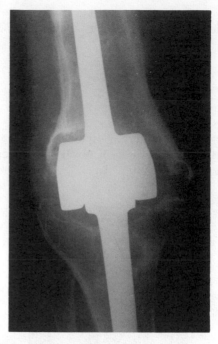

Fig. 27.22A Oxford meniscal knee replacement (unconstrained prosthesis).

Fig. 27.22B Shiers hinge knee arthroplasy.

patient is instructed in the pre-operative regime already discussed in the chapter on total hip replacement.

Day 1. Following surgery, the patient returns to the ward with the limb supported in a pressure bandage and back splint; the foot of the bed is elevated to minimise swelling and assist venous return.

Deep breathing exercises, bilateral vigorous foot and ankle movements and active exercises to the unaffected limb are given and the patient encouraged to practise them frequently. Static quadriceps contractions to the affected limb are supervised by the physiotherapist, with particular emphasis placed on obtaining full extension of the knee. Straight leg raising is encouraged when a satisfactory quadriceps contraction has been achieved. Dorsiflexion of the foot performed concurrently will reinforce the quadriceps contraction.

Day 2–day 5. When the wound drains have been removed, and the quadriceps contraction and straight leg raising is satisfactory, the patient commences weight-bearing wearing the back splint, at first with a walking aid if the patient is very disabled but progressing quickly to elbow crutches and then to walking sticks.

By the fifth day the patient is walking confidently taking weight through both feet using a three-point gait, already described in a previous chapter, progressing to full weight-bearing as soon as possible.

Day 5. The back-splint is removed and the pressure bandage reduced. Knee flexion is then commenced—some surgeons allowing only 30–40 degrees flexion until wound healing has occurred.

The back-splint is retained for weight-bearing until a satisfactory range of movement with adequate muscle control through the range has been achieved. Exercises to mobilise and strengthen are continued and as range of movement is gained and muscle power increases the back-splint is discarded altogether.

The sutures are removed between the tenth and twelfth day and the patient then attends the hydrotherapy pool for mobilising and stabilising exercises in water, further preparing the patient for increased weight-bearing and activity on dry land.

Progress varies with each patient, some attaining 90 degrees knee flexion with full extension of the knee and a normal pattern of walking with ease, while others require the encouragement, skilled handling and all the expertise of which the physiotherapist is capable. Depending upon progress the patient is discharged between 3–4 weeks after the operation.

Arrangements are made for those requiring further treatment to attend their local physiotherapy department. The patient is reviewed by the surgeons 4–6 weeks after discharge home.

OSTEOARTHRITIS OF THE ANKLE

This painful condition most usually occurs after a previous fracture, infection or rheumatoid arthritis. In early cases physiotherapy, analgesics and intra-articular injections may tide the patient over a few years. Other conservative measures include below-knee irons and splints made of lightweight polythene materials.

Operative treatment is usually arthrodesis of the ankle-joint (Fig. 27.23).

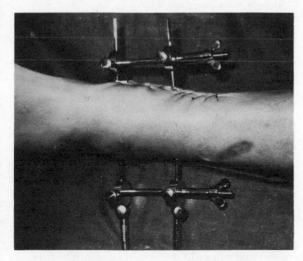

Fig. 27.23 Charnley arthrodesis of the ankle joint.

OSTEOARTHRITIS OF THE FOOT

Osteoarthritis of the sub-talar and transverse tarsal joints may follow injury, infection, rheumatoid arthritis or a congenital anomaly (e.g. calcaneo-navicular bar).

Conservative treatment includes physiotherapy, below-knee irons, adaptations to footwear and local steroid injections.

Operation may be a sub-talar arthrodesis, or a triple arthrodesis.

Osteoarthritis of the metatarsophalangeal joint of the great toe (hallux rigidus) is dealt with elsewhere (Ch. 15).

OSTEOARTHRITIS OF THE SPINE

Osteoarthritis in the small synovial joints of the spine is to be distinguished from osteophytosis of the vertebral bodies resulting from disc degeneration (Ch. 28).

The condition is characterised by pain in the neck or back accompanied by stiffness (Ch. 28).

Treatment. Early cases require general measures as already described with particular attention to weight reduction, correct posture and work surface heights. Physiotherapy is sometimes advised and many departments run special back schools. Exercises to strengthen the paraspinal muscles and those of the abdominal wall and pelvic floor are frequently helpful.

Supports. A plaster jacket may be applied as a temporary measure, and if the pain is relieved it may be replaced by a strong corset, a belt of the Goldthwait type similar to that shown in Fig. 28.12, a Jones spinal support, or some other form of spinal brace. For the cervical spine, a collar may be ordered (Fig. 28.19).

Manipulation under general anaesthesia may be advised, followed by active exercises.

Operative treatment. A spinal fusion may be performed if the osteoarthritis is localised, e.g. following a previous fracture.

OSTEOARTHRITIS OF THE JOINTS OF THE UPPER LIMB

Osteoarthritis of the joints of the upper limb is less common than that of the lower limb with the exception of the generalised osteoarthritis already mentioned, which principally affects the joints of the hands.

Treatment. In general treatment follows upon the lines already discussed for osteoarthritis affecting the lower limb.

Table 27.2 Comparison between rheumatoid arthritis and osteoarthritis.

Diagnostic features	Rheumatoid arthritis	Osteoarthritis
1. Age group commonly affected.	1. Childhood (Still's disease). 2. Adult life, usually before the 5th decade.	Middle-aged or elderly.
2. Joints affected.	Any or all joints in the body; tendency to subluxation, dislocation and ankylosis.	Commonly one weight-bearing joint, or spine. No ankylosis.
3. General health.	May be poor or very poor.	Usually good.
4. Weight.	Tendency to loss of weight.	Tendency to obesity.
5. X-ray findings.	Narrowed joint space, erosion of bone and justarticular osteoporosis	Narrowed joint space, formation of osteophytes, cysts, and sclerosis of bone.
6. Blood picture.	Anaemia sometimes present.	Normal.
7. Erythrocyte sedimentation rate.	Raised.	Normal.

It may be helpful for the nurse to compare in broad outline the diagnostic features of these two conditions.

BIBLIOGRAPHY

Adams G 1983 Girdlestone's operation. Nursing Mirror Clinical Forum, 13 July

Adams J C 1971 Outline of Orthopaedics. Edinburgh: Churchill Livingstone

Anderson M I 1972 Physiotherapeutic management of patients on continuous traction. Physiotherapy 58: 51–54

Apley A G 1977 A system of orthopaedics and fractures. London: Butterworths

Bradley D 1974 Checking a plaster—How and Why. Nursing Times, 1 August, 710: 1190

Bridgewater S E 1975 Charnley Hip Replacement. Nursing Times, 26 June, 1000

Brown P 1983 Clinical teaching opportunities (care of a patient before and after total hip replacement). Nursing Mirror, 8 June

Chivoff R T 1977 An overview of osteoarthritis. Geriatrics 32(6): 57–59

Copeman W S C 1970 Textbook of the Rheumatic Diseases. Edinburgh: E & S Livingstone

Donn M C 1974 Total hip replacement. Nursing Times, 24 October, 1654

Duthrie R B, Ferguson A B 1973 Mercer's Orthopaedic Surgery. London: Arnold

Farrell J 1977 Illustrated Guide to Orthopaedic Nursing. Oxford: Blackwell Scientific

Gunn D G 1975 Problems of middle age—Physical disorders—psychological disorders. Nursing Times, 4 December, 1952–5

Guy F M 1972 Implants used in orthopaedic surgery. Nursing Times, 20 April, 463

Haleen M A 1978 Peripheral arthropathies in the elderly. Nursing Times, 2 November, 1801

Helal B 1972 Joint replacement. Nursing Mirror, 1 September, 18

Irvine C M Complications after hip replacement. Nursing Times, 11 December, 71

King J 1978 Total Hip replacement. Theatre Nursing Care Study. Nursing Times 7(6): 1126

McFarland B 1962 Osteoarthritis of the hip. Nursing Times, 13 July, 890

MacRae R 1976 Clinical Orthopaedic Examination. Edinburgh: Churchill Livingstone

Menzies J 1982 The whole team won. Nursing Mirror, 30 June

Moskovitz R W 1973 Osteoarthritis: a new look at an old disease. Geriatrics 28: 121–128

Orpwood J 1981 Two hips for old. Nursing Mirror, Nursing Care Study, 9 August

Powell M 1973 Limb traction—some aspects of nursing management. Nursing Mirror, 27 July, 26

Ring P A 1965 Osteo-arthritis of the hip. Nursing Times, 15 January, 76

Roaf R, Hodkinson L J 1975 Textbook of Orthopaedic Nursing. Oxford: Blackwell Scientific

Rowe J W, Dyer L (eds) 1977 Care of the Orthopaedic Patient. Oxford: Blackwell Scientific

Shiers L G P 1973 Total replacement of knee joint. Nursing Times, 8 November, 61: 11

Short M 1973 Charnley Arthroplasty. Nursing Times, Nursing Care Study, 1 June, 22

Stauffer M A 1973 Charnley Arthroplasty. Nursing Mirror, 1 June, 136

Stone E, Pinney E 1978 Orthopaedics for Nurses. London: Ballière Tindall

Winkley D 1981 McKee-Arden total hip replacement. News Sheet of the British Association of Orthopaedic Nurses and the Association of Orthopaedic Physiotherapists, 6 March

Wong J 1983 Hip replacement. Nursing Mirror Clinical Forum, 13 July

28

Spinal disorders

LOW BACK PAIN

Low back pain remains one of the least understood areas in medicine. The fundamental problem is the lack of a solid scientific knowledge of the spine on which to base forms of treatment. Eighty per cent of the population will suffer from low back pain at some stage in their lives, and for 30 per cent this will be a recurring and debilitating problem.

The decision to intervene surgically is usually clear; the patient will be severely disabled and unable to conduct his or her life normally. As in deformity, all appropriate conservative measures will have been tried. The decision to operate is the final form of treatment. In 50 per cent of low back pain problems there is no known cause; this leaves the surgeon with two difficult problems:

1. Making a decision about the exact pathological lesion which is producing the pain.
2. Deciding on the correct operative technique.

The two preliminary requirements are the formation of a multi-disciplinary team approach and the structuring of a comprehensive assessment of the patient.

THE MULTI-DISCIPLINARY TEAM APPROACH

This is vital as most spinal problems are difficult to assess, needing thorough clinical evaluation from all members of the team. They are complicated in the adult by social, marital, employment and financial issues. It is often surprising how much greater the patients' real disabilities are when they have been assessed by a team of experts medical and paramedical. By combining all the information, a valuable decision can be reached. Team work is essential if the total patient management is to be successful. In Oswestry we are hoping to establish a clinical care co-ordinator, a nurse who would be able to liaise between clinics dealing with admission and surgery, thus giving the patient the security of continuous care by the same person.

CAREFUL COMPREHENSIVE ASSESSMENT

For all forms of spinal disorders detailed assessment includes:

1. A full clinical history including a family history and completion of a Disability Index Chart (Fairbank et al, 1980).
2. Full physical examination with the patient standing so that the physician can see whether there is any asymmetry; mobility is tested through a range of flexion extension and rotation movements. In cases of low back pain the anterior tenderness sign will confirm pathology in the lumbar spine (Fig. 28.1).

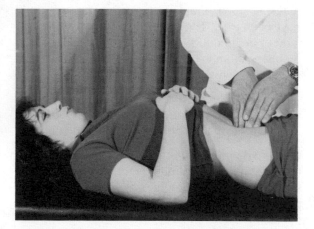

Fig. 28.1 Anterior palpation of the lumbosacral joint in patients with low back pain. The pain itself will often be reproduced and this is a valuable clinical diagnostic sign.

3. Neurological examination: testing of reflexes, motor and sensory impairment.
4. Relevant tests may include when appropriate:

radiographs, discograms, facet arthrograms, radiculograms, tomograms, myelograms, gait analysis (Fig. 28.2).

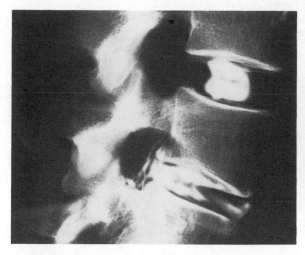

Fig. 28.2 The lateral X-ray to demonstrate the radiological investigation called discography. Dye is injected into the nucleus pulposus of the disc.
Note: Normal nucleus and abnormal nucleus.

ESSENTIAL BACKGROUND INFORMATION

The motion segment

There are usually 23 motion segments containing discs in the spine (Fig. 28.3) making up a unique flexible multi-articulated structure protecting the spinal cord.

Parts of the motion segment can be affected by a variety of pathological processes such as:

a. Vertebral body, e.g. fracture
b. Soft tissues, e.g. torn annulus fibrosus
c. Nerve, e.g. compression.

Abnormalities may occur in different areas of the motion segment. In due course abnormalities in one segment, e.g. abnormal growth, will affect the adjacent segments. Locating the exact mechanism of the motion segment that is at fault is crucial for diagnosis and effective treatment. Is the disc or the facet joint the primary problem or is it another area (Fig. 28.4)?

Pain referral

The most confusing aspect of spinal disorders is

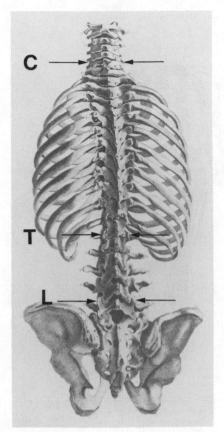

Fig. 28.3 There are 23 motion segments containing discs in the spine which are fairly susceptible to injury.
  C. Low cervical spine. T. Thoracic lumbar region. L. Low lumbar spine.

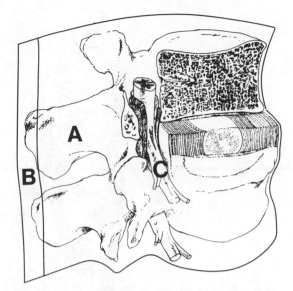

Fig. 28.4 The motion segment demonstrates two vertebral bodies connected by a disc and 2 facet joints. Three types of pain may be produced, termed A, B and C:
  Pain A: deep pain
  Pain B; spinal pain
  Pain C; pain due to nerve root decompression

the complex patterns of pain referral classically described by Kellgren (1939) (Fig. 28.5).

1. Pain in the leg can be referred from any part of a motion segment in the lumbar spine and does not necessarily indicate nerve root compression.
2. Abdominal or chest pain may be referred from a source in the spine.
3. Real abdominal and cardiac lesions can have pain referral to the spine and this can be a cause of diagnostic confusion and irrelevant surgery.
4. Groin pain is commonly referred from an involved motion segment and is often mistaken for uterine disease and results in a hysterectomy without relief of groin pain.
5. The outer half of the disc has a rich sensory nerve supply (Fig. 28.6) and tears of the annulus

are common in domestic and industrial accidents. Nurses are often victims of such tears when handling heavy patients. These tears will often produce leg pain but the radiculogram will be negative. This leads erroneously to surgical exploration for a hidden disc lesion. This sequence of events is very common and leads to increasing disability following the negative exploration, and makes the failed back-pain surgery patient one of the most afflicted sufferers in clinical medicine and they are far too readily dismissed as psychosomatic.

TYPICAL AREAS FOR SURGERY

A. Trauma
B. Degeneration

Trauma

There is a lot of disagreement about the place of spinal surgery in spinal injuries.

In spinal fractures gross instability will require stabilisation, the most popular method being double-Harrington rodding. It is vital that the spinal

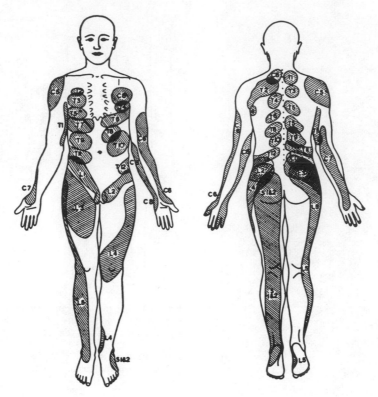

Fig. 28.5 Diagrams to illustrate patterns of deep pain, produced by injury to the various deep parts of the motion segment. Note that anterior pain may be due to irritation of the spine and may be confused with true abdominal pain leading to unnecessary laparotomy.

cord injured patient is handled in a special unit by a well-trained team of specialists.

Soft tissue injury is the most common cause of spinal pain. It is most disabling and difficult to diagnose because it is not apparent on a plain radiograph. A torn disc is unlikely to heal because of its poor blood supply; the nerves in the disc will make this a most painful lesion and it is best treated with fusion, the principle being that in obliterating most of the movement within the motion segment the pain will be relieved.

The commonest site for disc injury is the lowest two motion segments, that is lumbar 4–5 and the lumbo-sacral joints (Fig. 28.3). The thinnest part of the radius of the annulus fibrosus is posteriorly adjacent to the nerve root emerging from the intervertebral foramen. Continuing injury will tear more and more of the annular fibres; ultimately there will be a complete rent in the annulus, allowing extruded nucleus pulposus to compress the nerve

root and producing the classical leg pain. This ruptured disc syndrome is confirmed by radiculography and will require posterior spinal surgery, ideally a 'fenestration' or interlaminar approach permitting access to the inflamed compressed nerve root and allowing the ruptured disc to be removed with care, thus decompressing the nerve root. This is the most common spinal operation, but great care has to be taken in handling the nerve roots because of the high risk of nerve root scarring which seems to be associated with chronic intractable back and leg pain. Some patients seem more prone to nerve root scarring than others.

In a ruptured disc, in biomechanical terms, there is instability of the motion segment and there are valuable reasons why one should fuse this segment. The incidence of chronic low back pain several years after such surgery is quite high but opinion is still divided about the place of fusion of the motion segment in this situation.

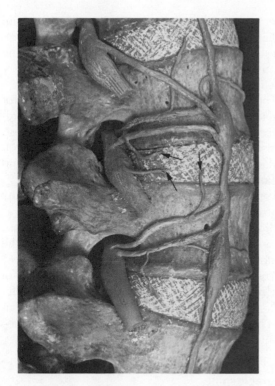

Fig. 28.6 A model of the lumbar spine to show vertebral bodies and discs and small nerve fibres entering the outer borders of the disc to produce a rich sensory nerve supply for its outer half.

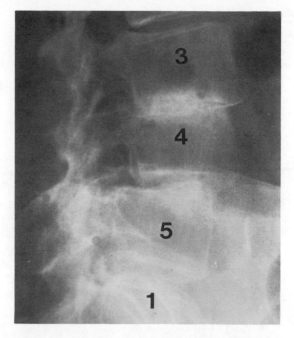

Fig. 28.7 A lateral X-ray to demonstrate degenerative spondylolisthesis at two levels in the lumbar spine, that is forward shift of one body upon another as a result of degeneration.

Degeneration

Degenerative changes begin within the motion segment in early adult life. The disc becomes desiccated and radial tears appear in the annulus fibrosus. The disc may narrow, producing overriding of the corresponding facet joints, which in due course become arthritic with loss of cartilage, osteophyte formation, etc. Narrowing of the motion segment produces reduction of the intervertebral foramen so that the emerging nerve root may be compressed. When these changes have taken place in the motion segment it is more vulnerable to minor injury which would not affect a normal motion segment. In the older age group marked degenerative changes in the facet joints at the lumbar 4–5 segment allow a forward shift of the body of 4 on 5, producing so-called degenerative spondylolisthesis (Fig. 28.7). This forward shift causes marked reduction of the spinal canal with compression of the dura mater and the nerve roots. It produces an intractable back and leg pain which may require decompressive laminectomy to relieve the symptoms.

Another degenerative lesion which is being seen more commonly with an ageing population is associated with marked osteoarthritis of the facet joints, producing large osteophytes which encroach on the space normally reserved for the spinal cord and nerve roots. In the cervical spine, osteophytes may encroach on the spinal canal and cause cord compression. In the lumbar spine these pathological changes produce 'spinal stenosis', which, if the symptoms of leg pain with walking become severe, will require decompressive laminectomy.

THE PRINCIPLES OF SURGERY IN SPINAL DISORDERS

1. Surgery should only be considered when conservative treatment has failed.
2. Surgery should only be undertaken after detailed and exhaustive preliminary investigations to define the exact pathological entity.
3. A brief summary of the surgical principles is shown in Table 28.1.

Table 28.1 Surgical principles

Cause	Principles of surgery
Compressed nerve root	Decompression (laminectomy)
Motion segment instability (trauma, disc degeneration, etc.)	Stabilise the segment (fusion)
Deformity or displacement of the motion segment	Reduction of the deformity and stabilise (fuse)
Discogenic lesion	Remove the disc and stabilise the segment
Facet joint arthritis	Stabilise the segment to eliminate motion which causes the pain
Torn annulus fibrosus	Rest to encourage healing. If this fails, fusion required (segmental motion produces pain)
Spinal stenosis	Laminectomy
Infected vertebral body, e.g.	(a) Chemotherapy
TB spine	(b) Excision of the infected tissue (anterior approach); replace defect with bone graft
Tumour	Remove the tumour (perhaps two-staged procedure), stabilise with bone graft and metallic implants (irradiate if necessary)

RATIONALE OF STABILISATION

There are numerous techniques of spinal fusion, posterior facet joint fusion, fusion of the transverse processes and interbody fusion. The surprising fact is that fusion in deformity and infection invariably has a high success rate, whereas in low back pain it remains a controversial issue. It is not surprising then that there are over 30 techniques for fusion in treatment of low back disorders.

The key factors are determining the exact pathological lesion and the precise motion segment which is causing the disability.

The failed back-surgery patient remains one of the largest problems in clinical medicine. The commonest causes of failure are surgery at the wrong level or for the wrong reason and damage to the nerve roots at the time of posterior exploration.

The cervical spine

The two commonest lesions requiring surgery in the cervical spine are:

1. disc disruption
2. cervical spondylosis.

The point of practical significance is that pain referred from the cervical spine can produce pain radiating to the head, eye (visual disturbance), chest, shoulder and entire upper limb, thus being commonly mistaken for migraine, coronary artery disease, frozen shoulder etc.

The most common surgical procedure is anterior cervical fusion: this involves disc excision with replacement by a bone graft taken from the iliac crest; post-operative in immobilisation involves a soft collar until the bone grafts are healed clinically and radiologically.

Less common is cervical spondylitic myelopathy (CSM) which produces local symptoms of pain as well as long tract signs (gait disturbance) because of pressure from the posterior osteophytes on the motor regions of the spinal cord.

The osteophytes may be removed at the time of anterior cervical fusion but many surgeons prefer to leave the osteophytes because the immobilisation of the joint by fusion and thus the loss of movement causes the osteophytes to regress with time.

Thoracic spine

Deformity is the most common lesion in the thoracic spine. Pain from thoracic disc lesions does occur but it is quite infrequent and will often produce compression of the spinal cord. Accurate diagnosis is essential. Laminectomy for treatment of the thoracic disc has a high incidence of paraplegia. The surgical treatment of the thoracic disc lesion is through an anterior approach, removal of the disc and stabilisation of the motion segment with a bone graft from the adjacent iliac crest.

General notes on nursing care

On admission the patient may be apprehensive or even in great pain; after a thorough physical examination, the surgeon will order drugs to relieve the pain, to induce relaxation and to ensure a good night's sleep. The patient is put to bed on a firm mattress supported throughout its length by a fracture board. Specific orders must be sought as to the extent of activity allowed; some patients may be allowed up at least once or twice a day for toilet purposes but, in general, strict recumbency is usually ordered and comprehensive nursing care is then required. In common with many of our

Case example

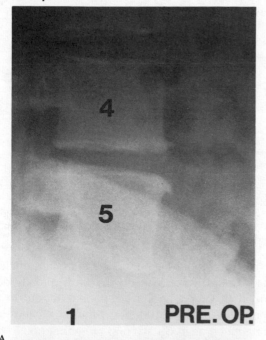

patients, these patients fall into the category of the very uncomfortable (Chs 2, 3 and 5). Many of them find the recumbent position very uncomfortable indeed and prefer to curl up in bed; those of heavy build appear particularly uncomfortable and are prone to abdominal upsets. Patients of above average height may require a seven-foot-long bed, especially if traction to the legs or pelvis is ordered. The bedclothes must be supported and a tilting mirror attached to the bed is helpful.

In the acute stage the patient will need help in washing the hands and face and the rest of his toilet must be carried out for him, including attention to the hair, teeth and nails, and strict daily attention to cleanliness of the external genitalia. Female patients are taught to use a urinal, especially if the back is very painful. Pressure areas, such as the sacrum, heels and elbows, should be inspected regularly and kept clean and dry. The patient may be allowed to raise himself by means of a trapeze for bedpans and for changing the bottom sheet but if the back is extremely painful he should be lifted

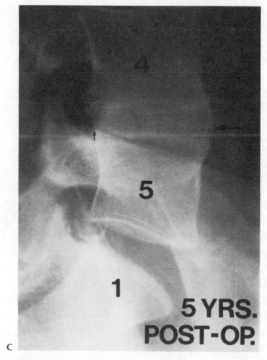

Fig. 28.8A–C Case example of a 35-year-old lady with intractable low back pain due to painful degeneration of the L4-5 segment. An anterior lumbar fusion was performed. When the bone graft had healed, the patient's symptoms were relieved and she could then lead a normal lifestyle:

X-rays demonstrate;
   A: the abnormal segment before surgery
   B: the bone graft in position 1 year after surgery
   C: the remodelling of the bone graft 5 years later

by two nurses while a third inserts the bedpan or straightens the sheet. The bowels must be regulated and many patients have difficulty of micturition in the early stages of recumbency, though this usually responds to simple measures and catheterisation is rarely necesssary. Vomiting and abdominal pain should be reported to the surgeon at once. Abdominal distension is often troublesome.

Later treatment. Static muscular contractions are ordered, progressing to more vigorous exercises as the condition improves. Special exercises are given for the spinal and abdominal muscles. Most patients require some form of support for the spine, and it is usual to apply a plaster jacket or spica, a leather and canvas belt of the Goldthwait type, or a strong corset before weight-bearing is attempted. Since this must often be worn for a long period, it must be a perfect fit, especially made for the individual patient, and he must understand its use and management before discharge from the hospital.

Individuals suffering from pain in the back, from whatever cause, *should always sleep on a firm mattress*. When the acute stage has passed the patient may practise 'bridging', i.e. the patient should flex the knees and lift the buttocks off the bed, while taking weight on the heels and shoulders, before rising each morning. The position is held for the count of 20; the object of the exercise is to contract the lumbar muscles before assuming the strain of the standing position.

Alternative methods of treatment

1. *Simple recumbency* as previously described may be sufficient in some cases, followed by exercises and weight-bearing in some form of support such as a plaster jacket, a canvas and leather belt, or a strong corset.

2. *A plaster jacket* is often ordered; application and nursing care are described in Chs 6 and 9.

A plaster spica may be ordered in cases where a plaster jacket does not give relief from pain, especially in low lesions, e.g. in the L5–S1 region. If sciatica is present the leg on that side is immobilised. Nursing care proceeds on the lines discussed in Chs 5, 9 and 10.

3. *Traction to the legs or pelvis* is often ordered.

Intermittent traction to the trunk and legs may be applied by means of a special apparatus in the physiotherapy department (Fig. 28.9).

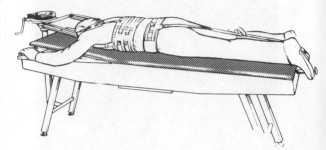

Fig. 28.9 A traction can be used in the Physiotherapy Department for rhythmical, intermittent or sustained traction in the treatment of low back pain. (Carter's Rosslyn Traction Couch.)

(a) *Continuous leg traction.* Preparation, including sedation, proceeds on the lines already described in Chs 3 and 9 for patients about to be immobilised on a plaster bed. Strapping extensions are applied as in Ch. 10 and are either tied to the elevated footend of the bed as shown in Fig. 10.14 (Pugh's traction) or attached to weighted cords as shown in Fig. 28.10 (weight and pulley traction). The exact amount of weight is decided by the surgeon and is largely governed by the weight of the patient and the severity of his condition. It is usual to increase the weight gradually during the first few days of fixation or even to delay application until the patient is accustomed to the supine position.

Nursing care proceeds on the same lines as described in Ch. 10.

(b) *Continuous pelvic traction.* This is applied by means of a well-fitting pelvic belt, from which canvas strips are attached to a wooden spreader, as shown in Fig. 28.11. Weights are attached to a cord running through slots in the spreader, and the foot of the bed is elevated. Very heavy traction can be applied by this means and is well tolerated by the patient.

Nursing care proceeds as before. The patient is able to move the legs freely without disturbing the traction force. Thin patients may require special attention to the iliac crests and sacrum, but if the belt is well-fitting, pressure-sores should not occur. Later treatment proceeds as described above. Some form of support for the back is usually ordered before weight-bearing is resumed.

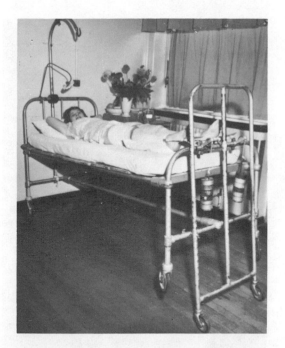

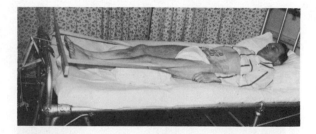

A

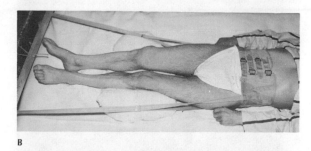

B

Fig. 28.10 Continuous leg-traction used in the treatment of a case of protrusion of an intervertebral disc. In this case the traction was increased gradually by adding weight until 6.5 kg was suspended from each leg. The patient made a good recovery.

4. *Manipulation of the spine*, with or without anaesthesia is sometimes advised.

5. *Goldthwait belt*. This is made on a cast of the patient's trunk (Ch. 7). A leather portion, strengthened by metal strips, supports the spine posteriorly, and a reinforced sail-cloth belt fastens in front either by lacing or by straps, as shown in Figs 28.12A–F. It is important that the support is long enough to support the lower rib-cage; groin straps prevent it from riding upwards.

A surgical corset is often ordered (Fig. 28.13) and may be obtained from a firm which specialises in this work such as Spencer, whose fitters will visit the patient and carry out any special instructions.

Fitting and care of a belt or corset. A well-fitting cotton vest is usually worn beneath a support. The patient lies supine and the support is unfastened at the front and rolled from sides to middle ready to be placed beneath him. An assistant helps the patient to raise himself and he is lowered on to the posterior part of the support. It is then fastened as tightly as possible; on standing, the straps or laces are again tightened. Instructions are sought

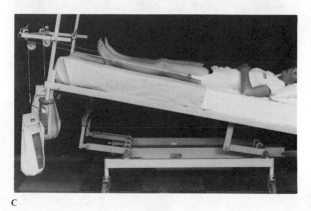

C

Fig. 28.11 A, B. Pelvic traction (see text). (With kind permission of the Royal Orthopaedic Hospital, Birmingham.) *Note:* An overhead pulley should be supplied (not shown here). **C.** This shows pelvic traction applied using a King's Fund bed.

as to whether (as is usually the case) it can be removed for toilet purposes. In some cases the support is worn continuously, even in bed; in others, it is discarded gradually until it can be dispensed with altogether.

Operative treatment

Preparation for operation is carried out most carefully and exhaustive tests are often conducted before surgery is finally decided upon. Investigations include special radiographs and a thorough

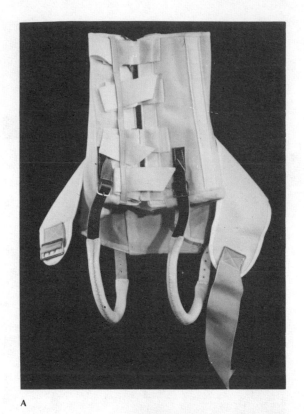

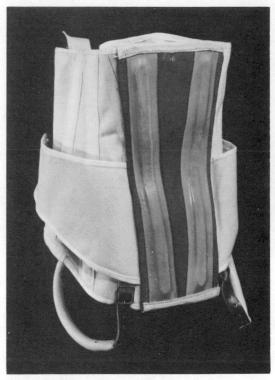

A

B

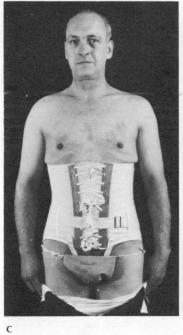

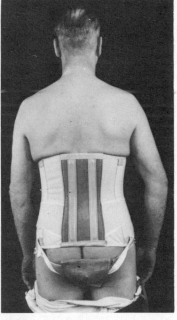

C

D

Fig. 28.12   A, B. Goldthwait belt, **C, D.** Goldthwait belt worn
for low back pain. **E.** Lumbo-sacral belt (Seton Products).
F. Tubigrip hip spica (Seton Products).

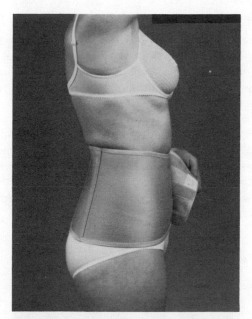

Fig. 28.12E

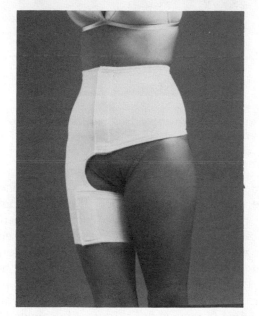

Fig. 28.12F

surgery. *Local skin preparation* varies from surgeon to surgeon.

Prophylactic anticoagulant therapy is frequently ordered.

Post-operative care. The patient is received on to a firm mattress supported by fracture boards and the usual post-operative care is given including observation of vital signs as for any other major operation; continuous drainage of the bladder by means of a catheter is sometimes ordered and it is common practice for fluids only to be given intravenously for the first few days. If bowel sounds are present a light diet is commenced and suppositories given on or about the 4th day.

Immobilisation and positioning depends upon the particular operation and the orders of the particular surgeon. Extensive spinal fusion may require fixation in a plaster bed though this is unusual nowadays. (Ch. 9); otherwise the patient lies flat in bed or on alternate sides with a pillow between the knees and will be log-rolled from side to side at regular intervals until he is allowed to turn himself by means of a trapeze. A careful watch is kept on the wound dressing (a Chiron drain is often used as shown in Ch. 27). Breathing exercises, quadriceps drill and exercises for the ankles and feet are performed regularly; any loss of sensation or motor power in the lower limbs is reported to the surgeon

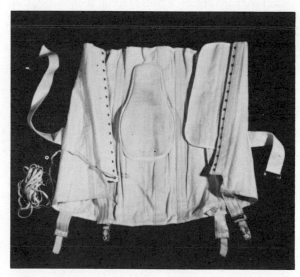

Fig. 28.13 Surgical corset for low back pain—note the lumbar pad: the corset is put on *in the lying position* and the laces tightened on standing.

physical examination which may include an electro-cardiogram; psychological tests may also be applied as already described. Examination of blood and urine and thorough cleansing of the whole body is carried out as for any major operation; a low residue diet is usually ordered and suppositories may be given on the evening before immediately as is any swelling or raised skin temperature in the calf of the leg which might indicate a deep vein thrombosis.

The toilet. In the early stages, the patient may be completely helpless and will require nursing care as already described for a patient in a plaster bed (Ch. 9). Female patients should be taught to use a special urinal (Fig. 5.4.A.) preferably *before* operation. Bedpans must be given in such a way that there is no strain on the spine. A slipper bedpan is shown in Fig. 5.4.B and in some cases a tray or kidney-shaped receiver or even an incontinence pad may be used instead; *whatever method used, faecal contamination of the wound dressing must be prevented.*

Activity is gradually increased but in general the patient is not allowed to sit up without assistance for the first two weeks. Sitting with the knees flexed over the edge of the bed is gradually introduced, but the long sitting position (i.e. with the knees straight) is strictly forbidden. If all goes well weight-bearing is permitted in two to four weeks. Exercises particularly for the muscles of the back and the abdomen, with postural training are continued, and a supporting belt or corset may be ordered. Patients are advised to avoid heavy lifting whilst in the stooping position for at least six months.

After spinal fusion the patient may be nursed in a plaster bed but this is unusual nowadays. A plaster jacket may be applied, and gradual weight-bearing commenced. The jacket is worn for a further six weeks and exercises to strengthen the spinal muscles are commenced. Later, a supporting belt may be ordered.

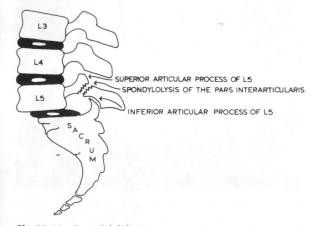

Fig. 28.14 Spondylolithesis.

Alternative treatment for cervical pain

Treatment as an out-patient may consist of a supporting collar, physiotherapy and reassurance.

Intermittent head-traction may be applied in the physiotherapy department by means of a head-suspension apparatus. Local heat, massage and exercises may also be ordered.

A collar is often ordered, which may be made of plaster of Paris, but more often of sorbo rubber, as shown in Fig. 28.15. Alternatively, one produced commercially may be used, such as those shown in Figs 28.17, 18 and 19. It is gradually discarded as the symptoms subside.

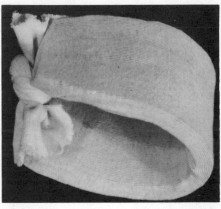

Fig. 28.15 Home-made sorbo-rubber collar. The ties should be long enough to cross at the back and fasten *in front*, not at the back as shown.

Treatment by continuous head-traction may be ordered in those cases which do not respond to the measures outlined above. It may be applied by means of a canvas head-harness applied as shown in Fig. 28.20, which is either attached to the elevated head-end of the bed or to a weighted cord running over a pulley attached to the head of the bed. This form of traction is extremely uncomfortable and constant nursing attention is required to prevent the chin from becoming sore. The harness is removed at four-hourly intervals for treatment of the skin, and permission is sought for it to be removed at meal times. Otherwise the patient may take fluids through a straw or bent glass rod.

Criles head-tractor may be ordered as an alternative method of treatment. This splint consists of a padded aluminium bar which is shaped to fit the

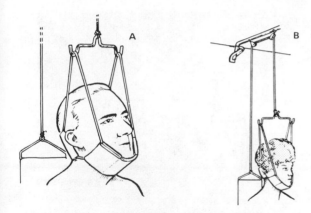

Fig. 28.16 **A.** Halter for intermittent cervical traction (Zimmer). This is made in one size only and is suitable for any patient—adult or child. The soft leatherette support pads are easily placed in position and hold the cords away from the neck. The apparatus adjusts automatically to give the correct degree of flexion and extension. The soft leatherette pads are sympathetic to the skin and provide a comfortable head halter. **B.** Home intermittent Traction Kit (Zimmer). This Home Traction Kit comprises: Overdoor Assembly, Spreader Bar, Watertight Bag, Traction Cord and Head Halter. The Home Traction Kit provides all the items necessary to apply hyperextension or flexion cervical traction for adult or child. It is suitable for patients who are able to apply traction to the physiotherapists' instructions.

occiput, and which is combined with a firmly buck-led padded forehead strap. Traction is exerted by weights fastened to the aluminium bar and the head of the bed is elevated to supply counter-traction. The traction force is exerted mainly on the occiput and to a lesser degree on the forehead; both these points will require frequent inspection and massage to prevent them from becoming sore. This type of traction is better tolerated by the patient than the

Glisson sling because the chin is left free for talking, eating, etc.

Physiotherapy for pain in the neck and back

In most diseases and pathological conditions, physiotherapists can only treat symptoms, the treatment having little, if any, effect on the underlying changes; in short, physiotherapeutic treatment cannot cure the condition, but on the other hand the pain felt by the patient as a symptom of neck or low back dysfunction can often be helped by physiotherapeutic techniques. There are many causes of neck and back pain; when pain arises from bones, joints or soft tissues such as ligaments, muscles and tendons, the exact diagnosis may be difficult to make; however the segmental level can often be pinpointed and specific treatment can help to relieve the symptoms.

The physiotherapist carries out an examination and assessment of the spine to discover the level and possibly, the structure causing the pain; this is done by observing and testing posture and movement. Movement is tested both actively and passively using physiological and accessory ranges. A painful restriction can be mobilised and restored to normal function. Muscle power is assessed and where necessary it is re-educated or strengthened by exercise. Work and leisure activities, together with rest and sleeping positions are discussed with the patient and advice is given on how these may be modified to help relieve pain.

When symptoms arise from more serious degenerative joint conditions or from disc disorders such as prolapse or herniation, surgery may be con-

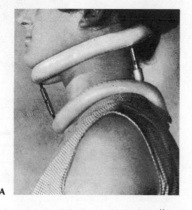
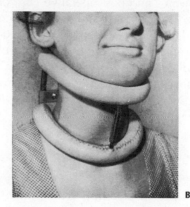

Fig. 28.17 **A, B.** Camp Victoria collar.

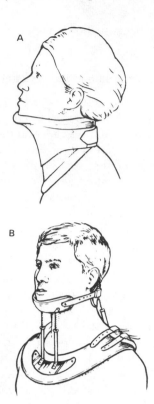

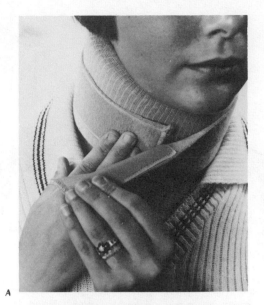

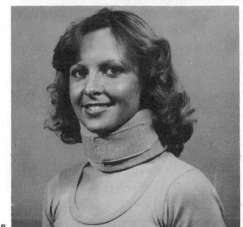

Fig. 28.18 **A.** Cervical collar with chinpiece (Zimmer). This cervical collar is supplied with an integral padded chinpiece to give positive positioning of the chin to occipit, minimum movement is allowed and chafing is eliminated. Made in white polythene with all contact parts covered in soft leatherette to ensure patient's comfort. Velcro is used to provide instant fixing. **B.** Cervical brace (Zimmer). This brace is leather-padded throughout with metal parts being made from painted aluminium and stainless steel. It can be used in cases where it is necessary to immobilise the head.

sidered; the role of the physiotherapist then concerns the general pre- and post-operative care of the patient related to the chest and maintenance of circulation, and more specific treatment depending on the type of surgery and on the affected level of the vertebral column.

An outline of physiotherapy for cervical and low back pain will now be given for both conservative and surgical management.

1. Cervical pain

Conservative management

Rest in a collar. When rest and support are needed, a temporary collar may be made out of Plastozote

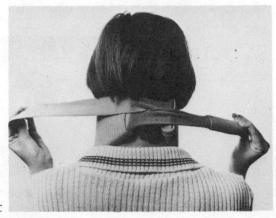

Fig. 28.19 **A–C.** This collar is available in three different sizes. (Seton Products.)

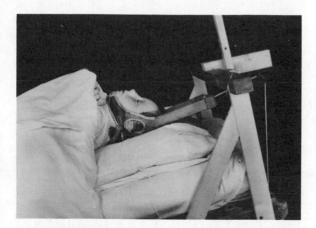

Fig. 28.20 Head traction by means of a Glisson sling. The head of the bed is raised to supply counter-traction.

Exercises. Postural re-education—correct head carriage, shoulder relaxation and freedom of neck movement is regained by active exercises. Strengthening exercises using proprioceptive neuromuscular facilitation techniques will develop isometric muscle control.

Advice. The patient is advised on 'neck life'. This modifies his home and work circumstances to help speed up resolution of neck problems.

Position of work surfaces and the use of space so that excessive neck movements are eliminated.

A 'butterfly' pillow is used to support the neck at night (Fig. 28.21). The patient is advised to avoid

for day wear and soft foam or felt for night wear (Fig. 28.15).

A patient wearing a collar is always advised to beware going out in the dark or going into a darkened room. Also he should not drive in a collar. Loss of proprioception from cervical joints and muscles leads to loss in ability to judge distance particularly laterally when driving. The additional loss of visual input in the dark can lead to accidents.

Relief of pain and muscle spasm. Any form of heat may be applied to relieve neck pain but hot packs, hot water bottles or small electrically heated pads are particularly valuable. A patient may use a hot water bottle at home, provided that sensation has been tested and care is taken in application; ice applications may be preferred in some cases.

Cervical traction. Intermittent or sustained traction may be given to help mobilise a painful neck and help relieve muscle spasm (Fig. 28.16); it is carefully localised to the affected level by positioning; referred pain down the arms responds well to cervical traction. *Mobilisation/Manipulation.* A segmental level of painful, restricted movement can be mobilised by a highly skilled, specially trained physiotherapist, using graded pressures to bring about localised movement. A manipulative thrust may be required to completely free a restriction particularly a 'locked' facet joint.

Soft-tissue techniques. Specific techniques using the hands, such as massage, can be used to mobilise the surrounding soft tissues to restore normal function.

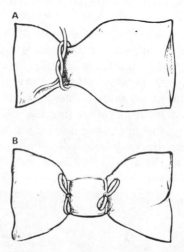

Fig. 28.21 The 'butterfly' pillow. Use a soft feather pillow; tie two pieces of ribbon or tape round the centre about 2–3 in apart; experiment will determine the exact situation of the ties. Place the pillow under your neck so that it is supported in the area between the two ties; the ends of the pillow will keep your neck in a good physiological position. **A.** Shows one tie being applied. **B.** Shows two ties in position; the neck rests in the area between them.

aggravating factors such as visiting the hairdresser, carrying heavy shopping; encourage the use of mirrors when driving a motor car. These are just some examples of adjustment of home and work circumstances, all of which obviously depend on the individual needs of the patient.

Surgical management. A patient undergoing surgery on the neck will require routine pre- and postoperative chest care and circulatory exercises regardless of the procedure carried out by the surgeon; most commonly, surgery to relieve pain in the cervical region will entail fusion of one or more vertebral segments; this will often be done from an anterior approach, fusing two vertebral bodies by means of a bone graft. This type of fusion leaves the posterior articulations and their supporting ligaments intact and stability is disrupted as little as possible. The patient may be allowed up wearing a supporting cervical collar within a few days.

Physiotherapy treatment in such cases will include gentle strengthening exercises for the arms if necessary. Relaxation of the shoulder girdle muscles and postural correction of neck position while wearing a supporting collar. Gentle active muscle strengthening and mobilising exercises for the neck may be required by some patients when fusion has occurred and the collar can be removed.

The 'halo' splint. Posterior fusion of the cervical spine usually requires post-operative immobilisation in a 'halo' splint (Fig. 28.22). Such patients will need help initially when they are allowed to get up. The heavy body plaster to which the halo is attached makes normal function difficult and much help and encouragement from nurses and physiotherapists may be needed for the patient to learn to carry out the activities of daily living; full

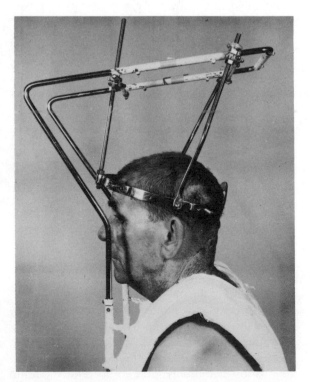

Fig. 28.22   'Halo' splint, applied after fusion of cervical spine.

range arm exercises are encouraged whilst wearing the plaster. Gentle strengthening for the neck and shoulder girdle muscles together with gentle neck movements may need supervision when the splint is removed.

2. Low back pain

Conservative management

Rest and back supports. In an acute attack of low back pain, the patient may need to rest in bed. The adoption of the 'Fowler position'—hips and knees flexed and supported may be found beneficial; the patient is taught to adopt this position. For the ambulant patient, a temporary back support may help when rest in bed is not possible; supports with elastic fastenings are easily fitted to most sizes of patients (Fig. 28.12).

Relief of pain and muscle spasm. Heat may help relieve pain by relaxing spasm of the paravertebral muscles; hot packs or electrically heated pads are most valuable; soft tissue manipulative techniques can also be used; and application of ice is used occasionally.

Lumbar traction. Lumbar traction is particularly useful in patients who suffer referred pain down the legs. In low lumbar segmental problems the traction will be applied with the patient lying in the 'Fowler position'. A sustained pull or intermittent pull may be used depending on how much movement is required at the affected level.

Mobilisation/Manipulation. The soft tissue lesions and facet joint problems which give rise to low back pain can very often be relieved by localised, accessory, oscillatory movements. These techniques, which are carried out by specially trained physiotherapists can include a specific thrust or manipulation when necessary to free a painful, restricted joint. They rely on meticulous examination, and assessment by palpation of the parts is most important. When correctly chosen and used, relief may be obtained within a few days.

Exercises. Exercises may be used to help regain spinal movements, but specific muscle groups often need to be strengthened. Isometric strengthening exercises, including the use of proprioceptive neuromuscular facilitation techniques are given, particularly for the abdominal muscles. Strong abdominal muscles act as a corset to protect the lumbar spine from excessive compression strain, particularly in lifting. At the same time, the back extensor and quadriceps muscles must also be strengthened. Hydrotherapy (Fig. 26.3) and swimming are very beneficial for back pain sufferers.

Posture. Postural re-education is often required and can be carried out together with the abdominal strengthening exercises; pelvic tilt and control is the key factor in postural correction (Fig. 28.23).

Lifting. All patients with low back pain must be taught correct methods of lifting. Strong abdominal muscles and quadriceps are essential so that the vertebral column can remain erect whilst the knees and hips are flexed allowing the stronger thigh muscles to do the work.

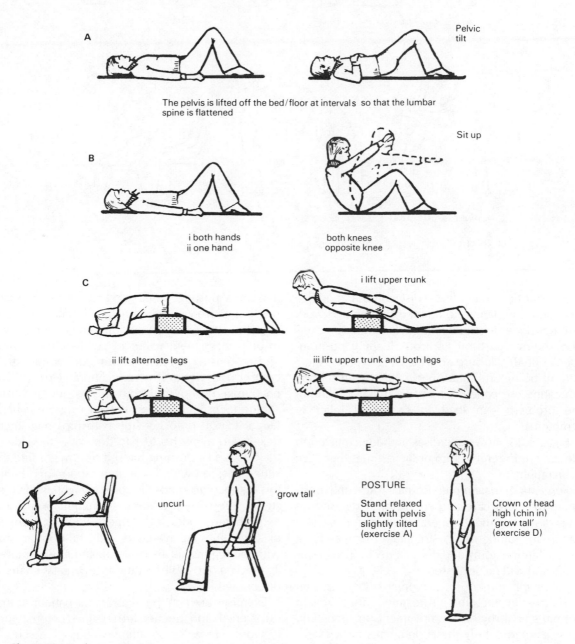

Fig. 28.23 Back care exercises.

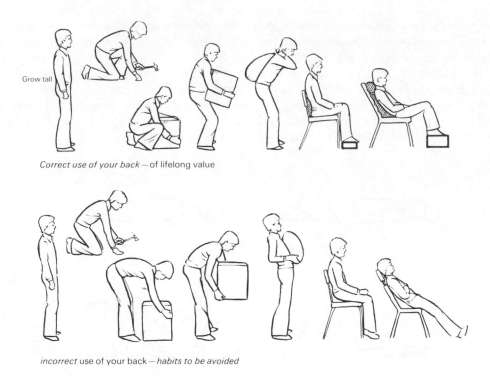

Grow tall

Correct use of your back — of lifelong value

incorrect use of your back — *habits to be avoided*

Fig. 28.24 Correct use of the back prevents problems.

Ergonomics. 'Back life'—discussion and advice to enable the patient to adapt his home and work circumstances to protect his back. Advice on exercise, lifting, postural control, sleeping position, special chairs, leisure activities (Fig. 28.24), etc., can all be incorporated into a 'back pain school' educating the patient so that an understanding of the problem can lead to successful relief of symptoms.

Fig. 28.23 shows exercises and advice given to the patient to remind him of the regimes that have been taught.

Surgical management. Routine pre- and post-operative chest care and circulatory exercises are given for all patients operated upon for the low back. An outline of physiotherapy regimes for a simple laminectomy and discectomy, and for a spinal fusion will be discussed.

Following surgery for a lumbar disc protrusion or herniation, the aims of treatment are to regain normal spinal rhythm in movement, to strengthen muscles (particularly the abdominals, back extensors and quadriceps), to re-educate normal lumbar and spinal posture, to teach correct lifting and ergonomics, with a view to return to full spinal function.

In the first few post-operative days, whilst still in bed, the patient will start gentle strengthening and mobilising spinal exercises, including pelvic control for postural re-education. He will be encouraged to log-roll from side to side and from supine to prone. When allowed to get up, he is taught to roll onto his side with hips and knees flexed and allow his legs to drop over the side of the bed whilst pushing himself up straight into the sitting position with his undermost arm and hand; this manoeuvre keeps the spine straight and avoids strain. The patient continues rehabilitation in the hydrotherapy pool and large swimming pool, if these facilities are available, and whilst progressing with the regime, is also encouraged to walk about as much as possible. Sitting in low easy chairs is discouraged.

Exercises are continued as an out-patient so that full strength and function are regained before return to work. He will also attend a 'back life school' as outlined under conservative management. The

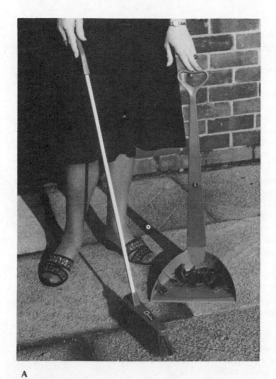

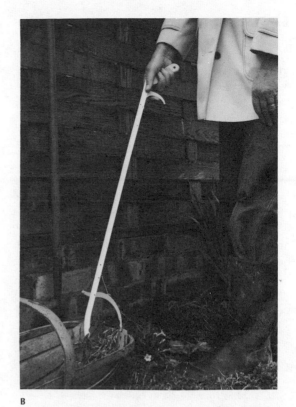

Fig. 28.25   A–C. 'Back savers'. Long-handled implements for housework or gardening. (By courtesy of the Disabled Living Foundation.)

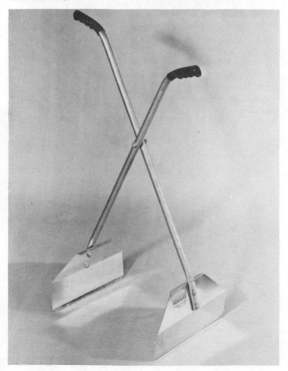

fundamental difference in the physiotherapy regime following spinal fusion is that spinal movement is prohibited initially until fusion is progressing. The patient will be taught static (isometric) exercises which strengthen the abdominal and back extensor muscles; actual movement is not allowed. He is taught to log-roll and how to get up out of bed as described above and encouraged to walk as much as possible. Flexion exercises are introduced very gradually and slowly depending on individual progress but full normal functions are gently and steadily encouraged until regained fully; swimming is particularly beneficial and the patient may attend a 'back life school' to learn ergonomics, including correct posture in walking, sitting and lying, and lifting techniques.

ULNAR NERVE COMPRESSION

Ulnar nerve compression at the elbow may be associated with a cubitis valgus deformity (Ch. 7), or with degenerative arthritis (Ch. 27). The patient complains of 'pins and needles' along the ulnar border of the hand and in the little and ring fingers.

Treatment is by operation either in the form of a decompression (Osborne) or by anterior transposition of the ulnar nerve.

MEDIAN NERVE COMPRESSION (CARPAL TUNNEL SYNDROME)

This is commonly seen in women, when the median nerve is compressed in the carpal tunnel at the wrist. The patient complains of pain and of 'pins and needles' in the thumb, index and middle fingers, characteristically at its worst in bed at night. The thenar muscles may be wasted.

Treatment is by application of a plaster nightshell, by injection of a steroid preparation or by operative division of the flexor retinaculum.

ACKNOWLEDGEMENTS

Figs 28.3, 28.5, 28.6, 28.7 and 28.8 have appeared in *Cash's Textbook of Orthopaedics and Rheumatology for Physiotherapists* and are reproduced by permission of the publishers, Faber and Faber Ltd.

BIBLIOGRAPHY

Adams John Crawford 1971 Outline of Orthopaedics. Edinburgh: Churchill Livingstone

Apley E Graham 1977 A system of orthopaedics and fractures. London: Butterworths

Armitage P 1938 Strategies for dealing with discomfort. Nursing Mirror, 30 March

Buchanan W Watson, Dick W Carson 1976 Recent Advances in Rheumatology, Pt. 1. Edinburgh: Churchill Livingstone

Copeman W S C 1970 Textbook of the Rheumatic Diseases. Edinburgh: E & S Livingstone

Cowell S 1984 Spinal fusion. Nursing Mirror, 31 October

Duthie R B, Ferguson A B Jnr 1973 Mercer's Orthopaedic Surgery. London: Arnold

Dyson R 1971 Spinal disc lesions. Nursing Mirror, 3 December, 133, 26

Fairbank J C T, Couper J, Davies J B, O'Brien J P 1980 The Oswestry low back pain disability questionnaire. Physiotherapy 66: 271–273

Farrell J 1977 Illustrated Guide to Orthopaedic Nursing. Oxford: Blackwell Scientific

Gunn D G 1975 Problems of middle age—Physical disorders—psychological disorders. Nursing Times, 4 December, 1952–5

Harrold A J 1971 Laminectomy for disc disorders. Nursing Times 8 April, 67–406

Kellgren J H 1939 On the distribution of pain arising from deep somatic structures with charts of segmental pain areas. Clinical science 4: 35–36

Kessel Lipmann 1969 Low back pain. Nursing Mirror, 21 March 22

Lenihan J et al 1983 Design in health care—taking the strain. Nursing Mirror, 29 June

McRae R 1976 Clinical Orthopaedic Examination. Edinburgh: Churchill Livingstone

Price B 1983 A pain in the back. Nursing Mirror, 13 July

Raistrick A 1981 Nurses with back pain—Can the problem be prevented? Nursing Times, 14 May

Roaf R, Hodkinson L J 1976 Textbook of Orthopaedic Nursing. Oxford: Blackwell Scientific

Rowe J, Dyer L (eds) 1977 Care of the Orthopaedic patient. Oxford: Blackwell Scientific

Stone E, Pinney E 1978 Orthopaedics for Nurses. London: Ballière Tindall

Tonfexis A 1980 That aching back. Time Magazine Cover Story, 14 July

29

Other rheumatic diseases

In the previous four chapters the most important types of rheumatic diseases have been dealt with, namely: rheumatoid arthritis, ankylosing spondylitis, osteoarthritis and degenerative disc disease. In this chapter other rheumatic diseases are discussed. Some occur commonly in orthopaedic practice; but others are seen less often.

In general, the cause of many of the rheumatic diseases is still unknown.

RHEUMATIC FEVER

This is a disease mainly of adolescent children, which primarily involves the joints but it is important to remember that the heart may be seriously affected. Fortunately it is much less common than it used to be; the incidence has dropped partly due to the widespread use of antibiotics and to improved standards of living.

Clinical features

Typically, *joint symptoms* appear some three weeks after a Group A β-haemolytic streptococcal throat infection. Joint pains are flitting in character, involving one joint for 24–48 hours and then moving to another; several joints may be involved. The severity of symptoms varies from mild aches to florid joint inflammation with pain, swelling, redness, heat, tenderness and marked restriction of movement of the affected joint. The symptoms and signs rapidly disappear from one joint only to appear in another the following day. Occasionally only one joint may be involved.

The temperature is raised and there is often tachycardia. The child may or may not be systemically ill with malaise, fretfulness, anorexia, etc.

The heart is not uncommonly involved and this is the most serious aspect of rheumatic fever. Tachycardia persists and the development of murmurs, with or without heart failure, an irregular pulse, pericarditis or e.c.g. changes indicate cardiac damage. In some cases the heart will recover, but in others the patient develops chronic rheumatic heart disease, the most common form being mitral stenosis.

The diagnosis is made on clinical grounds and is made easier if the patient develops a typical rash (erythema marginatum), nodules, or chorea. Laboratory findings such as a positive throat swab, raised erythrocyte sedimentation rate and anti-streptolysin titre (an antibody in the blood which indicates a streptococcal infection) support the diagnosis.

Treatment

This consists of complete rest in bed until the acute stage has passed, and then graded mobilisation. Rest in bed should be rigidly enforced if there is evidence of heart damage. A therapeutic course of penicillin is given at once and is followed by oral penicillin twice daily. Salicylate is given in adequate dose to relieve joint pain and occasionally cortico-steroids may be used. It is generally thought that both salicylate and cortisone merely suppress the acute manifestations of the disease but do not influence the occurrence or severity of heart disease.

Nursing management in rheumatic fever

This ranges from total care in the acute stage, when the patient is permitted to do nothing for himself, to carefully graded activities and finally, to complete self-care before discharge from hospital.

Progression is based on the following:

1. The temperature chart.
2. The result of a weekly erythrocyte-sedimentation rate test.
3. Clinical findings, i.e. general condition, joint pain, signs of cardiac involvement.

Stage I. Complete rest in bed means total dependency and total nursing care. The patient is nursed flat with one pillow; it is imperative that the bed is placed in a position where observation of the ward activities is allowed without exertion. The school teacher and occupational therapist, in common with other members of the team, must exercise ingenuity in providing suitable occupation. In the acute stage, especially where there is cardiac damage, the patient may not be permitted even to hold a book; page-turning devices and other aids are invaluable and full use is made of radio and television. The family is encouraged to participate in the care of the patient, for example a relative may visit at meal times to feed the child and to read to him, to play simple games or to give help with his toilet.

Daily nursing care proceeds on the same lines as for any other totally dependent patient and will not be described in detail. Care of the whole body, the pressure points, the hair, the nails, the mouth, and frequent changes of bed and personal linen without disturbance to the patient are carried out as part of the nursing routine. Painful joints are handled with the utmost care, and a regular turning routine may be necessary; splintage is rarely required but careful positioning by means of pillows, with a cradle to relieve pressure of bedclothes, is essential. Constipation is avoided and fluids are given freely, preferably by means of a bent straw. Female patients should be taught to use a urinal, to avoid the exertion involved in the frequent use of bedpans.

Observations. During nursing attention, observe the general condition, note reluctance to take food or fluids, undue fretfulness, lethargy or drowsiness. Note the appearance, the colour, the condition of the skin, any swelling or incipient deformity of joints; report these findings immediately.

Stage II. If there are no cardiac changes or other contraindications, e.g. changes in the ESR or the state of the joints, the patient is allowed two pillows and is allowed to feed himself with items of diet which can be held in his hand, e.g. bread and butter, cakes and sandwiches, and to wash his face with a wash-cloth passed by his nurse; at this stage, too, he is allowed to hold a book and the physician may allow a head-mirror fixed to the bed, as shown in Fig. 9.2.

Stage III. At this stage, the patient is allowed to sit up, to feed and wash himself and to participate in lessons and suitable games in the ward, but is *not* allowed out of bed.

Stage IV. The patient is allowed to sit out in a chair for gradually increasing periods each day.

Stage V. Ambulation progresses from a few steps daily, to a walk to the lavatory and finally outside the ward, deliberately increasing activities until the patient is up and about all day until his discharge home. Supervision with or without chemotherapy is continued indefinitely and the possibility of re-infection is borne in mind.

As already stated, progression is based on the clinical and other findings already described. Any adverse sign, such as rise of temperature or of erythrocyte sedimentation rate, or of joint or cardiac involvement is a set-back which necessitates regression to a previous stage in the programme. Though these stages are laid down as guidelines to the patient's care they are subject to the needs of the individual patient so that smooth and gradual progress from one stage to another according to tolerance requires the judgement, control and consideration of the individual patient which is the essential art of the practice of medicine and nursing alike.

GOUT

Gout is characterised by:

1. A raised serum uric acid level.
2. Acute attacks of arthritis.
3. Chronic arthritis.
4. Tophaceous deposits.
5. Renal disease, often with calculi.

Not all these features are necessarily present in any one individual. Indeed, a patient with a high serum uric acid level (hyperuricaemia) may never develop any of the clinical manifestations of gout.

Gout may be either *primary* or *secondary*. *Primary* gout is an inborn error of metabolism; *secondary* gout is a condition in which the level of uric acid in the blood is raised due to an acquired disease (such as leukaemia and polycythemia) and in which articular manifestations may occur.

Causation

In the primary form of the disease heredity plays a large part and hyperuricaemia is common in relatives of patients suffering from gout. It is important to define hyperuricaemia, and surprisingly enough, this is not an easy thing to do because of the varied results produced by different laboratories. The upper level of normal for men is usually taken as 7 mg per 100 ml (0.42 m mols per litre) and for women 6.5 mg per 100 ml. It is often wise to repeat the estimation before accepting the presence of hyperuricaemia. Although a great deal is known about the metabolism of uric acid there has been much controversy as to whether hyperuricaemia is the result of an excessive production or a decreased renal excretion. It is probable that both factors are concerned, too much uric acid being produced and too little excreted (due to a renal defect in handling it).

In most cases there is evidence of renal impairment resulting in a decreased amount of urate being excreted. It is also claimed that in a significant number of these patients there is also an increased rate of purine metabolism such that there is overproduction of uric acid. The inter-relationship of these two mechanisms has still to be defined but the former has been held to be of more importance in the typical cases of primary gout.

Genetic enzyme abnormalities have also been defined and shown to be responsible for producing hyperurinaemia. Such cases (e.g. the Lesch-Nyhan syndrome) are uncommon but have given a tremendous boost to our understanding of purine metabolism.

Course and pathogenesis

Some people with hyperuricaemia never develop clinical gout. In others there are attacks of acute gout and rather less than half of these develop chronic gout and tophaceous deposits. Chronic gouty arthritis may supervene in a joint previously affected by acute gout or may involve a joint which has never previously been affected clinically.

The mechanism of the acute attack of gout is not clearly understood but is thought to be related to the crystallisation of sodium urate from the body fluids. Chronic gout is associated with the deposition of urates in cartilage, epiphyseal bone, periarticular tissues and kidneys.

Clinical features

Acute attacks of gout usually commence after the age of 30 years. The joint symptoms are acute in onset, persist for several days and then disappear to leave a normally functioning joint. The most common joint involved is the first metatarsophalangeal joint, but it must be appreciated that other joints, especially those of the lower limbs, are sometimes the site of the first attack. There is severe pain and the area involved mimics cellulitis in appearance. Usually only one joint is involved. Further attacks occur within a year or two and the interval between attacks gets shorter.

As the disease progresses, in some patients, chronic deformities occur in several joints, whether they have been involved in an acute attack or not. This chronic gout may resemble rheumatoid arthritis. The longer the disease has been present, the greater the incidence of tophi. These are deposits of urates occurring in relation to joints and in subcutaneous tissues. They are frequently seen around the ears and in the fingers and toes (Fig. 29.1). Occasionally chalky deposits are extruded through the skin.

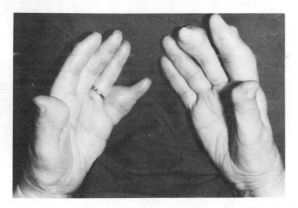

Fig. 29.1 Gout affecting the hands. Note the tophi causing swelling of the thumb and fingers.

Renal complications arise in about 15 per cent of patients. In particular, calculi are common and patients may eventually die of renal failure due to urate deposition. Hypertension is common.

The finding of urate crystals in a joint is confirma-

tory of gout even if the serum uric acid level is only slightly elevated.

X-rays reveal punched-out areas in the bone close to the articular surface.

Several factors may precipitate an acute attack of gout. These include trauma, over-indulgence (either dietary or alcoholic) and various drugs, especially the diuretics.

Treatment

During acute gout the patient should be on absolute rest in bed. Colchicine is known to relieve the acute attack and is given in a dose of 0.5 mg every two hours until the pain is relieved or until side effects appear. Unfortunately the drug commonly causes gastro-intestinal symptoms, particularly diarrhoea. An alternative drug is indomethacin which is very effective in terminating the acute attack.

After the acute attack has settled, there remains the problem of preventing further episodes. Uric acid is derived from purines and at one time it was common practice to give a low-purine diet. With the advent of uricosuric drugs (i.e. those that will increase the excretion of uric acid) and allopurinol (which inhibits the formation of uric acid) a strict dietary régimen is no longer necessary. However, it is still wise to avoid the factors known to precipitate acute attacks of gout and because of this such things as alcohol intake should be regulated and excessive fatigue, either mental or physical, should be avoided. At this stage the drugs commonly used are Benemid (0.5 g b.d. or t.d.s.), Anturan (400 mg daily) or Allopurinol (300 mg daily). Each of these drugs is capable of lowering the serum uric acid level and preventing further attacks of acute gout. Furthermore, they result in diminution in tophaceous deposits and probably protect the kidneys. They should be continued indefinitely. Benemid and Anturan increase the excretion of uric acid and paradoxically at the beginning of treatment may produce an acute attack of gout. Initially, therefore, they should be combined with one of the drugs used in the treatment of acute gout. Allopurinol inhibits the formation of uric acid and is becoming the drug of choice, especially in secondary gout or when there is evidence of renal involvement.

Occasionally surgical removal of tophi is required.

PSEUDO-GOUT

Pseudo-gout (crystal synovitis, or primary articular cartilage calcification with arthritis) is a condition in which one or more joints becomes painful, swollen and hot, rather as in gout or suppurative arthritis. X-ray examination shows the presence of calcification in the articular cartilage; and examination of the joint fluid reveals calcium pyrophosphate crystals. The serum uric acid is not elevated.

It is believed that the disease is a disorder of calcium metabolism leading to deposition of calcium pyrophosphate in the articular cartilage of joints. If such crystals are liberated into the synovial fluid, an acute crystal synovitis ensues. Hydroxyapatite crystals have also been implicated in some cases of pseudo-gout.

Treatment

This is symptomatic. Ultimately osteoarthritis supervenes in the affected joints.

NON-ARTICULAR RHEUMATIC DISEASES OF THE LOCOMOTOR SYSTEM

Supraspinatus tendonitis

The patient complains of the gradual onset of pain in the shoulder region, often following a minor injury. Physical examination, though revealing a full range of abduction in the shoulder, exhibits a painful arc between 70 degrees and 110 degrees. There may be tenderness over the insertion of the supraspinatus tendon into the greater tuberosity.

Treatment is by injection of a steroid preparation (with a local anaesthetic) into the tender area, supplemented by exercise. Calcification in the degenerate supraspinatus tendon sometimes occurs. If the calcium deposits rupture into the sub-acromial bursa, the pain becomes very severe, radiating down the arm and prohibiting shoulder movement. Morphine may be required for pain. Surgical removal of the calcific deposits may be undertaken using either irrigation through needles, or by operation if steroid injection does not work.

Bicipital tenosynovitis

The synovial membrane of the shoulder extends distally along the tendon of the long head of biceps. The tendon sheath sometimes becomes inflamed and painful, often after a strain.

Treatment is usually an injection of steroid followed by exercises.

Frozen shoulder (periarthritis of the shoulder, capsulitis)

This condition of a painful, stiff shoulder occurs after the age of 40 years, and often follows an injury to the joint; it may be preceded by supraspinatus tendonitis, bicipital tenosynovitis, and sometimes by a coronary thrombosis. All movements of the shoulder are limited in the acute stage by spasm, and in the chronic stage by fibrosis of the joint capsule.

Treatment is usually by exercises, often aided by the intra-articular or peri-articular injection of a steroid.

Polymyalgia rheumatica

This occurs in the elderly. There is severe muscle pain, often of the shoulder girdle, with little evidence of wasting. There is a very high erythrocyte sedimentation rate and subsequent loss of weight and general malaise are pointers to the diagnosis. The most dangerous aspect of this disease is the possibility of ocular involvement leading to blindness. Patients may subsequently develop a form of polyarteritis.

Treatment with corticosteroids is very effective and treatment may be withdrawn after about two to five years.

Tennis elbow

The pathological lesion is believed to be a degeneration in the origin of the extensor muscles (or in the orbicular ligament), superimposed upon which is an inflammation due to repeated movements of the wrist. It is characterised by pain on the outer side of the joint, and occurs in people whose work or recreation involves repeated movements of the forearm and wrist. The pain is referred down the back of the forearm, which is sometimes so severe as to prevent the patient lifting a shovel or using a hammer. There is tenderness over the lateral epicondyle of the elbow; and characteristically pain in the elbow is produced by resisting active dorsiflexion of the wrist.

Treatment. Most patients are relieved by one or more injections of hydrocortisone into the tender area on the lateral side of the elbow. Manipulation under anaesthesia may be advised followed by active exercises. Operative treatment is required only in a minority, and excision of the tender area or Z-lengthening of the extensor carpi radialis brevis (Garden) has been found to relieve symptoms when conservative measures have failed.

Golfer's elbow

This condition is similar to tennis elbow, but occurring as pain over the common flexor origin of the forearm muscles.

Treatment is by an injection of hydrocortisone.

Tenosynovitis of the long and short extensors of the wrist

The tendons of extensor carpi radialis longus and brevis lie together in a synovial sheath deep to the extensor retinaculum behind the wrist. In some people, unaccustomed and repeated actions of the wrist, e.g. painting or knitting, causes an inflammation of the sheath with pain and swelling on the back of the wrist.

Treatment is by a plaster, plastic or leather wrist support, or a steroid injection.

Stenosing tenosynovitis (De Quervain's disease)

This condition is due to fibrous constriction of the sheaths of the short extensor and the abductor of the thumb. There is pain centred over the radial styloid, which is exaggerated by abduction of the thumb. Palpation of the wrist may reveal a small nodule over the radial styloid process.

Treatment consists of a steroid injection or, occasionally, excision of the fibrous material.

Trigger finger

This occurs when a flexor tendon sheath becomes thickened and constricted and causes 'locking' of the finger in the fully flexed position. Often the finger cannot be extended except by main force,

when a distinct snap is heard as the extended position is reached.

Trigger thumb

A similar condition to trigger finger occurring in children, when the thumb becomes locked in flexion.

Treatment of both these conditions is by excision of the constriction in the tendon sheath.

Dupuytren's contracture

This is a progressive condition characterised by flexion deformity of the ring and little fingers and due to cord-like thickening and contracture of the palmar fascia (Fig. 29.2). It is most commonly seen in elderly men and is believed to be hereditary.

Treatment is operative and consists of excision

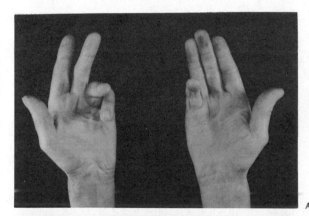

A

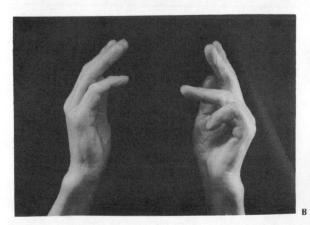

B

Fig. 29.2 A, B. A typical example of Dupuytren's contracture of the palmar aponeurosis.

of the contracted bands, sometimes followed by fixation in a plaster cast for about four weeks. Alternatively, a simple dressing and bandage is applied and physiotherapy is commenced early.

Lumbago

Severe pain unconnected with intervertebral disc protrusions may occur in the scapular and lumbar regions of the back. Sometimes such pain is due to fatty hernial projection through the deep fascia of the back, and which may be felt as exquisitely tender nodules (Copeman).

Treatment is by analgesics, heat, massage and occasionally by injection of the 'trigger' points by local anaesthetic or a steroid. If night disturbance is prominent, then small doses of anti-depressants help.

Plantar fasciitis

This is a painful condition of the heel at the site of attachment of the plantar fascia to the calcaneum. It may follow minor repetitive trauma or be associated with rheumatoid arthritis, ankylosing spondylitis, gout or Reiter's disease.

Treatment is by a sorbo-rubber pad fitted into the scooped out heel of the shoe, or by the injection of a steroid.

Bursitis

A non-suppurative painful inflammation of bursae is common and may follow a minor injury or occur spontaneously. Bursae frequently involved are: the olecranon bursa; ischial bursa (weaver's bottom); subcutaneous pre-patellar bursa (beat knee or house-maid's knee); subcutaneous infra-patellar bursa (parson's knee); semimembranous bursa; the Achilles bursa; and the bunion associated with hallux valgus.

Treatment is usually by rest of the part and sometimes by a steroid injection. Antibiotics are prescribed if the bursa becomes infected. Excision is sometimes performed.

Ruptured tendons

Over the age of 40 years degenerative changes occur in certain tendons which may then rupture during a minor strain. Such tendons include: Rotator cuff of the shoulder (Ch. 20); Long head of biceps (Ch. 20); Extensor pollicis longus (Ch. 20); common extensor tendons of the fingers (Ch. 20); Quadriceps tendon (Ch. 21); Tendo Achilles (Ch. 21); Plantaris.

SYSTEMIC DISORDERS OF CONNECTIVE TISSUE

This final section deals with some rare rheumatic diseases. They are seen more commonly in general medical than in orthopaedic practice, but are included here because they are rheumatic diseases which sometimes involve joints.

Dermatomyositis

This is an uncommon disease affecting skin, muscles and blood vessels. There are juvenile and adult types, the chief difference being that in adults 50 per cent of patients have underlying neoplastic disease. Skin lesions consist of periorbital oedema with heliotrope colouring around the eyelids, characteristic lesions on the dorsum of the small joints of the hands and nail fold telangiectases. Muscular weakness is very characteristic and usually the over-riding manifestation. Calcification in various sites is not uncommon. There may be a true arthritis present but this is not a prominent feature. Corticosteroids may be life-saving but immunosuppressives are being used increasingly. Surgery may be required for calcium deposits which are large and troublesome.

Polyarteritis nodosa

There are many forms of arteritis and this is not the place to attempt a classification. Essentially there is inflammation occurring in the walls of arteries and the clinical picture varies according to which vessels are involved. The following are some of the more common features: renal disease, hypertension, skin lesions (purpura, subcutaneous nodules), ischaemia of gut or abdominal viscera, muscle pain, joint pains and neuropathy. The kidneys are involved in most cases and renal failure is often responsible for death. Pyrexia and tachycardia are common. Anaemia may be present and the ESR is usually raised.

Treatment consists of corticosteroids in sufficient dosage to keep the patient as symptom-free as possible without giving rise to gross side effects. There is some evidence to suggest that steroids reduce the incidence of renal disease if given early.

Scleroderma (systemic sclerosis) (Fig. 29.3)

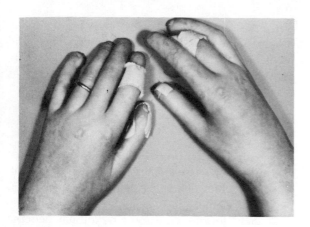

Fig. 29.3 Scleroderma affecting the hands.

The Raynaud phenomenon (Ch. 32) is the most common initial feature. When exposed to cold the hands become blue or white and as the circulation returns they are a diffuse red colour. This is associated with tingling and numbness and represents a hypersensitivity to cold. There are many causes of the Raynaud phenomenon and it may be quite a benign condition when occurring in the young. However, when its onset is in middle age, an underlying cause should always be suspected, in particular scleroderma. (When typical attacks occur in warm weather it is rather more suggestive of systemic lupus erythematosus.) This may continue for a number of years. Eventually ulceration of the fingers and calcium deposition in the subcutaneous tissues of the hands may occur. The calcium deposits are occasionally extruded through the skin. A further feature of the digital ischaemia is resorption of the terminal phalanges. Apart from this, the skin over the fingers and hands becomes tight so that it cannot be pinched up. The fingers and wrists become flexed, not due to joint disease,

but due to the fibrosis and contraction taking place in subcutaneous tissues. At a later stage the skin of the face may be involved, particularly around the mouth where it becomes tight, puckered and loses the normal movement associated with facial expression. The disease may remain confined to these sites, but not infrequently internal organs are involved, particularly the oesophagus (giving rise to dysphagia), lungs and kidneys—renal failure being one of the chief causes of death.

Treatment is unsatisfactory but it must be remembered that the disease runs a very long course, initially without much disablement in most cases. So many remedies have been advocated by different centres and have proved wanting, that there is no point in discussing them in this book. Treatment is largely symptomatic in the form of physiotherapy and avoiding exposure to cold.

Systemic lupus erythematosus

This disease is more common in women than in men and commonly occurs in the second or third decades. Although it may often carry a grave prognosis this is not always the case and there are a good many patients who have had a remission lasting for very many years.

Clinical features include the following: Fever, general malaise and weight loss. There is nearly always a rash at some stage of the disease. Typically it occurs in a 'butterfly' distribution on the face (cheeks and bridge of nose) and as erythematous patches around the finger-tips and on the palm of the hands and soles of the feet.

Arthritis may be present, usually in the form of a mild synovitis, often transient and migratory, as in rheumatic fever. Occasionally it may become chronic. Although the synovitis is mild, pain may be extreme.

Pleurisy and pericarditis may also occur.

Renal disease may resemble glomerulo-nephritis or present as a nephrotic syndrome.

Purpura is sometimes seen.

Neurological and psychiatric manifestations are sometimes present. In all cases, test for antinuclear antibodies (or other similar antibodies) will be positive at some stage except during remissions or as a result of treatment. The white cell count in the blood is lower than normal. Gamma globulin levels in the plasma are raised as is also the ESR. There may be splenomegaly and lymphadenopathy.

Of course, not all the possible clinical manifestations are always present in the one case and because of the varied nature of the presenting features the differential diagnosis can be extremely difficult. Treatment is by means of corticosteroids and sometimes, especially with renal involvement, the dose may have to be very high. If the dose cannot be maintained without serious side effects, cytotoxic drugs may be used.

BIBLIOGRAPHY

Buchanan W Watson, Dick W Carson 1976 Recent Advances in Rheumatology, Pt. 1. Edinburgh: Churchill Livingstone
Chen S C 1977 A tennis elbow support. Lancet 2: 894
Copeman W S C 1970 Textbook of the Rheumatic Diseases. Edinburgh: E & S Livingstone
Winchester I W 1960 The painful stiff shoulder. Nursing Times, 4 March, 281

SECTION | SIX

Care of the patient
with a condition
associated with
orthopaedic practice

30

Metabolic bone disease

INTRODUCTION

Bone is the tissue that provides mechanical stability to the body. Guarded by its strength are important organs such as the heart, lungs, and brain. Muscles rely upon bone to provide sufficient resistance for their action. As well as structural support, bone, especially in younger subjects, contains elements of the blood-cell forming system (marrow) and certain bones, such as the ossicles of the middle ear, have evolved highly specialised properties appropriate to their function. This chapter concerns itself, however, with bone diseases that are inherited and cause orthopaedic problems or that are acquired defects of bone cell activity.

BONE

Composition

The skeleton comprises about 10 per cent of the weight of a 70 kg adult man. Of the total skeletal weight, about 20 per cent is water, 60 per cent mineral and 20 per cent organic constituents. There are about 1.5 kg of calcium and 0.7 kg of phosphorus in the skeleton. Skeletal composition, however, is not constant throughout life. Teeth also contain calcium and phosphorus and, although the absolute quantities are not large, it serves as a reminder that teeth are often involved in disorders affecting bone and can manifest disease before it is suspected in bone.

The mineral phase of bone is in the form of hydroxyapatite. The process of mineralisation requires vitamin D, a collagen matrix on which the hydroxy-apatite crystal can be laid down, and a high local concentration of calcium and phosphate to allow formation of the crystal. Deficiency of vitamin D, defective collagen formation and inadequate concentrations of calcium and phosphorus all lead to abnormal bone and the ensuing diseases are described later.

Collagen is the main non-mineral constituent of bone comprising about 90 per cent of the organic phase. Collagen is found in skin, blood vessels and cartilage as well as bone, and several types are known to exist. Only type I collagen is found in bone. Collagen is a large protein synthesised by the osteoblast (see below) and is notable for its relatively high content of the amino acid hydroxy-proline. This is important because when collagen is broken down, hydroxyproline is released but cannot be used to make new collagen. Thus measurement of hydroxyproline (in urine) is a useful means of assessing bone degradation.

Other components of the organic phase of bone have been identified but their physiological significance is uncertain. They are important because inherited enzyme deficiencies can lead to their accumulation and cause bone deficiency.

Bone cells

Three types of cell are found in bone. The osteo-blast and osteoclast are relatively well understood but the function of the third, the osteocyte, is uncertain.

The osteoblast is responsible for making the collagen framework of bone and for the subsequent calcification. It is the source of the enzyme alkaline phosphatase in bone. Osteocytes are probably osteoblasts that have become incorporated into mineralised bone. Because these cells are often found lying in large holes (lacunae) it is thought that they cause localised breakdown of bone (osteolysis). Nevertheless they probably also contribute to the maintenance of the collagen matrix in bone.

The osteoclast has a completely different origin to the osteoblast. It is a large cell with several nuclei and produces enzymes that help break down the mineral phase of bone followed by the organic matrix. Whereas the osteoblast is derived from mesenchymal cells, the osteoclast comes from the same stem cell as the circulating white blood cells.

BONE TURNOVER

Bone is in a constant state of remodelling. The rate at which this proceeds is partially determined by hormones produced by the parathyroid glands, the thyroid (calcitonin) and the kidney (1,25-di-hydroxyvitamin D). These hormones are described in detail later. Other hormones are also important and excess or deficiency can lead to bone disease. Thus high levels of corticosteroid drugs (hydrocortisone, prednisolone) depress osteoblast function, whereas an increased rate of bone turnover is a feature of thyrotoxicosis. Oestrogens also play an important role in preventing bone loss.

Bone remodelling begins with osteoclastic resorption. Osteoblastic activity follows. Usually the two processes are coupled, so that resorption and formation take place at the same rate. Under some circumstances this process is uncoupled, leading to excess resorption or, less frequently, excess formation of bone. Turnover is more rapid in the softer cancellous bone than in the harder cortical (see below) bone, and resorption occurs at a rate of about 1 μm/day. After the age of 30 years bone density gradually falls in both sexes, although it is accelerated after the menopause because of oestrogen deficiency.

Bone growth and structure

In a young animal, bone grows both by expansion of the bone at the side (periosteal growth) and by elongation. The process of lengthening depends upon the growth plate at the end of the bone budding off cartilage cells. Cartilage cells are replaced in the body of the long bone by bone cells, resulting in gradual lengthening of the bone. The growth plate is easily damaged by trauma and its activity is affected by many drugs and hormones. Growth ceases and the growth plate fuses with the main body of the bone at various ages depending on the bone in question, though the majority fuse around the time of puberty, the process being hastened by the increase in the circulating levels of sex hormones at this time. The fusion of bones can be detected by X-rays and because growth plates fuse at specific ages the radiologist can often assess a patient's age accurately. This may be important in medico–legal work in a child whose chronological age is very different to the biological age. Disorders of the growth plate occur in many metabolic conditions and are discussed later.

Viewed with the naked eye two types of bone are visible in the post-pubertal subject: one form, cortical bone, is heavily calcified, and occurs largely in the limb bones. It is, for instance, the predominant bone of the shaft of the femur or tibia. Softer bone, cancellous or trabecular bone, is found in the vertebral bodies and the neck of the femur, although both structures have an outer casing of cortical bone. Because cancellous bone has a much higher remodelling rate than cortical bone, diseases that cause changes in this rate affect cancellous bone before cortical bone. The two types of bone have different mechanical properties. Although cancellous bone is softer, it may be able to bend further before breaking. Indeed, one study has suggested that fracture in osteoporosis is the result of losing bone matrix in excess of mineral, a process that renders the bone more brittle.

Mechanical factors and bone density

It is a common observation that disease or immobilisation will lead to loss of bone density and that destruction of the nerve to a limb will cause local bone loss. Coupled with observations that astronauts in space (where there is no gravity) lose bone rapidly, it is evident that, when there are no forces acting on bone, bone is broken down.

Hormonal factors and bone

In Fig. 30.1 are depicted the classic actions of the major calcium regulating hormones. Parathyroid hormone is a peptide that is responsible for stimulating both the osteoblast and osteoclast. In clinical situations bone resorption predominates and calcium is mobilised from the skeleton. Parathyroid hormone stimulates the formation of the active form of vitamin D, 1,25-dihydroxycholecalciferol $(1,25(OH)_2D)$, and it is through the action of $1,25(OH)_2D$ that intestinal absorption of calcium is increased. Parathyroid hormone also promotes phosphate excretion in the urine and this action has been the basis for several tests of parathyroid activity. Secretion of parathyroid hormone is stimu-

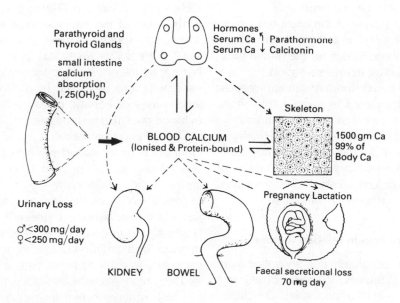

Fig. 30.1 Calcium metabolism.

lated by low serum calcium levels, and inhibited by high levels.

The second important calcium regulating hormone is 1,25-dihydroxycholecalciferol(1,25(OH)$_2$D). This hormone is synthesised from vitamin D by reactions in the liver and then in the kidney. The synthesis of 1,25(OH)$_2$D by the kidney is increased by high levels of parathyroid hormone and by low levels of serum calcium and phosphorus. Loss of kidney tissue, as in chronic renal failure, can cause serious bone disease because this hormone cannot be made.

Vitamin D is obtained either by the action of sunlight in the ultra-violet (UV) range on skin or from food. Very small amounts of ultra-violet light can cure vitamin D deficiency diseases, but for many people the diet is the most important source. Asians appear to be especially at risk of vitamin D deficiency although their response to UV light is equivalent to that of Caucasian (white) subjects. Dietary vitamin D is largely found in the fatty fish (halibut, mackerel) or in eggs. However, vitamin D is added widely to foodstuffs (e.g. margarine, breakfast cereals and beverages (e.g. Ovaltine)). Vitamin D is also a constituent of many health tablets and thus vegetarian diets prepared from raw vegetables and unsupplemented by vitamin tablets are the only diets likely to be deficient in vitamin D. Some Asian diets are also low in vitamin D, supplements of which may be required.

1,25(OH)$_2$D is a powerful stimulant of calcium absorption from the intestine and of calcium release from bone. It is also necessary for the proper functioning of the osteoblast in mineralisation.

Calcitonin is the third important calcium-regulating hormone. It is secreted by special cells in the thyroid gland, and is one of the oldest hormones known in the evolutionary process. Originally, it may not have been a calcium-regulating hormone, but has only acquired this action. Calcitonin tends to lower serum calcium levels and is stimulated by increasing calcium levels in the blood.

Calcium and phosphorus in relation to bone

Sufficient quantities of calcium and phosphorus are needed for bone synthesis. Whereas insufficient calcium may give rise to osteoporosis, deficiency of phosphorus can lead to osteomalacia.

The calcium intake of most western diets is low (about 300–400 mg/day) and only 30–50 per cent of this is absorbed. Phosphorus intake is usually adequate, and deficiency is more likely to occur because of excessive excretion by the kidney. Under these circumstances the kidney cannot reabsorb phosphorus ('renal phosphate leak') and this defect can either be inherited or acquired.

INVESTIGATIONS COMMONLY UNDERTAKEN FOR METABOLIC BONE DISEASE

It is impractical to describe all the procedures that may be undertaken in the course of investigating a metabolic bone problem. Nevertheless, there are some procedures commonly done, the value of which are readily understood.

Measurement of calcium and phosphorus and of the enzyme alkaline phosphatase in blood is best done on a fasting sample obtained without using a tourniquet. Calcium levels may rise if blood flow is impeded and phosphorus levels (and to a lesser extent calcium) are increased after a meal.

Low levels of calcium in blood may accompany deficiency of vitamin D or parathyroid hormone. Blood phosphorus levels are characteristically low in hyperparathyroidism, osteomalacia and rickets, and high in deficiency of parathyroid hormone. Deficiency of vitamin D also causes an increase in the level of the enzyme alkaline phosphatase. This is not a specific feature of vitamin D deficiency since the enzyme level may also increase after a bone fracture or in Paget's disease of bone. The enzyme is also produced by the liver and rises in some cases of hepatic disease. Vitamin D levels in blood may also be measured.

Urinary excretion of calcium and vitamin D deficiency may be increased in some cases of osteoporosis. When bone collagen is broken down the amino acid hydroxyproline is liberated and excreted in urine: its measurement provides a further estimate of bone turnover. Because collagen is also found in connective tissue it is widespread in meat and gelatin-containing foods. It is thus necessary to exclude meat, fish, jelly, cheesecake and ice-cream from the diet of a patient undergoing this test; otherwise hydroxyproline from ingested food may cause a falsely high result.

Other investigations often of value are microscopic evaluation of a bone biopsy which is usually taken from the iliac crest, and isotope bone scanning. The bone biopsy may reveal evidence of vitamin D deficiency, and the bone scan identify areas of increased bone activity.

DISEASES OF BONE

Vitamin D deficiency, rickets and osteomalacia

Vitamin D deficiency is manifested differently in children and adults, because the former are still growing and are laying down bone at the ends of the long bones. Since the growing ends of bones are the most active part of a skeleton, deficiency shows up there first. Vitamin D assists the calcification of newly formed bone matrix, and in the absence of vitamin D large seams of uncalcified bone matrix are found together with long shafts of noncalcified cartilage at the growing ends of bone in children. In adults the changes are termed osteomalacia and in children rickets.

Rickets is now very rarely caused by simple lack of intake of vitamin D or absence of exposure to sunlight. More commonly it is seen because intestinal absorption is too low (as in coeliac disease), because chronic renal failure has led to impairment of synthesis of the active form of vitamin D, or because of an inherited deficiency of an enzyme necessary to form $1,25(OH)_2D$. Rickets may also arise because of a deficiency of phosphorus but there are several important differences between this form and vitamin D deficiency rickets.

Rickets is characterised by failure to grow, painful joints and bones, muscle weakness and deformity of joints. Failure of the normal resorption of cartilage at the growing ends of bone leads to swelling and in the ribs causes a characteristic 'rickety rosary' along the costochondral junctions. Biochemical investigations show a low level of calcium and phosphorus in the blood, together with a high level of alkaline phosphatase. The low level of calcium (hypocalcaemia) may occasionally cause symptoms of tingling and tetany. Urinary calcium excretion is characteristically low. X-rays are diagnostic.

Diagnosis of the underlying cause is important, since recognition will indicate appropriate therapy.

In malabsorption, treatment of the underlying condition and supplementary vitamin D are necessary, whereas in chronic renal failure, calcitriol (1,25-dihydroxyvitamin D) is needed. This drug is, however, liable to cause high blood calcium levels and careful monitoring is necessary.

Rickets caused by a deficiency of phosphorus is known as 'hypophosphataemic rickets' or 'vitamin D resistant rickets'. The condition is usually inherited. Excessive phosphorus loss in the urine is the cause. Symptoms are similar to those for simple rickets, except that muscle weakness is not found. Some cases of rickets caused by a renal phosphate leak also show a generalised renal tubular defect and glucose and amino acids are found in the urine (Fanconi syndrome). Characteristically, blood calcium levels are normal, phosphorus very low, and alkaline phosphatase high. Urinary calcium is normal. In order to maintain normal growth extra phosphorus is needed and calcitriol is usually required. In spite of treatment, growth is often retarded, and in later life the spine may become stiff and cause backache.

Osteomalacia is the term given to the features of vitamin D deficiency after fusion of the growth plates. As well as the causes listed for rickets other conditions are relevant in adults (Table 30.1). The

Table 30.1 Causes of rickets (A) and osteomalacia (A + B)

A. Malabsorption
   Anticonvulsant drug (Phenytoin, Phenobarbitone)
   Chronic renal failure
   Lack of vitamin D in diet or little sunshine exposure
   Hypophosphataemia

B. Partial gastrectomy
   Late onset hypophosphataemia
   Tumours
   Obstruction to bile flow to intestine

elderly are a special risk group and 'aches and pains' in elderly subjects should always bring osteomalacia to mind. Elderly subjects may eat insufficient food to maintain vitamin D levels, or become deficient because they do not go outside sufficiently to allow vitamin D synthesis in skin. Osteomalacia is also frequently associated with intestinal malabsorption syndromes, the commonest being coeliac disease. Osteomalacia in any age group should be an indication for simple tests of intestinal absorption (e.g. xylose absorption; 3-

day faecal fat excretion). Some cases of liver disease are complicated by osteomalacia, because failure of bile salts to reach the gut (obstructive jaundice) leads to malabsorption of fat and fat-soluble vitamins (including vitamin D).

The Asian population also have a higher risk of osteomalacia. This may be related to their lower dietary intake of vitamin D. Moreover, absorption of calcium from the gut is reduced by consumption of chapattis which bind calcium and prevent absorption. The pigmented skin does not impair vitamin D synthesis by sunlight, and very low exposures to artificial UV light can cure osteomalacia in Asian subjects.

Other symptoms are vague but associated muscle weakness and some fractures of the femoral neck are complications of the process. Although serum calcium and phosphorus may be low, elevation of serum alkaline phosphatase is a more reliable test. Although bone X-ray changes can be diagnostic (Fig. 30.2) they may not be present and bone biopsy is usually necessary to confirm the diagnosis.

Treatment is directed towards management of

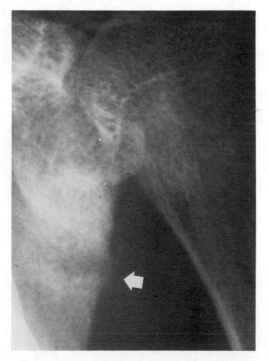

Fig. 30.2 A Looser's zone shown in X-ray of the lateral border of the scapula of a subject with anticonvulsant osteomalacia.

any underlying disorder. Simple osteomalacia will respond to 1000 iu vitamin D daily and calcium supplements are usually given to ensure adequate supplies for the mineralising bone.

A separate form of hypophosphataemic osteomalacia can affect adults. Sometimes osteomalacia may be associated with rare types of tumour or may precede the clinical appearance of the tumour by many years. Muscle and bone pain and muscle weakness are the predominant symptoms, and low levels of phosphorus in the blood the cardinal biochemical finding. Removal of the tumour can cure the osteomalacia, or, if there is no associated tumour, phosphorus supplements (Phosphate-Sandoz) are given.

INBORN ERRORS OF METABOLISM

Many of these are genetic defects causing deficiency of an enzyme; they may arise spontaneously or be inherited. Some give rise to a picture similar to that of rickets and are caused by excessive excretion of phosphorus in the urine. Unlike hypophosphataemic rickets, the excessive phosphorus excretion is part of a generalised 'leak' of inorganic molecules, glucose and amino acids by the kidney.

These disorders are found in patients attending orthopaedic hospitals because of the associated limb deformities. One such disease is Morquio's syndrome caused by an excessive deposition of a component of bone matrix. Similarly, bone structure may be weakened and lead to fractures as in homocystinuria.

Osteoporosis

Osteoporosis is one of the most common bone diseases and the process is responsible for most of the cases of fracture of the femoral neck or of compression fracture of the vertebrae.

Osteoporosis is probably not a homogeneous condition. Furthermore, it may be part of the ageing process since bone density declines after the age of 30 years in both sexes. Definition of osteoporosis is difficult; essentially it is a reduction in bone mass. Under the microscope the bone that is present is normal but is reduced in amount. The appearance on X-rays is more definitive, but the appearances are not specific to any particular pathological condition.

The usual laboratory investigations of calcium metabolism are not particularly helpful in osteoporosis. It is, however, essential to consider all the predisposing courses (see Table 30.2) and to be aware of other conditions (see Table 30.3) in which bone density may be reduced.

Table 30.2 Disorders associated with osteoporosis

Post menopause
Thyrotoxicosis
Cushing's disease (and corticosteroid therapy)
Malabsorption
Acromegaly
Diabetes mellitus

Table 30.3 Conditions in which osteoporosis is a feature

Homocystinuria
Osteogenesis imperfecta
Turner's syndrome
Myeloma
Leukaemia

Clinically, osteoporosis usually affects the spine or upper part of the femur. Typically, spinal compression fractures occur suddenly, often with little trauma, and cause acute pain which improves over 6–8 weeks. Height is lost following a compression fracture (see Fig. 30.3). The most frequent site of such a fracture is in the thoracic vertebrae, giving rise to the 'dowager's hump'. Fracture of the neck of the femur, another 'osteoporotic' fracture, also frequently occurs with minimal trauma. Spinal fractures often occur in a cluster, with the disease subsequently becoming quiescent.

Immobilisation is a particularly important cause of bone loss, because it is rarely remembered in practice. Acute experiments in volunteers have documented substantial bone loss in the course of a few weeks and on subsequent remobilisation the original bone density is not regained. Bed rest may therefore add to the problem of bone loss in osteoporotic subjects. In patients who are immobilised by disease, as in spinal injury, calcium loss from bone may be so great as to form stones in the kidney when it is excreted. Bone fracture in such patients may occur with minimal trauma.

The commonest cause of bone loss, and of clinical osteoporosis, is oestrogen deficiency after the menopause. Bone may be rapidly removed in the

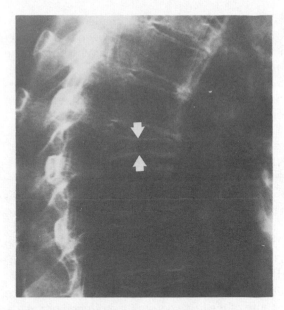

Fig. 30.3 Compression fracture (arrowed) of a vertebral body shown in an X-ray of the thoracic spine of a post-menopausal subject. The adjoining vertebrae are unaffected, but another, three vertebrae higher than the one arrowed, is beginning to collapse. Note that the spine is beginning to bend, a process which contributes to the loss of body height.

5–10 years after the menopause and this has led to patients continuing to take oestrogen therapy (in the form of the contraceptive pill) after the menopause. This is not without risk, since continuous use of oestrogen predisposes to uterine cancer.

Treatment of osteoporosis is difficult, largely because it is extremely difficult to increase bone density after the third decade of life. A list of treatments is given in Table 30.4. Calcium supplements are given to prevent any deficiency of calcium since calcium is not well absorbed in elderly subjects. Oestrogens have been discussed above, while anabolic steroids and calcitonin still await confirmation of their value. Sodium fluoride, a drug that stimulates osteoblastic activity, has been shown to be effective in preventing episodes of vertebral collapse.

Table 30.4 Treatment of osteoporosis

Calcium supplements
Vitamin D
Oestrogen
Anabolic steroids
Calcitonin
Sodium fluoride

Osteoporosis is the greatest challenge in metabolic bone disease today. Safe oestrogen therapy after the menopause, understanding how to maximise bone mass by the third decade of life and a clearer cognisance of the relationship between bone composition and bone strength will be major contributions to the management of this disease.

INHERITED DISORDERS OF BONE MATRIX

The foregoing sections describe how deficiencies of hormones or inorganic elements can affect bone. In addition there are disorders, present from birth, in which a metabolic pathway is blocked. Some of these abnormalities have been well worked out, others are ill understood. As a group they are rare, but form an important part of orthopaedic practice because of the bone deformity produced or the fragile bones that result. Although a wide variety of inherited disorders can give rise to orthopaedic problems only in relatively few is this aspect the most prominent part of the disease.

Homocystinuria is caused by deficiency of an enzyme concerned in the metabolism of the amino acid homocystine. It is readily diagnosed biochemically by finding this amino acid in urine. Clinical manifestations include mental deficiency, a tendency to thrombosis and dislocation of the lens. Although some bones can be large, vertebrae can appear flattened and osteoporotic on radiological examination. The tendency to thrombosis is the most important aspect of the disease, and is especially frequent after surgery. Since surgery may be undertaken to correct an orthopaedic condition in homocystinuria, prophylaxis against thrombosis is important. Some cases of homocystinuria are improved by vitamin B6 therapy.

Morquio's disease is the most frequent of a group of diseases known as the mucopolysaccharidoses to be seen in an orthopaedic clinic. Other types are more common, but in these the associated mental deficiency dominates the clinical picture. Patients with Morquio's disease have normal intelligence. The underlying defect causes accumulation of one of the components of bone matrix. The diagnosis is made by examining the urine for this component. The clinical picture (Fig. 30.4) is dominated by short stature, genu valgum and barrel

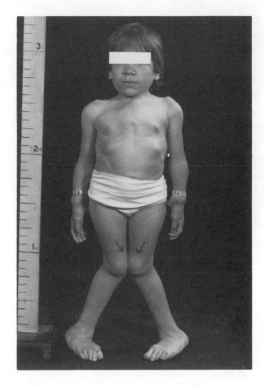

Fig. 30.4 Morquio's disease. Note the genu valgum and barrel chest.

chest. Surgery may be required to correct limb deformity. The most dangerous aspect of Morquio's disease is instability of the upper cervical spine. Thus the spinal cord is at risk of compression, especially during surgery, and cervical fusion may be considered.

Osteogenesis imperfecta is another rare bone disease caused by defective synthesis of collagen, and is important because recognition may necessitate genetic counselling. The disease constitutes a spectrum from severe fractures at birth, through a condition resembling osteoporosis in young people, to a redisposition to fractures in post-menopausal women. Only the most common features are considered here.

The brittle bones in osteogenesis imperfecta can easily be fractured and recurrent fractures in a child or multiple fractures in a child not suspected of having suffered 'battering' could arouse suspicion. Additional features include blue sclerae, deafness and early dental caries. A significant number of patients with scoliosis have osteogenesis imperfecta. Chest infections often compound the problems.

Laboratory investigations are not helpful, although in some centres it is possible to delineate the defect in collagen synthesis in a skin biopsy.

Treatment is difficult, and is confined to orthopaedic procedures to repair fractures and rehabilitation. There is no medical treatment for the primary disease, but chest infection can be treated and dental care advised.

PAGET'S DISEASE OF BONE

This is characterised by deformity of the bone consequent upon an abnormally high rate of bone turnover. The disease may be widespread or confined to a single bone. The bone is very cellular with many active osteoblasts and osteoclasts. The rapidity of the process does not allow normal bone to be formed, thus causing structural weakness of the bone, and affected bones tend to enlarge, a situation that is associated with many of the clinical problems encountered.

The incidence of Paget's disease rises with age, it being rare below the age of 40 years. It is slightly more often found in males and there is a pro-

nounced variation in the geographical distribution. In England the disease tends to be distributed in clusters with the North West having a relatively high incidence. Worldwide, it is rare in Japan and the author has never encountered a case in a negro. There appears to be familial clustering, although no definite genetic mode of transmittance is known. A viral aetiology has been proposed, but there is little evidence for this hypothesis.

In the past the most common presentation of the disease was pain. Nowadays it is frequently discovered incidentally because a high level of alkaline phosphatase is found in the blood when tests are requested for symptoms unconnected with Paget's Disease. Nevertheless pain is the symptom with which patients most frequently present. The pain may be in a bone or associated with a joint. In the latter case, swelling and deformity of the bone is the most important element. Deformity can also be severe (Fig. 30.5) and cause limb shortening. It is remarkable, however, how minimal may be the pain in the presence of severe deformity and radiological change. The complications for which help is most frequent are pain, either in bone or joint, limb deformity, nerve compression (usually caused by enlargement of a vertebra or

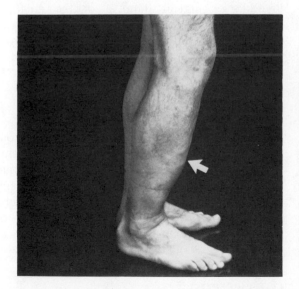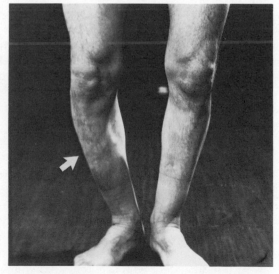

Fig. 30.5 Paget's disease of bone. Note the curved deformed leg (patient's right leg). Such bones are often warm because blood flow is increased. Extensive involvement of bone with Paget's disease may require such a large flow of blood that heart failure ensues.

of the temporal bone round the auditory nerve) and fracture. Rare complications are neoplastic change and heart failure.

Clinical examination of bones in the limbs reveals that the affected bones are warm and deformed. The bone is often enlarged. Pain and limitation of movement are found on examining a joint where one of the bones has Paget's disease. If nerve compression occurs the signs depend on the site of the pressure.

The alkaline phosphatase level in blood and hydroxyproline output in urine are both elevated. Scanning with ^{99}Tc methylene diphosphonate demonstrates areas of increased isotope uptake where the bone is affected by Paget's disease, and shows increased blood flow in the bone. The X-ray appearances are diagnostic.

Treatment of Paget's disease depends on the symptoms. Pain is initially treated with analgesics such as aspirin. Otherwise there are three main drugs used. Calcitonin (100 MRC units subcutaneously daily) relieves pain, reduces bone blood flow and lowers alkaline phosphatase and urinary hydroxyproline. Resistance to the action of calcitonin may develop and usually courses are restricted to 9–12 months. Diphosphonates are drugs that suppress bone resorption and have a similar clinical effect as calcitonin. The only available drug in this category is EHDP (Didronel) and this may also inhibit the calcification process in bone. A course of treatment is therefore restricted to 6–9 months. Calcitonin and EHDP may be used in combination. A particularly useful drug where rapid pain relief is required is mithramycin. This has to be given by daily intravenous injection (10 mcg/kg for 10 days) but can be toxic and daily liver function tests must be done.

Although these forms of treatment are useful for pain and may reduce blood flow in affected bone, their value in reducing bone size, preventing fractures, lowering the incidence of neoplastic change or improving the structural properties of bone are uncertain. Although some cases of improvement of symptoms of nerve compression after calcitonin administration are known, surgical relief is often required. Pre-treatment with calcitonin may diminish the considerable bleeding caused by surgery to the vascular bone affected by Paget's disease but it is difficult to render such bone sufficiently structurally sound to secure a prosthesis (e.g. artificial hip joint).

HYPERPARATHYROIDISM

Hyperparathyroidism is caused either by primary overactivity of one or more parathyroid glands or by chronic stimulation of the parathyroid glands by a low serum calcium level (secondary hyperparathyroidism). Such a condition arises out of chronic osteomalacia or chronic renal failure. In the latter the parathyroid glands may become autonomous and continue to secrete parathyroid hormone even though the serum calcium is rendered normal (tertiary hyperparathyroidism).

The bone lesion of primary hyperparathyroidism is most frequently recognised either because of recurrent renal stones or because a high blood calcium level is found incidentally. Serious hyperparathyroidism is now usually encountered as a complication of chronic renal failure. Bones may become painful and X-rays show dense bone (sclerosis) and erosions of the phalanges. In chronic renal failure many of the features are linked to a deficiency of the active form of vitamin D, 1,25-dihydroxyvitamin D (calcitriol), which is made in the kidney. In this case use of calcitriol may reverse the changes. Otherwise, as in primary hyperparathyroidism, surgical removal of the enlarged gland(s) is necessary. Post-operatively, serum calcium levels may fall rapidly leading to tetany. Infusion of calcium and oral calcitriol is indicated in these circumstances.

HYPOPARATHYROIDISM

This disorder, caused by deficiency of parathyroid hormone or resistance to its action, usually presents in general medical, neurological or ophthalmic clinics. The low serum calcium level causes tetany and convulsions, psychoneuroses and cataracts. Bone turnover rate is reduced in the absence of parathyroid hormone and the incidence of clinical osteoporosis is thought to be lower.

OSTEOPETROSIS

Bone may be unusually fragile if there is excess mineral present as well as too little. Excess of mineralised bone is termed osteopetrosis. Two main types exist, the infantile and the adult.

The infantile form is rarely seen in orthopaedic practice today. This is because the defect appears to be related to the osteoclasts, a cell derived from the bone marrow, and the most successful therapy is bone marrow transplantation in special centres. Clinical features of this form include enlargement of the liver and spleen, delayed growth, small head, mental retardation and entrapment of the optic and facial nerves because of overgrowth of bone around these nerves. If bone marrow transplantation is unsuccessful, calcitriol may be of value. Even with treatment the prognosis remains poor.

The adult form is inherited in a dominant fashion and is therefore relatively common. The clinical picture is very variable and suspicion is aroused by recurrent fractures and a positive family history. There is no specific therapy.

ECTOPIC CALCIFICATION

Occasionally bone may form in soft tissues. Commoner causes are shown in Table 30.5. Myositis

Table 30.5 Causes of ectopic bone formation

Myositis ossificans
Tumoral calcinosis
Trauma
Paraplegia
Dermatomyositis
Scleroderma

ossificans often occurs on the inner aspects of the thighs and horse riding has been suggested as a predisposing factor. Calcification in dermatomyositis follows the inflammatory response in the skin and muscles and a similar process is responsible in scleroderma. The calcification in paraplegia may be related to high local levels of calcium and phosphate from resorbing bone.

Treatment is difficult. Calcification associated with dermatomyositis may improve round puberty.

TALL STATURE

This is usually a problem in girls and referral may be made to an orthopaedic clinic for surgical treat-

ment. Detailed endocrine investigations are required to exclude chromosomal disorders in males, pituitary disorders, thyroid overactivity, hypogonadism and constitutional conditions such as Marfan's syndrome and cerebral gigantism. It is usually possible to predict final adult height from data about current bone age and parental height in non-endocrine cases. If final adult height in a female will exceed six feet, treatment is indicated. Oestrogen in high dose, with a progestogen to initiate menstrual bleeding, is used. The rapid feminisation is alarming to many patients and the side-effects (e.g. thrombosis, jaundice) sufficiently unpleasant to cause many physicians not to use them. Moreover, treatments are now being reported which promise to be more reliable and less hazardous.

NURSING CARE IN METABOLIC BONE DISEASE

Many of the investigations described for the diagnosis and treatment of metabolic bone disease are undertaken and samples collected by the nursing staff. Attention to detail is extremely important because specimens lost may lead to incorrect interpretation of a test. Accurate measurement of height and weight is also of great importance.

Many patients with metabolic bone disease are in pain and are not keen to move. Attention to pressure points is important under these circumstances. Such procedures as emptying the bladder or opening the bowels may be uncomfortable and prevention of constipation may help the patient.

BIBLIOGRAPHY

Gordon G S 1976 Clinical management of the Osteoporoses. Aylesbury, Bucks: HM & M Publishers
Jaffe H L 1972 Metabolic Degenerative and inflammatory diseases of bones and joints. Philadelphia: Lea and Febiger
Nordin B E C 1973 Metabolic Bone Disease. Edinburgh: Churchill Livingstone
Rasmussen H, Bordier P 1974 The physiological and cellular basis of metabolic bone disease. Baltimore: Williams and Wilkins

31

Tumours of bone

The classification and terminology relating to bone tumours is very complicated, so that no attempt will be made to describe all aspects of these conditions; rather, we will confine ourselves to a brief, simplified discussion of some of those which are seen in orthopaedic practice; fortunately, primary bone tumours are extremely rare.

A tumour usually occurs as a lump or swelling; sometimes this lump or swelling is easily seen, but it might be situated deep in the body and grow to a large size before it is noticed; in bone, it may be obvious only on X-ray examination. A tumour is often referred to as a *new growth* or *neoplasm*; we are all familiar with the word *cancer*, which is used as a general term meaning a new growth of a serious nature in any part of the body.

Classification

Tumours are broadly classified as follows:

1. *Simple or benign* tumours are those which remain encapsulated and localised and do not spread to other parts of the body.

2. *Malignant tumours*, on the other hand, not only invade the host tissues but spread to other parts via the bloodstream and lymphatic system, to lay down subsidiary lesions which are called 'secondaries' or 'metastases' so that even if the original growth is removed, e.g. by amputation of a limb, secondary deposits may already be disseminated to vital structures such as the lungs or brain and results in death.

There is also the possibility that a tumour which

Table 31.1 Benign and malignant tumours

Tumour	Cell of origin	Host tissue	Classification
Osteoma	Osteoblast	Bone	Benign
Osteoid osteoma	Osteoblast	Bone	Benign
Osteosarcoma	Osteoblast	Bone	Malignant
Osteoclastoma	Osteoclast	Bone	Benign or malignant
Chondroma	Chrondroblast	Cartilage	Benign
Chondrosarcoma	Chondroblast	Cartilage	Malignant
Fibroma	Fibroblast	Fibrous tissue	Benign
Fibrosarcoma	Fibroblast	Fibrous tissue	Malignant
Ewing tumour	Unknown	Marrow	Malignant
Reticulum cell sarcoma	Reticulum cell	Marrow	Malignant
Multiple myeloma	Plasma cell	Marrow	Malignant

is believed to be benign may in time become malignant; moreover tumours in bone may be secondary to primary disease in another part of the body.

Classification by cells or origin

Tumours are named according to the cells of the tissues from which they originate, although the exact cellular origin may be difficult to establish, as also is variation in malignancy or in potential malignancy. Some examples of benign and malignant tumours and of their cells of origin in bone are listed below:

Cause

The cause of tumours is not clearly understood, but various factors are associated with their formation, including heredity, injury, exposure to sunlight, infection, metabolic and hormonal disturbances, irradiation and assimilation of irritant substances, e.g. cigarette-tobacco smoke, oil and tar.

The formation of a tumour is due to the failure of the cells of origin to behave in a normal manner and to follow recognisable patterns; in malignant disease, it is as if certain cells had taken the law unto themselves, to become the enemies of their host, whose tissues they invade, infiltrate and eventually destroy.

Clinical features

These vary with the site of the tumour. There may be obvious swelling, local tenderness, or deformity, with limitation of joint movement, pain in the part, or evidence of pressure on neighbouring structures, e.g. nerves. Sometimes a tumour is found during treatment of an injury, or it may be the cause of a pathological fracture, as in Paget's disease (Ch. 30), a condition which, together with some other is known to be predisposing to malignant disease. Pathological fractures are dealt with by internal fixation of the fracture, particularly in the aged. If secondary deposits are already present there may be generalised signs and symptoms, for example, metastases in the lungs may give rise to symptoms of respiratory distress.

X-ray examination may reveal the presence of a local abnormal mass or cavity, or there may be evidence of secondary deposits, e.g. in the lungs. Serial X-rays, which show the rate of growth and behaviour of the neoplasm and of the surrounding tissues are used to determine the prognosis and subsequent treatment.

Other important investigations include biopsy, sternal marrow puncture, and examination of the blood and the urine.

Microscopical examination of suspected tissues may reveal the presence of abnormal cells; the degree of deviation from normal may also indicate the degree of malignancy and influence the prognosis.

OUTLINE OF TREATMENT

Treatment is related to the type of tumour, the prognosis, the age and general condition of the individual patient, and to the site of the lesion.

1. *Radiotherapy* by means of external radiation, e.g. by radioactive cobalt beam or by the linear

accelerator, is used to halt the progress of the disease and to relieve pain, particularly in inoperable cases, for example, in lesions of the spine. Neoplasms of the spine may result in paraplegia.

2. *Hormonal therapy* is also used as a means of halting the progress of the disease and relieving the symptoms. *Chemotherapy*. This represents the most significant modern development in the treatment of malignant primary bone tumours. Drugs used include methotrexate with vinocristine or methotrexate alternated with doxorubicin. Since these drugs are potentially lethal they are used only under the careful supervision of a specialist oncologist working in collaboration with the orthopaedic surgeon; admission to a specially designated centre is required, usually at intervals of a few weeks for at least a year.

It has been reported that use of these drugs has improved the survival rate amongst patients and that they may represent the eve of a breakthrough in the management of a hitherto almost untreatable condition (Corkery, 1978).

3. *Other forms of treatment* include measures to improve the general condition, e.g. treatment of anaemia or of respiratory disease.

4. *Orthopaedic treatment*. Amputation or disarticulation of a limb has already been mentioned; management is discussed in Chapter 32. Other measures include internal fixation of pathological fractures, and physiotherapy to improve muscle tone and the range of movement of joints. Splintage such as a caliper or back-support is sometimes ordered.

Some notes on nursing care will be found at the end of this chapter.

BENIGN TUMOURS

In general these do not endanger life and may require no treatment unless they grow to such a size as to be a disfigurement, or to press upon vital structures, or to interfere with the function of a limb. On the other hand, the possibility of malignant change in a tumour believed to be benign necessitates periodic examination. Treatment then depends upon the site of the tumour, and excision of the part may be advised. Some individual benign tumours are listed below:

Osteoma is a slowly growing tumour of the face or skull which usually presents as a lump. Solitary exostoses occur in limb bones. Multiple hereditary exostoses occur in association with diaphyseal aclasia. *Treatment* consists of surgical removal.

Osteoid osteoma may occur at any site in the skeleton and pain is usually the presenting feature. *Treatment* consists of surgical removal.

Chondromata arise most frequently as cartilaginous tumours of the bones of the hand (enchondroma), or as a protuberance towards the end of the long bones (enchondroma) and are often associated with diaphyseal aclasia. *Treatment* is by surgical removal.

Benign osteoclastoma (giant-cell tumours) occurs in the epiphyseal region, commonly around the knee joint; there is pain, and expansion of the overlying bone giving a 'soap-bubble' appearance on an X-ray film. *Treatment* is by curettage and bone-graft and sometimes by block excision.

MALIGNANT TUMOURS

Some of these are listed below; they are treated by wide excision of the part or by amputation or disarticulation of a limb; tumours in bone may in fact be metastases from a primary lesion elsewhere, for example, carcinoma, which arises from epithelial tissue, may be seen in bone as secondary deposits from lesions in the breast, prostate gland, kidney or lung.

Osteosarcoma (osteogenic sarcoma) occurs in the long bones of young people, especially in the femur or tibia of males aged from 5 to 20 years. The onset is often sudden, with pain in a long bone, sometimes associated with trauma of a trivial nature. *Treatment*. Lesions of the tibia are treated by amputation at mid-thigh level; femoral lesions are treated by disarticulation of the hip or by hindquarter amputation. *Radiotherapy* may halt the disease process, but metatastic spread to the lungs and other vital organs is common, and the disease is often rapidly fatal, though recent advance in high-energy radiation treatment applied to the primary lesion in the limb may enable the surgeon to postpone amputation for a period of 6 months; if at this point in time secondary deposits have not occurred at other sites (notably the lung) amputation may be advised. This regime may be adopted on humanitarian grounds to postpone a mutilating amputation in a young subject whose life expectancy might well be only a few months.

Chondrosarcoma is the cartilaginous counterpart of the osteosarcoma and occurs in young subjects. *Treatment* is similar to that of osteosarcoma.

Fibrosarcoma causes symptoms similar to those of osteosarcoma. *Treatment* is by wide resection of the part or by amputation. Radiotherapy is not used.

Malignant osteoclastoma (malignant giant-cell tumour) is the malignant counter-part of the benign giant-cell tumour. Diagnosis is established by biopsy. *Treatment* is by amputation.

Ewing's tumour is notable because it is characterised by a periosteal reaction similar to that seen in osteomyelitis, so that 'onion-layers' of new bones are laid down around the affected area; this is usually the femur or tibia, and as in sarcoma, it is a disease of young people. *Treatment* is by amputation and radiotherapy.

Reticulum-cell sarcoma occurs in long bones, causing pain and sometimes, pathological fracture. *Treatment* is usually by high-energy radiation.

MULTIPLE MYELOMATOSIS

This is a malignant disease arising from abnormal plasma cells, and originating in the marrow cavities of cancellous bones, such as the spine, sternum, ribs, pelvis and skull. It is a disease of the middle-aged and elderly; there is generalised osteoporosis of the skeleton, and punched-out cavities may be present in individual bones. An important diagnostic sign is the presence of an abnormal protein substance in the serum (globulin) and in the urine (Bence Jones protein) and abnormal plasma cells in sternal marrow. Presenting symptoms include bone pain, which may be of sudden onset, and there is a strong tendency to pathological fracture. As the disease progresses, there may be anaemia, a raised erythrocyte-sedimentation rate, and complications associated with deposits of abnormal protein material in the kidneys, the heart and the alimentary tract, leading to disturbance of renal and cardiac function and eventually to amyloid disease. There may also be deposits in nerves and in joint capsules which interfere with the function of a limb, together with a tendency to chest infections and to abnormal bleeding.

Treatment is largely symptomatic, but corticosteroids, chemotherapy (urethane) and radiotherapy have all been found useful.

METASTATIC CANCER OF BONE

Secondary deposits can arise in any part of the skeleton from primary lesions in the breast, lung, kidney, prostate or thyroid gland and less commonly from reticuloses such as leukemia and Hodgkin's disease. *Treatment* includes splintage, radiotherapy, hormonal therapy and chemotherapy, internal fixation of bone lesions and rarely, amputation.

NOTES ON NURSING CARE

It goes without saying that a patient undergoing specific orthopaedic treatment for a bone tumour requires the same high standard of nursing care related to his condition, his symptoms, and to the progress of his disease as has already been discussed in foregoing chapters, and imaginative treatment of symptoms as they arise, the relief of pain, and the maintenance of activity whenever possible are self-evident. But there is another important aspect; it is distressing for all concerned to accept the fact that a young patient must lose a limb because of an osteosarcoma, even though we know that it is a life-saving measure. The surgeon will choose the method of informing the patient and his family of his decision to amputate a limb and his reasons for so doing; sometimes several interviews are required so that decisions are made known gradually; on the other hand, some patients demand to know 'the worst' and it is for the surgeon to decide how much or how little the patient and his family is told. We must seek specific instructions as to how we ourselves will answer questions which might be put to us, so that the patient is not given conflicting information. Many patients will face amputation of a limb and even the fact that their days are probably numbered with amazing courage, and prefer to be told the truth so far as it is known. But there are others from whom it is kindest to withhold information regarding the true nature of their illness; in any case the decision as to what the patient and his family is told does not lie with us but with the surgeon in charge of the case.

Patients may be admitted to orthopaedic wards because of multiple myelomatosis or metastatic carcinomatous disease of the skeleton which eventually invades vital structures until death supervenes. Such patients are often cachetic and emaciated, and may have distressing symptoms associated with secondary deposits, for example, cough and respiratory embarrassment from invasion of the lungs, or mental confusion from invasion of the brain. In spite of these complications the patient may linger for many weeks; it is our duty to ensure for him not only unremitting physical care but such mental comfort and peace as lies in our power, not forgetting that this also includes his family and friends.

BIBLIOGRAPHY

Corkery Patrick H 1978 Tumours of the bone. Nursing Mirror, 20 June, 15
Deeley T J et al 1973 A Guide to Radiotherapy Nursing. Edinburgh: Livingstone Nursing Texts
Deeley T J et al 1974 A Guide to Oncological Nursing. Edinburgh: Churchill Livingstone
Jacobs Philip 1972 Tumours of bone. Nursing Times, 14 December, 1572
Proceedings of a National Symposium. Care of the Dying. HMSO 1972 London: 29 November: Her Majesty's Stationary Office
Stuart E 1972 Amputation for osteogenic sarcoma. Nursing Times, 16 November 68: 1453

32
Peripheral vascular disorders

Patients suffering from peripheral vascular disorders are sometimes seen in orthopaedic practice, so that brief notes on these conditions and on their treatment and nursing care are included here.

PERIPHERAL CIRCULATION

The peripheral circulation is controlled by the autonomic nervous system by means of sympathetic nerves, which travel with the peripheral nerves supplying various parts of the limbs. Their function is to control vasomotor activity in response to different stimuli, for example, the normal response to exposure to cold is *vasoconstriction*, while heat causes *vasodilation*; certain chemical changes also influence these functions, in that the capillaries in the extremities are the site of intense activity in physiological processes, notably in the interchange of oxygen and carbon dioxide, in carrying nutriments to the tissues, and in the elimination of waste material. For this reason, any disturbance of capillary blood flow in the peripheral parts of the limbs leads to impoverishment of tissue requirements, alteration in local temperature and eventually, to local death of the fingers or toes, with gangrene which may be a menace to life.

Disturbance in capillary blood flow

This may be due not only to lack of vasomotor control, but to an actual obstruction of the lumen of an artery or vein, as for example, in trauma, arteriosclerosis, and in embolism; but in some conditions these factors occur together; for example, a patient suffering from diabetes mellitus may also suffer from hypertension and arteriosclerosis, so that his peripheral circulation is disturbed not only by imperfect metabolism in the tissues due to his diabetic condition, but also to mechanical obstruction due to thickening and occlusion of the arteries.

In brief, therefore, peripheral vascular insufficiency is due to the following:

1. Disturbance of vasomotor control.
2. Occlusion or partial occlusion of the blood-supply caused by trauma, by organic disease or by arterial embolism, as in thyrotoxicosis, mitral stenosis and sub-acute bacterial endocarditis.

In general, patients suffering from peripheral vascular disease require treatment in orthopaedic hospitals only when the condition is so far advanced that gangrenous extremities require amputation; treatment of the underlying organic disease of the cardiovascular or endocrine system requires medical treatment which is outside the scope of this book. On the other hand, in an orthopaedic hospital, pre-operative treatment to improve the general condition, to choose the optimum site for amputation, and to prepare the patient for operation and for subsequent rehabilitation requires continuation of medical care, and of nursing measures which will be discussed later in broad outline.

SYMPTOMS AND SIGNS OF PERIPHERAL VASCULAR DISEASE

These include the following:

1. *Unnatural coldness* of the extremities, despite a warm environment.
2. *Alteration in skin colour:* unnatural pallor, mottling, cyanosis, or reactive hyperaemia.
3. *Pain* which is not always associated with activity, and yet not relieved by rest; pain may be worse at night and only relieved by hanging the affected limb over the side of the bed.
4. *Intermittent claudication* is a sharp, cramp-like pain in the calf muscles occurring during activity, and which is relieved at once by rest; it is due to a reduced blood-supply to the muscles of the calf.

5. *Diminished arterial pulsation*.
6. *Trophic changes* in the skin indicate ischaemia from disturbance of circulation; the skin may be puffy and thickened at first, but later becomes tense, thin, shiny, hairless and prone to indolent ulceration and infection.
7. *Gangrene* indicates severe occlusion of the blood-supply. It may be 'dry' in the presence of chronic arterial obstruction; or 'wet' in the presence of acute arterial obstruction or chronic venous occlusion.

The line of demarcation is taken to mean the border between the area of gangrene and that of comparatively healthy tissue, with a tendency to spontaneous separation at this site.

8. An important feature related to the nursing care of patients suffering from peripheral vascular disease is that there is always disturbance of the body's normal powers of resistance and adjustment to alterations in surrounding temperature. There is also lowered resistance to the effects of trauma, to infection, to operative interference, and to physical and mental stress.

RAYNAUD'S DISEASE

Raynaud's disease is a paroxysmal vasopasm affecting the digital, palmar and plantar arteries so that the fingers or toes become at first, blue or white, and then cyanosed, with pain, stiffness, and loss of function; the condition is often bilateral and the cause is unknown; in severe cases, ulceration and gangrene eventually occur. Treatment is by sympathectomy.

Chilblains (perniosis) indicate a constitutional hypersensitivity of small skin vessels to exposure to cold. Other conditions due to exposure to cold include frost-bite and 'trench-foot' or 'immersion foot' which occur, as their names suggest, in the course of wars or of disasters at sea.

PERIPHERAL ARTERIOSCLEROSIS

This occurs in a condition called atherosclerosis, when lesions called atheromata develop in the arterial walls and undergo changes which lead to hardening and narrowing of the arteries; atheromata are frequently the seat of thrombosis, and depending on the vessel affected, may deprive a vital organ of its blood and so result in disability or death (notably in the coronary and cerebral arteries) or cause arterial insufficiency in a limb. No single cause of atheromata has been isolated, but disturbances of blood pressure and metabolism and variations in environmental factors such as exercise and diet are all believed to contribute to the condition. Occasionally local dilatation of an artery forms an aneurysm.

THROMBO-ANGIITIS OBLITERANS (BUERGER'S DISEASE)

This is an inflammatory condition affecting the peripheral arteries and veins; it is of doubtful aetiology, and affects mainly young males, particularly those of the Jewish race; it is associated with excessive smoking. There is coldness and pallor of the extremities, and severe pain which is not relieved by rest; mild trauma may lead to ulceration and gangrene. Treatment is symptomatic.

DIABETES MELLITUS

Diabetes mellitus is a metabolic disease due to intrinsic disease of the pancreas, leading to insufficiency of insulin control of the metabolism of carbohydrate, protein and fat, and characterised by hyperglycaemia, glycosuria and ketonuria. Neglect of treatment leads to ketosis, acidosis, coma and death. The total treatment of the diabetic will not be described here; summarised briefly, it includes the following:

1. Strict dietary control.
2. Insulin (or substitute) therapy, where necessary.
3. Education of the patient so that he understands the nature of his illness and of its treatment, including strict life-time habits directed to dietary measures, self-administration of insulin (or other drugs), routine daily urine testing, recognition of the onset of complications and the institution of appropriate measures to combat them.

In general, a patient suffering from this condition is seen in orthopaedic practice only as a result of disease or injury unrelated to his diabetic condition, or because gangrene of an extremity has complicated the course of his disease.

OUTLINE OF TREATMENT OF PERIPHERAL VASCULAR DISEASE

The aim of treatment is primarily to preserve the limb, and to avoid complications leading to its loss or those which threaten life itself.

Treatment is therefore influenced by the age, sex, and occupation of the patient and must include the adoption of a way of life commensurate with the condition, including protection from cold, from repeated minor trauma, including burns, and from overexertion. This means, for example, that the outdoor manual worker may have to change his occupation and the housewife must exercise special care in handling domestic equipment. In all cases, scrupulous care of the skin of the affected extremities is essential; the application of local heat, e.g. from a hot water bottle, is forbidden, as is the use of tobacco, which produces transient vasoconstriction.

Physiotherapy may be ordered, in the form of diathermy, special baths, and special exercises (Buerger's) to increase peripheral blood flow.

OUTLINE OF TREATMENT AND NURSING CARE IN HOSPITAL

Complete rest in bed, with all its implications in nursing care, is usually ordered; the affected extremity is kept at rest, supported on a pillow, either in the horizontal position or a little below it; it is never elevated except on the order of the doctor. The limb is exposed to the air and the room temperature is kept at a constant level; sometimes a heat-cradle is used to produce reflex vasodilation in the affected limb. Infected lesions, if present, are treated by rest and application of wet compresses; strong antiseptics are never used since they may cause further devitalisation of tissue. Handling of the limb and dressing techniques are carried out with the utmost gentleness.

Chemotherapy is often ordered.

Pain is treated by means of analgesics; alcohol injections into peripheral nerves are sometimes used for persistent pain.

Operative treatment includes embolectomy, thromboendartectomy, excision of the affected vessel and graft replacement, or some form of by-pass replacement. Lumbar sympathectomy is sometimes advised. In diabetes with gangrene, local resection of the gangrenous area is often effective. In those cases where progressive gangrene and spreading infection threatens the life of the patient, amputation (Ch. 33) is the only remedy.

Gangrene of the extremities due to interference with circulation from tight bandages, splints or plasters

This subject is of special significance to the orthopaedic nurse.

The importance of constant vigilance and observation of the extremities in patients whose peripheral circulation may be impeded by an orthopaedic appliance such as a plaster cast has already been stressed. Special vigilance is required in those cases where the circulation is already known to be inadequate, as, for example, in poliomyelitis, cerebral palsy, and spina bifida, and in those cases where bandages, splints or plasters are applied post-operatively or in the treatment of recent injuries.

In particular, exercise special care and vigilance in those cases where although the circulation appears to be normal, the patient has an anxious expression and complains of incessant pain; it is better to seek the surgeon's permission to release tight bandages or plasters than to risk permanent loss of function or loss of the limb itself.

Pressure sores (bed sores, decubitus ulcers.) These are due to local gangrene of tissue which have been devitalised by pressure; the importance of *prevention* by frequent change of the patient's position has already been stressed throughout this book.

Venous thrombosis and embolism

Venous thrombosis

Preventive measures include provision of anti-embolic stockings, active exercises and abstention from smoking. An excellent discussion of this topic appeared in the *Nursing Mirror* (Turner & Turner, 1982).

Thrombosis of a deep vein in the leg may occur as a result of inactivity, and especially as a complication of surgery; disorders of the circulatory system previously referred to in this chapter predispose the patient to this complication.

Clinical features of deep vein thrombosis include pain in the calf, especially on dorsiflexion of the foot (Homan's sign), local tenderness and rise of temperature.

Treatment consists of rest in bed and the administration of anticoagulants, e.g. heparin and Dindevan; these drugs are sometimes given prophylactically.

Venous embolism

A thrombus (or local 'clot') may become detached from its venous bed and escape into the circulation as an embolus, which if carried to the pulmonary vessels may result in death.

Clinical features include pain in the chest, nausea, syncope, rise of temperature and haemoptysis.

Treatment includes complete rest with intensive nursing care, the administration of anticoagulant drugs, of analgesics, and of oxygen where indicated; this may result in resolution of the embolus with spontaneous recovery. Embolectomy is occasionally performed.

These brief notes are included to emphasise the importance of *observation* of the patient and of prompt reporting of any sign of this serious condition.

BIBLIOGRAPHY

Abramson D I 1974 Vascular disorders of the extremities. 2nd ed. Hagerstown, Maryland: Harper and Row
Allen E V 1962 Peripheral vascular disorders. 3rd ed. Philadelphia: Saunders
Datta Pradip K 1982 A case for critical selection. Nursing Mirror, 3 March
Datta Pradip K 1982 The last resort. Nursing Mirror, 10 March
Hetherington H 1981 Peripheral vascular disease. A nursing care study. Nursing Times, 23/30 December
Hierton T 1972 Amputation in the treatment of arteriosclerotic gangrene or pre-gangrene. Journal of Bone and Joint Surgery 54B, (4), 759

Hobbs J T 1977 Treatment of venous disorders. MTP Press

Holling H E 1972 Peripheral vascular disease: diagnosis and management. Philadelphia: Lippincott

Kakkar V V 1977 The prevention of acute pulmonary embolism. British Journal of Hospital Medicine, July, 32

Miller G A H 1977 The management of acute pulmonary embolism. British Journal of Hospital Medicine, July, 26

Morris G K, Mitchell J R A 1977 The aetiology of acute pulmonary embolism and the identification of high risk groups. British Journal of Hospital Medicine, July, 6

Oakley C 1977 The diagnosis of acute pulmonary embolism. British Journal of Hospital Medicine, July, 15

Turner A, Turner J 1982 An unexpected killer. Nursing Mirror, 25 August

33

Amputations

Loss of a limb is a serious mutilation and in general is only undertaken as a life-saving measure, as for example, in the presence of vascular insufficiency, severe injuries, infection or malignant disease. Roaf and Hodkinson (see Bibliography) give an excellent account of the modern approach to this problem.

In Western countries, peripheral vascular disease is the most important condition which requires the skills of the amputation surgeon and the prosthetist, whereas in the developing world trauma still plays a large part in the question of amputation. Nevertheless in the developing world, too, peripheral vascular disease is still a considerable problem.

It is noticeable that many patients undergoing amputation for peripheral vascular disease are elderly, but despite this, advances in operating techniques and especially in investigations such as those using ultra-sound devices and radio-isotope uptake (Ch. 4) mean that the surgeon is able to plan the operation to give the maximum length of stump and the most satisfactory prosthesis.

Psychological preparation is essential and it is helpful for the patient to talk to others who have lost a limb (Farrell, 1977).

INDICATIONS FOR AMPUTATION

The following are indications for amputation:

1. Injuries.
2. Infection, e.g. gas gangrene, chronic osteomyelitis.
3. Malignant disease, e.g. osteosarcoma (Ch. 31).

4. Peripheral vascular disease, as in thrombo-angiitis obliterans and diabetic or senile arteriosclerosis (Ch. 32).

5. Paralysis of a limb, particularly where there is deformity, loss of sensation and trophic changes.

6. Deformity which seriously interferes with function.

In the upper limb, where *mobility* is the primary functional demand and therefore the primary objective of treatment, every effort is made to save as much as possible, particularly in the case of the hand, where even remnants, particularly of the thumb, are often more useful for function than any artificial device. In the lower limb, however, *stability* is the primary need and therefore the primary objective.

THE IDEAL STUMP

The ideal amputation stump is of the optimum length, firm, smooth, well-muscled, free from tension, from contractures and from adherent scars and other skin blemishes, and with free, controlled movement in all directions.

At operation, the skin is cut in flaps to cover the end of the stump, the flaps being equal in length so that the operation scar lies distally and away from the weight-bearing area, which in most modern protheses is side-bearing rather than end-bearing in relation to the stump. The muscles, which are severed below the site of bone division, are either sutured to bone (myoelesis) or joined to their antagonists, which improves the function and the circulation of the stump (myoplastic amputation). Vascular stasis in the stump may lead to ischaemia, and amputation at a higher level may then be advised.

SITES OF ELECTION FOR AMPUTATION

IN THE UPPER LIMB

Forequarter amputation, which includes the whole arm, the scapula and the outer end of the clavicle may be required as a radical procedure in the presence of malignant disease.

Disarticulation of the shoulder may be advised in severe injuries.

Upper arm amputation is sometimes advised in the treatment of brachial plexus lesions; it is preceded by arthrodesis of the shoulder. The site of election for amputation is usually 15–20 cm from the acromion process.

Disarticulation of the elbow is usually performed at a site 15–18 cm below the olecranon process.

Amputation of the fingers or thumb. Sometimes this is a necessary emergency procedure in crush injuries or open fractures; the need to salvage any part of the digits which may serve a useful function has already been mentioned, but in the case of those which are stiff, painful, useless and perhaps ankylosed in extension, amputation is usually advised.

IN THE LOWER LIMB

Hindquarter amputation may be required in the presence of malignant disease and includes not only the hip-joint but the corresponding one-half of the pelvis.

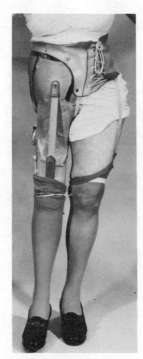

Fig. 33.1 Hindquarter amputation, showing apparatus for walking.

Disarticulation of the hip is usually performed through the lesser trochanter of the femur.

Mid-thigh amputation; the site of election is chosen so that the stump measures 25–30 cm from the greater trochanter.

Disarticulation of the knee provides a good stump and is often chosen for elderly people.

Gritti-Stokes amputation uses the patella to form part of the weight-bearing surface.

Below-knee amputation is usually performed at a level of 12–15 cm below the knee.

Syme's amputation, when the limb is divided just above the ankle joint, is often advised for severe injuries to the foot. It is usually successful because the skin of the heel which is already accustomed to weight-bearing is used to cover the end of the stump.

Amputation of all the toes ('pobble operation') is sometimes advised in cases of rheumatoid arthritis or of peripheral vascular disease. A special insole is worn post-operatively, which is carefully moulded to support the foot and which carries a cork toe-block covered with sponge rubber.

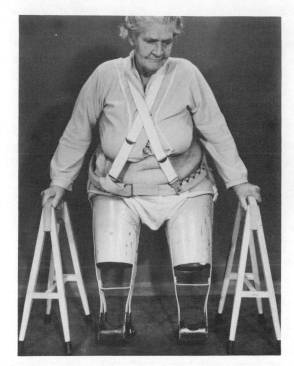

Fig. 33.2 Bilateral above-knee amputation: short 'penguin' prothesis.

PREPARATION FOR OPERATION

The success of an amputation depends not only upon the operation, subsequent care and expert fitting of the appropriate prosthesis, but upon the co-operation of the patient in learning to use it to the full and in adjusting himself to it in relation to his life and work, so that preparation includes not only physical aspects but investigation of family circumstances, home conditions and occupational possibilities. Each patient requires individual consideration when planning the future programme; for example, in young, vigorous, well-muscled subjects the correct use of a conventional prosthesis and a return to a full active life is the aim of treatment. On the other hand, in the elderly patient a less ambitious programme with modification of conventional prostheses is usually acceptable (Fig. 33.2). As in other conditions, children require special consideration related to growth of the limb and to their educational and recreational needs and from the first, the parents are included in the rehabilitation programme.

Preparation includes not only skin preparation but where possible, intensive exercises to strengthen the muscles of the limb, to improve the posture, the general musculature, the circulation and the respiratory state. Treatment of associated conditions such as anaemia may be required, so that the general health is maintained at a high level.

Psychological preparation is important; where possible the patient should visit a limb-fitting centre where he will meet other amputees and learn that loss of a limb will not necessarily interfere seriously with his life and work.

POST-OPERATIVE NURSING CARE

In addition to the régime which is standard practice in post-operative care, the patient is nursed in a divided bed and the stump is observed continuously. At one time it was common practice to fasten a tourniquet to the foot-rail of the bed where it could not be seen by the patient but where it served as a constant reminder to the nursing staff of the danger of reactionary or secondary haemorrhage. This practice has been discontinued, though this does not mean that observation is no longer necessary; staining of blood through the dressing is treated by the prompt application of a firm, thick dressing and bandage and the doctor is summoned; sometimes ligation of a bleeding vessel is required. Blood-transfusion, chemotherapy and sedatives may be ordered, and breathing exercises are commenced as soon as possible.

Position of the stump

In some cases, a modified plaster spica enclosing the distal joint is ordered; otherwise, at the earliest possible moment, the stump is laid flat on the bed and it is most important that flexion-abduction contracture is avoided, since this will hamper subsequent efforts to use a prosthesis; in no circumstances should the stump be flexed over a pillow; traction by means of skin extensions attached to a weight and pulley is occasionally ordered. The above-knee stump should be held close to the sound leg to prevent abduction contracture. Flexion contracture of the knee in a below-knee amputation is prevented by the application of a back-splint which projects below the end of the stump.

The stump is handled only with the utmost gentleness, and for the first two or three days the patient is often completely confined to bed and requires nursing care relative to every patient who has undergone major surgery. As soon as possible, however, he is encouraged to move about the bed and to use an overhead pulley and some patients may be allowed up in a wheel-chair in a few days, particularly in the case of elderly patients. As in other conditions, general management is influenced by the age and the general condition of the individual patient. *Chronic oedema* must be prevented by elevation of the part and by support, if ordered.

After about 48 hours, the drain is removed without disturbing the rest of the wound and as soon as healing takes place, measures to prepare the stump for the fitting of a prosthesis are commenced.

Bandaging the stump

At one time this was considered of vital importance in shaping the stump; nowadays however the surgeon shapes the stump at the time of operation and will give specific orders in this connection. In case bandaging should be ordered the conventional method is described below. At least three 15 cm crepe bandages are required for an above-knee stump; the patient should lie flat and may assist in the procedure; place the end of the bandage longitudinally on the front of the stump with the free end towards the trunk; carry it firmly but gently over the centre of the end of the stump and up the back of the 'thigh' to the gluteal fold, then carry it back over itself and over the stump end to overlap its fellow in such a way as to compress the right lateral aspects of the 'thigh'; the next turn compresses the left lateral aspect, and the bandage is then continued in turns which cross on the outer side of the stump from below upwards and which continues over the pelvis in the form of a spica; the bandage is carried up into the groin in front and to the level of the gluteal fold posteriorly; it is *essential* that it is applied *firmly* and *evenly*, but not tightly, leaving no gaps, so that the stump is compressed (but not squeezed) from below upwards along its entire length and in all its dimensions. It is important to remember that a bandage which is too tight may interfere with circulation and do more harm than one which is too loose. The bandage is renewed morning and evening or, if necessary, even more frequently.

In some cases a temporary prosthesis is fitted immediately since a well-shaped socket will itself mould the stump efficiently (Fig. 33.3).

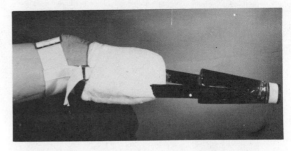

Fig. 33.3 Below-knee amputation: 'instant' prosthesis applied immediately after operation.

When healing is complete the skin of the stump is kept immaculately clean and dry; 'stump socks' are ordered and a clean one is applied daily. Constant vigilance is required to prevent flexion-abduction contracture in an above-knee stump and flexion contracture of the knee in one below this level. Incipient flexion contracture at the hip or knee joint is prevented by strict attention to posture at all times; all patients should spend part of each day lying in the prone position.

Exercises are commenced at the earliest possible moment and in uncomplicated cases of leg amputation, early ambulation on crutches is usually ordered. Since loss of a limb interferes with balance this has to be regained. Sometimes a temporary home-made prosthesis such as that shown in Fig. 33.3 is ordered, particularly in the case of elderly patients, who are often allowed out of bed in a wheel-chair at an early stage. Again, strict attention to the posture of the stump whether abed, afoot or in a wheelchair is essential, together with intensive exercises for the stump and for the whole body.

In upper limb amputations, early activity is encouraged and a prosthesis is fitted at the earliest possible moment so that the patient does not come to rely solely on the sound limb; a prosthesis for the upper limb is shown in Fig. 33.4. Attachments are fitted to enable the patient to carry out different functions ranging from the ordinary acts of daily living, such as eating, to more specialised skills related to employment. Artifical arms may be activated either manually or by means of carbon dioxide gas released from a cylinder (Fig. 33.4) (Heidelberg arm), or by amplification of electrical currents produced by the patient's own muscles (myoelectric arm). Roaf and Hodkinson (see Bibliography) describe a power-operated arm developed in Moscow.

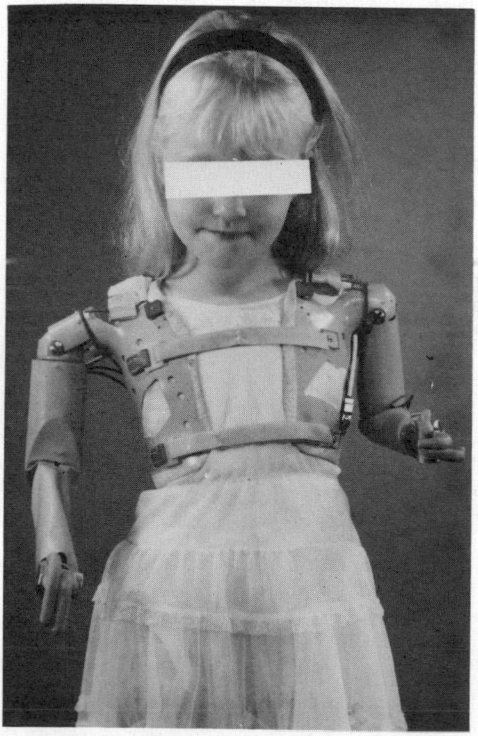

FITTING OF PROSTHESIS

The type of limb chosen varies with the age, sex, occupation, length and shape of the stump, and with the physical and mental endowment of the individual patient. Sometimes a simple appliance is chosen to begin with, which may later be exchanged for, or supplemented by, a more elaborate prosthesis for occupational or cosmetic purposes.

IMPORTANCE OF THE ROLE OF THE PROSTHETIST (LIMB-FITTER)

The prosthetist is always asked to see the patient with the surgeon before operation, because success depends upon team-work between the surgeon and other members of the hospital team, the prosthetist and the patient. It is essential that the prosthesis chosen fits the life-style of the patient; for example, a conventional patella-bearing prothesis may be suitable for a farmer in a Western country but it is useless for one working in a muddy paddy-field. Doctors and prosthetists in developing countries are working out prosthetic devices which are most suitable for the environment and financial resources of their own people. Once the operation has been performed and the patient is ready for the fitting of a prosthesis, the prosthetist emerges as a key member of the team and successful rehabilitation depends not only upon the perfect fit and alignment, the manoeuvrability and efficiency of the limb, but upon the ability of the patient to use it. As already stated, older patients, especially those no longer at work, may not require such an elaborate prosthesis or so much emphasis on its correct

Fig. 33.4 CO_2 powered prosthesis for congenital absence of arms. (With kind permission of the Princess Margaret Rose Hospital, Edinburgh.)

use as in the case of young persons, in whom not only the function but the appearance of the limb is important; for them, every effort is made to prevent or correct faulty use of the prosthesis, and in successful cases the use of an artificial limb may go practically unnoticed. Everything depends, however, upon the common-sense, powers of perseverance and will-power of the individual patient and, in the case of children, on the intelligent co-operation of the patient's parents.

COMPLICATIONS

Infection, ischaemia, oedema and the importance of prevention of contractures have already been mentioned. Patients wearing an artificial limb must avoid obesity, since bulging of excess tissue over the upper end of the prosthesis leads to excoriation of the skin or to interference with the circulation in the stump. Skin lesions on weight-bearing surfaces are avoided by strict attention to hygiene and to cleanliness.

Pain in the stump may result from an ill-fitting limb or one in faulty alignment with the trunk; sometimes a painful neuroma requires treatment by percussion, or ischaemia may require lumbar sympathectomy.

The phantom limb is sometimes troublesome; if the sensation that the absent limb is still present is not accompanied by pain, the condition usually clears up on fitting of an artificial limb and subsequent rehabilitation. If pain is also present, however, perhaps with other unpleasant sensations, the condition tends to persist and local treatment such as percussion or more radical measures such as intrathecal injections of phenol may be required.

Physiotherapy in lower limb amputations

In ideal circumstances, the physiotherapist's assessment and treatment of a patient with an amputation of the lower limb starts before the operation. However, circumstances may preclude this in some cases, e.g. in traumatic amputation: There are two major groups of patients who undergo amputation:

1. Patients with peripheral vascular disease, neoplasm or a gross deformity or diseased joint, who may have a lower limb amputation carried out as an elective procedure. Such patients will have been admitted for assessment and a physiotherapeutic assessment of functional ability and the need for specific post-operative re-education can be made.

2. Major trauma to the lower limb may require amputation as a primary life-saving procedure; obviously in such cases, the physiotherapist will not see the patient until after the operation; these patients may also have other major injuries which may present additional problems in rehabilitation; in addition, the age and general condition of the amputee will vary considerably.

The level of a lower limb amputation may be:

Symes amputation—through the ankle joint;
below-knee;
through-knee;
mid-thigh (also called above-knee).
The two most common levels are below-knee and mid-thigh.

Teamwork between the surgeon, nurse, physiotherapist, prosthetist, and last but not least, the patient, is very important. The loss of a limb is a deep psychological shock and a positive attitude to the future will help lessen this. Surgery is only the first stage of rehabilitation towards full function with an artificial limb; however, preoperative assessment ensures realistic goals set by members of the team, for example, in an elderly patient, restricted function may have to be accepted, but that does not mean that the patient cannot be helped to enjoy life.

The stages of fitting of a prosthesis can be somewhat prolonged and it may be some months before the definitive prosthesis can be fitted. However, the rehabilitation regime works towards having the stump ready for the final limb as soon as possible.

An outline of pre- and post-operative physiotherapy, together with later treatment including walking re-education will be given. These aims can be applied to both below-knee and mid-thigh amputation but will be discussed with particular reference to one at mid-thigh level.

The presence of a normal knee joint is very important; re-education is much easier in a below-knee amputation than in one above the knee; loss of the knee joint is a great disadvantage because of corresponding loss of sensory input regarding proprioception, and the difficulties in retraining balance mechanisms to compensate for this loss. The intact proprioceptive input from the knee joint is a major reason for the success in rehabilitation of the below-knee amputee, who, in addition does not have to face the problems of adjusting to variations in mechanical knee-joints when being fitted with a prosthesis.

The aims of pre-operative physiotherapy treatment

These are:

1. To gain the patient's confidence and appreciation of the importance of physical preparation.
2. Prevention of post-operative complications, e.g. chest or circulatory complications.
3. Preparation for crutch walking, including exercises for the sound limb, arms and the joints of the affected leg above the level of surgery.
4. Instruction in crutch walking—balance and stabilisations on the sound leg if the condition of the patient is suitable.
5. Correction of posture, if necessary.

The type of surgery carried out at operation is important. If a myoplastic technique is used, the re-education of the stump muscles is different from that when a standard amputation is employed. The standard stump shape is conical and the loss of muscle tone makes bandaging to prevent oedema a vital procedure; when a myoplastic technique is carried out however, opposing muscle groups are sutured using a physiological tension technique which helps these muscles to hold the stump in the neutral position post-operatively. Stump bandaging is less important provided the patient is encouraged to carry out active muscular contractions in the stump, and the shape of a myoplastic stump is rounded and U-shaped rather than conical.

When stump bandaging is necessary, nurses and physiotherapists work together, re-applying the bandage as and when necessary according to the surgeon's orders; where necessary, the patient is also taught to bandage the stump himself.

If, for any reason, a patient with a mid-thigh amputation cannot wear his pylon or limb for a length of time, stump bandaging may be required to prevent oedema and help maintain the shape of the stump and therefore correct fit of the socket of the prosthesis (Fig. 33.5 A and B).

The aims of post-operative physiotherapy

These are;

Prevention of post-operative complications.
Continuation of exercises for all limbs, particularly the arms in preparation for crutch walking.
Prevention of contractures and preparation of the stump for fitting of prosthesis.

An amputation is a major surgical procedure and the usual post-operative regime of breathing exercises to prevent chest complications and aid general circulation are carried out. In most cases and especially where the patient suffers from peripheral vascular disease, these exercises are vital. The patient continues the general activities practised pre-operatively; these are often functional aids to nursing procedures. The patient helps strengthen his arms and prepare them for taking weight on crutches, by pushing down on extended arms and lifting his buttocks off the bed. Similarly the patient is encouraged to move freely around the bed and roll from side to side using his arms and sound leg.

After operation, the first important step in preparing the stump for the prosthesis is to prevent the formation of contractures which would give a flexed, abducted stump in the mid-thigh amputee and a flexed stump in the below knee. This is best done by co-operation between the nurses, physiotherapist and patient. *Pillows should never be placed under the stump or proximal joint*; the patient is encouraged to lie flat, with only one pillow under his head, for periods during the day and is taught to correct his own posture; as soon as the general condition permits; it is essential that the patient turns into prone-lying two or three times daily.

When the drainage tube has been removed (if one has been used) specific stump exercises can be started; these are best done in side-lying so that full extension of the hip and active adduction and 'holding' can be practised against gradually increased resistance; the proximal joint is exercised through its full range of movement.

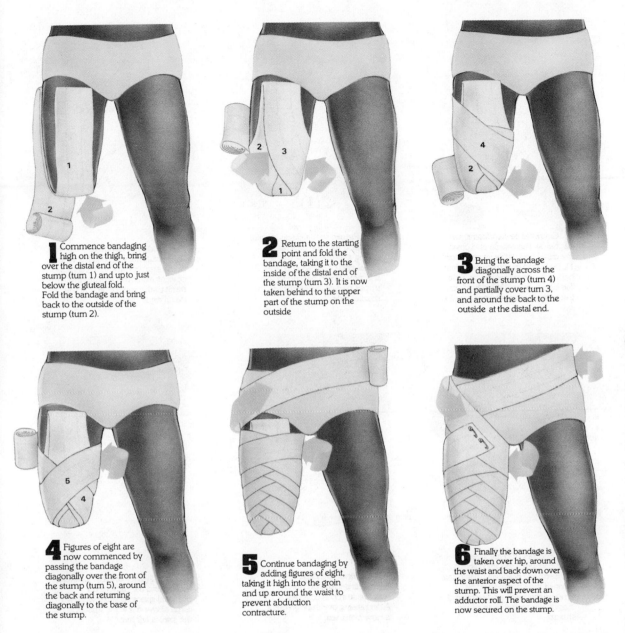

1 Commence bandaging high on the thigh, bring over the distal end of the stump (turn 1) and up to just below the gluteal fold. Fold the bandage and bring back to the outside of the stump (turn 2).

2 Return to the starting point and fold the bandage, taking it to the inside of the distal end of the stump (turn 3). It is now taken behind to the upper part of the stump on the outside

3 Bring the bandage diagonally across the front of the stump (turn 4) and partially cover turn 3, and around the back to the outside at the distal end.

4 Figures of eight are now commenced by passing the bandage diagonally over the front of the stump (turn 5), around the back and returning diagonally to the base of the stump.

5 Continue bandaging by adding figures of eight, taking it high into the groin and up around the waist to prevent abduction contracture.

6 Finally the bandage is taken over hip, around the waist and back down over the anterior aspect of the stump. This will prevent an adductor roll. The bandage is now secured on the stump.

Fig. 33.5   A. Shows bandaging technique for an above-knee stump. (Courtesy of Seton Products.)

When the surgeon allows the patient to get up out of bed, balance retraining can be started using parallel bars. When the patient can safely take weight on the sound leg he transfers his weight to his arms and learns to walk in parallel bars, progressing to crutches as soon as possible. A natural posture and rhythm are encouraged whilst walking and these involve correct positioning of the stump, which is moved in opposition to the sound leg when walking and held in natural alignment when standing. The patient is not allowed to walk on his crutches in the ward until the physiotherapist considers it is safe for him to do so; he is usually allowed to go home when he is competent to use his crutches to walk on all surfaces, to go up and down stairs in safety, to dress and use the lavatory

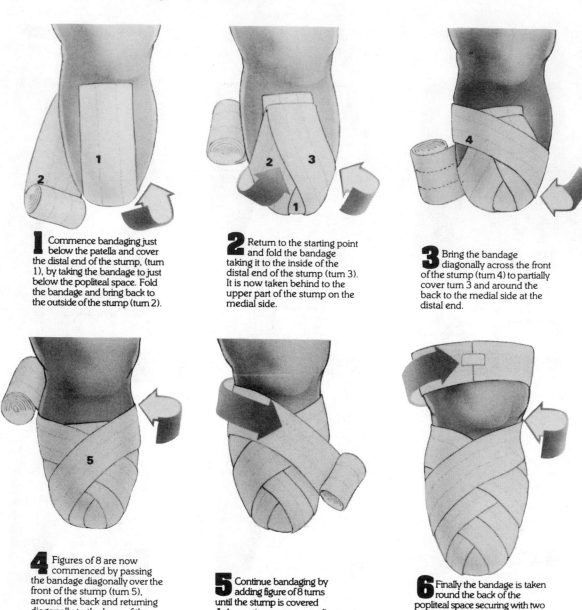

1 Commence bandaging just below the patella and cover the distal end of the stump, (turn 1), by taking the bandage to just below the popliteal space. Fold the bandage and bring back to the outside of the stump (turn 2).

2 Return to the starting point and fold the bandage taking it to the inside of the distal end of the stump (turn 3). It is now taken behind to the upper part of the stump on the medial side.

3 Bring the bandage diagonally across the front of the stump (turn 4) to partially cover turn 3 and around the back to the medial side at the distal end.

4 Figures of 8 are now commenced by passing the bandage diagonally over the front of the stump (turn 5), around the back and returning diagonally to the base of the stump.

5 Continue bandaging by adding figure of 8 turns until the stump is covered A decreasing pressure gradient is now obtained.

6 Finally the bandage is taken round the back of the popliteal space securing with two turns above the knee, ensuring the joint is left free.

Fig. 33.5 B. Shows bandaging technique for a below-knee stump. NB The bandage used in this illustration is 'Elset S' (Courtesy of Seton Products).

with minimum aid. He continues his treatment by home exercises or by attending as an out-patient. This is very important whilst waiting for his pylon (temporary prosthesis).

Walking with a prosthesis

There are many different types of artificial limbs and the type chosen is the one most suited to the patient's age and capabilities. He is fitted firstly with a pylon, which usually has a rocker bottom and a stiff knee; the patient first stands using parallel bars, wearing the pylon over a stump sock with the pelvic band and shoulder straps comfortably adjusted. The important points in stance and balance are explained to ensure the patient takes

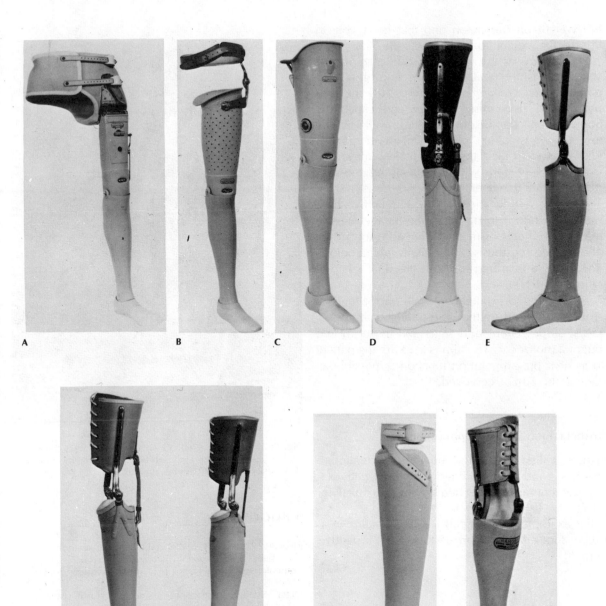

Fig. 33.6 **A.** Canadian tilting table leg for hemipelvectomy, hip disarticulation or very short above-knee amputation. **B.** Light metal limb for above-knee amputation with pelvic band suspension, conventional socket, and finger tip operated gait control of the knee. **C.** Light metal limb for above-knee amputation with metal suction socket. **D.** Light metal leg for through-knee amputation. Knee-bearing with ring-catch locking knee joints. **E.** Light metal leg for below-knee amputation. Polycentric joints. **F.** Light metal legs for below-knee amputation. Ball-bearing uni-axial knee-joints. **G.** Patella tendon bearing (PTB) leg. All plastic, with articulated ankle. **H.** Child's wooden leg for below-knee amputation. (J. E. Hanger and Co., Ltd.)

full weight on the pylon and that he is able to transfer the weight from one foot to the other.

He progresses to weight transference in the standing position and then takes steps along the parallel bars; walking sticks are usually the next progression depending on age and capability. Some patients can be encouraged to walk without any aid whilst others clearly will never manage without two sticks; the aged patient may only manage a few steps with a walking aid and may need to adapt to wheelchair life.

Walking re-education with the definitive limb requires a return to basics in the parallel bars to master the mechanism of the knee flexion in the above-knee prosthesis. For patients with a below-knee patella-bearing prosthesis this final rehabilitation is much easier.

All patients are taught to walk with a natural stride length and rhythm and to negotiate all surfaces, slopes, steps and stairs and to get in and out of a motor car. The aim is to return the patient to as near pre-amputation function as possible as soon as this can be achieved.

Artificial limbs in developing countries

In the so-called developing countries, conventional prostheses must be modified to suit the patient's requirements and enable him to earn his living (Fig. 33.7).

For example, an artificial limb terminating in a rubber foot enables a farmer to work in a paddy-field.

Conclusion

This brief and simplified description of amputations and prostheses is intended to give the nurse a working knowledge which she can apply to patients seen in orthopaedic wards. In common with other patients, rehabilitation includes not only the physical state but socio-economic facets as well. The fitting of artificial limbs and the rehabilitation of the amputee is in fact a complex subject involving techniques of surgery, physiotherapy, prosthetics and subsequent rehabilitation which are outside the scope of this book.

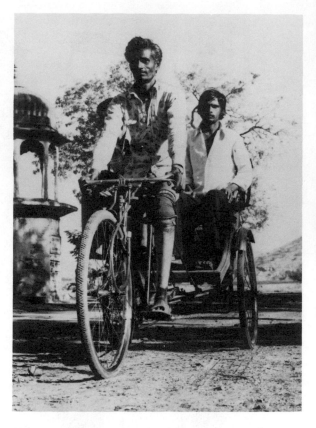

Fig. 33.7 An artificial limb suited to his needs gives greater mobility and new hope to the worker in a developing country. (Courtesy of WHO/RR Centre Jaipur, India.)

BIBLIOGRAPHY

Biffen M F, Fulford E 1969 Rehabilitation of lower limb amputees. Occupational Therapy, 28 December
Computerised artificial arm 1973 Nursing Mirror, 31 August, 29
Datta P K 1982 A case for critical selection. Nursing Mirror, 3 March
Datta P K 1982 The last resort. Nursing Mirror, 10 March
Davis B C 1974 Rehabilitation of the lower limb amputee. Nursing Mirror, 7 June, 138: 70
Farrell J 1977 Illustrated Guide to Orthopaedic Nursing. Oxford: Blackwell Scientific
Harding J M 1974 Amputation of the lower limb. Nursing Times, 4 July, 70: 1025
Iveson-Iveson J 1981 Amputation. Nursing Mirror, 24 June
Jones C 1974 Above knee amputation. Nursing Mirror, 7 June, 138: 77
Lamb D W 1969 Amputation surgery and rehabilitation. Nursing Mirror, 3 January, 26
Little J M 1971 An immediate prosthesis. Nursing Mirror, 1 October, 133: 17
McVittie C K 1975 Traumatic amputation of right arm. Nursing Mirror, 28 August, 141: 47

Moncur S D 1969 Rehabilitation of a lower limb amputee. Nursing Times, 20 March, 372

Parkes C M 1975 Reaction to the loss of a limb. Nursing Mirror, 2 January, 140: 36

Roaf and Hodkinson 1975 Textbook of Orthopaedic Nursing. Oxford: Blackwell Scientific

Rowe J, Dyer L 1977 Care of the orthopaedic patient. Oxford: Blackwell Scientific

Southcombe A 1982 Hindquarter amputation. Nursing Care Study. Nursing Mirror, 10 November

Stuart E 1972 Amputation for osteogenic sarcoma. Nursing Times, 16 November, 68: 1453

Tuh J 1981 The Jaipur Limb. Geneva: World Health Organization

Van de Ven C M C 1981 An investigation into the management of bilateral leg amputees. British Medical Journal, 12 September, 283

Wood M A 1969 Dundee Limb Fitting Centre. Nursing Times, 30 January

Wood M A 1974 Nursing care of the elderly lower-limb amputee. Nursing Mirror, 7 June, 138: 66

SECTION | SEVEN

Rehabilitation of the
orthopaedic patient

34

Rehabilitation 1: general considerations

Rehabilitation can be defined as the total process of preserving or restoring an individual to the highest level of physical and socio-economic independence which he can reach. Though this process is generally regarded as one of *restoration of function*, it is important for the nurse to recognise the element of *prevention* of conditions leading to loss of function. This point is stressed because of the tendency to regard rehabilitation as 'someone else's business', as a terminal event in the patient's treatment or something to be turned to when all else has failed.

The process of rehabilitation is described here under two headings as follows:

1. *Preventive rehabilitation* in the community and in the hospital, and

2. *Restorative (or medical) rehabilitation* as practised in a special centre.

PREVENTIVE REHABILITATION

This takes place:

1. *In the community*, by means of measures which promote positive health, including environmental factors, health teaching, maternal and child care, control of communicable diseases and special arrangements for the care of vulnerable groups of people, e.g. the mentally and physically handicapped and the aged. *Exercise therapy* for elderly patients in a community setting is discussed by Copple (1983). Prevention of accidents in the home, the school, the sports field, in factories, on

farms and on the roads is also part of preventive rehabilitation, as is the availability of medical aid, the training of first-aid workers and provision of rapid transportation to hospital.

2. *In the hospital*, preventive rehabilitation begins with prompt and effective treatment and nursing care in the accident centre, casualty or out-patient department, and continues in the operating theatre and in the ward; the rôle of the nurse in this connection will be discussed later. Patients with orthopaedic conditions often require the ser-vices of the physiotherapist, and often, those of the occupational therapist and social worker as well. Some will require certain aspects of the spe-cial resources offered by a purpose-built medical rehabilitation centre, but if treatment and nursing care is successful, only a minority will require the whole gamut of the expensive facilities offered by such an establishment.

In the main, our patients fall into two groups:

1. *The temporarily disabled*, i.e. those who are expected to make a complete recovery in the fullness of time and to suffer no significant per-manent physical handicap.
2. *The permanently disabled*, i.e. those with a phy-sical handicap which cannot be cured; obvious examples are the paraplegic and the amputee.

Many patients with orthopaedic conditions belong to the first group, as will have been noted in the pages of this book. An important aim of treat-ment is to prevent a patient belonging to the first group from entering the second; but if he does, then the varied resources of the rehabilitation or retraining centre are used to help him to overcome his permanent disability and if necessary, to retrain him for new work in a suitable environment.

RESTORATIVE (MEDICAL) REHABILITATION

Rehabilitation services as offered by a hospital and/or special centre will now be discussed.

The medical rehabilitation centre

Rehabilitation centres were first established by Sir Robert Jones in the First World War, when the majority of patients were healthy vigorous young men who had sustained injuries in battle and who required intensive programmes of physical exercise to fit them for an early return to active service. From these centres grew the sophisticated estab-lishments we know today, where programmes are designed for all age-groups and sections of the population.

A rehabilitation centre may be a separate estab-lishment with residential accommodation, or, part and parcel of a hospital so that patients are trans-ported thence from their wards or attend as out-patients. The centre generally provides not only facilities for gymnastics and sport, including swim-ming, conventional physiotherapy and occupa-tional therapy departments, but 'daily living units', part of which resemble a normal home and where the patient can practise the ordinary skills he must acquire before discharge from hospital.

In addition, there may be workshops for orthotics and prosthetics, for retraining for employment or for the practice of skills in leather, wood or metal; the craft taught might be purely diversional, and devoted to making objects of varying decorative or useful value, or to more ambitious skills such as splint-making, radio assembly, or watch-repair-ing, always supposing that skilled tuition and super-vision is available.

The rehabilitation team

The team is usually led by the doctor, but each member takes his/her place as leader according to the activity involved.

All team members share in making an assessment of the patient in preparation for programmes in occupational therapy, physiotherapy, orthotics/prosthetics, speech therapy and medico-social work. It is important to appreciate the fact that *rea-listic assessment* of the patient is essential; no reha-bilitation programme will replace what was not present before, whether it is a missing limb or a subnormal level of intelligence; the establishment of realistic aims is an important element in the team management of the disabled patient.

The nurse's rôle in assessment of the patient. Nurses have been found to be deficient in this rôle. In a research project, Lee & Aitken (1983) report that when asked to assist in the assessment of patients for rehabilitation programmes 'the nurses were inaccurate in their predictions about difficulty with self-care, work problems, and emotional, family and financial problems'. The same report, however, does mention the 'complex nature of disability' and goes on to say 'In the absence of routine occupational therapy and social work assessment of all patients admitted to orthopaedic trauma wards, it might be thought that it is in these areas that nurses would have a distinctive contribution to make to the overall care and rehabilitation of patients. If so, there is a clear need to find ways of enabling nurses to assess and predict patients likely problems more accurately.' The report concludes, 'they might then contribute more to multi-professional decision-making about treatment and referral in rehabilitation, and thus help to improve the overall recovery of patients from their injuries'.

Wilson-Barnett (1981) discusses the nurses rôle in recovery from illness and suggests that: 'Much more active involvement with the patient is fundamental to the success of recovery planning'.

Where indicated, the team makes a study of *forms of gainful employment* which are suited to patients suffering from physical handicaps; they work in conjunction with doctors and medico-social workers inside the hospital, and outside, with family doctors, with community nurses, with Disablement Resettlement Officers, with Careers Advisers, with representatives of local government, and with employing authorities in finding suitable employment for the handicapped person, and suitable means, including transport, whereby he can be trained to follow it. Sometimes adaptation of machinery enables a handicapped person to work in a factory, or modifications such as ramps may be required to allow a patient to enter his place of work in a wheel-chair.

Rehousing, or alterations to existing housing may be required so that a handicapped person can live at home; in many cases, members of the rehabilitation team will visit the home to advise on adaptations (for example, the kitchen or bathroom Figs 34.1, 34.4). There are appliances to enable the handicapped person to look after bodily needs (Figs 34.2A and B) and aids for dressing (Fig. 34.3A). In this connection excellent advice is given in an article by Bush (1984) listed in the Bibliography. Figure 34.3B shows how a simple adaptation of the telephone can dramatically improve opportunities for communication for the one-handed.

The use of aids. It must be stressed once more however that aids are not recommended unless and

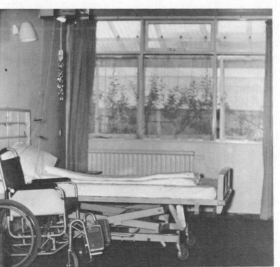

Fig. 34.1   A, B. Part of the purpose built flat for assessment and training disabled persons in the activities of daily living. (From Mary Marlborough Lodge, Oxford.)

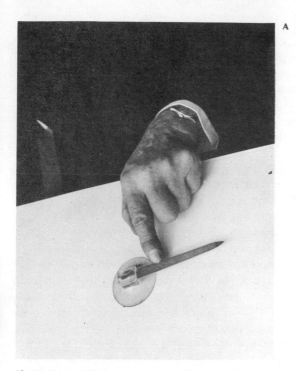

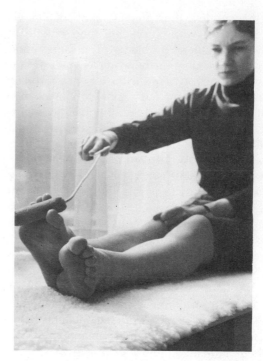

Fig. 34.2   A, B. Toilet aids for care of hands and feet. (Courtesy of Disabled Living Foundation.)

until attempts to teach the patient to use ordinary every-day equipment have failed.

Social problems. For some of our patients these may be as great or greater than physical ones; there may not be easy solutions but many patients are helped by discussion of their difficulties—'a trouble shared is a trouble halved'.

Other members of the team include, besides the nurse, the physiotherapist, the occupational therapist, the medico-social worker, an orthotist/prosthetist, a speech therapist, and in the case of children, a schoolteacher. Sometimes the team includes a psychologist, or vocational guidance counsellor, or physical training instructor and/or instructors in specialised skills such as metal work. In general, as we have seen, the physiotherapist takes care of the function of the lower limbs, and teaches walking and stair-climbing, often in a realistic situation, as for example, in a model bus, and the occupational therapist devotes herself to skills of the upper limb, as in feeding, shaving, making-up the face and attending to the hair and teeth. In practice, the work of both therapists tends to overlap and there may be other members of the team whose work is helpful to both, such as the art therapist and the school-teacher, not forgetting the librarian and the hospital chaplains.

Members of the team in the community, of equal importance to those in the hospital, are the general practitioner, the health visitor, the community nurse, members of the welfare and voluntary services and others too numerous to mention, including the home-help.

The place of the nurse in the rehabilitation team

In the community the nurse has a vital role, firstly in *prevention* of physical disability by health education and by case-finding with early recognition of conditions leading to disability, and secondly, in the care of disabled persons in their homes.

In hospital, the special function of the nurse begins with the reception of the patient in the accident centre, casualty or out-patient department where her work supports that of the doctor in giving prompt and effective treatment and in the prevention of complications which might lead to temporary or permanent disability. To give a simple

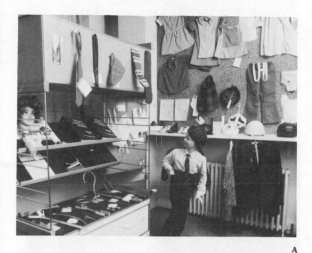

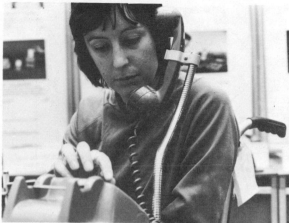

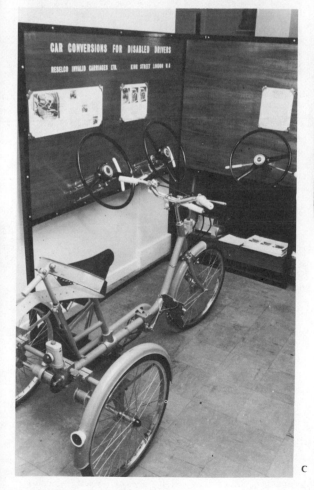

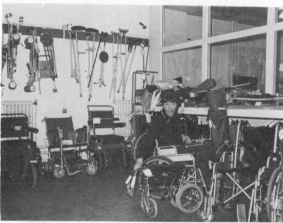

Fig. 34.3 Advice on adaptation on aids to clothing and to communication and mobility can be obtained from the Disabled Living Foundation.

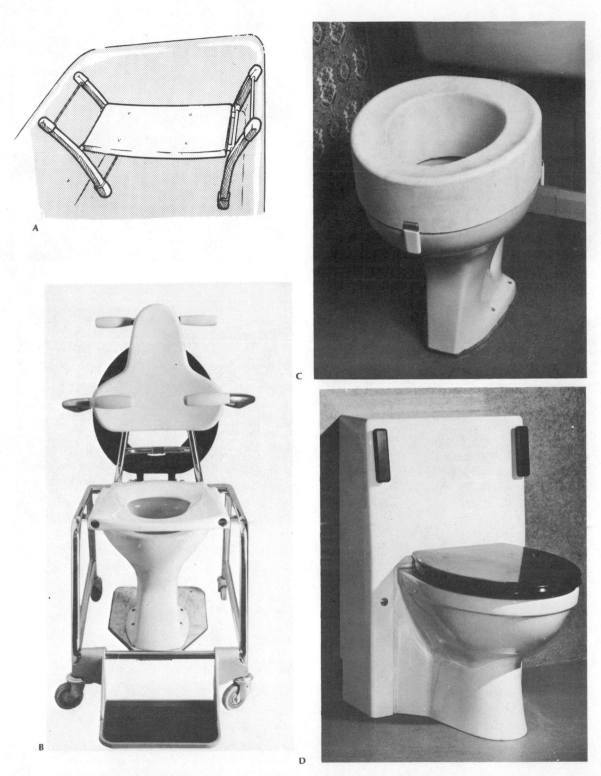

Fig. 34.4 **A.** Adjustable bath seat (Home craft); **B.** Toilet Chair (Mecanaid); **C.** Raised toilet seat. (Courtesy Disabled Foundation.) **D.** The 'Closomat' toilet comprises flushing, warm water washing, and warm air drying, all operated by one simple lever (elbow or foot pedal). (Courtesy of 'Closomat' (Great Britain) Ltd.)

example, stiffness of the shoulder must be prevented during treatment of a Colles' fracture (Ch. 20). In the operating theatre, her duties include not only assisting the surgeon but attending to all aspects of theatre technique in relation to prevention of wound infection (Ch. 8). In the ward, in the same context, a high standard of hygiene is required. *The nurses responsibilities in the prevention of the complications of rest in bed* have already been discussed in Chapter 2. These are most important in the prevention of both temporary and permanent disablement. Another vital aspect of her work is the *prevention of complications* which may not only lead to disability but which, in the severely disabled patient, might actually prevent or retard rehabilitation for home-life and work. For example, as we have seen in Chapter 23, a paraplegic patient can be successfully rehabilitated provided he has no pressure sores, joint contractures or severe urinary tract infection; similarly, the amputee (Ch. 33) can be fitted with a prosthesis and taught to use it so that it is almost unnoticeable provided that his stump is free from contractures, oedema, infection and skin disorders.

Another important function of the hospital nurse is to so arrange her patient's day as to fit in all the activities he needs for his rehabilitation within the pattern of his general care. She must understand *the aim* of the activities he is following so that treatment given by other members of the team can be followed up in a purposeful manner in the ward. Moreover in many cases the ordinary acts of daily living are used as a basis for rehabilitation; in fact they are the first skills to be learned in preparation for discharge from hospital; for example, a housewife with a disability must first of all be independent of aid in management of her person, and will then progress to learning how best to manage her home (Fig. 34.5).

There is a strong temptation for the nurse either to regard the patient following an intensive rehabilitation programme as 'out of her hands' and no longer deserving of her care and attention, or, to be reluctant to 'let him go', particularly if he has a serious handicap and has previously been heavily dependent upon her, as for example, the paraplegic patient. Both these attitudes are mistaken; in both cases the patient is still dependent upon his nurse for his general care and welfare and for pursuing

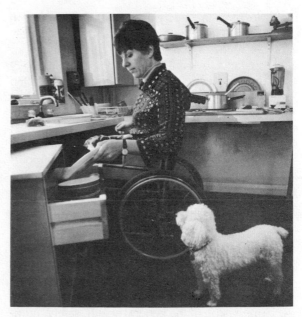

Fig. 34.5 Wheelchair living. (Please see text.)

the policy of active rehabilitation within the ward; for example, it does not help the patient being taught to feed, wash or dress himself in the rehabilitation centre if on his return to the ward continuous practice of these skills is not insisted upon; *it is often more troublesome and time-consuming to help patients to help themselves than to do things for them.* Then there is the patient who regards the hospital ward as a haven of rest and believes that if a nurse is present he is entitled to her services; he does not appreciate the fact that the activities advised for him are for his benefit and not for hers. Because of these factors, patients undergoing intensive rehabilitation programmes directed to teaching self-care are often best treated in wards or sections of wards devoted to this purpose, and where the equipment and furnishings resemble those found in normal homes, for example, divan beds of normal height.

The role of the nurse in the special medical rehabilitation centre

Since rehabilitation of the physical state relies heavily on the skills of the physiotherapist, occupational therapist, or the orthotist/prosthetist, the rôle of the nurse may seem at first glance to be vague and uncertain. In some centres however, the nurse may develop a satisfying professional rôle; in others, her skills may be wasted and she is merely a figure-head, or worse still, a 'pair of hands' or a tea-maker; in some, she may be deliberately excluded because, it is said, her training is slanted towards giving service to the patient rather than teaching him and helping him to do things for himself. If this is true, the nurse's training is defective; or, the team-leader has failed to include her as an equal in discussions with other team-members regarding assessment of the patient's abilities, the goals and objectives of his treatment and the means to be used to achieve them.

In brief, the nurse's duties could include:

1. General management of the unit.
2. Assisting with the initial and periodic assessment of the patient's abilities and progress.
3. Coordination of patient's activities.
4. Supervision of the general health, safety, nutrition, hygiene and comfort of the patient.
5. Specialised nursing functions such as skincare, wound dressings, catheter management, bladder and bowel training.
6. Working with medical and para-medical staff in teaching patients self-care and activities of daily living.
7. Teaching patients' relatives.
8. Cooperation with the social worker in dealing with patients' difficulties.
9. Acting as liaison officer with community nurses and others; home visiting.
10. Assisting the medical and para-medical staff to maintain an atmosphere of optimism and encouragement, with emphasis on the things that the patient can do rather than on those that he can not.
11. Show leadership in cooperative attitudes towards other staff, patients, relatives and outside agencies.
12. Teaching other nursing staff, student nurses and ancillary workers the concept of rehabilitation as part and parcel of the total and comprehensive care of the patient.
13. Instituting or assisting with research projects aimed at improving patient care.

The patient's place in the team would appear too obvious to mention, yet it is vital that he understands that the efforts of the other members of the team cannot succeed without his wholehearted cooperation. The patient who for some reason is reluctant to face a long haul and make a conscious effort often requires special consideration with regard to finding some facet of the activities offered which will fire his interest and enthusiasm and lead him not only to self-help, but to some degree of self-forgetfulness. Each patient requires careful assessment, steady progression in activity and constant encouragement in a warm, cheerful, friendly atmosphere; the will to succeed must spring from the hopeful attitudes of all those with whom the patient comes in contact, and whose interest and concern can be his inspiration.

Social activities and sports (Fig. 34.6) can form part of rehabilitation programmes; television, films,

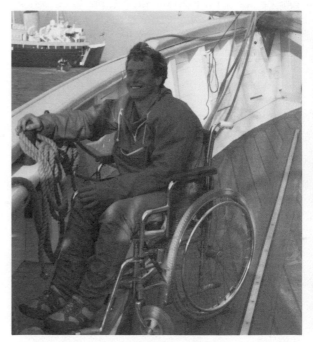

Fig. 34.6 One of the voyage crew on the Jubilee Sailing Trusts' chartered brigantine Soren Larsen in Cowes week, photographed in his own wheelchair. Note the wheelchair deck track behind him for which the Trust has specially made chairs for use at sea (Royal Yacht Britannia in background) (Courtesy of Jubilee Sailing Trust.)

concerts, table-tennis, darts, card games and bingo sessions are all popular pastimes. *Visitors* are encouraged, and *outings* are an essential feature of a return to normal life. Lethargy, boredom and inertia lead only to despair; on the other hand, *controlled rest* is important and definite times should be set aside each day for rest periods; adequate sleep must be ensured.

Rehabilitation of the patient's family

This is of vital importance in every case, especially if the patient has some permanent handicap. Ordinary people without medical or nursing knowledge cannot cope with a heavily handicapped member of the family, day in and day out, without adequate preparation. Again, careful assessment of the situation, including home locality, housing, availability of home help, transport, contact with the family doctor and community nurse, and assessment of the financial position of the family is essential. Sometimes the burden of caring for the patient will fall on the shoulders of one individual and he or she has no-one with whom to share it, as for example, the wife who must care for an invalid husband. Sometimes it is advisable for the members of a family to spend days, weekends, or even nights in the hospital or special centre in order to be fully aware of the patient's requirements. The question of medical or nursing help, the loan of equipment, and transortation must all be explored before the patient is finally discharged. Arrangements for covering family holidays and social occasions are also very helpful; many families will care happily for a handicapped member if they are given an occasional rest.

Conclusion

Rehabilitation of patients suffering from a wide variety of orthopaedic conditions is part and parcel of comprehensive patient care. It is a complex network which requires the special skills of a large number of people. As in all our endeavours, *teamwork* is the key to successful treatment, and this brief survey is intended to give the nurse a bird's-eye view of the work of other members of the team and to lead her to a better understanding of her own rôle and of the needs of her patient.

BIBLIOGRAPHY

Ansell Barbara, Lawton Sheila 1978 Your home and your rheumatism. London: Arthritis and Rheumatism Council.
Bleakley Rachel (ed.) 1974 Despite Disability. Reading: Educational Explorers
Boxall J et al 1982 The seven ages of disability. Nursing Times Supplement, August
Bush T 1984 The sense of well-being. Nursing Times, January
Callaghan W 1981 Aids for the disabled. Nursing Times, June
Central Office of Information 1965 Rehabilitation and care of the disabled in Britain. Reference Division, Central Office of Information. London. No: R.P.F. 4972/65 Classification 14C
Chartered Society of Physiotherapy 1975 Handling of the Handicapped. London: Woodhead Faulkner
Consumers' Association 1974 Coping with disablement. London: Consumers' Association
Davies Eira M 1975 Lets get moving. Mitcham, Surrey: Age Concern—National Old Peoples Welfare Council
DHSS & Welsh Office 1977 Help for Handicapped People. Leaflet HB1 March Aids for the Disabled. Leaflet HB2 September 1977. London and Cardiff. Issued jointly by the Department of Health and Social Security and the Welsh Office.
Disability Aids Directory 1983 Nursing Times Community Outlook, February
Disabled Living Foundation 1971 How to adapt existing clothing for the Disabled. London: Clothing Project Staff
Family Welfare Association 1978 Guide to the Social Services. London: MacDonald and Evans
Fanshawe E et al 1978 Disability without handicap. Nursing Times, 17 August, Supplement 3
Foott et al 1976 Kitchen sense for disabled or elderly people. London: William Heinemann Medical Books Ltd for the Disabled Living Foundation
Forbes Gillian 1971 Clothing for the handicapped child. London: Disabled Living Foundation
Hunt Paul (ed.) 1966 Stigma—the experience of disability. London: Geoffrey Chapman
Lee R, Aitken Cairns 1983 Predicting problems. Nursing Times, October
Nicholls P R J 1971 Rehabilitation of the Severely Disabled. Vol. 2 Management. London: Butterworth
O'Connor B T, Nichols P R J 1970 Rehabilitation in Orthopaedics. London: Annals of Physical Medicine
Robinson Wendy 1973 Sport and recreation for the physically handicapped. Nursing Times, 12 July, 895
Stewart W F R 1975 Sex and the physically handicapped. Horsham, Sussex: National Fund for Research into Crippling Diseases
White A S et al 1972 The easy path to gardening. London: Readers' Digest
Wilson-Barnett J 1981 Recovering from illness: Looking down the road to recovery. Nursing Mirror Feature, 27 May
WHO Technical Report Series 1969 WHO Expert Committee on Medical rehabilitation. 2nd report. Geneva No: 419
World Health Organization 1980 International Classification of Impairments, Disabilities and Handicaps. Geneva

35

Rehabilitation 2: special considerations

OCCUPATIONAL THERAPY IN ORTHOPAEDICS

The traditional picture of the role of the Occupational Therapist as a provider of diversional activities for long stay patients has fortunately almost disappeared. Whereas the undoubted value of diversional activity is not disputed, it is now often undertaken by Occupational Therapy Helpers working under supervision; this releases the Occupational Therapist to carry out specific and purposeful treatment. Recent advances in orthopaedic surgery and treatment mean that the Occupational Therapist has had an increasingly large role to play in ensuring that the patient becomes independent in personal care, for example, those with fractures or osteoarthritis.

Occupational Therapy for this type of patient falls into three sections:

1. Assessment of ability and practice in activities of daily living.
2. Specific activities to increase muscle power and the strength or range of movement of joints.
3. Assessment of progress and preparation for return to home and work.

All patients awaiting hip or knee surgery, or those with lower limb fractures should be interviewed by the Occupational Therapist on admission; a full social history should be taken and presenting problems should be noted.

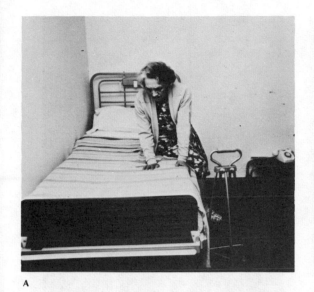
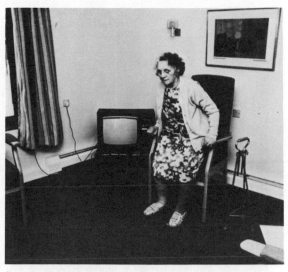

A   B

Fig. 35.1 A, B. Assessment of a patient's ability to get in and out of bed and chair. *Note:* The patient shown is wearing soft bedroom slippers. If possible, these should be discarded for the bootee type of slipper, or, better still, flat-heeled comfortable shoes which give good support to the feet.

The points covered include:

Type of housing—semi-detached, flat etc.
Access and number of steps and stairs.
Type of heating.
Position of toilet and bathroom.
Persons living with the patient and the amount of help they can give. Other help received, i.e. Meals on Wheels, Home Help, Social Services.
Hobbies and interests.
Ability to dress.
Transfers—bed, chair, toilet and bath (Fig. 35.1A, B).
Mobility.
Housework and cooking.
Laundry and shopping.
Transport.

By writing a short report on the patient's case sheet, nurses, physiotherapists and medical staff can all see the existing problems, if any, and those likely to arise in the future.

Activities of daily living. It is very tempting for the nurse or for any member of the treatment team to assist a patient struggling to get dressed, or to take him to the toilet rather than letting him walk there by himself; because time is so often limited on a busy ward. However, in many cases it should

be remembered that a patient will not be able to cope adequately at home unless he is able to carry out these basic activities himself.

The use of aids to function. Co-operation with nursing staff cannot be emphasised too much. The nurse must be aware of the aids issued to the patient and how to use them, so that she can make sure that the patient continues to use them during the time that the therapist is not present, i.e. evenings and weekends.

Dressing practice is usually carried out on the ward and aids such as stocking gutters, long shoe horns, and elastic laces may be used (Fig. 35.2A, B and C).

Many wards now have Hi-Lo beds, and high seat geriatric chairs and this, of course, helps the patients to help themselves. Patients will also be taught to get in and out of bed correctly and how to get out of a chair. Some patients will require a raised toilet seat and/or rails or other bath aids. Fortunately, many wards are now fitted with these aids.

Patients living alone will need to be able to manage in the kitchen; the majority of Occupational Therapy Departments have a kitchen where they can first of all make a cup of tea progressing to preparing a meal; aids such as trolleys, high

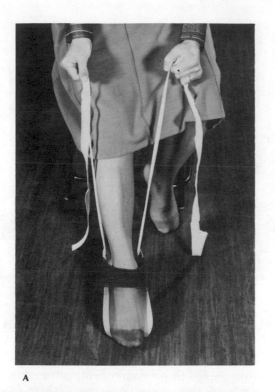

A

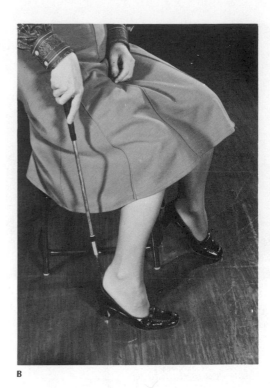

B

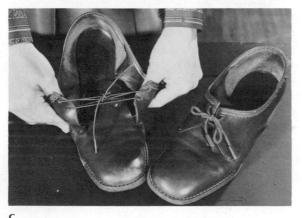

C

Fig. 35.2 A, B. A stocking gutter and long-handled shoe horn are useful aids for those who cannot reach their feet. **C.** Shoes are more easily put on if elastic laces are supplied.

stools and teapot tippers may need to be provided (Fig. 35.3).

If there is any doubt that a patient may not be able to manage the therapist may take him home for part of the day so that she can assess him in his own setting. Steps may need to be replaced by ramps, or the legs of beds or chairs raised before discharge is possible. Some aids or adaptations may need to be referred to the Social Services Department and the therapist will arrange this.

A patient who cannot return home may have to wait for a place in a Welfare Home; this can take many months and as the requisite for entry is that the patient is independent in personal needs it is up to both therapist and nurse to see that the patient does not deteriorate and continues to dress and transfer without help.

In some cases, a follow-up visit to the patient's home is needed if there is uncertainty as to his ability to manage, or if aids, adaptations and com-

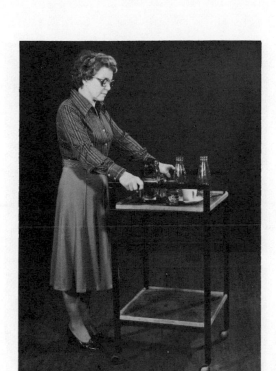

Fig. 35.3 A trolley of suitable height can be used as a walking aid.

munity services have been requested. If there is a community occupational therapist, then the case can be handed over to her. If not, then the hospital based Occupational Therapist will visit and make out a report. It can be very advantageous to the nurse if she can accompany the therapist as she will gain great insight into home conditions and learn how patients cope with their problems. We tend to forget that many houses are still without proper sanitation—outside toilets and earth closets are often seen, particularly in old property. We should also remember that we all have different standards and that however untidy or dirty a house may be, it is the patient's home and he may like it that way.

Specific Treatment. After fractures or certain types of surgery, a patient may be left with weak muscles, stiffness and/or limited range of movement in one or many joints, and these will need to be strengthened.

Both the occupational therapist and the physiotherapist work towards this common end by using different methods and types of treatment; best results are obtained by working together, for example, the patient with a hand injury might have wax treatment from a physiotherapist first, followed by occupational therapy while the hand is most supple.

The physiotherapist teaches the patient walking, with perhaps sticks or crutches, but at the same time the occupational therapist and the nurse ensure that he continues the walking pattern taught and does not regress to using a wheelchair.

Upper limb injuries; for example—hand injury, finger amputation, fracture or dislocation (Fig. 35.4A, B).

Hand dominance must be first ascertained and then the joints are measured using the unaffected side as a comparison. If the patient is a wage earner then a break-down of the work can be done, because treatment must be directed towards getting the patient back to home and work as soon as possible. Canework, mosaics and stool seating still play their part as useful methods of treatment; one of their values is that often they will be new activities for the patient to learn and so can be taught in the particular way the therapist chooses to encourage a particular range of movement or form of hand dexterity; also, a pleasing end product means that the patient often works harder and tends to forget his injury. Remedial games such as draughts which are made out of cotton reels or large different shaped blocks can either be played on a flat surface or in an elevated position to increase the range of movement in the elbow or shoulder. By using different shapes hand/eye coordination can be taught and concentration and perseverance built up where necessary.

Many Occupational Therapy Departments have a heavy workshop section employing trained technicians, who often work with the occupational therapists in the final stages of treatment. Activities here include wood and metal work and tools can be adapted to suit different grips if necessary. Items that can be made can either be purchased by the patient when completed or he can help to make aids for the department, i.e. dressing sticks, sock sticks and kitchen trolleys.

Lower limb injuries. For example, fracture, patellectomy and menisectomy, knee-joint replacement. If a patient has been immobilised for a long time or has had surgery to the knee, there will be

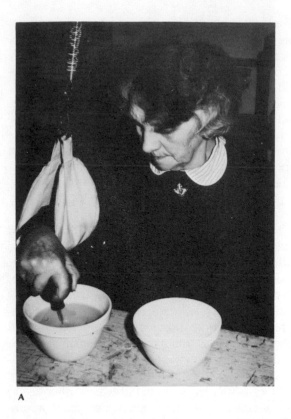

A

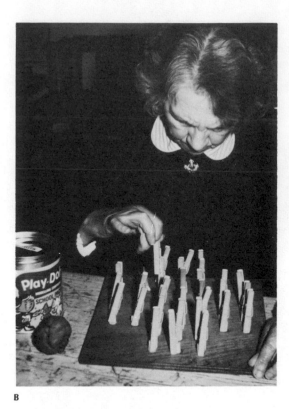

B

Fig. 35.4   A, B. Squeezing a syringe in water, manipulating Play-doh or peg-solitaire are all used to increase manual dexterity and strength.

some loss of muscle power and range of movement. Standing tolerance and balance may also be affected. A printing press can be adapted by using a pulley circuit so that flexion and extension of the knee joint may be obtained. This is especially useful for meniscectomy patients where there is an initial 'extension lag', i.e. inability to achieve full extension. The occupational therapist also uses other machinery such as lathes, ankle fretsaws and electric cycles—all of which can be altered to help increase strength and range of movement in the hip and knee joints. The cycles differ from those used in the Physiotherapy Department in that they have a fretsaw blade and so resistance can be added by cutting out a jigsaw or book rest in plywood. Bowls and candlesticks can be made on the lathe (Fig. 35.5).

Gardening and other similar outdoor activities can be used towards the end of the patient's treatment and heavy workshop activities can be directed to increase standing tolerance (Fig. 35.6).

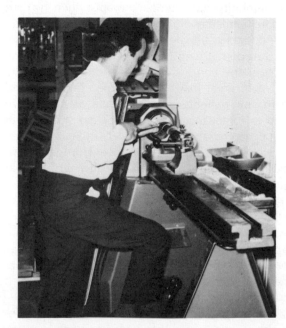

Fig. 35.5   By turning a wooden candlestick on the lathe, further resistance to hand movement can be added.

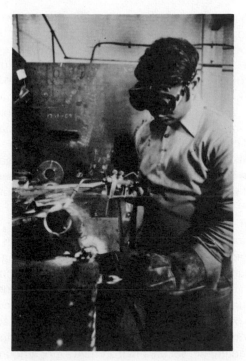

Fig. 35.6   A welder whose right hand has been amputated has a special attachment for his prosthesis which enables him to return to full employment.

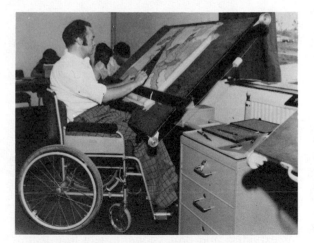

Fig. 35.7   Work from a wheelchair is made possible by a drawing board supplied under the Special Aids Scheme.

Assessment and preparation for return to work. Many patients will be able to return to home duties or to their jobs without any problems. However, there will always be the man or woman who will be unable to go back to their particular work and will need help in this area. Some patients will eventually be able to return to their old jobs but will need to build up to a full day's activities in hospital; this will often be done on an out-patient basis. The occupational therapist can assess a patient's concentration, use of initiative, memory, perseverance and motivation by observing him perform certain activities. Psychological factors often play a large part and the therapist must be aware if there is any compensation claim pending as this will often influence a patient's attitude to his treatment. Where possible the therapist will try to simulate the job situation as closely as possible in the Occupational Therapy Department (Fig. 35.7), and contact with the employer will often have to be made at any early date.

The occupational therapist works closely with the Disablement Resettlement Officer (DRO) whose job it is to try and help the patient back to work by any means within his power; the patient may be advised to attend an Employment Rehabilitation Centre, designed to assess a patient's aptitude in learning new skills and also to help him build up the work habit in a simulated industrial atmosphere (Fig. 35.6).

If a particular aptitude is discovered then the DRO will arrange for the patient to attend a training centre and will help him to find a job later. (Please see Retraining and Job-Replacement of the Orthopaedically Disabled at end of this Chapter.)

As it will be seen by this brief synopsis, the work of the occupational therapist is very varied and is essentially practical. Together with all members of the treatment team it should always be directed at resettling the patient back into society to fulfil a useful and purposeful role.

SOCIAL WORK WITH ORTHOPAEDIC PATIENTS

No matter how welcoming are our hospitals, clinic and staff, treatment of an orthopaedic condition is rarely an enjoyable experience or one which would have been undertaken, if the patient had the choice! For most people, it is an experience shot through with anxiety, pain or discomfort, and accompanied by considerable personal and social upheaval. The more permanent or long-lasting the condition, the more profound are likely to be its social consequences. It is often impossible to separate the orthopaedic problem from its psycho-social implications and it is therefore with this latter problematic area that the hospital-based social worker concerns herself.

In general the social worker concentrates on the personal, emotional and social implications of illness or disability and her work is primarily to provide support, advice, guidance and practical help to individuals and their 'relevant others' (i.e. families, friends, anyone involved in the patient's life). She is also, however, part of the multi-disciplinary hospital team and, as such, contributes her particular expertise and professional insight to a team's assessment of the *total* needs of the patient; in this way, the patient can be seen as a *whole* person and his socio-psychological integrity preserved during his 'career' as an orthopaedic patient. The social worker can help to stimulate within the medical setting an awareness that the physical and psychological are often inseparable, that the ability to benefit fully from orthopaedic—or any other medical—treatment is closely linked with the patient's coping skills, his personal make-up and with the social influences prevailing on his life at that time.

Put simply, it is obviously much harder for staff to motivate an elderly patient after, say, a fractured femur, if she has been recently widowed and feels that she has little to return home to. She will perhaps need support and counselling to work through the grieving process; sometimes the social worker will need to contact family, neighbours or other agencies to mobilise practical avenues of support before discharge. The whole medical and paramedical team will treat the patient more effectively if they know a little about her home and social circumstances.

With spinal disorders, the low back pain sufferer may be admitted to hospital after years of social stress, exacerbated by failed medical treatment and having been told that his pain is 'all in his head'. Pain and the inability to live as fully as he did formerly affects his employability, his financial and social status, his interpersonal relationships, so that he frequently becomes depressed, sometimes suicidal, or conversely, almost hysterically anxious and obsessed with his condition and treatment.

With some patients the social worker's main task is to iron out some of the practical difficulties associated with admission. Since it is now accepted that, whenever possible, a parent should be encouraged to accompany a child admitted to hospital, the social worker can sort out accommodation and provide non-medical information for the parent, thus lessening the trauma for both parent and child.

All in all, the social worker helps to bridge the gaps between home and hospital, between patient and family, and between individual and community.

In social work with the disabled, however, it is important not to overlook the wide age ranges, the varying degrees of impairment and the differing personal and social skills which the patients bring to the situation; the disabled are not a homogeneous group. The social worker must bear in mind that the problems (if any exist) are of individual adaptation to impairment and also the result of a hostile or apathetic social environment—no amount of emotional fortitude will enable a paraplegic wheelchair-user to go shopping independently if the only access to the shopping precinct is via a long flight of steps. Disability brought about by an orthopaedic condition is therefore a matter of *personal* acceptance and coping, plus a *socially* imposed disadvantage. The social worker's task must thus be to help the impaired individual to locate resources, both emotional and practical, to enable him to live as full a life as he or she would wish.

Much of the social worker's brief is contained in statute. The Seebohm Committee's recommendations formed the basis of the Local Authorities Personal Social Services Act, 1970, which created Social Services Departments as they exist today. The committee's particular thoughts on services for the disabled are contained in the Chronically Sick and Disabled Persons Act, also of 1970. This act imposes two duties on local authorities: to inform themselves of the numbers and needs of the handicapped in their areas, and to publicise services available. Section 2 of the Act outlines such services, such as social work support, practical assistance in the home, help with meals, provision of aids and adaptations, recreational facilities etc.

In some respects it becomes a social worker's job to alleviate and help counteract some of the high costs of the impairments brought about by an orthopaedic condition. For some the costs may be minimal—the young person who fractures tibia and fibula in a motorcycle accident may soon be back to normal, so that he or she may need little more than information on Statutory Sick Pay. For others, however, the costs are heavy. Pain, for those suffering from rheumatoid or osteoarthritis, brings irritability and depression, which taxes relationships with spouse, children and others, bringing tension or social isolation. The enforced dependence brought about by crippling conditions may bring with it its own form of grieving. Sometimes there is accompanying physical humiliation with loss of control over body functions. Often the patient faces devaluation by society or in his own eyes, with the loss of former employment, loss of financial status and income, or of familial rôles etc. In addition, he or she may be patronised or treated as if a child, particularly if wheelchair-bound (and therefore without easy eye contact with others) or elderly; an amputee soon realises that the general public uncomfortably averts its eyes and a tetraplegic becomes a victim of the 'Does he take Sugar?' syndrome. No amount of social work support can directly shield the recipient from such hurtful repercussions but, by sharing them with the social worker, the patient may be helped to face or challenge such attitudes and trials.

In actual terms the social worker's task is so varied as to be almost indefinable but, briefly, it regularly covers some of the following areas:

(i) The social worker is sometimes asked simply to 'be there' and give time to the patient through the chaos of fear, panic, bewilderment, anger or frustration following, say, admission after an R.T.A. or an accident involving a spinal injury. For some people the fear of hospital procedures and equipment alone may cause great anxiety, particularly halo-femoral traction, drips, Stryker beds, leg lengthening apparatus etc. Sometimes the mother who has recently learned that her young child needs major orthopaedic surgery may need a shoulder to cry on away from the ward.

(ii) Practical problems arise before admission. If a mother is admitted to hospital, arrangements must be made for dependent children. Problems of travel and visiting, with the considerable expense which these involve, can also be discussed. Admission frequently poses financial problems—advice on keeping up financial commitments such as mortgage repayments etc., can be given by the social worker.

(iii) If the social worker is to help the patient mobilise all available resources to cope with a future life affected by an orthopaedic condition, she must, with the patient's permission, gather information about the former life-style and assess whether or how this will be changed by the disability. She will try to help patient and family understand and cope with any change, particularly if denial of the new limitations is the first reaction. Sometimes, in the case of a high and complete spinal cord lesion, the adjustment of life expectancies will be considerable, for example in terms of future sexual potential. Whether the patient is married or single, he or she will need basic facts and information, plus the chance to discuss what this means in terms of their own sexual life in the future. In some cases no amount of counselling will help spouse or family members to accept the degree of impairment or necessary change, and the inevitable outcome here is withdrawal or divorce.

(iv) Reactions to a disability by the patient's family cover the whole spectrum of possible emotions. For some the shock may be intense but short-lived and the patient's spouse, parent or friend may be quickly engaged in helping to make realistic plans for the future. Occasionally, however, the young teenager or adult finds himself overwhelmed by the reactions of a well-meaning but over-protective parent after, for example, the trauma of a spinal cord injury—the 'swaddling clothes syndrome'— so that the patients' attempts to regain normal independence are hampered. Conversely it may be that the patient becomes accustomed to playing a 'sick' role, and develops a learned helplessness, which has its own secondary gains. In both extremes the social worker's skills are needed to stimulate a more balanced approach, so making a more complete rehabilitation possible.

(v) The social worker should also possess as wide a knowledge as possible of available resources for practical help, developing an almost encyclopaedic knowledge of DHSS benefits, charitable, voluntary and statutory funds and agencies etc. She will frequently be the first person to put the patient in touch with solicitors, where relevant, so that he may discuss issues of compensation after an R.T.A., industrial or criminal injury, and she can pass on information about legal aid.

(vi) A major area of work is in acting on behalf of a patient to help plan discharge. Social services provide aids and adaptations for a wide variety of situations, from bath and toilet aids for the permanently and substantially handicapped to help with a home extension to provide ground floor accommodation for the wheelchair user. Sometimes no amount of aids will make housing suitable and the social worker must then advise about alternative accommodation in, for example, a Local Authority warden-controlled flat or a disabled person's bungalow. Support in such situations may include provision of meals-on-wheels, home help, attendance at a day centre or club, or day care in a welfare home. Occasionally, the choice for the elderly may be application for admission to a welfare home (Part 111 accommodation), while many families may benefit from some of the respite care schemes available, according to area, such as those offered by Family Support Groups, 'Rent-a-Granny' schemes etc.

The family with a severely handicapped child may be offered participation in schemes offering help via foster 'aunts and uncles', or be introduced to the variety of services offered by the Joseph Rowntree Family Fund.

(vii) Lastly, and again with the patient's permission, the social worker can alert community social workers and voluntary workers to the particular difficulties that the patient may face on discharge. It is particularly helpful when the social worker from the patients' home area can visit the patient in hospital to get to know him and help him plan the future.

In conclusion, it is important to remember that, depending on the condition, its severity and permanence, the social worker's task is to help the patient cope with the emotional and social adjustment which accompany physical treatment or change. She should also bear in mind that the condition— no matter how severe—need not necessarily touch the emotional and intellectual core of the patient's being—it is his *relationship* with the world that changes in some way. The delicate task of the social

worker is to facilitate the smoothest passage possible to that new relationship.

RETRAINING AND JOB-PLACEMENT OF THE ORTHOPAEDICALLY DISABLED

Retraining and job-placement of the orthopaedically disabled is initiated and co-ordinated through the Disablement Resettlement Officer (DRO) or Disablement Adviser who, with the help of the Manpower Services Commission, is able to complete the rehabilitation process. The DRO is responsible for those patients who are unemployed, whilst the DA is responsible for assisting those patients who are employed, to return to suitable employment with their employers. Fortunately there are few patients so severely disabled that they will never be able to do work of some kind. We will consider them under two headings:

1. *Patients with a temporary disability.* Quite often orthopaedic patients have been employed in manual or craft occupations which require use of all four limbs, e.g. agriculture. Those with a temporary disability are nearly always able to return to their former employment. The DA negotiates with the employer for a return to part-time work, suggesting ways of arranging light duties and monitoring the patient's progress. At the same time the DA acts as liaison officer between the doctor and the patient when he is seen at a clinic until a full return to work is accomplished.

2. *Patients with a permanent disability.* These present more serious problems and, if it is obviously impossible for a patient to return to his former employment, the DRO is required to give vocational guidance. The choice depends on the disability, patient's age (which may range between 16–65 years), previous employment attainments, education, disposition, home location and local opportunities available.

DRO's assessment

All patients must, on realisation of their handicap, wonder if they will ever be able to do any work again and thus be an independent member of society. Quite naturally they are often negative in their own assessment of the situation and it is therefore essential that both nursing staff and the DRO or DA concentrate on persuading them to think positively in terms of what they can do, rather than what they can not. A paraplegic has the use of his upper limbs and there are many jobs which entail the constant and precise use of them, thus allowing this type of disabled person to do a good job. The DRO or DA will interview the patient, obtain information regarding the physical and domestic circumstances, employment and educational attainments, physical and mental abilities, and from this basis, gives advice on the type of employment best suited to the individual.

Practical employment assessment and rehabilitation

Sometimes it is advisable for the patient to receive practical employment assessment, not only to ascertain his abilities but also to help him regain confidence in his abilities. This can be done to some extent in the Occupational Therapy Department of a hospital or in a Local Authority Rehabilitation Unit, but mainly is more successful if completed at an Employment Rehabilitation Centre (ERC). There are 27 ERCs throughout the country, two of which are residential. At an ERC the patient undergoes a practical assessment, in an industrial and commercial environment, in clerical and commercial sections, engineering machinery operations, general fitting, horticulture, bench fitting, electrical and other assembly work and general fitting. These activities are used for assessment of the patient's strength, limb dexterity, retention of instruction, motivation, initiative and academic ability. These facilities are available for patients of school leaving age, as are facilities for remedial education. The average length of an ERC course is eight weeks but each patient is assessed individually so the length is dependent upon the individual's progress. From the recommendations of the DRO and/or ERC, the patient should be able to make positive progress in his search for suitable employment. However, before embarking on his new career, it may be necessary for the patient to receive appropriate training to enable him to be accepted into that trade or profession.

Training for alternative employment

The scope for training for alternative suitable employment extends from the semi-skilled operative level to that at management level. There are five types of establishments where training can take place and the choice will depend on the disability, training required, age and domestic circumstances of the patient (now referred to as the trainee). The five categories of training establishments are listed below, together with details of the level of training and type of trainee catered for:

1. *Skill centres.* (Formerly known as Government Training Centres). Skill centres are where most craft skills are taught, e.g. bricklaying, welding, joinery and electronics. They are very similar to small factories, equipped with the very latest equipment and machinery which are laid out to represent normal working conditions. Even the working hours are the same as in the average job.

2. *Residential training colleges.* These colleges are designed to cater for the more severely disabled or those who are unable to attend a skill centre. They are fully residential and teach the craft trades as at skill centres plus some additional commercial courses, e.g. Office Studies and Draughtsmanship. They also provide Further Education courses for the disabled juvenile and practical employment assessment, as found in the ERCs.

3. *Colleges of Further Education.* If a trainee wishes to attend a clerical, commercial, arts or management level vocational course, then it is probable that he will be able to attend a College of Further Education for his training. There are numerous colleges which have arrangements with the Manpower Services Commission for disabled trainees to undertake their courses under the sponsorship of the latter. Some courses are better catered for at these specialised colleges, e.g. agricultural, horticultural and computer programming. Again some of the colleges offer residential accommodation.

4. *Individual training with an independent employer.* Some trainees are suitable for training in an occupation for which the required training is not catered for by any of the previously mentioned establishments. Similarly, trainees may not be able to attend any of the other training establishments because of their disability, location or

domestic circumstances. So as not to lose the opportunity for such training, the DRO is able to arrange such a course with a local employer who is qualified and suitable to give the required training. Two examples of trades often taught under this scheme are floristry and butchery. One advantage of this method is that the trainee is guaranteed 6 months employment following completion of training.

5. *Training colleges run by Trusts and other voluntary bodies.* There are many such colleges which cater for many different types of disabled people and training. They are mainly designed for the disabled school-leaver. An example of such a college is the Derwen College for the Physically Handicapped at Gobowen, Oswestry. At the Derwen College the trainee can receive training in upholstery, surgical splint manufacture and repair, office studies and other occupations.

6. *Special schemes to help the disabled compete in the employment field.* On completion of the appropriate training, the disabled person is ready to be placed into suitable employment; when trying to secure it, the DRO can further assist the disabled jobseeker to complete the rehabilitation process. So often we take for granted the ability to travel to work, to gain access to and exit from the place of employment, and to operate equipment and use basic machinery. To the disabled person, inability to perform these normal activities can represent a barrier to being accepted as suitable for employment.

The DRO is able to assist the disabled jobseeker in the following ways:

1. *Assistance with fares to work.* Because of the severity of the disability, the patient is not able to travel by public transport and if not the owner of a car can be housebound. The alternative is to travel by taxi which will result in substantial expense being incurred. The DRO can arrange for financial assistance for this method of travelling to and from work.

2. *Grants for adaptations to premises and equipment.* It may be necessary for the employer's premises to be adapted or structurally altered to enable access and exit for the disabled. Also existing equipment may need to be adapted for use by the disabled employee. Again the DRO can arrange

for financial assistance with this, either in part or whole and give advice to the employer on how these adaptations should be carried out. Examples of these adaptations are provision of ramps, accessible toilets and external lifts.

3. *Special aids.* Even when found employment the disabled employee may require special equipment to ensure independence in his work (Figs 35.6 and 35.7). If this is not already available the DRO can arrange for such equipment to be purchased and loaned to the disabled employee whilst in employment. Examples of these are electric typewriters for tetraplegic patients and those with rheumatoid arthritis; adjustable chairs and desks for spinal and hip disabilities; a special work bench and a mini-hydraulic-hoist for a paraplegic. (N.B. The draft copy for this section was typed by a tetraplegic patient using an electric typewriter.)

4. *Setting up business on own account.* The DRO can arrange for grants to be made available to certain severely disabled people to set themselves up in business if all other resettlement possibilities have failed (Fig. 35.8).

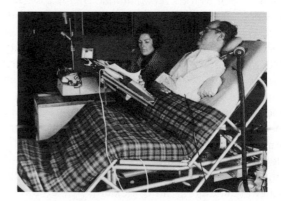

Fig. 35.8 'Business as usual.' This disabled gentleman is a sales representative who works from home with the help of 'Possum' adaptations for use of typewriter and telephone.

Sheltered employment

A small minority of disabled people are so severely disabled that they are unable to work under normal conditions. For them the answer may be found in sheltered employment; facilities being provided either through sheltered workshops, run by either Remploy Ltd., Local Authorities or Voluntary Bodies; or Sheltered Industrial Groups. The latter arrangement allows the disabled person to work in a normal employment environment. The selection of people for sheltered employment, it should be noted, is a matter for agreement between the relevant organisation and the DRO who is responsible for introducing the disabled person concerned.

Conclusion

The nurse spends more time with the patients than anyone else and is aware that rehabilitation is only complete when the patient is fully resettled within the community. Obtaining suitable employment is an essential element of that complete rehabilitation, so that the DRO and/or DA can play an important role; he knows what attainments and abilities are required for most types of employment and industry, is able to relate this to disability and advise employers accordingly. He is in continual communication with employers about possible vacancies and is often approached by employers when one of their employees becomes disabled. This often allows the employee to keep their employment, even though in an alternative job, by using some, if not all of the previously described facilities. The nurse should always be ready to refer patients to the DRO or DA if he/she feels that the patient may have an employment problem, however small. He can then communicate with the doctors and other members of the hospital team about the prognosis and make a preliminary assessment of what might be required. Most training centres, sheltered workshops and all Rehabilitation Centres are open to visitors and nurses should always feel free to approach the DRO or DA for the purpose of arranging a visit. This not only allows nurses to see part of the rehabilitation process but also gives them some insight into working conditions in factories and offices; this leads them to a better understanding of a patient's working life.

REHABILITATION OF A SPECIAL GROUP

Congenital conditions resulting in permanent disability in the adolescent

There are a considerable number of patients in this group, which includes those suffering from cerebral palsy, muscular dystrophy, spina bifida and other, rarer, conditions. The need for specialised help increases with the age of the patient and they require, in many instances, education in special units (Special schools) where trained staff, including nursing staff, are available at all times. At school-leaving age continuation of specialised help in the form of further education and vocational training is very often necessary to give these young people the opportunity of acquiring maximum independence. Care within the community is the ideal if the necessary facilities are available but this is rarely so and then use must be made of specialised units.

Independence is the cry from all disabled adolescents; unfortunately this cannot always be attained because of the severity of the disease but even in these cases relative independence improves the quality of life, making it more enjoyable and acceptable. If independence is to be acquired, continuing support is needed and this will involve the specialised unit, the family, medical care and other ancillary services and, in particular, Social Services who have a statutory responsibility for community care.

It is in units such as Derwen College for the Disabled that young handicapped people of school-leaving age can be given specialised help in order to acquire maximum independence. The help takes the form of:

a. Preliminary assessment
b. Instruction with the aim of acquiring maximum social and daily living competence
c. Continuing further education with the addition of a vocational training.

a. *Assessment.* Increasing emphasis is now placed on the assessment of the young disabled and, in fact, it is now statutory under the Education Act 1981 to report annually (to be called a 'Statement') on all young people with special educational needs, with or without physical handicap, from pre-school age to the age of 19. It is essential to assess the young handicapped accurately before commencing a period of further education and vocational training. If they are to attain the maximum benefit, obviously they will require guidance with the object of becoming socially independent and eventually capable, wherever possible, of open employment, thus giving satisfaction to the individual as well as financial independence.

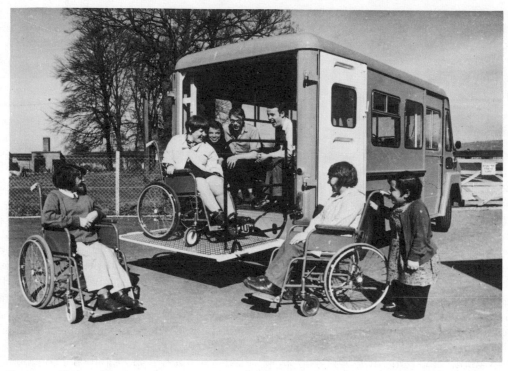

Fig. 35.9 All aboard for an outing in specially adapted bus. (Courtesy of Mr J. G. Kendall, Derwen College.)

Assessment is time-consuming and at Derwen College for the Disabled a period of three months is devoted to this. Its value lies in the information collected concerning the social competence and the vocational potential of the person and, as a result, allows a programme to be drawn up which takes account of all the problems, so that the disabled person can pursue a period of further education and vocational training which will lead to a full and independent life.

b. *Acquiring maximum social and daily living competence.* This need varies enormously from person to person. The teaching of social competence is a team effort in which every staff member—doctor, nurse, houseparent and teacher—must be involved. To acquire the ability to overcome all the problems of 'daily living' specialised help is needed, not only in learning new methods of meeting particular problems but also by adapting equipment and accommodation so that help is minimal or even unnecessary.

c. *Further education and vocational training.* Further education and vocational training assist the handicapped to function at their maximum level. Where there is some degree of illiteracy and enumeracy further education is essential; at the same time it can help in other directions and so supplement the learning of a particular trade or craft. The vocational training undertaken must be right for the individual disabled person and so the necessity for assessment cannot be over-emphasised, including the interests, the potential and the degree of handicap of the individual concerned. The ultimate aim of this whole period of further education and vocational training is a successful and correct work placement and this can be at differing levels from an Adult Training Centre through sheltered employment to open employment. Dame Agnes Hunt was very well aware of the problems of the 'crippled' adolescent who, because of permanent handicap, found difficulty in obtaining work. It was due to this great foresight that she founded the Derwen College with the object of teaching skill to the young disabled and so allowing them to become employable, working alongside the non-handicapped on equal terms.

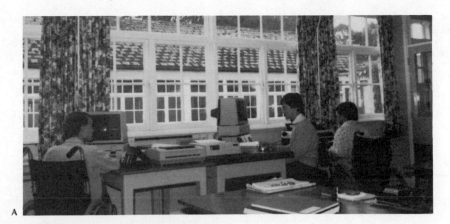

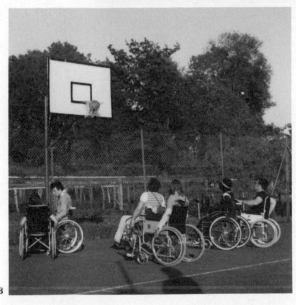

Fig. 35.10A, B   A. Students at the Derwen College at work. **B.** At play. (Courtesy of Mr J. G. Kendall, Derwen College.)

The future. It has been stated recently that if disabled students are to achieve their true potential they need a measure of positive discrimination in their favour; equality of opportunity is not enough. This is admirable and would be a great step forward if it was acceptable but at present it must remain a hope for the future. In the meantime the principle of teaching independence advocated by Dame Agnes Hunt will continue to prevail into the foreseeable future.

BIBLIOGRAPHY

Bleakley Rachel (ed.) 1974 Despite disability—career achievement by handicapped people. Reading: Educational Explorers

Central Council for the Disabled: Access for the Disabled (A series of booklets in a guide to access to public places and facilities in many large towns and cities). Published by The Central Council for the Disabled, 34 Eccleston Square, London SW1

Central Council for the Disabled: Holidays for the Physically Handicapped. Published by the Central Council for the Disabled

The Disablement Income Group: An ABC of Services and General Information for Disabled People—Published by The Disablement Income Group, 180 Tottenham Court Road, London, W1

Hooker Susan 1976 Caring for Elderly People. London: Routledge and Kegan Paul

Hunt Agnes DBE RC 1938 This is my life. Glasgow: Blackie

Hunt Paul (ed.) 1966 Stigma—the experience of disability. London: Geoffrey Chapman

Kuyendall J 1981 The vulnerable adolescent. Nursing Mirror Clinical Forum, October

Morris Alfred, Butler William 1972 No Feet to Drag. London: Sidgwick & Jackson

Rowe J, Dwyer L 1977 Care of the Orthopaedic Patient. Oxford: Blackwell Scientific

Rudinger E (ed.) 1974 Coping with disablement. London: Consumers' Association, publishers of WHICH?

Watson-Jones R 1948 Dame Agnes Hunt. Journal of Bone and Joint Surgery 30: 709–713, November

Wilmot Phyllis 1971 Consumer's Guide to The British Social Services. Harmondsworth: Penguin

Index